White Lesions

Newborns
A. *Flat*
1. Piebaldism, 242-243
2. Ash leaf macules, 243-245
3. Hypomelanosis of Ito, 246-247
4. Superficial hemangioma, 187-193, 309-310
5. Postinflammatory hypopigmentation, 249-250
B. *Raised*
1. Milia, 168-170, 299
2. Microcomedones of acne, 15-16
3. Molluscum contagiosum, 115-116

Infants and Children
A. *Flat*
1. Pityriasis alba, 249
2. Tinea versicolor, 71-72
3. Vitiligo, 247-248
4. Postinflammatory hypopigmentation, 249-250
5. Scleroderma (morphea), 264-266
6. Lichen sclerosis et atrophicus, 266-267
7. Ash leaf macules, 243-245
8. Piebaldism, 242-243
9. Waardenburg's syndrome, 242-243
10. Chediak-Higashi syndrome, 251
11. Hypomelanosis of Ito, 246-247
12. Halo nevus, 258
B. *Raised*
1. Microcomedones of acne, 15-16
2. Milia, 169-170
3. Keratosis pilaris, 41-42
4. Molluscum contagiosum, 115-116

Brown Lesions

Newborns
A. *Flat*
1. Mongolian spot, 253, 255, 309, 312
2. Café au lait spot, 252, 254-255, 312
3. Junctional nevus, 257, 260-261, 312
4. Nevus of Ota, 253-254, 255
5. Freckles, 251, 254-255
6. Lentigo, 251-252, 254-255
7. Postinflammatory hyperpigmentation, 254, 255
8. Transient neonatal pustular melanosis, 302-303
9. Linear and whorled hypermelanosis, 254-255
B. *Raised*
1. Congenital melanocytic nevus, 255-257
2. Skin tags, 318

Infants and Children
A. *Flat*
1. Freckles, 251, 254-255, 260
2. Café au lait spot, 252, 254-255
3. Junctional nevus, 257, 260-261
4. Mongolian spot, 253, 255, 312
5. Postinflammatory hyperpigmentation, 254, 255
6. Tinea versicolor, 71-72
7. Diffuse endocrine hyperpigmentation, 261-262
8. Incontinentia pigmenti, 280-281
9. Becker's nevus, 257, 258, 260
10. Nevus of Ota, 253-254, 255
11. Lentigo, 251-252, 254-255
B. *Raised*
1. Intradermal nevus, 260-261
2. Dermatofibroma, 173-174
3. Spindle and epithelioid cell nevus, 260-261
4. Urticaria pigmentosa, 208-210
5. Juvenile xanthogranuloma, 177-178
6. Blue nevus, 258-260
7. Skin tags, 318
8. Melanoma, 258-261
9. Lentigo, 251-252, 254-255
10. Flat warts, 111, 112-113
11. Pyogenic granuloma, 178-179, 199
12. Hemangioma, 187-193

Yellow Lesions

Newborns
1. Carotenemia, 12
2. Sebaceous gland hyperplasia, 299-300
3. Sebaceous nevus, 314-315
4. Juvenile xanthogranuloma, 177-178
5. Mastocytomas, 208-210
6. Goltz's syndrome, 282-283

NOTE: In a baby with jaundice any skin lesion containing fluid may be yellow.

Infants and Children
1. Jaundice, 12
2. Juvenile xanthogranuloma, 177-178
3. Urticaria pigmentosa, 208-210
4. Sebaceous nevus, 314-315
5. Mastocytomas, 208-210
6. Carotenemia, 12
7. Xanthomas
8. Necrobiosis lipoidica diabeticorum, 177
9. Goltz's syndrome, 282-283

Red Papules and Nodules

Newborns
1. Erythema toxicum, 302-303, 305
2. Furunculosis, 50-52
3. Insect bites, 77-88
4. Erysipelas, 205
5. Pyogenic granulomas, 178-179
6. Acne, 19, 164, 304
7. Epidermal nevus, 313-314
8. Candidiasis, 73-75, 305
9. Congenital syphilis, 57-59

Infants and Children
1. Insect bites, 77-88
2. Acne, 15-25
3. Viral exanthems, 89-118
   a. Rubella, 92-93
   b. Rubeola, 89-92
   c. Infectious mononucleosis (Epstein-Barr virus), 97-98
   d. Herpesvirus, 106-108
   e. Parovirus B19, 94-96
   f. Echovirus, 96-97
4. Urticaria, 202-210
5. Scarlet fever, 49-50
6. Erythema multiforme, 155-157
7. Erythema marginatum, 210-211
8. Erythema annulare, 210
9. Furunculosis, 50-52
10. Candidiasis, 73-75
11. Keratosis pilaris, 41-42
12. Early lesion of papulosquamous disease, 119-143
    a. Pityriasis rosea, 125-127
    b. Guttate psoriasis, 119, 123, 124, 125
    c. Acute parapsoriasis (PLEVA), 128-130
13. Neurofibroma, 174-175
14. Keloids and hypertrophic scars, 173-174
15. Shagreen patch, 244
16. Angiofibromas, 243
17. Pyogenic granulomas, 178-179
18. Granuloma annulare, 175-176
19. Secondary syphilis, 57-59, 128-129
20. Tinea corporis, 67-68
21. Cellulitis, 46-48
22. Bony fracture
23. Angioedema, 202-206
24. Cold panniculitis, 180
25. Lupus panniculitis, 132-134

(Lyme

87

D1349103

Continued on inside back cover.

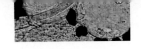

Third Edition

Color Textbook
of Pediatric
Dermatology

WILLIAM L. WESTON, MD
Professor, Departments of Dermatology and Pediatrics,
University of Colorado;
Head, Pediatric Dermatology,
The Children's Hospital and University of Colorado Hospital;
Denver, Colorado

ALFRED T. LANE, MD
Chair, Department of Dermatology;
Professor of Dermatology and Pediatrics,
Stanford University;
Service Chief, Pediatric Dermatology,
Stanford University Hospital and Clinics,
Lucile Salter Packard Children's Hospital at Stanford;
Palo Alto, California

JOSEPH G. MORELLI, MD
Associate Professor,
Departments of Dermatology and Pediatrics,
University of Colorado Health Sciences Center,
Denver, Colorado

with 557 illustrations

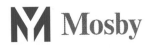

An Affiliate of Elsevier Science

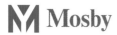

An Affiliate of Elsevier Science

Acquisition Editor: Elizabeth M. Fathmann
Editorial Assistant: Paige Mosher Wilke
Publishing Services Manager: Pat Joiner
Project Manager: Karen M. Rehwinkel
Designer: Mark A. Oberkrom

THIRD EDITION

Mosby, Inc.
An Affiliate of Elsevier Science
11830 Westline Industrial Drive
St. Louis, Missouri 63146

Printed in China

International Standard Book Number 0-323-01821-1

03 04 05 06 TG/RRD-W 9 8 7 6 5 4 3 2

Dedication

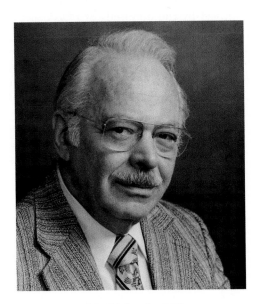

Alvin H. Jacobs, MD
1913–2001

This book is dedicated to the memory of Alvin Jacobs, MD. Two score years ago, there were less than five pediatric dermatologists in the United States. The effect that these "pioneers of pediatric dermatology" had on the understanding of skin diseases in children has been exponential. Doctors Nancy Esterly, Sam Weinberg, and the late Sid Hurwitz are recognized for their major contributions to the field. The authors praise all the pioneers and re-dedicate this textbook to another "pioneer"—Alvin Jacobs, MD—who promoted pediatric dermatology to primary care physicians like no other. He will always hold a special place in our memory. In its formative years, pediatric dermatology struggled to find its way as a field of medicine. Al Jacobs was always there to listen, to help, and to guide. Any pediatrician worth his or her salt knows the name of Alvin Hirsch Jacobs, MD. He presented hundreds of lectures on pediatric dermatology to national, regional, and local meetings, with never a negative comment. We can think of no others in the field who can match that accomplishment. His seminars on neonatal dermatology were classic; often they were the most popular sessions at national pediatric or dermatology meetings. Those who heard Al Jacobs talk know they heard the master. There are thousands of pediatricians whose first and often only formal teaching in pediatric dermatology came from Al Jacobs.

We decided to dedicate this book to Al Jacobs for another aspect of his professional career: his work behind the scenes in pediatric dermatology. For a complete appreciation of his contributions we must first examine the man. He was born in Reno, Nevada, and spent his boyhood among the ponderosa pines and broad valleys below the Comstock lode. This was still the Wild West, an invigorating life for an ambitious young man. After receiving the gold medal at graduation from the University of Nevada in 1933, he ventured east to the famous Johns Hopkins University School of Medicine, where he received his medical degree in 1937. After internship in Pittsburgh, he spent a year in child neurology at the Neurological Institute of New York. He returned west for training in pediatrics and infectious disease at San Francisco County Hospital, then served as chief resident in pediatrics at Stanford University. It was then June 1942, his country was at war, and Dr. Jacobs joined the Navy and was assigned to Navy Medical Research Unit Number 1. By 1946 he was a Lieutenant Commander and ready to return to the practice of pediatrics. In his private practice of pediatrics in San Francisco, Al quickly recognized that 20% of his patients had primary skin complaints and that he was poorly prepared to deal with them. He found his colleagues in pediatrics similarly unprepared and decided to remedy the situation. After a year's fellowship in dermatology at Stanford he joined the Stanford faculty and established a career in pediatric dermatology that has spanned five decades. Until his death on November 9, 2001, he was Professor of Dermatology and Pediatrics, Emeritus (active) at Stanford University.

Al Jacobs was a founder of the Society for Pediatric Dermatology and served as its first president. In many ways Al Jacobs was to pediatric dermatology what George Washington was to the establishment of the United States. It is so crucial that the leaders at the founding have the wisdom and vision to create an organization that will grow and be flexible enough to accommodate the changes needed in future generations. The advice and counsel of Al Jacobs was critical for the field of pediatric dermatology.

It was Al Jacobs the man who endeared himself to so many in pediatrics and pediatric dermatology. He avoided the arrogance that often accompanies positions of importance in academic medicine and remained the kind, considerate, warm man who always had time to listen to your needs or your problems. It was his accessibility that made the field of pediatric dermatology accessible for all who are interested. Who could resist that big smile beneath the cookie-duster moustache or those kind, twinkling eyes? Any personal encounter with Al Jacobs made you feel you were with your best friend. When you have a moment to reflect on your own careers, remember that big smile and what it meant to pediatric dermatology.

It is said that the fulfillment of life is to love, be loved, and have useful work. Al Jacobs loved his charming wife, Opal; his children and grandchildren; and his chosen field of pediatric dermatology. In turn, he was loved by the hundreds of physicians whose lives he touched.

This book is also dedicated to our families: Dr. Janet Atkinson Weston, Betsy and Kemp Weston; Maureen, Amy, Andy, Jeremy, Jordan, and Matthew Lane; Laura Wilson, Reed and Stefan Morelli.

William L. Weston, MD
Alfred T. Lane, MD
Joseph G. Morelli, MD

Preface

The third edition of *Color Textbook of Pediatric Dermatology,* as is characteristic of many third editions, is more polished than previous editions. The focus of this third edition is to meet the specific needs of the clinician responsible for the primary care of children. To accomplish this, there are many upgrades in this edition. We have increased the number of color photographs and replaced those in the second edition that did not reproduce well. We incorporated the latest information regarding the pathogenesis of skin diseases to completely revise some chapters and add important conditions to others. We added the latest references and greatly expanded the popular patient instruction sheets on the advice of our colleagues in primary care. We rely heavily on our colleagues in pediatrics and primary care of children to advise us on what to include in the book and on what aspects of the previous editions were not clearly explained. Many of the changes in this edition are the direct result of our learning the pediatric dermatology strengths and weaknesses of our primary care colleagues.

Although each of us wrote specific sections, every section was reviewed by all three. Each of us strongly believes that a textbook should not be written from other textbooks, but rather from original articles. Thus this edition was written as a unique resource, as was the last. We all believe that the book should be written in the simplest, most understandable and most usable manner for the clinician. We have tried to hold to these beliefs, even as we incorporated the latest information, including the multitude of recent genetic discoveries, by explaining their importance in the pathogenesis of disease and including phenotype-genotype correlations when they explain the disease. Specific patient instructions are invaluable in the success of any treatment plan. Thus we increased to 17 the specific Patient Education Information sheets provided in the appendix. These are written in easy understandable terms for your patients. These sheets may be copied and used in your practice.

We retained a number of useful features that were included in the previous edition. The Problem-Oriented Differential Diagnosis Index was retained on the inside of the front and back covers to allow the busy clinician rapid access when the diagnosis is not clear. A concise formulary specific for pediatric patients is still available in the appendix. All of the useful tables throughout the text were retained and several new ones added. The same organization for each disease was retained. We have tried to provide the busy clinician with concise, decisive information.

Without the encouragement of our own mentors, this book would not be possible. We have rededicated this third edition to Alvin Jacobs, MD, who, at a time when the world had less than a handful of pediatric dermatologists, had the vision to create a new discipline. He provided the impetus to so many young people hesitant to enter the uncertain world of a discipline yet undefined. Along with Dr. Jacobs, a tribute to the other three founders of the Society for Pediatric Dermatology is included. We recognize that the basis for the discipline of Pediatric Dermatology comes from Drs. Jacobs, Sam Weinberg, Sid Hurwitz, and Bill Weston. We also recognize the many early contributions to the discipline from Drs. Nancy Esterly and James Rasmussen. A special tribute to Dr. Jacobs appears on the dedication pages. We thank all the officers and members of the Society of Pediatric Dermatology, who provided us with collegiality, clinical expertise, scientific interest, and nurture. We trust that with this book we are in some way again repaying the great debt we owe our colleagues.

A special debt is owed to Drs. Robert Goltz, W. Mitchell Sams, and Lowell Goldsmith for their guidance, protected time, and generous support of our careers. We hope that we may be as supportive of those young people interested in skin disorders of children.

William L. Weston, MD
Alfred T. Lane, MD
Joseph G. Morelli, MD

Contents

Color Textbook
of Pediatric
Dermatology

CHAPTER ONE

Structure and Function of the Skin

A firm understanding of normal skin structure and function is necessary for recognition and treatment of skin disease. Those providing medical care for children should apply the principles of skin biology to the pediatric patient and master essentials of embryology and development.

THE EPIDERMIS
Keratinization

The epidermis functions as a barrier, preventing penetration from outside and retaining substances inside.[1,2] Over 95% of epidermal cells are keratinocytes. The process of keratinocyte replication and maturation is called *keratinization*. The major keratinocyte proteins are keratins, which provide scaffolding to determine keratinocyte shape. Keratin pairs form intermediate filaments by combining an acidic keratin with a basic keratin.[1,2] In basal keratinocytes, long keratins 5 and 14 provide the tall structure. As differentiation occurs, the long keratins are replaced by short keratins 1 and 10 and the cells flatten. The process of keratinization begins with proliferation of new keratinocytes in the region of the basal cell layer, near the dermal-epidermal junction (Fig. 1-1). As keratinocytes differentiate, they accumulate granules called *keratohyaline granules* in their cytoplasm, and the type of keratin bundles within the cells becomes thicker. Within the granular layer the cells lose their cylindrical and cuboidal shapes and begin to flatten as they go through the process of terminal differentiation or programmed cell death (apoptosis).[1-4] Cell nuclei are lost and the keratinocytes flatten like stacks of plates. This final layer is called the *horny layer,* or *stratum corneum.* The stratum corneum cells accumulate like bricks on a wall, separated by intercellular lipids, which function like mortar. The thick corneocyte membranes are created by the formation of an inner protein envelope including the proteins profilaggrin, involucrin, and epiligrin.[1-4] The intercellular and cell-surface lipids are an integral part of the epidermal barrier function.[1,3]

Individual keratinocytes are bound together by desmosomes and adherens junctions. The desmosomes contain membrane glycoproteins desmocollins and desmogleins, and cytoplasmic proteins desmoplakins, periplakin, and plakoglobin.

The process of keratinization is continuous within the skin. The newly formed keratinocytes of the basal layer mature and are shed from the skin over an interval of approximately 28 days. Skin diseases may be associated with variation in the speed and process of keratinization.

Epidermal Barrier

It is said that the skin is the interface between humans and their environment. Indeed, the most important functions of the epidermis are to provide a skin barrier against microorganisms and irritating chemicals and to impede the exchange of fluids and electrolytes between the body and the environment. This barrier function resides in the stratum corneum, where the terminally differentiated keratinocyte develops a tough cell envelope beneath the plasma membrane.[1,3-5] The process of envelope formation involves biochemical processing of involucrin, the major cytoplasmic protein precursor of the cell envelope. The epidermal barrier is completed by extracellular lipid layers surrounding the terminally differentiated keratinocytes.

Although the skin, including the epidermis and dermis, is 1.5- to 4.0-mm thick, the epidermal barrier is only 0.05- to 0.1-mm thick. By the daily shedding of one to two cell layers of stratum corneum, or scale, the epidermal barrier prevents excessive colonization of the skin surface. In addition to continuous shedding, the flattened stratum corneum cells are tightly adherent to each other, so that to obtain entrance into the lower epidermis and dermis, chemicals or microorganisms must pass between tightly compacted epidermal cells.

The water content of the environment greatly influences the epidermal barrier (see Chapter 22). Both an excessive and an inadequate water content in the

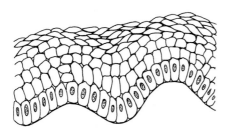

Fig. 1-1 Normal epidermis. The germinative layer with prominent nuclei is at the base of the epidermis and within the same compartment as the fully differentiated cells. As these basal cells differentiate, they migrate up toward the skin surface, shed their nuclei, become flattened, and are shed from the skin surface.

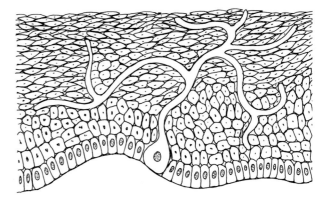

Fig. 1-2 Melanocyte-keratinocyte unit. The dendritic melanocyte, shown here as a clear cell with many branches, provides melanin pigment to many keratinocytes.

epidermal barrier will cause microscopic and macroscopic breaks in the barrier.

In response to friction or other forms of repeated trauma, such as exposure to ultraviolet light (UVL) or chemical injury, stratum corneum is formed in amounts greater than usual, as can be noted on the palms and soles. The stratum corneum is thinnest over the eyelids and scrotum.

Pigmentation and Ultraviolet Light

Four biochromes in the skin are responsible for clinical pigmentation: melanin, betacarotene, oxyhemoglobin, and reduced hemoglobin.[1,6-8] The brown-black pigment melanin is the dominant pigment of the skin. It is the pigment closest to the observer's vision and darkest in color. In dark-skinned individuals, it is difficult to recognize yellow pigment (betacarotene), red pigment (oxyhemoglobin), and blue pigment (reduced hemoglobin). Melanin is produced by the pigment-forming cell, the melanocyte, which is located in the epidermis. Different skin regions contain different numbers of melanocytes. For example, three times as many melanocytes are found in the epidermis of the forehead as in the abdominal skin.[1] Numbers of melanocytes per unit area of skin are the same despite racial differences in pigmentation.

Each epidermal melanocyte has dendritic cytoplasmic extensions that make contact with 35 to 45 epidermal cells. This melanocyte-keratinocyte unit (Fig. 1-2) is responsible for clinical pigmentation. The brownish-black polymer melanin is produced within the melanocytes in special membrane-bound

organelles called *melanosomes*. It is dependent on stimulation of the melanocortin 1 receptor (MC1R) by melanocyte stimulating hormone (MSH).[6,7] Polymorphisms in the MC1R determine skin and hair color; certain polymorphisms stimulate the red phaeomelanin pathway rather than the brown-black eumelanin pathway.[6-8] The enzymes, including tyrosinase, that are crucial for melanin production are contained within the melanosome membrane. Melanosomes develop in stages. Tyrosinase and other enzymes convert the colorless chemical tyrosine to an oxidized quinone compound, which in turn becomes polymerized into the brownish-black compound melanin. Clinical pigmentation depends on the stage of the melanosome produced and dispersion of melanosomes from melanocytes to keratinocytes. Keratinocytes actively phagocytize the melanosomes. In black skin, there are single units of advanced-stage melanosomes, whereas in lighter-skinned persons, the melanosomes are aggregated and of earlier developmental stages. Thus the major difference in black and white skin is the stage of melanosome development and the ability to transfer and disperse melanin pigment, not the number of melanocytes per unit area of skin.

The function of melanin is to protect the deoxyribonucleic acid (DNA) structure of epidermal cell nuclei from damage by UVL irradiation. Melanin dispersed within the cytoplasm of keratinocytes forms a protective cap over the keratinocyte nucleus when the keratinocytes are exposed to UVL (Fig. 1-3). Melanin pigment is lost by the daily shedding of stratum

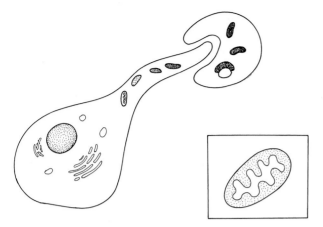

Fig. 1-3 Melanin production and transfer. Melanosomes *(inset)* are organelles formed in the rough endoplasmic reticulum and Golgi area of melanocytes. Their membranes contain the enzyme tyrosinase, which is responsible for the formation of the brown-black polymer melanin. At the end of the dendrite, the melanocytes are shown transferring pigment to the keratinocyte, where the melanin moves to form a cap of the keratinocyte nucleus as protection against ultraviolet injury.

Table 1-1	Biologic Effects of Ultraviolet Light	
Ultraviolet (UV) group	**Wavelength (nm)**	**Biologic effects**
UVC	200-290	Cytotoxic (bactericidal, retinal injury)
UVB	290-320	Sunburn, sun tanning, systemic lupus erythematosus, skin cancers
UVA	320-400	Drug photoallergies, porphyria, phytophotodermatitis, psoralen photoaging, PUVA therapy

PUVA, Psoralen ultraviolet A-range.

corneum cells. Melanin within the dermis, such as that found in dermal melanocytic birthmarks, has no such mechanism available for its elimination.

UVL from the sun increases melanin pigmentation by first oxidizing preformed melanin, increasing cross-linking of the melanin polymer and darkening the color. This effect occurs within minutes after exposure and is called *immediate pigment darkening.* During the 4 to 6 days after UVL exposure, both increased melanin production and melanin transfer to keratinocytes produce tanning.

Sunlight

The sun produces UVL of numerous wavelengths, which, based on their biologic effects, are arbitrarily divided into three groups: ultraviolet A (UVA), ultraviolet B (UVB), and ultraviolet C (UVC) (Table 1-1). Incoming UVL from the sun is scattered by small molecules in the atmosphere and absorbed by the ozone layer; all UVL below 290 nm is absorbed, so that virtually no UVC reaches the earth's surface.

Sunburn is caused by wavelengths of light from 290 to 320 nm. Photons of UVL are absorbed by electrons of chemicals with double bonds and ring structures, such as nucleic acids, DNA, and proteins, producing excited electron states within these molecules or free-radical formation. Betacarotene and melanin act by stabilizing the free radicals and are natural photoprotective chemicals found in skin. About 10% of UVB passes through the epidermis and reaches the dermis. The erythema and pain of sunburn are mediated via prostaglandins and other mediators.

The sunburn wavelengths of UVL are blocked by window glass. The tanning and thickening of the epidermal barrier that result from exposure to sunlight impair the penetration of UVL into the lower epidermis and dermis. Wavelengths of light from 320 to 400 nm (UVA) are responsible for the photosensitivity seen in the many drug photoallergies and psoralen phototoxicity. Light of these wavelengths passes through window glass and also is emitted from fluorescent lamps such as those used as in overhead lighting in schools.

Epidermal Basement Membrane

The junction between the epidermis and dermis is the epidermal basement membrane. This structure is composed of complex protein-cell and protein-matrix interactions among the basal keratinocyte, the lamina lucida, the lamina densa, the sublamina densa, and dermal collagens.[9,10] Keratins in the basal keratinocyte attach into the electron-dense plaques associated with the hemidesmosomes. Anchoring filaments extend from the hemidesmosome to dermal collagen fibers and have attachment sites to laminin

5 as well.[9,10] The complex basement membrane anchoring interactions resists shearing forces to the skin and provides strength.

Bullous pemphigoid antigen 1 is associated with the cytoplasmic portion of the basal cell hemidesmosome, and bullous pemphigoid antigen 2 is a transmembrane portion of the hemidesmosome. Laminins 5 and 6 are associated with the anchoring filaments. Laminin 1, nidogen, and type IV collagen are associated with the lamina lucida and lamina densa. The long anchoring fibrils of the sublamina densa are composed of type VII collagen. Integrins are extrahemidesmosomal attachments to the lamina densa.

Autoantibodies against basement membrane structures or genetic defects of these structures cause a variety of diseases. Correlation of the function of specific structures of the basement membrane and disease-associated defects has helped to increase understanding of the epidermal-dermal junction.

THE DERMIS

The dermis is composed predominantly of collagen fibers and elastin fibers enclosed in a gel continuum of mucopolysaccharides.[1,10-13] This fibrous complex gives the dermis its great mechanical strength and elasticity, allowing the skin to withstand severe frictional stress yet still be extensible over joints. Elastin, collagen, and mucopolysaccharide gel are all produced and secreted by fibroblasts. Types I, III, IV, and VII are the predominant collagens in the skin. Although the principal mass of the dermis consists of collagen fibers and is acellular, numerous other elements are present, including mast cells, inflammatory cells, blood and lymph vessels, and cutaneous nerves. These elements are responsible for regulation of heat loss, the host defenses of the skin, nutrition, and other regulatory functions.

Collagen, Elastin, and Mechanical Properties

Most of the mechanical strength of the skin is derived from the fibrous protein *collagen,* a macromolecule with a large hydroxyproline content.[1,11,12] Mature collagen structure becomes rigid with cross-linking of adjacent protein chains, and young collagen that is without significant cross-linking fails to limit skin distention. Defective collagen results in extensive and excessive distensibility of the skin, as seen in Ehlers-Danlos syndrome, or severe blisters, as seen in recessive dystrophic epidermolysis bullosa. Elastin fibers, which are composed of both an amorphous and a fibrillar portion, are responsible for the reversible distensibility that allows the skin to be restored to normal size after stretching.[1,13] Defective elastin production results in extreme wrinkling and redundant skin, as seen in cutis laxa.

Cutaneous Vasculature

Cutaneous arteries course through the subcutaneous fat and give rise to two vascular plexuses that run parallel to the epidermis. These vascular plexuses contain arteriovenous shunts to divert blood from the skin and provide nutrition to it, to regulate heat loss, and to participate in the defense against foreign substances. The epidermis contains no blood vessels and receives its nutrition via the diffusion of plasma into the intercellular epidermal spaces. The stratum corneum has no such nutritive process.

Heat Regulation and Sweating

Skin is important in the control of body temperature. Heat generated in organs and muscles is rapidly transported to the skin vasculature.[1,14,15] The cutaneous circulation acts as a radiator. Varying the rate and volume of blood flow through the skin controls heat loss from this radiator. The blood flow is controlled by the autonomic nervous system. Heat from the skin surface is lost by evaporation of water in the form of eccrine sweat. Heat loss or gain by convection or radiation depends on environmental temperature. At comfortable temperatures, body heat can be regulated by the cutaneous vasculature alone, without sweating. In hot, dry environments the core body temperature may rise slightly but is stabilized by heat loss via sweating. In hot, humid environments evaporation of water from the skin surface is restricted, and heat gain occurs in the child's body. If this condition is allowed to continue, high fever, dehydration, and sodium depletion may occur. With exercise and heat gain, sweating is critical to maintaining body temperature.[14,15] In children born with deficient numbers of eccrine sweat glands (hypohidrotic ectodermal dysplasia), heat gain occurs during hot weather, overheating, or exercise, and recurrent high fever is often a presenting feature of the condition.

Cutaneous Nerves

Sensory nerve endings in the skin can elicit all of the principal sensations: touch, pain, itch, warmth, and cold. The skin is supplied by both myelinated and unmyelinated branches of spinal nerves.[1,16,17] Nerve branches enter the dermis from the subcutaneous fat and form both a superficial and a deep nerve plexus. Unmyelinated branches from either plexus terminate in nerve endings that may be simple or specialized. Terminals from a single axon may serve an area as broad as 1 cm^2 and overlap with nerve endings from other axons. Inflow of cutaneous sensory information is strongly controlled and modulated by the cerebral cortex. The skin has a high sensitivity to rapid mechanical stimulation, with positional movements of less than 1 μm detectable. Sensations of cold persist continuously when skin temperature is below 30° C, and sensations of warmth persist continuously when it is above 37° C.[1] Changes in temperature of 0.03° C can be detected, especially if the skin temperature changes faster than 0.007° C/sec. Thermal sensitivity is highest on the face. At temperatures below 18° C and above 45° C, pain is produced. Pain may also be induced by pressure greater than 50 g/mm^2 and by disruption of skin.[17] A number of chemicals injected into the skin may also elicit pain. Itch is a sensation related to pain and is greatest close to transitions of mucous membranes. Histamine is considered to be the most important mediator of itch, but many other mediators are capable of producing this sensation. Itch may be exclusively central rather than cutaneous in some conditions, such as cholestasis.[18]

HOST DEFENSES OF THE SKIN

When breaks in the epidermal barrier occur, microorganisms invade the upper epidermis. Plasma proteins, such as complement proteins and immunoglobulins that normally bathe the intercellular epidermal space, initiate an inflammatory response. Cutaneous vasodilation (erythema) occurs early after this initial process, with diffusion of more plasma proteins, followed by the migration of neutrophils, T lymphocytes, B lymphocytes, and monocyte-macrophages into the dermis and later the epidermis. Such cells initially accumulate around dermal blood vessels but may migrate to the epidermis through the dermal-epidermal junction and between epidermal cells. For example, in impetigo large numbers of neutrophils accumulate just beneath the stratum corneum. Mast cells containing histamine, heparin, and platelet-activating factors are located around cutaneous blood vessels and play a regulatory role in the immune response of the skin by their influence on cutaneous vascular responses.

The initial response of the skin to invasion by microorganisms consists primarily of migration of neutrophilic leukocytes, but by 18 to 24 hours it is characterized by the appearance of lymphocytes and monocyte-macrophages in the dermis. Microorganisms or foreign substances not initially destroyed by neutrophils are presumably further digested by macrophages or destroyed by direct lymphocytotoxicity. A rich lymphatic system is also found in the dermis, and foreign substances are carried to regional lymph nodes, where specific immune responses are generated by T lymphocytes and B lymphocytes. Some antigen recognition probably occurs in the skin because antigen-processing cells (Langerhans cells) are found in the epidermis, and direct Langerhans–T lymphocyte contact occurs that may be important in the recognition of foreign antigens.

The epidermal barrier remains the primary defense of the skin, but microorganisms that pass through the barrier are destroyed within the midepidermis as the skin defenses attempt to keep them out of deeper tissue.

EPIDERMAL APPENDAGES

Epidermal appendages, which are modifications of epithelium, include hair follicle structures, sebaceous glands, nails, and the apocrine and eccrine sweat glands. Hair follicles are formed under the direction of several genes, including the hairless gene involved in the rare congenital atrichia.[19]

Hair Growth

The hair growth cycle has three phases: the growing phase, *anagen;* the regressing phase, *catagen;* and the resting phase, *telogen.*[1,19,20] The cells of anagen hairs have a high mitotic rate and are among the most rapidly replicating cells in humans. The hair growth originates from the hair bulb, which is located in the lower dermis.[1,19,20] The delta and notch genes may be involved in initiation of hair growth, along with ectodysplasin, a protein involved in ectodermal dysplasias.[19] Human scalp hair grows about 1 cm per month. When growth of the hair ceases, the catagen phase occurs, resulting in cessation of mitosis, apoptosis, and upward migration of the hair bulb into the middermis.[19,20] The hair shaft becomes clubbed at the bottom, causing the catagen hair to become a telogen hair (also called *club hair*). The telogen hair remains in the follicle for 2 to 3 months and is pushed out when the new hair grows.

There are great differences in the hair growth cycle among the different hair types found in the various body regions. It is believed that fibroblast growth factor 5 regulates the duration of the anagen phase.[19,20] Ambisexual hair follicles are common to both sexes and are androgen dependent. At puberty, androgen converts vellus hairs to terminal hairs in the axilla and the lower pubic triangle. Conversely, conversion of terminal scalp hairs to vellus hairs occurs in the temporal area of the scalp at puberty. Male sexual hair is responsive to high androgen levels, which convert vellus hairs to terminal hairs in the beard area, ears, sternum, and upper pubic triangle. In the occipital and bifrontal areas of the scalp, androgen levels result in a conversion from terminal to vellus hairs, resulting in androgenetic alopecia.

Hair cycles are asynchronous and vary within body sites. In the scalp at any point in time, about 85% of the hairs are growing (anagen), 14% are resting (telogen), and 1% are regressing (catagen). Newborns convert most of their hairs to telogen hairs within the first 6 months of life. Some newborns take several months to develop new anagen hairs, resulting in a "bald" baby. Other infants develop new anagen hairs so rapidly that they appear not to lose their hair. After acute febrile diseases children or adults can have many hairs convert from anagen to telogen with a subsequent period of months with markedly thinned hair (telogen effluvium). Curly hair is in part regulated by the transcription factor DLX (distal-less) and fibroblast growth factors.[19]

Sebaceous Glands

Sebaceous glands are present everywhere on the human skin except for the palms, soles, and dorsa of the feet. Generally they are associated with hair follicles and empty through a short duct into the canal of the hair follicle.[1,21] The sebaceous sweat glands are holocrine glands that produce sebum, a semiliquid mixture of glandular cell debris containing glycerides, free fatty acids, wax esters, squalene, cholesterol, and cholesterol esters. The largest and most numerous sebaceous glands are found on the face, scalp, chest, and back.

Sebum production is androgen dependent and begins at puberty in skin regions with abundant sebaceous follicles.[1,21] Sebaceous gland volume, sebaceous cell size, and secretory capacity are all directly androgen dependent. Obstruction of the sebaceous gland is associated with acne in humans.

Eccrine Glands

Humans have 2 to 5 million eccrine glands. These glands function to cool the body through evaporative heat loss of eccrine sweat. In addition, these glands may help to moisten the frictional surfaces of the skin.

Apocrine Glands

Apocrine sweat glands are in the axilla, mons pubis, areola of the breast, circumanal area, and the scalp. They are located deep in the subcutaneous tissue and usually open into a hair follicle. Apocrine glands secrete a yellowish, sticky fluid after puberty. The secretion is produced in response to stress or sexual stimulation. In lower animals, these glands function as sexual attractors and territorial markers.

Nails

Nails are formed by the fifth fetal month.[1,24] The nail matrix contains epithelial cells responsible for the production of the nail plate. The nail matrix occupies an area beneath the proximal nail fold, a portion of which may be seen as the lunula. Fingernails grow approximately 1 cm in 3 months, and toenails grow slower. Newborn nails are spoon-shaped and thin and may remain so until 2 or 3 years of age.

SUBCUTANEOUS FAT

The subcutaneous fat lies just beneath the dermis and is composed principally of lipocytes. It serves as a cushion to trauma, a heat insulator, and a highly important source of energy and hormone metabolism. Premature infants have poorly developed subcutaneous tissues, contributing to thermal instability and metabolic difficulties.

DEVELOPMENT OF SKIN
Periderm

Knowledge of the structure and function of developing fetal skin is invaluable in understanding abnormalities observed in newborn and infant skin. The single layer of ectodermal cells overlaying the developing fetus interacts with the mesoderm below to form the epidermis and dermis, respectively.[1,24] Through this interaction the appendages develop, and the unique properties of skin at different body sites result. Homeobox and lateralizing genes are critical in the proper timing and orientation of skin.[19]

Between 4 and 5 weeks gestation, the single layer of ectodermal cells of the fetal epidermis is covered by a layer of flattened cells called the *periderm*. The periderm cells expand across the developing epidermis by active mitosis, becoming rounded bulging cells uniformly covered by microvilli. The stratum corneum forms beneath the periderm cells during the fifth to sixth month. At this time periderm cells regress and become shrunken remnants that slough into the amniotic fluid and become one component of the vernix caseosa.

From the morphologic characteristics it is suggested that a transport function exists for periderm cells. The periderm may transport fluids, electrolytes, and sugars into the developing embryo.

Epidermal Development

After 8 weeks gestation an intermediate cell layer develops between the basal cells and the periderm.[1,24] In time this layer stratifies and adds additional cell layers. By 24 weeks gestation, granular and cornified cells are present on almost all regions of the body. From this time until birth, the stratum corneum matures and thickens so that at birth, the term infant's skin barrier function is comparable to that of an adult. The premature infant's barrier function is more deficient the earlier the premature birth.

The sequence of development of the keratins, the development of the basement membrane zone, the development of the desmosomes, hemidesmosomes, and the antigens of the epidermis have been catalogued.[1,24] The epidermis follows a sequence of development that is being intensively studied to understand the cellular interactions of normal development and the errors that occur in skin diseases.

Cells That Migrate Into the Epidermis

Although the epidermis is ectodermal in origin, cells from other sources migrate into the epidermis. Langerhans cells are present within the epidermis by 6 weeks gestation, but they may not be functionally mature until after 12 weeks gestation.[1,24] The melanocyte is derived from the neural crest and migrates to the epidermis before the twelfth gestational week. By 16 weeks gestation melanocytes with melanosomes capable of synthesizing melanin are noted, and by 20 weeks gestation the epidermis has its full complement of melanocytes. Merkel cells appear in the epidermis of the fingertips, glabrous skin, and nail beds by 12 weeks gestation and serve as special sensory organs. These cells may develop within the epidermis rather than being an immigrant cell as previously thought.

Epidermal Appendages

Hair follicle or sweat gland development begins earlier in the scalp, palm, and sole than in other body areas. The hair germ begins in the scalp by 12 weeks gestation as a proliferation of keratinocytes above a collection of fibroblasts.[1,19,24] These cells proliferate and invaginate into the dermis, forming the hair peg and the subsequent hair follicle. Granular cells are present within the hair follicle after 14 weeks gestation, a full 6 to 10 weeks before they are seen in the interfollicular skin. Hair grows at an oblique angle to the skin surface such that hair will erupt caudally, causing the hair to point downward.

Anlagen of eccrine glands may be present on the sole as early as 10 weeks gestation. The eccrine gland secretory coil forms on the sole at about 16 weeks gestation, and the secretory and myoepithelial cells differentiate at 22 weeks gestation. The sebaceous gland primordia develop off the hair follicle after 16 weeks gestation. Steroid hormone stimulation of sebaceous glands is so great that these glands are considerably larger in the third trimester fetus than those of a child. Apocrine glands, the last of the appendages to develop, first appear during the sixth month of fetal development.

Nails and volar pads

Development of the fetal nail, the volar pads, skin ridges, and sweat glands are tied together in the developing digit.[1,24] These structures form simultaneously at 8 weeks gestation, just after the digits separate from one another. By 12 weeks gestation the proximal and distal nail folds have formed, and the volar pads are formed from mounds of mesenchyme and an increased intermediate layer of the epidermis. The distal nail fold is the first epithelial structure to keratinize, beginning at 12 weeks gestation. A nail plate covers the nail bed by 17 weeks gestation. Primary dermal ridges appear at 12 weeks gestation, and secondary dermal ridges at 16 weeks gestation.[24] Sweat gland buds appear in the fingertips at 12 weeks gestation, but sweating does not occur until after 32 weeks gestation.

Influences of the Dermis on Epidermal Growth and Differentiation

The fetal dermis plays an overwhelmingly predominant role in transformation of the ectoderm into epidermis and maintenance of controlled epidermal appendage development. The continued interaction between the epidermis and dermis maintains the continued presence of the thickened skin of the palms and soles or the thinner skin of the face. The epidermal appendages are maintained by epidermal-dermal interaction, and once full-thickness injury occurs, the re-formed scar tissue appears unable to regenerate new appendages. Skin diseases associated with thickening or thinning of the epidermis may be associated with abnormal epidermal-dermal communications.

The Dermis

The primordial dermis begins as a cellular mesenchyme that is watery and without fibrous structure.

By 6 weeks of age a fine meshwork of collagen fibrils underlies the dermal-epidermal junction and adheres to the dermal mesenchymal cell surfaces.[1,24] Extracellular collagen increases with age, and fibrils associate into collagen fiber bundles. Cells of the dermis become spaced farther apart, and their elongated axes become oriented parallel to the skin surface. The fine collagen network persists at the dermal-epidermal junction and ensheaths epidermal appendages as they project downward. The dermis increases in thickness from 0.1 mm at 7 weeks to 0.7 mm by 20 weeks of gestation. As the epidermal appendages project deeply into the dermis at 16 weeks gestation, the dermis organizes two distinct regions: the papillary dermis with fine fibrillar collagen and the reticular dermis with large collagen bundles. By 20 weeks gestation, the fetal dermis is similar to that of the adult in structure, although still smaller in total thickness. Preliminary studies have demonstrated the 8-week-old fetus to contain fibronectin and types I, III, and V collagen within the dermis. By 14 weeks, recognizable fibroblasts, mast cells, endothelial cells, Schwann cells, and histiocytes are found in the fetal dermis.[24] By 60 days of gestation, anchoring filaments are associated with the basal lamina at the dermal-epidermal junction. At 22 weeks, the elastin fibers form, but well-developed elastin fiber networks are not observed until after 32 weeks, and the adult form of mature elastin fibers does not occur until after 2 years of age.

Few rigorous studies have been performed on the other components of the dermis, including vasculature, lymphatics, and nerves. Fat initially forms with discrete areas within the dermis at 16 to 18 weeks, then demarcation of a distinct fat layer that coincides with the development of hair follicles and their projection into the lower dermis.

Overall, newborn epidermal, hair, sweat, and sebaceous structures are nearly identical to adult structures. The dermis is less mature than adult dermis, being thinner with less organization of collagen and elastin fibers, with a less organized vascular network and cutaneous nerves.[24] The newborn dermis appears as a transition between fetal and adult structures.

REFERENCES

1. Goldsmith LA: *Physiology, biochemistry & molecular biology of the skin,* ed 2, New York, 1991, Oxford University Press.
2. Blumenberg M, Tomic-Canic M: Human epidermal keratinocyte:keratinization processes, *EXS* 78:1, 1997.
3. Gandarillas A et al: Evidence that apoptosis and terminal differentiation are distinct processes, *Exp Dermatol* 8:71, 1999.
4. Ishida-Yamamoto et al: Programmed cell death in normal epidermis and loricrine keratoderma: multiple functions of profillaggrin in keratinization, *J Invest Dermatol* 4:145, 1999.
5. Aeschlimann D, Thomazy V: Protein crosslinking in assembly and remodeling of extracellular matrices: the role of transglutaminases, *Connect Tissue Res* 41:1, 2000.
6. Schallreuter KU: A review of recent advances on the regulation of pigmentation in the human epidermis, *Cell Mol Biol* 45:943, 1999.
7. Rees JL: The melanocortin receptor (MCIR): more than just red hair, *Pigment Cell Res* 13:135, 2000.
8. Cohn BA: The vital role of the skin in human natural history, *Int J Dermatol* 37:821, 1998.
9. Erickson AC, Couchman JR: Still more complexity in mammalian basement membranes, *J Histochem Cytochem* 48:1291, 2000.
10. Aumailley M, Rousselle P: Laminins of the dermo-epidermal junction, *Matrix Biol* 18:19, 1999.
11. Uitto J, Bernstein EE: Molecular mechanisms of cutaneous aging: connective tissue alterations in the dermis, *J Invest Dermatol* 3:41, 1998.
12. Bella J, Berman HM: Integrin-collagen complex: a metal-glutamate handshake, *Structure* 8:R121, 2000.
13. Debelle L, Tamburro AM: Elastin: molecular description and function, *Int J Biochem Cell Biol* 31:261, 1999.
14. Galloway SD: Dehydration, rehydration and exercise in the heat: rehydration strategies for athletic competition, *Can J Appl Physiol* 24:188, 1999.
15. Armstrong LE, Maresh CM: Effects of training, environment and host factors in the sweating response to exercise, *Int J Sports Med* 19:S103, 1998.
16. Kanda T: Pathological changes in human unmyelinated nerve fibers: a review, *Histol Histopathol* 15:313, 2000.
17. Schmidt R et al: Mechano-insensitive nociceptors encode pain evoked by tonic pressure to human skin, *Neurosci* 98:793, 2000.
18. Jones EA, Bergasa NV: Evolving concepts of the pathogenesis and treatment of the pruritus of cholestasis, *Can J Gastroenterol* 14:33, 2000.
19. Van Steensel MA, Happle R, Steijlen PM: Molecular genetics of the hair follicle: the state of the art, *Proc Soc Exp Biol Med* 223:1, 2000.
20. Paus R, Muller-Rover S, Botchkarev VA: Chronobiology of the hair follicle: hunting the "hair cycle clock," *J Invest Dermatol* 4:338, 1999.
21. Cunliffe WJ et al: Comedogenesis: some new aetiological, clinical and therapeutic strategies, *Br J Dermat* 142:1084, 2000.
22. Tomita K et al: Congenital ectopic nails, *Plast Reconstr Surg* 100:1497, 1997.
23. Mayeaux EJ Jr: Nail disorders, *Prim Care* 27:333, 2000.
24. Holbrook KA: Embryogenesis of the skin. In Harper J, Oranje A, Prose N (editors): *Textbook of pediatric dermatology,* London, 2000, Blackwell.

CHAPTER TWO | Evaluation of Children With Skin Disease

The language of dermatology frequently inhibits students, house officers, and practitioners dealing with children from using the correct terminology for skin disease.[1] It is neither proper nor helpful to simply use the term *rash*.[2] This chapter describes the correct approach to the presenting features, signs, and initial laboratory findings when evaluating children with cutaneous disease. Morphology is the key to diagnosis of skin problems, and the student of dermatology should become expert in recognizing and describing morphologic features. The description of primary lesions should be memorized. Particular attention should be paid to the presence of *vesicles, pustules, scaling*, and *color changes*. These four morphologic features will allow the identification of the major morphologic groups, which is essential for proper diagnosis and differential diagnosis.[3] A problem-oriented algorithm is included in this chapter to allow determination of the morphologic groups of skin disease by their cutaneous appearance. Mastering this information will aid in communication with others delivering medical care to children.

MEDICAL HISTORY

The history obtained regarding a child's skin condition should be considered in the same fashion as a general medical history. The onset and duration of each symptom should be recorded. Associated systemic symptoms should be sought, along with a thorough review of systems. A past medical history, complete family history, and information on recent medications should also be obtained.

Health care advice is sought for children for three major concerns regarding their skin: itching (pruritus), scaling, and cosmetic appearance.

Pruritus

Persistent itching in the skin often provides the impetus to seek medical attention. The examiner should note whether the itching is localized or generalized and whether it is associated with skin lesions. Itching without skin lesions suggests biliary obstruction, diabetes mellitus, uremia, lymphoma, or hyperthyroidism. If the pruritus is associated with skin lesions, dermatophytosis, scabies, and the many types of dermatitis should be considered.

Scaling

Normally one cell layer of stratum corneum, composed of flattened nonviable remnants of keratinocytes packed with protein (keratin), is shed daily. This is not usually visible. Acute injury and resultant separation of 10 to 20 cell layers of stratum corneum result in clinically visible white sheets of scale, such as that seen in desquamation after a sunburn or thermal burn. Overproduction of stratum corneum by proliferating epidermis, as in psoriasis, results in visible accumulation of excess surface scale. The scale in psoriasis is thick in contrast to thin (pityriasis) scale.

Cosmetic Appearance

Parents may be concerned about the appearance of a child's skin, particularly any color change. A history of the time of appearance of skin lesions, sequence of color changes, and course of skin changes should be obtained.

EXAMINATION OF THE SKIN

The evaluation of skin lesions requires careful inspection of the entire cutaneous surface, and many skin diseases are diagnosed only by their morphologic appearance.[4] Examination of the skin should consist of identification of the primary lesion (the earliest lesion to appear), the size or range of the primary lesion in millimeters, secondary changes, and a description of the color, arrangement, and distribution of lesions. Often, however, one sees children with secondary skin changes without primary lesions. For correct diagnosis, a rigorous search should be made for a primary lesion. To properly evaluate the primary lesion, both visual inspection and palpation are required. Palpation should determine whether the lesion is hard or

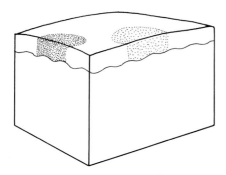

Fig. 2-1 A *macule* is a color change in the skin that is flat to the surface of the skin and not palpable (e.g., a tan macule, café-au-lait spot, white macule, vitiligo).

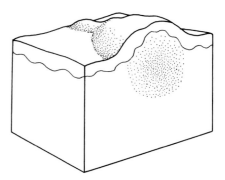

Fig. 2-3 A *nodule* is a raised, solid lesion with indistinct borders and a deep palpable portion. A large nodule is termed a *tumor* (e.g., rheumatoid nodule, neurofibroma).

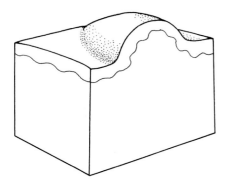

Fig. 2-2 A *papule* is a solid, raised lesion with distinct borders 1 cm or less in diameter (e.g., lichen planus, molluscum contagiosum).

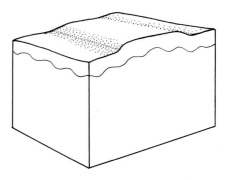

Fig. 2-4 A *wheal,* an area of tense edema in the upper dermis, produces a flat-topped, slightly raised lesion (e.g., urticaria).

soft, and whether it moves with the skin or the skin moves over it.

Primary Skin Lesions (The Morphology of Skin)

1. A *macule* (Fig. 2-1) is a color change in the skin that is flat to the surface of the skin and not palpable (e.g., a tan macule, café-au-lait spot, white macule, vitiligo).
2. A *papule* (Fig. 2-2) is a solid, raised lesion with distinct borders 1 cm or less in diameter (e.g., lichen planus, molluscum contagiosum).
3. A *plaque* is a solid, raised, flat-topped lesion with distinct borders and an epidermal change larger than 1 cm in diameter (e.g., psoriasis).
4. A *nodule* (Fig. 2-3) is a raised, solid lesion with indistinct borders and a deep palpable portion. A large nodule is termed a *tumor* (e.g., rheumatoid nodule, neurofibroma). If the skin moves over the nodule, it is subcutaneous in location; if the skin moves with the nodule, the nodule is intradermal.

5. A *wheal* (Fig. 2-4), an area of tense edema in the upper dermis, produces a flat-topped, slightly raised lesion (e.g., urticaria).
6. A *vesicle* (Fig. 2-5) is a raised lesion filled with clear fluid (e.g., varicella, herpes simplex) that is less than 1 cm in diameter.
7. A *bulla* is a raised lesion larger than 1 cm and filled with clear fluid.
8. A *cyst* (Fig. 2-6) is a raised lesion that contains a palpable sac filled with solid material.
9. A *pustule* (Fig. 2-7) is a raised lesion filled with a fluid exudate, giving it a yellow appearance (e.g., acne, folliculitis).

Size of the Primary Lesion

The size or range of sizes of the primary lesion or lesions should be measured in millimeters and recorded. To expedite the examination, measure certain landmarks on the examining finger to estimate lesion size.

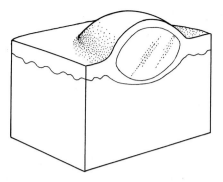

Fig. 2-5 A *vesicle* is a raised lesion filled with clear fluid (e.g., varicella, herpes simplex) that is less than 1 cm in diameter. A *bulla* is a raised lesion larger than 1 cm and filled with clear fluid.

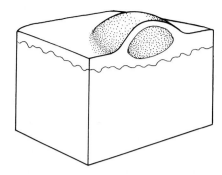

Fig. 2-7 A *pustule* is a raised lesion filled with a fluid exudate, giving it a yellow appearance (e.g., acne, folliculitis).

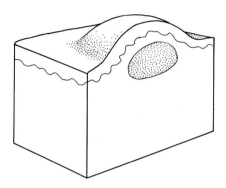

Fig. 2-6 A *cyst* is a raised lesion that contains a palpable sac filled with liquid or semisolid material (e.g., epithelial cyst).

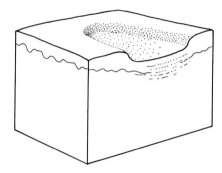

Fig. 2-8 In *atrophy* the skin surface is depressed because of thinning or absence of the dermis or subcutaneous fat (e.g., atrophic scar, fat necrosis).

Secondary Changes

1. *Erosions and oozing.* A moist, circumscribed, slightly depressed area represents a blister base *(erosion)* with the roof of the blister removed (e.g., burns, dermatitis). Because the action of chewing or sucking easily removes the thin blister roof (oral mucosa lacks a stratum corneum), most oral blisters present as erosions (e.g., aphthae, herpes simplex stomatitis).
2. *Crusting* represents dried exudate of plasma combined with the blister roof, which sits on the surface of skin after acute dermatitis (e.g., impetigo, contact dermatitis).
3. In *scaling*, whitish plates are present on the skin surface (e.g., psoriasis, ichthyosis). *Desquamation* refers to peeling of sheets of scale after an acute injury to skin (e.g., burn, toxic drug reaction, scarlet fever).
4. In *atrophy* (Fig. 2-8), the skin surface is depressed because of thinning or absence of the dermis or subcutaneous fat (e.g., atrophic scar, fat necro-

sis). If the epidermis is thinned, it appears as fine wrinkling.
5. *Excoriations* are oval to linear depressions in the skin with a complete removal of the epidermis, exposing a broad section of red dermis. Excoriations are the result of fingernail removal of the epidermis and upper dermis.
6. *Fissures* are characterized by linear, wedge-shaped cracks in the epidermis extending down to the dermis and narrowing at the base.

Disruption of the Skin Surface

The presence of weeping, crusting, cracking (fissures), or excoriations is characteristic of disruption of the skin surface.[2] Disruption is seen in eczematous lesions but is absent in papulosquamous lesions and is an important feature in distinguishing the two.

Mobility of Skin

When grasping the skin between thumb and forefinger, the skin should be mobile. Excessive stretching indicates a type of Ehlers-Danlos syndrome; immobility suggests scleroderma (see Chapter 19).

Color

The color of a skin lesion should be described as skin-colored, brown, red, yellow, tan, or blue. Particular attention should be paid to whether the red or red-brown lesion completely blanches (e.g., petechiae do not blanch). Red or red-brown color in skin is dependent on the pigment oxyhemoglobin, which is found in red blood cells within superficial cutaneous blood vessels. Compressing the superficial vascular plexus by direct pressure forces red blood cells into deeper vascular channels, and blanching of the skin is observed. If the skin does not blanch with pressure, red blood cells are outside the vascular channels and located in the adjacent dermis.

Melanin is the dominant pigment in the skin. Because it is located in the outer layer of skin closest to the observer's eye, melanin may obscure other pigments located in deeper layers. In dark-skinned infants and children, one must use a disciplined approach to detect erythema, cyanosis, or jaundice. First, determine the normal skin color, then compare the involved skin area with the normal skin. Erythema will appear dusky red or violet. Cyanosis will appear black. Jaundice will appear diffusely darker, and one must examine the sclera to detect the presence of this disease. Carotenemia will appear golden-brown. The examiner may observe melanin as brown, blue-black, or black shades.

Arrangement of Lesions

1. *Discrete* lesions are distinct and discretely separated from one another.
2. *Linear* lesions are found in a straight line (e.g., lichen striatus).
3. Special attention should be given to *curvilinear*, *whorled*, or *parallel linear* lesions. These indicate genetic mosaicism and such arrangements follow the embryonic lines of Blaschko. The gene mutation is limited only to the affected area, and the remainder of skin does not contain the abnormal gene (e.g., epidermal nevus, nevus sebaceous, hypomelanosis of Ito).[3] The presence of genetic mosaicism should prompt the examiner to assess visual and neurologic abnormalities.[3]
4. *Annular* lesions are found in a circular arrangement (e.g., granuloma annulare).
5. Vesicles, papules, or nodules found closely adjacent to each other in a localized skin area are considered to be *grouped* (e.g., herpes simplex, herpes zoster).

Distribution of Lesions

It is useful to note whether an eruption is generalized, acral (hands, feet, buttocks, and face), or localized to a specific skin region, such as a dermatome.

RECORDING OF SKIN LESIONS IN THE HEALTH RECORD

Skin lesions should be described in an orderly fashion: distribution, arrangement, color, secondary changes, and primary lesion (including size). For example, guttate psoriasis could be written as generalized, discrete, red, scaly, 3- to 6-mm papules. If altered, mobility of skin, hair changes, or nail changes should also be recorded.

THE PROBLEM-ORIENTED ALGORITHM

After mastering the description of skin lesions the clinician can prepare a logical series of steps toward a correct diagnosis, even if the disease is initially unrecognized. Lynch has developed a problem-oriented algorithm for the nondermatologist (Fig. 2-9).[5] It can be applied to infants and children with skin disease, where it has been found to be most useful. Lynch's algorithm defines morphologic groups of dermatologic disease, which will allow the differential diagnosis and eventual correct diagnosis of a skin condition. These groups and the chapters in which they are found are listed in Table 2-1 (see also the Problem-

---

Table 2-1   Groups of Dermatologic Disease

Morphologic group	Chapter
1. Vesiculobullous diseases	4, 5, 7, 8, 9, 11, 18
2. Pustular diseases	3, 5, 6
3. Skin-colored papules and nodules	7
4. White lesions	16
5. Brown lesions	16
6. Yellow lesions	7, 16
7. Inflammatory papules and nodules	3, 5, 6, 7, 9, 18
8. Vascular reactions	13
9. Papulosquamous diseases	9
10. Eczematous diseases	4, 18
11. Hair changes	14
12. Nail changes	15
13. Immobile and hypermobile skin	19

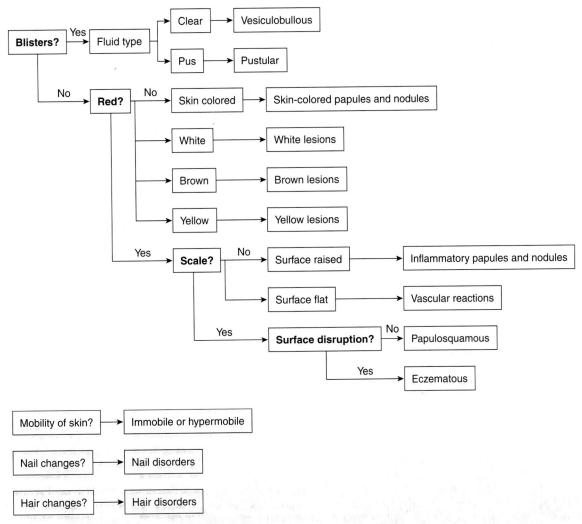

Fig. 2-9 The problem-oriented algorithm. (*From Lynch PJ:* Dermatology for the house officer, *ed 3, Baltimore, 1994, Williams & Wilkins.*)

Oriented Differential Diagnosis Index, located inside the front and back covers of this book).

The problem-oriented algorithm requires that three initial objective findings be determined:

Are blisters present?

Are the lesions red?

Are the lesions scaling?

A series of 11 additional determinations completes the algorithm.

The detection of blisters is the crucial initial step in this diagnostic exercise.[5] If even a single blister is detected, no matter what form of other skin lesions may be observed, the clinician should consider first the possibility of a blistering disease and proceed to determine whether the blister fluid is clear or pustular. If

no blisters are observed, it should be determined if the skin lesions observed are red. If they are not red, the clinician should determine whether they are skin-colored or another color such as brown (which includes blue-black or black shades), yellow, or white.

The algorithm is particularly helpful if lesions are red.[5] If the skin lesions observed are red, it should be determined whether the individual lesions themselves are scaling or nonscaling. If they are red and nonscaling, it should be determined whether the surfaces of individual lesions are dome-shaped papules or flat. If lesions are red, nonscaling, and flat, vascular reactions should be considered. If lesions are red or raised, it should be determined whether they are firm or compressible. If compressible, vascular lesions should be considered. If firm, the morphologic group called *inflammatory papules and nodules* should be considered. If lesions are red and scaling, it should be decided whether there is surface disruption. If lesions have surface disruption, eczematous lesions should be considered. If they are red, scaly, dome-shaped papules, papulosquamous lesions should be considered.

Changes in skin mobility should be determined. This includes skin that can be stretched excessively or is fixed to the underlying fascia or deeper structures and cannot be moved. Finally, any changes to hair or nails should be described.

Starting with the three initial determinations, and then adding up to 11 more, one can place the skin disease observed into one of 13 morphologic groups. Grouping the skin disease observed in this fashion increases the likelihood of finding a precise diagnosis. Determining the proper diagnosis can be done using the Problem-Oriented Differential Diagnosis Index.

LABORATORY FINDINGS
Exfoliative Cytology

Exfoliative cytology is indicated in any blister-forming disease to detect acantholytic cells (pemphigus) or epidermal giant cells (herpes simplex or herpes zoster). Scrape the blister base with a No. 15 blade and place the sample on a glass microscope slide. Allow it to dry, and then apply Wright's or Giemsa stain and examine under the 40× objective of a microscope.[6,7]

Skin Biopsy

Any skin tumor, palpable purpura, persistent dermatitis, or blister that is not diagnosed by morphologic appearance should be examined by biopsy for a histopathologic diagnosis.[6]

Punch Biopsy

The biopsy site should be cleansed with alcohol and then intradermally injected with 0.1 to 0.2 ml of lidocaine 1% using a tuberculin syringe and 30-gauge needle.[6,7] A 4-mm biopsy punch should be pressed firmly downward into the skin, which is stretched perpendicular to wrinkle lines. The punch is rotated until the soft subcutaneous fat is penetrated. The specimen is removed with forceps and scissors and placed in buffered formalin 10% for histologic examination.[6,7] For immunofluorescence testing, the specimen should be obtained from perilesional skin and frozen at −70° C or in liquid nitrogen, or placed in special skin immunofluorescence transport media.

Shave Biopsy

After local anesthesia is achieved as previously described, a small elevated lesion may be shaved off with a sterile No. 15 blade or razor blade.[6]

Fungal Scraping

Any red, scaly skin or scaly scalp should be scraped to evaluate the possibility of dermatophyte infection, which can mimic a wide variety of skin disorders (see Chapter 6). Fine scales are scraped from the edge of a lesion onto a glass slide.[6] A drop of 20% potassium hydroxide (KOH) added to the scale will dissolve the stratum corneum cells but not the hyphae. A coverslip is placed on the slide, and the scrapings are examined under the 10× objective of the microscope for long, thin, branching hyphae or spores.

Hair Examination

Hairs pulled from the scalp should be placed on a glass microscope slide, covered with histologic mounting media such as Histoclad or Permount and a coverslip, and examined under the 4× objective of the microscope. Immersion oil is also helpful, but aqueous solutions are not used unless searching for fungus.

REFERENCES

1. Burton JL: The logic of dermatological diagnoses, *Clin Exp Dermatol* 6:1, 1981.
2. Hubert JN, Callen JP, Kasteler S: Prevalence of cutaneous findings in hospitalized pediatric patients, *Pediatr Dermatol* 14:426, 1997.
3. Happle R: Loss of heterozygosity in human skin, *J Am Acad Dermatol* 41:143, 1999.
4. Lookingbill DP: Yield from a complete skin examination: findings in 1157 new dermatology patients, *J Am Acad Dermatol* 18:31, 1988.
5. Lynch PJ: *Dermatology for the house officer,* ed 3, Baltimore, 1994, Williams & Wilkins.
6. Oranje AP, Folkers E: The Tzanck smear: old, but still of inestimable value, *Pediatr Dermatol* 5:127, 1988.
7. Arndt KA: *Manual of dermatologic therapeutics. II. Procedures and operations,* Boston, 1989, Little, Brown.

CHAPTER THREE | Acne

ACNE VULGARIS
Clinical Features

The common variety of acne, acne vulgaris, is the most prevalent skin condition observed in the pediatric age group. The common forms of acne occur during two major ages: the newborn and the adolescent. Neonatal acne is a response to maternal androgen and first appears at 2 to 4 weeks of age, lasting until age 4 to 6 months. The lesions are primarily on the face, upper chest, and back, in a distribution similar to that in adolescent acne. The individual lesions seen are the same as described for adolescent acne. An oily scalp or face is often seen. It is believed that severe adolescent acne will develop in infants with severe forms of neonatal acne.[1] Persistence of neonatal acne beyond 12 months of age may be associated with endocrine abnormalities.[2]

Early lesions of acne in the form of microcomedones develop in 40% of children ages 8 to 10 years, primarily on the face. Acne vulgaris peaks in late adolescence and may continue until the late twenties or early thirties. Many authorities believe acne is one of the earliest signs of puberty.[3,4] Eventually 85% of adolescents will develop acne. Acne occurs in sebaceous follicles (Fig. 3-1). There are several types of follicular channels present in skin. The sebaceous follicles have large, abundant sebaceous glands and a small vellus hair. They are located primarily on the face, upper chest, back, and penis (Fig. 3-2).

Obstruction of the sebaceous follicle opening produces the clinical lesions of acne.[5] If the obstruction occurs at the follicular mouth, a wide, patulous opening develops that is filled with a plug of stratum corneum cells. This is the *open comedone, or blackhead* (Fig. 3-3). Open comedones are the predominant clinical lesion in early adolescent acne. The black color results from oxidized melanin within the stratum corneum cellular plug, not from dirt. Open comedones do not often progress to inflammatory lesions.

Obstruction of the sebaceous follicle just beneath the follicular opening in the neck of the sebaceous follicle produces a cystic swelling of the follicular duct just beneath the epidermis. The stratum corneum produced accumulates continuously within the cystic cavity. This is seen clinically as the *microcomedone* (*closed comedone,* or *whitehead*) (Fig. 3-4). These microcomedones may be the precursors to inflammatory acne. Children 8 to 10 years of age often have microcomedones for many months before red papules or pustules are observed. If open and closed comedones are the predominant lesions seen in adolescent acne, it is designated as *comedonal acne.*

Inflammatory lesions in acne prompt the adolescent to seek medical attention. These lesions include firm red papules, pustules, nodules, cysts (Fig. 3-5), and, rarely, interconnecting draining sinus tracts. Most adolescents will have a mixture of microcomedones, red papules, pustules, and blackheads at the time of examination. Inflammatory acne can be classified as mild, moderate, or severe. Mild inflammatory acne consists of a few to several inflammatory papules, pustules, and no nodules. Patients with moderate inflammatory acne will have several to many inflammatory papules, pustules, and a few to several nodules, whereas those with severe inflammatory acne will have numerous and/or extensive inflammatory papules, pustules, and many nodules.[5] Excoriation of acne papules and microcomedones is common and scarring may result. Usually, multiple shallow erosions or crusts are found.

Adolescents with cystic acne require prompt medical attention because ruptured cysts or sinus tracts result in scar formation. New acne scars are highly vascular and have a red or purplish hue. Such scars eventually regain normal skin color after several years. Acne scars may be depressed beneath the skin level, raised, or flat to the skin. In adolescents with a tendency toward keloid formation, keloidal scars can occur after acne lesions, particularly over the sternum. Hypertrophic scars may also occur, even in those without keloids. In typical adolescent acne several different types of lesions are present at one time, such as open and closed comedones (Fig. 3-6), inflammatory papules (Fig. 3-7) and pustules (Fig. 3-8), excoriated lesions (Figs. 3-9 and 3-10), and nodulocystic acne (Fig. 3-11). Neonatal acne (Fig. 3-12) is characterized by inflammatory papules on the face and chest, with all of the lesions in a similar stage.

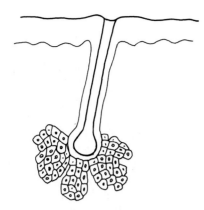

Fig. 3-1 Normal sebaceous follicles. Large sebaceous glands excrete sebum into cylindrical sebaceous channel.

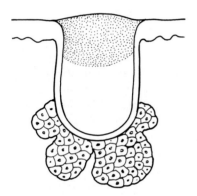

Fig. 3-3 Open comedone. Wide, patulous opening of sebaceous channel with plug of stratum corneum cells in follicular mouth.

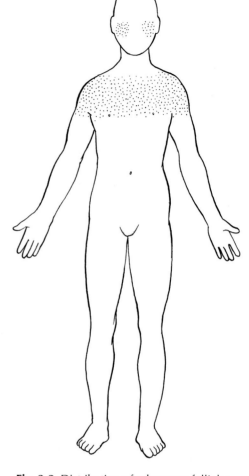

Fig. 3-2 Distribution of sebaceous follicles.

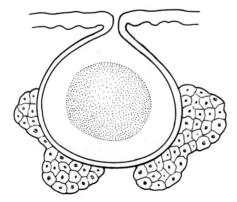

Fig. 3-4 Microcomedone (closed comedone). Obstruction of the follicular channel just beneath the opening.

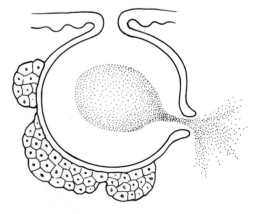

Fig. 3-5 Inflammatory papule. Overgrowth of bacteria and rupture of the wall, producing a foreign body reaction surrounding the follicle.

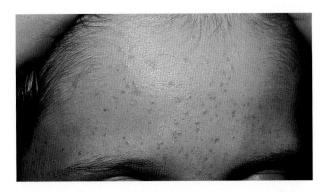

Fig. 3-6 Comedonal acne. Multiple microcomedones on the forehead of an 8-year-old female.

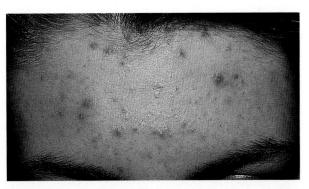

Fig. 3-7 Mild inflammatory acne. Several inflammatory papules.

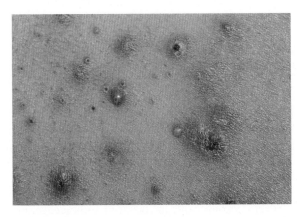

Fig. 3-8 Severe inflammatory acne. Extensive papules/pustules on the back.

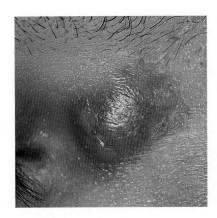

Fig. 3-9 Excoriated acne. Oozing from red papule that has been squeezed.

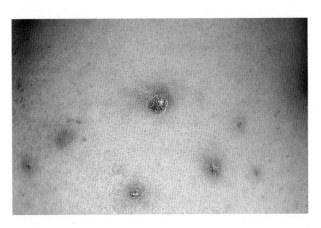

Fig. 3-10 Excoriated acne. Atrophic scar from attempted fingernail removal of acne lesion.

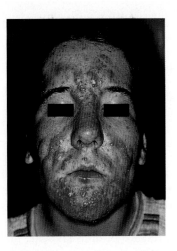

Fig. 3-11 Nodulocystic acne. Deep nodules and cysts on the face of an adolescent.

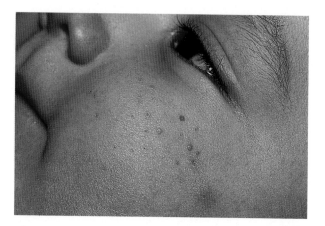

Fig. 3-12 Neonatal acne on the face of a 3-month-old infant.

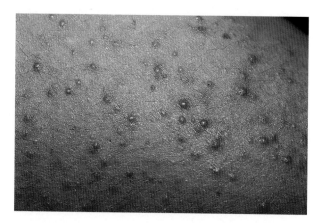

Fig. 3-13 Steroid acne. Pustules all in the same stage on the back of an adolescent treated with systemic steroids.

Box 3-1   Drugs Responsible for Acne

Androgens
Adrenocorticotropic hormone (ACTH)
Glucocorticoids
Hydantoins
Isoniazid

Drug-induced acne should be suspected if all of the lesions are in the same stage at the same time, with involvement of the abdomen, lower back, arms, and legs (Fig. 3-13) in addition to the usual acne areas (Box 3-1).[6] The presence of unusual acne, hirsutism, premature pubarche, or androgenic alopecia, especially when associated with obesity and/or menstrual irreg-

---

Box 3-2   Differential Diagnosis of Acne

ADOLESCENT
Rosacea
Steroid rosacea
Flat warts
Angiofibromas of tuberous sclerosis
Molluscum contagiosum

NEWBORN
Miliaria
Nevus comedonicus

---

ularities, should prompt an endocrine evaluation.[7,8] The most common causes of hyperandrogenism in females are functional ovarian and functional adrenal hyperandrogenism. Laboratory screening for hyperandrogenism is evaluated by obtaining blood levels of free testosterone, dehydroepiandrosterone, and androstenedione. If any of these are elevated, the source of the excess androgens can then be determined by measuring the response of free testosterone, dehydroepiandrosterone, and cortisol to dexamethasone suppression testing. Treatment options for hyperandrogenism include oral contraceptives, low-dose glucocorticoids, and antiandrogens.

Several variants of acne occur in adolescence. Frictional acne from headbands, football helmets, baseball caps, tight bras, or other tight-fitting garments occurs predominantly under the skin area where the garment is worn. Oil-based cosmetics may also be responsible for a predominantly comedonal acne, and hair sprays and oil-based mousse produce acne along the scalp hair margin.

Differential Diagnosis

Conditions to be considered in the differential diagnosis of acne are listed in Box 3-2. Rosacea in children can be confused with acne vulgaris. In addition to acne papules and pustules, prominent telangiectasia and a persistent flush to cheeks, nose, or chin are observed. In many instances rosacea in children results from the use of potent topical glucocorticosteroids on the face (Fig. 3-14).

Nevus comedonicus, which may be confused with neonatal acne, is a birthmark consisting of a linear arrangement of open comedones. It is present from birth and is usually unilateral. The anatomic abnor-

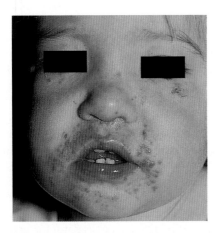

Fig. 3-14 Perioral dermatitis aggravated by topical steroid use. Toddler with perioral red papules and pustules from prolonged daily therapy with topical steroid.

mality of nevus comedonicus may also result in obstruction of the sebaceous follicle, with resultant red papules, pustules, or cysts, with inflammatory lesions restricted to the birthmark.[9] Miliaria may also mimic neonatal acne, although the lesions are transient, lasting less than 48 hours, in contrast to neonatal acne lesions, which persist for weeks.

Flat warts occurring on the face are sometimes confused with acne. They are papular, flat-topped, and skin-colored to slightly darker. The angiofibromas seen in tuberous sclerosis may be confused with acne. They are erythematous, soft papules seen in the nasolabial folds and on the cheeks and chin. The onset of these lesions is typically at 5 or 6 years of age. The absence of comedones is an important clue to the diagnosis of angiofibroma, as is the presence of leaf-shaped white macules, seizure disorders, and connective tissue nevi.

Molluscum contagiosum may occasionally be mistaken for acne lesions, but careful inspection will reveal the central umbilication at the top of the papule characteristic of this disease.

Pathogenesis

It is accepted that the primary event in acne is obstruction of the sebaceous follicle. Ordinarily the lining of such follicles contains one to two layers of stratum corneum cells, but in acne the stratum corneum is overproduced. This phenomenon is androgen dependent in adolescent acne. The sebaceous follicles contain an enzyme, testosterone 5α-reductase, which converts plasma testosterone to dihydrotestosterone (DHT). DHT is a potent stimulus for sebaceous follicle cell nu-

clear division and, subsequently, of excessive cell production. Thus obstruction requires the presence of both circulating androgens and the converting enzyme. The interplay of circulating and skin factors is believed to be crucial to the genesis of clinical acne. After the production or the administration of androgens, one would expect a delay of 2 to 4 weeks until cellular proliferation occurs and follicular obstruction appears. This, indeed, is what is seen in androgen-induced acne and acne vulgaris. The majority of patients that have only acne vulgaris do not have endocrinologic abnormalities.

The pathogenesis of inflammatory acne is not well understood. Undoubtedly, manipulation of a closed comedone could lead to rupture of the cavity contents into the dermis, with a subsequent inflammatory response (see Fig. 3-5). Spontaneous inflammation also occurs in obstructed follicles, but the reasons are unclear. A currently attractive hypothesis is that overgrowth of gram-positive bacteria in the obstructed follicle, either *Propionibacterium acnes* or *Staphylococcus epidermidis,* might produce bacterial chemotactic peptides, enzymes, or other factors that initiate inflammation. Although overproduction of sebum frequently accompanies acne, sebum or metabolites of sebum are unlikely as a cause of inflammation in acne as presently understood. Rupture of the comedonal contents into the dermis induces a foreign-body reaction, which may heal with fibrosis.

Treatment
Topical keratolytic agents

The mainstay of antiacne therapy is the use of potent topical keratolytic agents applied to the skin to relieve follicular obstruction.[10-12] Two classes of potent keratolytic agents—retinoids and those agents that possess both antibacterial and keratolytic properties—have been found to be the most efficacious agents for the treatment of acne. The retinoids include retinoic acid and the retinoid-like compound adapalene. The other class includes benzoyl peroxide and azelaic acid. The agents may be used alone once daily, or in combination. If retinoic acid or adapalene is used, they should be applied to the acne-bearing areas of the skin once daily in the evening. If combination therapy is used, an agent from the other class should be applied in the morning. Because the two classes of keratolytics work by different mechanisms, they are synergistic. Topical keratolytic regimens will control 80% to 85% of adolescent acne. Retinoic acid, adapalene, and benzoyl peroxide are most effective in the gel forms; lotions and solutions, particularly the over-the-counter (OTC) preparations, have less efficacy. Azelaic acid is available only in the cream form. Dryness to the skin from using an alcohol-acetone–containing gel may be severe. The adolescent will often not use the prescribed gel medication because of the dryness experienced. Alternative strategies designed to reduce dryness are use of a noncomedogenic moisturizer such as Moisturel, Purpose lotion, or Neutrogena Moisture after application of the gel; use of the gel every other day; or use of the cream preparations. Topical keratolytic therapy is recommended as the primary therapy for comedonal and mild papular forms of acne. Continuous use for several months is often required. There is debate as to whether tretinoin should be avoided in pregnancy because of the potential of photoisomerization to isotretinoin, but a recent retrospective study did not demonstrate an increase in birth defects in children whose mothers used tretinoin in the first trimester of pregnancy.[13] For papular acne, benzoyl peroxide gel or azelaic acid should be used once or twice daily; for comedonal acne, retinoic acid or adapalene should be used once daily as initial therapy. If no improvement occurs over 4 to 6 weeks, the other form of keratolytic can be added. In inflammatory acne, topical keratolytics plus oral antibiotics are recommended as initial therapy. Topical keratolytics are not used when oral retinoids, such as isotretinoin, are required.

Antibiotics

Topical antibiotics are used to avoid systemic side effects caused by systemic antibiotics. Antibiotics are less effective given topically than systemically and at best are equipotent to 250 mg of oral tetracycline taken once a day. Clindamycin phosphate 1% is the most efficacious of all topical antibiotics. Some percutaneous absorption may rarely occur with this drug, resulting in diarrhea and colitis. Topical erythromycin 1%, 1.5%, and 2% solutions, 2% ointment, and 3% gel are quite effective, as is 1% meclocycline cream; topical tetracycline 1% or 2.2% is minimally efficacious (Tables 3-1 and 3-2).

Topical antibiotics are most useful for maintenance therapy after improvement from the use of oral antibiotics is observed. Oral antibiotics can be discontinued and improvement maintained with topical antibiotics plus topical keratolytics.

Oral antibiotics that are concentrated in sebum, such as tetracycline, minocycline, doxycycline, and erythromycin, are very effective in inflammatory acne. The usual dose is 500 mg to 1 g of tetracycline or erythromycin or 100 to 200 mg of minocycline or doxycycline taken daily divided into two doses. Tetracycline should be taken on an empty stomach for reliable absorption. Doxycycline is the most photosensitizing. Oral antibiotics should be continued for 1 to 3 months until the acne lesions are suppressed. Topical keratolytics

Table 3-1 Quick Guide to Initial Acne Therapy

Clinical appearance	Treatment
Comedones only (Fig. 3-6)	Once daily: Retinoic acid 0.025% cream or adapalene 0.1% gel or benzoyl peroxide 5% gel or azelaic acid 20% cream
Red papules, few pustules (Fig. 3-7)	Retinoic acid 0.025% cream or adapalene 0.1% gel in the evening, plus benzoyl peroxide 5% gel or azelaic acid 20% cream in the morning
Red papules, many pustules (Fig. 3-8)	Retinoic acid 0.025% cream or adapalene 0.1% gel in the evening, plus benzoyl peroxide 5% gel or azelaic acid 20% cream or a topical antibiotic in the morning, plus oral antibiotics twice daily: either tetracycline or erythromycin 500 mg or minocycline or doxycycline 50 to 100 mg
Red papules, pustules, cysts, and nodules (Fig. 3-11)	Retinoic acid 0.025% cream or adapalene 0.1% gel in the evening, plus benzoyl peroxide 5% gel or azelaic acid 20% cream in the morning (or substitute a topical antibiotic morning and evening), plus oral antibiotics taken twice daily: either tetracycline or erythromycin 500 mg or minocycline or doxycycline 50 to 100 mg

should be used in combination with oral antibiotics. Therapy for a period of at least 4 to 6 weeks is required for clinical improvement. Routine laboratory monitoring is unnecessary during antibiotic therapy.[14]

Oral retinoids

The oral retinoid isotretinoin (13-*cis*-retinoic acid) has been very efficacious in nodulocystic acne resistant to standard therapeutic regimens (see Fig. 3-11). It is not recommended that isotretinoin be used as the drug of first choice for acne.[15] The precise mechanism of action is unknown, but decreased sebum production, follicular obstruction, and skin bacteria, in addition to general antiinflammatory activities have been described. The initial dosage is 40 mg once or twice daily (0.5 to 1.0 mg/kg/day) for 4 months, then the drug is stopped. Isotretinoin is neither designed for nor efficacious in the treatment of comedonal acne or other mild forms of acne. Side effects include dryness and scaliness of the skin, dry lips, and occasionally dry eyes and nose. Up to 10% of patients experience mild hair loss, but it is reversible. Elevated levels of liver enzymes and blood lipids have rarely been described. Oral retinoids are the most efficacious treatment of severe cystic acne. Teratogenicity restricts the use of isotretinoin in females of childbearing potential.[16,17] The isotretinoin teratogen syndrome is characterized by malformations of the central nervous system, and has been reported in 25% of women who became pregnant while taking isotretinoin. Usage in young women of childbearing age is not recommended, and a negative pregnancy test should be obtained before the drug is considered, with careful adherence to the guidelines provided by the manufacturer, including monthly contraceptive counseling

Table 3-2   Selected Acne Treatment Products

Product	Form	Size
TOPICAL KERATOLYTICS (apply once or twice daily)		
Retinoic acid (tretinoin)		
Retin-A	0.025% cream	20 g, 45 g
	0.05% cream	20 g, 45 g
	0.1% cream	20 g, 45 g
	0.01% gel	15 g, 45 g
	0.025% gel	15 g, 45 g
	0.1% micro gel	20 g, 45 g
	0.1% lotion	30 ml
Adapalene	0.1% gel	15 g, 45 g
Benzoyl peroxide	5% and 10% gel	45 g, 90 g
Azelaic acid	20% cream	30 g
TOPICAL ANTIBIOTICS (apply twice daily)		
Clindamycin phosphate	1% solution	60 ml
Meclocycline sulfosalicylate	1% cream	20 g, 45 g
Erythromycin	2% solution	60 ml
SYSTEMIC ANTIBIOTICS (one or two capsules twice daily)		
Tetracycline hydrochloride		250- and 500-mg capsule
Erythromycin		250- and 500-mg capsule
Minocycline		
Doxycycline		50- and 100-mg capsule
		50- and 100-mg capsule
ORAL RETINOIDS (40-mg capsule twice daily for 16-20 weeks)		
Isotretinoin (Accutane)		10- and 40-mg capsule

and pregnancy tests. Patients should be encouraged to enroll in the pregnancy prevention program of the manufacturer. Treatment for longer than 4 months is not recommended. At least a 4-month rest period from the drug is recommended before a second treatment course is considered.

Other acne treatments

There is no convincing evidence that dietary management, mild drying agents, abrasive scrubs, oral vitamin A, ultraviolet light, cryotherapy, or incision and drainage have any beneficial effects in the management of acne. Oral contraceptives have been shown to be effective in the treatment of acne vulgaris.[18,19]

Other types of oral hormonal therapy should be reserved for patients with documented endocrine abnormalities or hirsutism. Topical antiandrogens are now under investigation, but so far have been demonstrated to be only modestly effective.[20,21]

Factors That Aggravate Acne Vulgaris

Acne can be aggravated by a variety of external factors, resulting in further obstruction of partially occluded sebaceous follicles. Avoidance of oil-based cosmetics, hairstyling mousse, face creams, and hair sprays may alleviate the comedonal component of acne 4 to 6 weeks after use of the cosmetics is discontinued. A list of nonacnegenic cosmetics and moisturizers is found in Box 3-3.

Box 3-3 Nonacnegenic Cosmetics and Moisturizers

COSMETICS
Allercreme
  Matte-Finish Makeup
  Waterbase, Oil-Free
Almay
  Fresh-Look Oil-Free Makeup for Oily Skin
  Smooth Coverup Makeup for Blemish-Prone Skin
  Oil Control Makeup
  Teen Oil-Free Makeup
Charles of the Ritz
  T-Zone Controller
Chanel
  Teint Pur Oil-Free Makeup
  Teint Pur Matte
Clarion
  Oil-Free Liquid Makeup
Clinique
  Pore Minimizer Makeup, Fragrance- and Oil-Free
  Stay True Makeup, Fragrance- and Oil-Free
  Stay True Oil-Free—designed for sensitive skin—
    SPF 15
Coty
  Glowing Finish
Covergirl
  Fresh Complexion, 100% Oil-Free
Dermage
  Sheer Foundation Base
  Opaque Foundation Base
  Sunscreen Foundation Base
Elizabeth Arden
  Extra Control Makeup
Estee Lauder
  Tender Matte Makeup, Fragrance- and Oil-Free
  Lucidity Makeup

Simply Sheer
  Fresh Air Makeup Base, Oil-Free
  Demi-Matte Makeup, Fragrance- and Oil-Free
Lancome
  Maquicontrol, Oil-Free Liquid Makeup
L'Oreal
  Mattique Illuminating Makeup
Mary Kay Cosmetics
  Oil-Free Foundation, Fragrance- and Oil-Free
Maybelline
  Shine-Free Oil-Control Liquid Makeup
  Shade of You Oil-Free Makeup
Max Factor
  Shine-Free Makeup
Monteil
  Habitat Natural Light Makeup
Nuskin
  No Colour Oil-Free Moisturizing Finish
Physician's Formula
  Oil-Control Matte Makeup
Revlon
  Spring Water Matte Makeup
  Color Style Natural Color Oil-Free Makeup
Shisheido
  Pureness Oil-Control Makeup
Ultima II
  The Nakeds: The Foundation Oil-Free Formula

MOISTURIZERS
Moisturel
Cetaphil lotion

Change of habits, such as not wearing tight-fitting garments, may be helpful. Stopping drugs that induce acne should be attempted, if possible.

Patient Education

Acne therapy requires that adequate time and explanation accompany any treatment program. It is important to explain the mechanism of acne and the treatment plan to the adolescent patient. The clinician should specifically explain that not much improvement can be expected for 4 to 8 weeks. Time should be set aside at the first visit to answer the patient's questions about acne. The clinician should be certain to inquire what the patient's peers, relatives, and others have advised. Written patient education handouts (see p. 333) and lists of useful moisturizers and cosmetics (see Box 3-3) are extremely valuable. The presence of excoriations should prompt an explanation regarding how attempted fingernail removal of acne usually results in scars that are permanent (see Figs. 3-9 and 3-10). Suggestions as to relieving the nervous habit are useful.

Follow-up Visits

Follow-up visits should initially be every 4 to 6 weeks. The criterion for ideal control is a few new lesions every 2 weeks. The clinician and patient should not expect to completely prevent any new acne lesions from appearing. The clinician should also re-explain what the prescribed medications are intended to achieve and question the patient to determine whether the medications are being used properly. At the first visit a baseline evaluation grading comedones, papules, pustules, and cysts in each affected skin region should be entered on the patient's record to assist with objective measurement (Tables 3-3 and 3-4). At each subsequent visit the same scoring system should be used for comparison. Objective and subjective evaluations are more likely to differ than correlate in acne patients, and the clinician must rely on objective findings to properly evaluate response to therapy. Most authorities recommend treatment with oral antibiotics for at least 1 to 3 months. At the follow-up visit a decision to stop oral antibiotics is made when 90% improvement in red papules and pustules is observed and documented by the scoring system listed in Tables 3-3 and 3-4. When oral antibiotics are stopped, improvement can be maintained by twice-daily application of topical antibiotics. At each follow-up visit, the clinician should emphasize that therapeutic response is slow in acne and is evaluated over weeks to months, not days. He or she

Table 3-3 Grading System for Acne

Location	Baseline grade* (date)	Follow-up Grade*		
		1 (date)	2 (date)	3 (date)
Face				
Comedones				
Papules				
Pustules				
Cysts				
Chest				
Comedones				
Papules				
Pustules				
Cysts				
Back				
Comedones				
Papules				
Pustules				
Cysts				

*0 = no lesions; 1 = 1-19 lesions; 2 = 20-39 lesions; 3 = 40 or more lesions. Grade each category (comedones, papules, pustules, cysts) for each location (face, chest, back).

Table 3-4 **Evaluation of Acne Patients (Example)**

Location	Baseline grade* (10/1/00)	Follow-up Grade* 1 (11/3/00)	2 (12/8/00)	3 (1/28/01)
Face				
Comedones	2	1	1	0
Papules	1	1	0	0
Pustules	0	0	0	0
Cysts	0	0	0	0
Chest				
Comedones	0	0	0	0
Papules	0	0	0	0
Pustules	0	0	0	0
Cysts	0	0	0	0
Back				
Comedones	1	1	1	1
Papules	2	2	2	1
Pustules	1	0	0	0
Cysts	0			

*0 = no lesions; 1 = 1-19 lesions; 2 = 20-39 lesions; 3 = 40 or more lesions. Grade each category (comedones, papules, pustules, cysts) for each location (face, chest, back).

should also be certain that the red-purple scars, which require 6 to 12 months to fade, are not the lesions that determine alterations in treatment strategy. Scars are not influenced by antibiotics or keratolytics.

PERIORAL DERMATITIS AND STEROID ROSACEA
Clinical Features

Erythema, slight scaling, telangiectasia, and red papules characterize these closely related conditions.[22,23] In perioral dermatitis and steroid rosacea, lesions are found in the nasolabial folds, just beneath the nose, and on the chin (see Fig. 3-14). Often lesions begin as red macules with a slight scale and are misdiagnosed as dermatitis. A topical steroid is used, and the lesions get progressively worse, with redder, telangiectatic skin and red papules or pustules seen. Frequently the child received the steroid from a relative in the health care field or used an OTC steroid. Superpotent topical steroids are most often associated with steroid rosacea after a few weeks of use, but low-potency steroids, if used daily over many weeks, will also induce the condition. Infants and adolescents are most often involved, although the exact prevalence is not known.

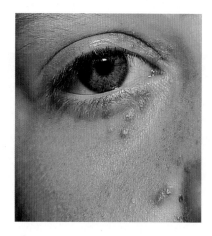

Fig. 3-15 Lower eyelid lesions in a child with perioral dermatitis.

Occasionally, pustules and red papules will be found on the lower eyelids in addition to the perioral skin (Fig. 3-15). Rarely the perioral lesions will have a granulomatous histology and reveal closely spaced, skin-colored micronodules in a perioral distribution.[24,25]

Differential Diagnosis

At the onset of disease, a dermatitis such as seborrheic or contact dermatitis is suspected, although careful examination will not detect disruption of the skin surface. This misdiagnosis leads to therapy that worsens the condition. Acne vulgaris may also be restricted to the perioral skin, but the presence of comedones, which are usually absent in rosacea, will help differentiate. Rarely, tinea faciei (see Chapter 6) will involve perioral skin. Scrapings for microscopic identification of fungus and fungal culture will differentiate.

Pathogenesis

Although many authorities believe that perioral dermatitis and steroid rosacea are related to acne, the pathogenesis is unclear. Sebaceous gland hyperplasia, obstructed sebaceous follicles, and prominent telangiectasias are pathologic features. In steroid rosacea the role of topically applied steroids is well established, although the exact mechanism is unknown. Although there is speculation that yeast species have a role, it is as yet unproven.

Treatment

The treatment protocols used for common acne are effective in perioral dermatitis and steroid rosacea. Topical steroid preparations must be discontinued, recognizing that the condition will worsen for about 1 week. In mild cases topical keratolytics or topical antibiotics alone will suffice. With many red papules and pustules present, oral erythromycin for 4 to 6 weeks may be required.[22] Topical metronidazole 0.75% gel has also been shown to be effective.[23]

Patient Education

Many patients are reluctant to stop topical steroids, because their skin is improved for 2 or 3 hours after each application. The clinician should insist that topical steroids be stopped and advise that the child's skin will worsen for 1 week before it begins to improve. Patients should be cautioned not to use steroids to treat the predicted worsening. It is important to emphasize that this is a form of acne, and treatment is similar to acne treatment. Providing advice that only certain children are susceptible is useful. Patient handout instructions for Perioral Dermatitis can be found on p. 342.

Follow-Up Visits

A visit in 4 weeks to evaluate the response to therapy is recommended.

REFERENCES

1. Chew EW, Bingham A, Burrows D: Incidence of acne vulgaris in patients with infantile acne, *Clin Exp Dermatol* 15:376, 1990.
2. Lucky AW: A review of infantile and pediatric acne, *Dermatol* 196:95, 1998.
3. Lucky AW et al: Predictors of severity of acne vulgaris in young adolescent girls: results of a five-year longitudinal study, *J Pediatr* 130:30, 1997.
4. Lucky AW et al: Acne vulgaris in early adolescent boys, *Arch Dermatol* 127:210, 1991.
5. Brown SK, Shalita AR: Acne vulgaris, *Lancet* 351:1871, 1998.
6. Fung MA, Berger TG: A prospective study of acute onset steroid acne associated with administration of intravenous corticosteroids, *Dermatol* 200:43, 2000.
7. Rosenfield RJ, Lucky AW: Acne, hirsutism, and alopecia in adolescent girls: clinical expressions of androgen excess, *Endocrinol Metab Clin North Am* 8:347, 1993.
8. Lucky AW: Hormonal correlates of acne and hirsutism, *Am J Med* 98:89S, 1996.
9. Vasiloudes PE, Morelli JG, Weston WL: Inflammatory nevus comedonicus in children, *J Am Acad Dermatol,* 38:834, 1998.
10. Thiboutot D: New treatments and therapeutic strategies for acne, *Arch Fam Med* 9:179, 2000.
11. Russell JJ: Topical therapy for acne, *Am Fam Phys* 61:357, 2000.
12. DeGroot HE, Friedlander SF: Update on acne: current opinion *Pediatrics* 10:381, 1998.
13. Jick SS, Terris BZ, Jick H: First trimester topical tretinoin and congenital disorders, *Lancet* 341:1181, 1993.
14. Driscoll MS et al: Long-term oral antibiotics for acne: is laboratory monitoring necessary? *J Am Acad Dermatol* 28:595, 1993.
15. Azurdia RM, Sharpe GR: Isotretinoin treatment for acne vulgaris and its cutaneous and ocular side effects, *Br J Dermatol* 141:947, 1999.
16. Anonymous: Accutane-exposed pregnancies—California, 1999, *MMWR* 49:28, 2000.
17. Dai WS, LaBraico JM, Stern RS: Epidemiology of isotretinoin exposure during pregnancy, *J Am Acad Dermatol* 26:599, 1992.
18. Williams JK: Noncontraceptive benefits of oral contraceptive use: an evidence-based approach, *Int J Fertil Womens Med* 45:241, 2000.
19. Thorneycroft IH et al: Effects of low-dose oral contraceptives on androgenic makers and acne vulgaris, *Contraception* 60:25, 1999.
20. Battman T et al: RU 58841, a new specific topical antiandrogen: a candidate for the treatment of acne, androgenetic alopecia and hirsutism, *J Steroid Biochem Mol Biol* 48:55, 1994.
21. Lookingbill DP et al: Inocoterone and acne, *Arch Dermatol* 128:1197, 1992.
22. Weston WL, Morelli JG: Steroid rosacea in prepubertal children, *Arch Ped Adol Med* 154:62, 2000.
23. Laude TA, Salvemini JN: Perioral dermatitis in children, *Semin Cutan Med Surg* 18:206, 1999.
24. Frieden IJ et al: Granulomatous perioral dermatitis in children, *Arch Dermatol* 125:369, 1989.
25. Smitt JH, Das PK, Van Ginkel JW: Granulomatis perioral dermatitis (facial Afro-Caribbean childhood eruption [FACE]), *Br J Dermatol* 125:399, 1991.

CHAPTER FOUR | Dermatitis

Dermatitis is inflammation of the superficial dermis and epidermis, leading to disruption of the skin surface. The characteristic disruption of the skin surface is recognized as crusting, weeping, excoriation, and cracking (fissures). The terms *dermatitis* and *eczema* are used interchangeably, although eczema was initially used to refer to blistering dermatitis, being derived from a Greek term meaning to boil over. Dermatitis may vary in intensity from an acute condition, with vesicle formation, oozing, and crusting, to a chronic form, with epidermal thickening; a shiny, flattened epidermal surface; and exaggerated skin creases. In an intermediate form, called *subacute dermatitis*, both vesiculation and epidermal thickening are present. *Acute dermatitis* implies an intense stimulus, whereas *chronic dermatitis* suggests a stimulus of low potency repeatedly occurring over time. All forms of dermatitis characteristically involve the epidermis, with inflammation and disruption of epidermal integrity.

The categories of dermatitis are traditional and imprecise. Except for irritant, allergic contact, and dry skin dermatitis, the pathogenesis is unknown. Therefore it may be best simply to describe the lesions as dermatitis rather than to apply modifying adjectives, such as atopic, when the etiology is unclear. Some traditional terms are used in this section to avoid confusion with the previous medical literature.

ATOPIC DERMATITIS
Clinical Features

Atopic dermatitis is a hereditary disorder characterized by dry skin, the presence of eczema, and onset under 2 years (Box 4-1).[1-5] The term *atopy* was first employed in 1923 by Coca and Cooke to denote inherited human hypersensitivity as exemplified by asthma and hay fever. A variety of terms have been used in literature to designate the condition. *Atopic eczema, allergic eczema, Besnier's prurigo, eczema,* and *circumscribed neurodermatitis* are terms less acceptable and less widely used than atopic dermatitis. Children with more severe atopic dermatitis are more likely to have respiratory manifestations, such as allergic rhinitis or extrinsic asthma.[1,3-5] Very rarely does a patient have all three.

The diagnosis of atopic dermatitis is a clinical one. The clinical appearance of atopic dermatitis may represent a phenotype resulting from different mechanisms. There is no single diagnostic criterion for the phenotype we appreciate as atopic dermatitis; rather, a combination of features must be considered. The major features listed in Box 4-1 are useful in the diagnosis. Although many other features may be noted, such as facial pallor, Denny's lines under the eyes, intolerance to wool or occlusive clothing, associated ichthyosis, cataracts, elevated serum immunoglobulin E levels, and eosinophilia, they are not considered diagnostic of the disease or necessary for the diagnosis.[3-5]

Atopic dermatitis usually begins before age 2 and commonly begins before the age of 6 months. At the onset the distribution is primarily on the scalp, face, trunk, and extensor surfaces of the arms and legs (Fig. 4-1). Frequently the dermatitis seen in the first months of life is a subacute dermatitis characterized by thickened skin and oozing. The exact prevalence is unknown, but most authorities agree it is from 5% to 15%, with regional variations.[1,2] It is the most common dermatitis of childhood.

Itching has long been recognized as a significant feature of atopic dermatitis. It commonly occurs in paroxysms and can be severe. In most patients itching is most severe in the evening, and scratching continues while the child is sleeping. The threshold for itching in atopic dermatitis patients is lowered, and their itching is more prolonged than that in normal persons. Scratching frenzies may be reported. The propensity for itching and the resultant trauma from

---

Box 4-1 Cardinal Diagnostic Features of Atopic Dermatitis in Children

Presence of a dermatitis
Dry skin
Onset under age 2 years
History of flexural dermatitis

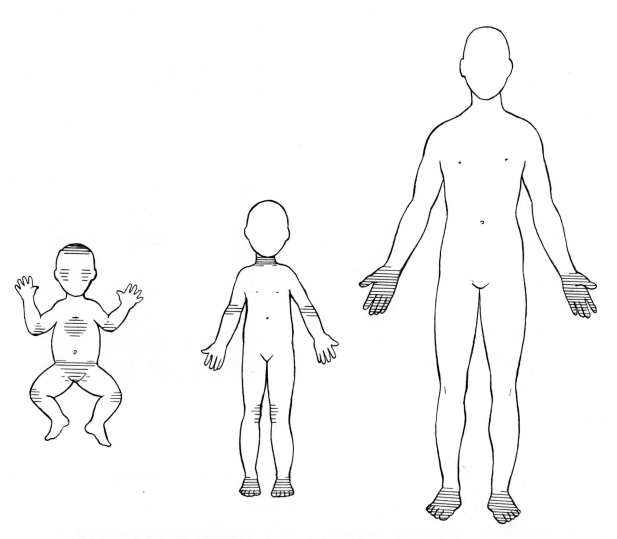

Fig. 4-1 Age-dependent distribution of atopic dermatitis. Involvement of the face, scalp, trunk, and extensor surfaces of extremities as seen in infants, flexural skin in toddlers, and hands and feet in preteens and adolescents.

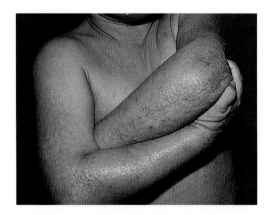

Fig. 4-2 Itching frenzies may be severe.

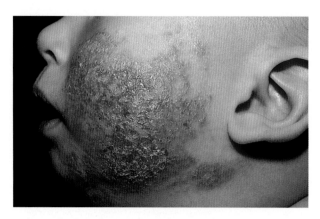

Fig. 4-3 Acute dermatitis of the cheeks with oozing and crusting in an infant with atopic dermatitis.

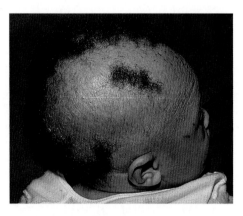

Fig. 4-4 Alopecia associated with atopic dermatitis; note the lichenification of the face and scalp.

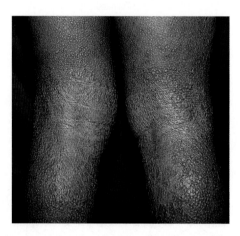

Fig. 4-5 Flexural involvement of popliteal fossa in atopic dermatitis.

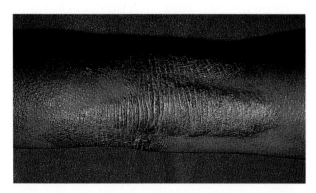

Fig. 4-6 Lichenification of the popliteal fossa from chronic rubbing of the skin in atopic dermatitis.

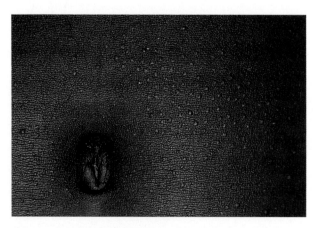

Fig. 4-7 Follicular hyperkeratosis seen on the abdomen of an adolescent with atopic dermatitis.

scratching are central to the genesis of atopic dermatitis (Fig. 4-2).

The distribution of dermatitis is largely age dependent (see Fig. 4-1).[1-5] Infantile atopic dermatitis, distributed largely on the cheeks (Figs. 4-3 and 4-4), face, trunk, and extensor surfaces of extremities, evolves into the childhood phase, with dermatitis on the feet and in the flexural areas, such as the antecubital fossa, popliteal fossa (Figs. 4-5 and 4-6), and neck. By adolescence the distribution has become that seen in older adults, with bilateral involvement of the flexural areas and hand dermatitis. Involvement of the eyelids is common in all phases of atopic dermatitis and may help to make the diagnosis. Foot dermatitis is common in school-age children, and adolescents and may be associated with atopic dermatitis or juvenile plantar dermatosis (JPD).

The primary clinical lesion of atopic dermatitis has not been described. In fact, many observers believe that all visible skin lesions in atopic dermatitis are secondary to scratching, as observed in sparing of protected skin areas such as the diaper area.[3-5] Intense erythema and oozing are observed on the face and scalp in infancy but are otherwise absent except in patients with secondary bacterial infection.[3-5] During exacerbation, dark-skinned patients may demonstrate follicular papules (Fig. 4-7), especially on the trunk. In black skin, hyperpigmented, lichenified nodules are commonly found on the lower arms and legs in addition to flexural involvement (see Fig. 4-6).

Dry skin is a constant feature with atopic dermatitis.[3-5] Patients with atopic dermatitis have reduced water content of the stratum corneum despite greater water loss through the skin and decreased water-binding ceramides on the skin surface. Dry skin and horny follicular papules (keratosis pilaris) are common findings, particularly on extensor surfaces. Secretion of sebum and sweat may be suppressed in some patients with atopic dermatitis. Microscopic fractures of the stratum corneum during drying result in loss of the epidermal barrier and increased susceptibility to irritants and infection. There is little doubt that dryness of the skin during the winter months in cool climates is a significant factor in exacerbation of atopic dermatitis. Dry, slightly scaly, hypopigmented patches seen in mild atopic dermatitis are called *pityriasis alba* (Fig. 4-8). In pityriasis alba, histology shows mild inflammation.

There are a number of factors that aggravate atopic dermatitis (Box 4-2). Children with atopic dermatitis may be extremely sensitive to certain contact

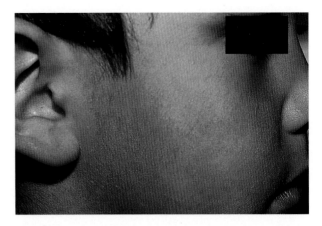

Fig. 4-8 Hypopigmented, slightly scaly patch of mild dermatitis on cheeks is referred to as *pityriasis alba*.

Box 4-2   Factors That Aggravate Atopic Dermatitis
Drying of the skin Soaping of the skin Sweating Contact sensitivity Stress and anxiety Secondary bacterial infection Secondary herpes simplex virus infection

irritants. They may experience bouts of itching and subsequent exacerbation of dermatitis when wool or an irritant chemical contacts the skin. Detergents and frequent soaping of the skin often result in prolonged itching. Sensitivity to contactants may partially explain localization of dermatitis in certain areas, particularly on the hands and feet.

Emotional stress indisputably leads to increased scratching. This occurs frequently in children, from either heightened awareness of itching or a habit of scratching. The child experiences transient relief after a scratching frenzy. Atopic dermatitis worsens during such episodes.

Secondary skin infection with bacteria such as *Staphylococcus aureus* may worsen the dermatitis (Figs. 4-9 and 4-10) and worsen itching.

Differential Diagnosis

Differential diagnosis should include any disorder manifested by dermatitis. Thus contact dermatitis of

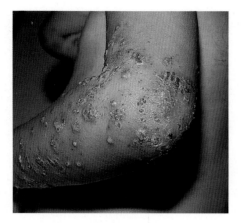

Fig. 4-9 Secondarily infected atopic dermatitis with multiple pustules and areas of crusting.

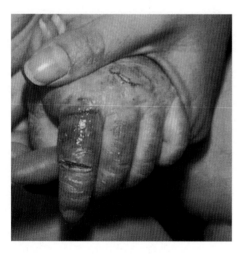

Fig. 4-10 Fissures and many breaks of the skin in atopic dermatitis, with secondary bacterial infection.

the primary irritant and allergic type, seborrheic dermatitis, nummular eczema, scabies, molluscum contagiosum dermatitis, JPD, polymorphous light eruptions, the dermatitis of human immunodeficiency virus (HIV) infection, or the hereditary immunodeficiencies and tinea constitute the major considerations in the differential diagnosis of atopic dermatitis in childhood. In infants, seborrheic dermatitis may be impossible to distinguish from atopic dermatitis.

Pathogenesis

Although there are a number of hypotheses as to the mechanism of the generation of atopic dermatitis in children, the exact pathogenesis is unknown. There is

| **Box 4-3** | **Systemic Therapy for Atopic Dermatitis** |

1. Use of hydroxyzine (1 mg/kg in a single daily dose) may decrease the sensation of pruritus. One dose given 1 hour before bedtime may be most effective. For severe pruritus, addition of cetirizine 2.5 mg for children under 6, or 5 mg for children over 6 years in the morning is helpful.
2. For crusted, oozing, infected-appearing lesions, antistaphylococcal oral antibiotics are beneficial (e.g., dicloxacillin, 12 to 25 mg/kg/day, or cephalexin, 25 to 50 mg/kg/day) three to four times a day for 10 to 14 days.
3. For eczema herpeticum, oral acyclovir 20 mg/kg/day for 5 days.

no evidence to substantiate food or other allergies as the cause of atopic dermatitis.[6,7] Substances involved in both epidermal barrier function and immunity, such as the serine protease inhibitor SPINK-5 and interleukin-4 mutations, have recently been implicated in the pathogenesis.[8-10] Atopic dermatitis has been associated with various forms of both antibody and cellular immunodeficiency, abnormal β-adrenergic receptors and responses, food allergies, and aeroallergens such as house dust mites, but there is no convincing evidence to substantiate any of these hypotheses.[6] The dermatitis can be exacerbated by drying or soaping of the skin, sweating, frictional irritation of the skin, or epicutaneous application of a contact irritant or allergen.

Treatment

Atopic dermatitis is a chronic disease that is frustrating for both child and parents. It may be disruptive to family dynamics and an economic burden on the family.[4,5] Weeks of effective control can be followed by a sudden, severe relapse. It is tempting for the clinician to focus on one or several factors as causes and to regard their elimination as curative. The patient or the family should be told that there is no immediate cure for atopic dermatitis but that spontaneous remissions do occur, and that this disorder can be controlled by therapy.

Initial therapy should be simple. The mainstays of initial therapy are topical steroid ointments and oral antihistamines (Box 4-3). Topical steroid ointments

---

Box 4-4 Topical Steroids for Use in Childhood Atopic Dermatitis

LOW POTENCY
Hydrocortisone 2.5%
Desonide 0.05%

MODERATE POTENCY (START WITH MODERATE POTENCY)
Fluocinolone acetonide 0.025% (Fluonid, Synalar)
Mometasone furoate 0.1% (Elocon)
Triamcinolone 0.1% (Kenalog, Aristocort)

Box 4-5 Instructions for Wet Dressings

MATERIALS NEEDED
1. Prescription for moderately potent steroid ointment or cream.
2. Two pairs or more of cotton or mostly cotton sleepers or long johns.
3. Warm water in a sink or basin.

TECHNIQUE
1. Apply steroid ointment to affected area.
2. Wet one pair of cotton sleepers in warm water.
3. Wring out thoroughly until barely damp.
4. Place damp sleeper on child and then put the dry sleeper over the damp one.
5. Be certain room is warm enough (not too hot) and child does not chill.

DURATION OF TREATMENT (USE 1 OR 2)
1. Use overnight for 5 to 10 nights.
2. Change every 6 hours for 24 to 72 hours (e.g., reapply steroid; redampen damp sleepers).

Box 4-6 Instructions for Topical Maintenance Care of Atopic Dermatitis

1. Wet the skin for 5 to 10 minutes twice a day.
2. Towel off the beads of water and quickly apply the steroid preparation to wet skin twice daily. Apply the steroid only on the area of dermatitis.
3. Apply a lubricant to the entire body immediately after the topical steroid has been applied. The lubricant may be applied over the steroid if the steroid is a cream. The lubricant should be applied twice a day while the skin is still wet.
4. Reapply the lubricant throughout the day if the skin appears dry.
5. As the skin improves, continue the lubricant twice a day or more frequently. Decrease the topical steroid to once a day, or less frequently as needed. You may also be able to decrease the potency of the topical steroid.
6. With further improvement, the frequency of wetting the skin and lubrication can be decreased.

Secondary bacterial infection by *S. aureus* or *Streptococcus pyogenes* resulting from the frequent breaks in the skin and the excoriations caused by scratching is treated with systemic antibiotics (see Figs. 4-9 and 4-10 and Box 4-3).[12] Staphylococcal septicemia has been reported.[12]

Secondary infection by herpes simplex virus may result in widespread vesicles and fever (see Chapter 8). Eczema herpeticum should be treated with oral antiherpes agents (see Box 4-3).

Once improvement has been accomplished, parents may substitute lubricants for the steroid ointments to improve skin barrier function.[13,14] Also, patients and family should be instructed to pay careful attention to avoidance of factors that aggravate atopic dermatitis, which are listed in Box 4-2. On the follow-up visit, maintenance care instructions may be instituted (Boxes 4-6 and 4-7). Busy households may find it impractical to follow the frequent bathing instructions listed in Box 4-6, and infrequent bathing strategies outlined in Box 4-7 may be employed.

Dry skin can be managed by rehydration of the skin with water and covering the skin generously with a lubricant. Irritant contact sensitivity can be managed by

(Box 4-4) should be applied twice daily, and an antihistamine taken before bedtime for a 2-week period. If the dermatitis is severe, wet dressings can be used overnight (Box 4-5). Parents may exhibit an irrational fear of topical steroids, but careful studies of daily long-term use of moderate-strength steroids show no adverse effects.[11] If lichenification is present, topical steroid ointments should be used daily for 4 to 6 weeks on the thickened areas.

Box 4-7   Alternative Instructions for Maintenance Care of Atopic Dermatitis for Busy Households

1. Reduce bathing to every 3 or 4 days.
2. Apply moisturizer several times a day to dry skin.
3. Use antihistamines such as hydroxyzine at bedtime for itching as necessary.
4. If flareup occurs, retreat as described in Boxes 4-4 and 4-5.

Box 4-8   General Instructions for Long-term Management of Atopic Dermatitis

Keep the skin lubricated
Wear loose-fitting cotton clothing
Keep fingernails trimmed short
Avoid overheating of skin
Always use a soap substitute
Limit time of soap-substitute exposure to the skin and pat dry—don't rinse off

---

decreasing bathing to every third or fourth day and by washing infants without soap when possible. When using soap, contact with the skin can be limited by rinsing the child quickly after the soap has been applied. A soap substitute, such as Cetaphil or Moisturel cleansers, may be used. These are applied to the skin, then gently patted dry with a soft cloth instead of being rinsed off.

Sweating and heat intolerance can be managed by avoiding occlusive clothing, airtight occlusive dressings such as Saran Wrap, and overheating (Box 4-8). Direct contact with wool clothing, home cleaning agents, or irritating chemicals should be avoided.

Stress and anxiety can be difficult to manage. Stress increases the sense of pruritus. Parents usually do not intentionally accelerate stress for their children, and all stresses cannot be removed. The stress and anxiety of the atopic dermatitis condition may require therapeutic intervention and discussion with parents who already blame themselves for the child's condition. The clinician should emphasize to the parents that the primary problem is the skin condition. Re-

moval of stress may be beneficial, but treatment of the skin is most important.

Relief of itching is the cornerstone of therapy for atopic dermatitis. Itching may be relieved by removal of the factors aggravating atopic dermatitis, or by the use of topical glucocorticosteroids of low or moderate potency or antihistamines.

Management of acute severe dermatitis

Steroids and wet dressings. Acute weeping dermatitis is best treated by the application of wet dressings, the methodology for which is outlined in Box 4-5. Patients with this type of dermatitis often have multiple excoriations, crusting, and secondary bacterial infection; thus the use of wet dressings in combination with systemic antibiotics is necessary. It may be difficult to treat such patients successfully without the use of antibiotics. A moderate-potency steroid ointment (see Box 4-4) should be applied to affected areas and covered with a damp cotton dressing followed by a dry cotton dressing. A handout on patient instructions for application of wet dressings is provided in the appendix on p. 350. The keys to successful wet dressings are to thoroughly wring out the clothing until it is barely damp and to be firm with the child. Systemic antistaphylococcal antibiotics should be administered to treat secondary infection, and oral antihistamines can be used to relieve pruritus. Therapy should be simple, and the routine use of lubricants is not recommended in the initial care of acute severe dermatitis.

Long-term management of atopic dermatitis

In addition to the methods of skin care listed in Boxes 4-4 and 4-7, cetyl alcohol lotion cleanser can be used as a soap substitute or in place of the bath. The child should be bathed only once a week, and a lubricant cetyl alcohol lotion should be applied liberally to the body three or four times per day. Additional lubricants can be applied throughout the day as needed.

Topical steroids and lubricants are discussed in detail in Chapter 22. Boxes 4-4 and 4-8 give a short list of commonly used products. In very humid climates lotions and creams may be effective. In drier climates greasy lubricants and ointments are more effective.

Referral for special therapy

Children who are not responding to treatment may be referred to a dermatologist for further treatment. Often, therapeutic failures result from not following the treatment plan or the presence of unrecognized and untreated secondary bacterial infection or scabies. A detailed history of the treatment times and individuals responsible for treatments will be useful in ascertaining compliance. Simplifying the regimen may be all that is necessary for success.

Topical tacrolimus ointment may be effective in older children with limited areas of skin involvement, such as chronic facial dermatitis.[15] The high cost and burning and stinging on application limit its use.[16] Tars are effective in the treatment of atopic dermatitis, but they stink and stain. Phototherapy with narrowband ultraviolet B (UVB) or UVA1 sunlamps, or photochemotherapy with psoralen and ultraviolet light (PUVA) may be efficacious in children with atopic dermatitis who have failed standard therapy. Phototherapy should be supervised by trained, experienced dermatologists. In severe cases, systemic immunosuppression with cyclosporin may help.

Alternative therapies

Although many parents or physicians are convinced that foods induce exacerbation of atopic dermatitis, scientific evidence to reproduce dermatitis by foods is unconvincing for most children. This should not become an emotional issue between parents and the treating physician. Restrictive diets have no long-term benefits in atopic dermatitis and may result in nutritional deficiency if too restrictive.[17] Evening primrose oil, desensitization shots, interferon, Chinese herbs, and a number of other remedies have been advocated, but there is no compelling evidence for their efficacy or long-term safety. Oral steroids may produce temporary benefits, but high doses are required, and they have no role in management of a chronic disease because of side effects with long-term use.

Patient Education

It is helpful to instruct the child and parents in the method of application of the topical medications (see patient education handouts for Atopic Dermatitis [Eczema], p. 334, and Wet Dressings, p. 350). A clinician may choose to explain that the child has "immature, sensitive" skin and that heredity plays a role in determining this tendency but the cause is not known. The clinician should emphasize to the parents the extreme pruritus associated with this condition. The severity of the itching sensation is so great that the child will produce painful, deep excoriations in an effort to relieve the pruritus. It should be stressed that a cure is not possible, but that good control can be achieved, so that the child can live a comfortable and

---

> **Box 4-9   Lubricants Useful for Atopic Dermatitis**
>
> Hydrophilic petrolatum (Vaseline)
> Aquaphor
> Cetyl alcohol cream (Cetaphil)
> Eucerin
> Moisturel
> Vanicreme

---

normal life. Measures to prevent further skin irritation are also helpful (see Box 4-3), especially soap avoidance, as is emphasis on the factors aggravating atopic dermatitis, particularly secondary bacterial skin infection. The patient and the parents should be told that the principle underlying good control is the liberal use of lubricants (Box 4-9) to restore moisture to the skin and protect it from contactants. Using lubricants in this manner avoids the necessity for high-potency topical glucocorticosteroids and long-term steroid medications. The clinician should not make the patient or parents feel guilty if a flare of the eczema occurs. Active treatment should be immediately reinstituted. Therapy should be directed at relieving pruritus, not focusing pressure on stopping the child from scratching.

Follow-up Visits

The first follow-up visit should be within 10 to 14 days so that therapy can be reviewed. It is often helpful at this time to have the parents or child demonstrate how medication is applied and to determine how much was used. Have the medication brought back for each visit so that you can document the quantity used. Evaluation of the response to antihistamines and the need for antibiotics can be completed at the first follow-up visit. Thereafter, monthly visits will suffice until the patient is using lubricants only, after which he or she should be reevaluated every 3 to 6 months. Clinicians should be certain patients and their families know that they will be available when flares occur, and the children should be examined for secondary infection at the visit related to the flare-up.

CONTACT DERMATITIS

Contact dermatitis, or dermatitis resulting from substances coming in direct contact with the skin, is divided into two subtypes: primary irritant contact dermatitis and allergic contact dermatitis.

Primary Irritant Contact Dermatitis

Strong chemicals that penetrate the epidermal barrier readily, weaker chemicals that penetrate a faulty epidermal barrier, or substances that remove intercellular lipids produce inflammation of the skin (primary irritant contact dermatitis). The form most commonly seen in pediatrics is diaper dermatitis. Dry skin dermatitis and JPD are other forms commonly seen in children.

Diaper dermatitis

Clinical features. The exact incidence of diaper dermatitis is unknown, but roughly 20% of all infants under age 2 years are believed to develop this condition at any time.[18,19] Four clinical forms are recognized. The most frequently observed is chafing dermatitis, in which involvement of the convex surface of the thighs, buttocks, and waist area is common (Fig. 4-11). Chafing diaper dermatitis most frequently is observed at 7 to 12 months of age, when the baby's urine volume exceeds the absorbing capacity of the diaper, including the superabsorbant diapers. In the second form the dermatitis is limited to the perianal area. This form is particularly observed in newborns or in children who have experienced diarrhea. The third form is characterized by discrete shallow ulcerations scattered throughout the diaper area, including the genitalia. In the fourth form, beefy-red confluent erythema involving the inguinal creases and the genitalia, with satellite oval lesions about the periphery, is seen (Fig. 4-12). This fourth form is observed when secondary invasion with *Candida albicans* occurs. Despite major differences in clinical appearance, all four forms share a similar pathogenesis.

Differential diagnosis. Atopic dermatitis or the other forms of dermatitis may begin in the diaper area. Rarely, psoriasis, Langerhans cell histiocytosis, or the eruptions associated with hereditary immunodeficiencies or HIV infection may occur in this area. In perianal forms of diaper dermatitis, perianal cellulitis must be distinguished and a bacterial culture obtained.

Pathogenesis. Diaper dermatitis is a result of prolonged contact of urine and/or feces with diaper-area skin.[18-20] Feces are responsible for perianal distribution, urine for thigh and waistband lesions. Airtight

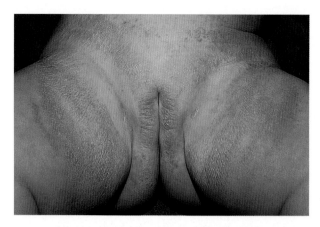

Fig. 4-11 Chafing type of diaper dermatitis.

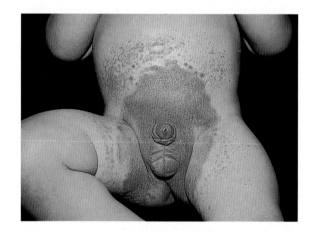

Fig. 4-12 Candidiasis in the diaper area. A positive culture for Candida can be obtained from satellite pustules.

occlusion of feces and urine by diaper covers increases the penetration of these alkaline substances through the epidermal barrier. Prolonged contact with water is central to the genesis of the dermatitis. Ammonia by itself is not responsible for the dermatitis. If diaper dermatitis is present for longer than 3 days, there is likely to be secondary *C. albicans* invasion of the inflammatory areas of the skin.

Treatment. The basis for all treatment programs is to remove the contactants (urine and feces) from the skin surface and eliminate maceration by keeping the diaper area dry.[21] Lubrication of diapered skin with a greasy ointment decreases the severity of diaper dermatitis and may protect the skin from urine and feces. Very frequent diaper changes, followed by application of ointment, limits maceration and decreases recurrences. Diaper changes several hours after the baby goes to sleep for the night and reducing fluids just before bedtime may be beneficial. Plastic and rubber pants should be avoided when possible. Letting the diaper-area skin air dry when practical may be helpful, but moisture and maceration followed by dry air or hot, dry air such as from a hair dryer should be avoided. When contamination by urine and feces occurs, the skin should be rinsed gently with warm water. A minimum of soap should be used in this area. Care should be taken to not "over treat" the diaper area, because excessive washing and drying techniques can produce an irritant dermatitis.

Candidiasis in the diaper area requires topical antiyeast therapy such as nystatin or an imidazole. Use of topical steroid creams or ointments for diaper dermatitis is discouraged because of the development of striae or granuloma gluteale infantum.[22] Until toilet training is achieved or diaper care procedures are changed, recurrences may be frequent. The incidence of diaper dermatitis decreases with eight or more diaper changes per day.

Patient education. Reducing the amount of contact of urine and feces with skin is essential. Very frequent diaper changes and lubrication of the skin constitute the best prevention, with careful attention to overnight care. Having the baby sleep on a rubber sheet without a diaper cover may be helpful. Determining the person actually responsible for diaper changes during the daily routine is very helpful in planning a therapy program. In the 7- to 12-month-old, the parent should check the diaper for wetness several hours after bedtime and change the baby if wet. Restriction of fluids in the hour just before bedtime may also be helpful for the toddler. Parents should be told that successful toilet training is the ultimate cure.

Follow-up visits. The routine visits for pediatric care are sufficient for follow-up, but in cases of severe diaper dermatitis, a revisit in 2 days may be useful.

Dry skin dermatitis
Clinical features. A dry, rough skin surface with rectangular scales that have erythema on the scale borders is seen in dermatitis caused by dry skin. Horny follicular papules on the proximal extremities and buttocks (keratosis pilaris) are also usually seen. Occasionally the dermatitis will coalesce, and the patient will present with diffuse erythema (Fig. 4-13).

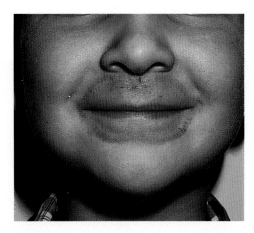

Fig. 4-13 Lip-licker dermatitis associated with constant licking of dry lips.

Differential diagnosis. The differential diagnosis includes all other forms of dermatitis, the ichthyoses, and scabies. Children with atopic dermatitis have very dry skin.

Pathogenesis. Environmental humidity of less than 30% is the most important factor. Frequent soaping of the skin, removing skin lipids with alcohol or acetone, or the use of drying lotions predisposes children to dry-skin dermatitis. Disrupting the skin surface by drying induces release of tumor necrosis factor alpha (TNF-α) and interleukin-1 by keratinocytes, with subsequent inflammation.

Treatment. Therapy is designed to restore moisture to the skin by liberal use of water followed by application of lubricants. Generally, application of water-in-oil emulsions (see Chapter 22) two or three times per day is sufficient.

Patient education. The value of a home humidifier in an area of low environmental humidity and of avoiding frequent soaping of the skin is important to convey to the patient or family (see patient education handout on Atopic Dermatitis [Eczema], p. 334). Children with dry skin require daily lubricant therapy.

Follow-up visits. One visit in 4 weeks' time to evaluate the therapy program is often sufficient.

Juvenile plantar dermatosis
Clinical features. Redness, cracking, and dryness of the weight-bearing surface of the foot are characteristic of JPD. The great toes are often the first area involved.

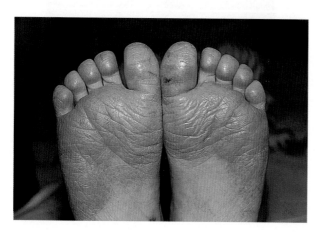

Fig. 4-14 Red, shiny distal sole and toes associated with juvenile plantar dermatosis.

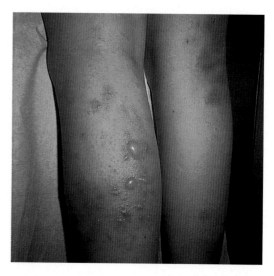

Fig. 4-15 Allergic contact dermatitis caused by poison ivy, with blister formation.

Involvement of the entire forefoot may occur that can mimic tinea pedis (Fig. 4-14). Involvement is usually quite symmetric. Many, but not all children with JPD may exhibit features of atopic dermatitis.

Differential diagnosis. Tinea pedis often mimics JPD. However, JPD is quite common in preadolescence, whereas tinea pedis is uncommon; JPD involves weight-bearing areas, whereas tinea pedis involves the instep. Direct microscopic examination of scale with potassium hydroxide (KOH) and fungal culture will help to distinguish the two conditions. Allergic contact dermatitis usually involves the dorsum of the foot rather than the weight-bearing surface.

Treatment. The use of ointment bases such as Aquaphor or petroleum jelly applied two or three times per day is most useful. The ointment should be applied as soon as shoes are taken off to avoid heat and humidity in a shoe and xerosis in bare feet. Socks may need to remain over lubricated feet to prevent slipping and greasing of floors. Attempts to dry the feet often aggravate the condition because the feet are already dry and chapped. Topical glucocorticosteroid ointments of moderate potency may be required if inflammation is severe.

Patient education. Emphasis that this is neither a fungal infection nor the result of excessive sweating of the foot is important. The patient should recognize that the excessive dryness is similar to chapping of the skin.

Follow-up visits. A visit 2 weeks after therapy is begun is most useful in evaluating compliance and response to therapy.

Allergic contact dermatitis

Clinical features. The exact incidence of allergic contact dermatitis in children is unknown, but some authorities estimate it at 5% to 10% of all dermatitis.[23-26] By age 5, 10% to 20% of children have already been sensitized to at least one contact allergen, and sensitization is likely to have occurred in infancy.[27,28]

In childhood, allergic contact dermatitis usually presents as acute dermatitis with erythema, vesiculation, and oozing (Fig. 4-15). The dermatitis is limited to the area of contact with the external substance, such as the metal snaps on pants,[29] or the stem or leaf of a plant[30] (Fig. 4-16). Less often, children are exposed repeatedly to weaker chemical allergens, resulting in development of the features of subacute or chronic dermatitis (Fig. 4-17). Usually the contactant is obvious, although considerable detective work is occasionally required to determine the cause. Once the response occurs and dermatitis is generated, as seen with a strong allergen such as poison ivy, it lasts for 3 weeks, even though the child has not had repeated exposure to the allergen.

Distribution of the dermatitis may provide an important clue to the contact allergen (Fig. 4-18). For example, one may see involvement of the dorsa of the feet in shoe dermatitis; of the subumbilical skin, earlobes, neck, wrists, and fingers in metal allergy (e.g., caused by nickel); of the face and eyelids in cosmetic

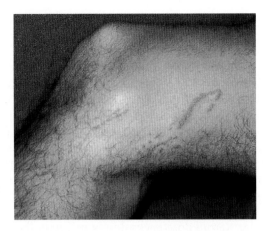

Fig. 4-16 Allergic contact dermatitis on the legs secondary to poison oak; note the linear pattern where the leaf has brushed against the leg.

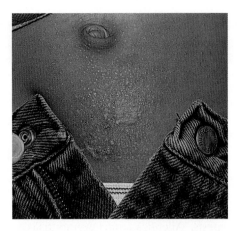

Fig. 4-18 Allergic contact dermatitis to nickel caused by metal snap on blue jeans.

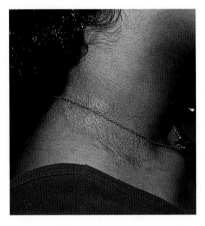

Fig. 4-17 Chronic dermatitis of neck from nickel allergy caused by necklace.

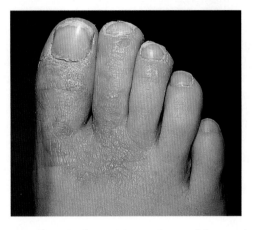

Fig. 4-19 Chronic dermatitis on dorsa of feet and toes caused by potassium dichromate allergy from chronic exposure to leather tennis shoes.

allergy; of the axilla in deodorant allergy; of the ear canal from medication; of the perioral area from toothpaste or lipstick; or of areas of clothing from exposure to formaldehyde (Box 4-10). Once sensitization occurs, repeated exposure to the antigen may result in a widespread papulovesicular dermatitis or so-called *"id reaction."* This is particularly observed in nickel allergy.[23,25,29]

Differential diagnosis. Although all other forms of dermatitis may mimic allergic contact dermatitis, it is usually localized to one area of skin. A sudden onset of dermatitis limited to the hands or feet in children and adolescents is most likely to be contact dermatitis (Fig. 4-19). Patch testing (described under Follow-up visits) may detect the chemical allergen and help

---

Box 4-10   Common Sources of Contact Allergens in Children

Plants: poison ivy, oak, and sumac (urushiol)
Clothing snaps, earrings, bracelets (nickel)
Shoes (potassium dichromate and rubber additives)
Topical medications, creams, lotions (neomycin, thimerosal, formaldehyde, quaternium 15 and other formaldehyde-releasing preservatives, wool alcohol [lanolin]
Perfumes, soaps, cosmetics (balsam of Peru, colophony, 'fragrances')

distinguish allergic contact dermatitis from other forms of dermatitis.

Pathogenesis. Allergic contact dermatitis is a form of cell-mediated immunity. The process is divided into two distinct but interrelated phases: the sensitization phase and the elicitation phase.[23,25] The antigens involved in allergic contact dermatitis are incomplete antigens called *haptens* (Box 4-11). The hapten applied to the skin surface penetrates the epidermis, combines with the antigen-binding site of the epidermal Langerhans cell, and is carried via the lymphatics to the regional lymph node. There the antigen is processed by macrophages and presented to T lymphocytes. Recognition occurs, as does proliferation of the T lymphocytes specifically programmed to recognize that antigen. These T lymphocytes leave the lymph node and enter the bloodstream, migrating back to the skin. The sensitization phase takes 5 to 7 days to complete in the case of strong chemical allergens; with weak allergens, it may take from weeks to months.

In the elicitation phase, antigen-specific T lymphocytes are present in the skin. The next time the allergen comes in contact with the skin surface and penetrates the epidermis, the T lymphocyte combines with the allergen in the skin and releases inflammatory mediators, causing erythema and the accumulation and activation of mononuclear cells, which results in the dermatitis. This phase begins 6 to 18 hours after the antigen is applied.

A great variety of chemicals are responsible for causing allergic contact dermatitis, varying from the simple metal nickel to complex chemicals such as dinitrochlorobenzene. Common sources of contact allergens in children are listed in Box 4-10. However, they have certain features in common, as seen in Box 4-11.

Treatment. Antiinflammatory agents such as glucocorticosteroids are the therapy of choice in allergic contact dermatitis. In localized areas topical glucocorticosteroid ointments of moderate potency (see Box 4-4 and Chapter 22) applied three times per day may clear the dermatitis and decrease the discomfort. In generalized skin involvement, or in acute vesicular involvement, wet dressings and topical glucocorticosteroids for 2 to 3 days give dramatic relief. This is followed by application of moderate-potency topical glucocorticosteroids three times per day until the pruritus resolves. When the face or genital area is involved, or when greater than 10% of the skin surface is involved, oral glucocorticosteroids are used, such as prednisone, 1 mg/kg in a single dose every morning for 1 week and then tapered over 7 to 14 days. The popular steroid dose packs do not maintain their antiinflammatory effects for a sufficiently long time and often result in a rebound exacerbation of acute allergic contact dermatitis.

Patient education. Knowledge and avoidance of the offending antigen are central to the care of the child with allergic contact dermatitis. Poison ivy/oak dermatitis is the most common allergic contact dermatitis in the United States.[23,25,26] The next most common is nickel allergy. Nickel allergy often begins in infancy.[23,25,27,29] Other common contact allergens such as fragrances[30] are listed in Table 4-1. The clinician should emphasize that treatment requires 2 or 3 weeks.

Follow-up visits. In 3 to 4 weeks, after the allergic dermatitis has subsided, epicutaneous (patch) testing (Fig. 4-20) to identify the offending allergen may be desirable in children in whom the cause is obscure. This is not necessary in acute poison ivy or plant-related dermatitis. Epicutaneous testing has been standardized and is reliable in detecting the suspected allergen. The test is made on the upper back. The suspected antigens are placed on the chambers, and vertical rows of three to five strips are placed on the upper back and firmly secured with nonirritating occlusive tape. The area is taped securely, so that it is airtight, and the patches are left on for 48 hours without allowing the area to become wet. The patient removes the patches and tape, and the tests are read 72 to 96 hours after initial application. Erythema and vesiculation are observed in an allergic reaction, the same clinical and histologic features that are seen in allergic contact dermatitis. In allergic reactions the papules extend beyond the chamber margins, whereas they are limited to the chamber in irritant reactions. The angry back syndrome of hyperreactivity has not been reported in children. Standardized allergens have

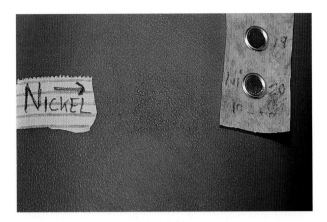

Fig. 4-20 Removal of the patch test after 48 hours in child with positive reaction to nickel.

Table 4-1	Most Prevalent Allergens in Children	
Allergen		**Sensitized (%)**
Plant (poison oak, ivy)		80*
Nickel		10
Neomycin		8
Potassium dichromate		8
Thimerosal		3
Balsam of Peru		2
Formaldehyde		1
Quaternium 15		1
Colophony		1
p-tert-Butylphenol formaldehyde		1
Wool (lanolin) alcohol		1

*In endemic areas of North America.

been developed by the North American Contact Dermatitis Group and may be obtained from the American Academy of Dermatology. Prepackaged patch testing materials such as TrueTest (Allerderm Laboratories) have been safely used in children.[27] Patch testing should be performed by a physician experienced in the interpretation and pitfalls of the procedure.

SEBORRHEIC DERMATITIS
Clinical Features

Chronic dermatitis accompanied by overproduction of sebum may occur on the scalp, face, midchest, or perineum in two age groups: the neonate and the adolescent. The scalp appears greasy, with accumulation of scales entrapped in the sebum. In some infants it is limited to the scalp, with a greasy accumulation of scales adherent to the scalp (seborrhea capitis). Many infants also have flexural dermatitis as seen in atopic dermatitis. Infants with a tendency to have seborrheic dermatitis may have severe worsening of their dermatitis if they develop persistent diaper dermatitis. In adolescents, erythema and greasy scales in the nasolabial folds and the scalp may be seen. In HIV-infected patients, seborrheic dermatitis may be an early sign of acquired immunodeficiency syndrome (AIDS). Widespread infantile seborrheic dermatitis associated with failure to thrive and recurrent infections should bring to mind a hereditary immunodeficiency disorder.

Differential Diagnosis

Because physiologic overproduction of sebum occurs in many infants during the first 6 months of life, any dermatitis occurring at this age may be mistakenly called seborrheic dermatitis. There is considerable confusion over whether it is necessary to distinguish between atopic dermatitis, contact dermatitis, and seborrheic dermatitis in infants. Most infants with dermatitis eventually demonstrate features consistent with atopic dermatitis, especially if the involvement of the extremities and trunk accompanies the more characteristic lesions of the scalp and face. Scabies may also mimic seborrheic dermatitis in this age group, and identifying mites by scraping unscratched burrows will confirm scabies. Seborrheic dermatitis with petechiae is often seen in Langerhans cell histiocytosis, and this diagnosis may also be excluded by skin biopsy. The hereditary immunodeficiency diseases, such as Leiner's disease, severe combined immunodeficiency, and the immunodeficiency that accompanies HIV infection, may be considered by the presence of signs and symptoms of failure to thrive, severe pulmonary or gastrointestinal infection accompanying the eruption, or the appropriate immunologic or serologic evaluation.

Multiple carboxylase deficiency and other biotin-responsive dermatoses also mimic seborrheic dermatitis, and serum biotin levels may be required to confirm the diagnosis.

Seborrheic dermatitis limited to the scalp (seborrhea capitis) must be distinguished from the diffuse form of tinea capitis caused by *Trichophyton tonsurans* and from cradle cap. A KOH examination of scalp scrapings plus a fungal culture will distinguish tinea capitis, whereas the absence of redness characterizes cradle cap.

Adolescent seborrheic dermatitis occurs in the nasolabial folds, midface, postauricular area, scalp, and chest. It may be difficult to distinguish from atopic or contact dermatitis, perioral dermatitis, or psoriasis.

Pathogenesis

Although seborrheic dermatitis has been attributed to excessive sebum accumulation on the skin surface, the mechanism is unknown. Overgrowth of *Pityrosporum orbicularis* occurs in sebum-rich environments and some authorities believe the host response to these yeasts may account for the inflammation. Similarly, the pathogenesis of the seborrheic-like dermatitis of immunodeficiency or HIV infection is unknown. Although there are many carboxylase enzymes in skin, and biotin may be a cofactor for many skin enzymes, the mechanism of dermatitis is unknown.

Treatment

Topical steroid ointments of low potency applied twice daily for several days and then occasionally will often clear the dermatitis and treat recurrences. Keratolytic or antifungal shampoos on the scalp are useful in some patients but will be painful if they wash into the infant's eyes, and they may worsen the dermatitis. Tear-free shampoos may be adequate. The shampoo can remain on the scalp for several minutes while the scalp is lightly scrubbed with a soft brush or toothbrush to remove the scale and crust. The low-potency topical steroid ointment can be applied immediately after shampoo. This process can be repeated daily until adequate improvement or resolution occurs. Oral biotin therapy should be considered if biotin-responsive dermatoses are suspected. On the face, topical steroids should be of low potency and used twice daily for several days and then moisturizers substituted. If perioral dermatitis is suspected, antiacne therapy as outlined in Chapter 3 is used.

Patient Education

Patients and parents should be advised that the cause of this disorder is unknown. Although it is tempting to use rigorous methods to remove scale from the scalp, it is unnecessary. Gentle therapy repeated several days in a row is more effective.

Follow-up Visits

A visit in 1 week to review diagnostic tests and to evaluate response to therapy is recommended. If the lesions remain thick and crusted, the diagnosis of seborrheic dermatitis is probably incorrect and requires reevaluation of the condition. Thereafter the child should be seen only if the dermatitis does not resolve.

NUMMULAR DERMATITIS
Clinical Features

Symmetrically distributed areas of dermatitis 1 to 10 cm in diameter are seen primarily on the extremities in this condition (Fig. 4-21). The Latin word *nummulus*, meaning "little coin," is used to describe the shape of the lesions. Two forms occur in children: the wet form, with oozing and crusting (Fig. 4-21), and the dry form, with erythema and scaling. Both forms are persistent, lasting for months if untreated. Most patients volunteer that the lesions are intensely pruritic, and they frequently are scratching the affected skin. Occasionally, a patient will deny touching the lesions.

Differential Diagnosis

Nummular dermatitis is important because it frequently mimics two common pediatric conditions: impetigo and tinea corporis. The wet form is frequently confused with impetigo, and multiple courses of antibiotics are given before the diagnosis is suspected. Biopsy of the lesion readily distinguishes it from impetigo. The dry form can be distinguished from tinea corporis by a KOH examination of skin scrapings or a fungal culture. At times, nummular lesions will occur in otherwise typical atopic dermatitis or contact dermatitis. Presence of lichenification confirms rubbing and scratching of the lesions when the patient's history suggests absence of trauma to the lesions.

Pathogenesis

The cause is unknown, but recently mercury compounds have been implicated in a few patients.[31]

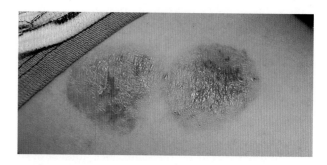

Fig. 4-21 Two oozing coin-shaped areas of dermatitis in nummular eczema.

Treatment

The treatment is the same as for atopic dermatitis, although often high-potency topical steroids are required. A sedating antihistamine in the evening and a nonsedating antihistamine in the morning will reduce the pruritus. Lesions are difficult to resolve, and treatment programs require considerable effort before improvement is seen. From 4 to 6 weeks of therapy are required to reverse the thickening.

Patient Education

Patients should be informed of the chronicity of nummular eczema and its tendency to recur. They should be told the cause is unknown.

Follow-up Visits

The child should be seen initially in 2 weeks to evaluate the initial response to therapy, and bimonthly follow-up for 6 to 12 months may be required.

KERATOSIS PILARIS, LICHEN SPINULOSUS, FOLLICULAR MUCINOSIS
Clinical Features

Keratosis pilaris is a common skin condition in childhood.[32,33] In keratosis pilaris, prominent follicular plugs are noted over the extensor aspects of the extremities, the buttocks, and the facial cheeks (Figs. 4-22 and 4-23). Individual lesions represent plugs of stratum corneum in individual follicular openings. Dermatitis may surround the plugs. The affected skin surface feels rough and dry. Keratosis pilaris on facial skin is often accompanied by telangiectatic erythema, especially on the cheeks and occasionally the eyebrows.[32] Keratosis pilaris is worsened by drying of skin and is frequently associated with dry skin, ichthyosis vulgaris, and atopic dermatitis. However, some children may present with extensive keratosis pilaris with no evidence of the other conditions. In these children keratosis pilaris is extensive and often involves the forearms, lower legs, and much of the face. Keratosis pilaris lesions often improve in a humid climate and become more extensive in a drier climate.

Lichen spinulosus represents grouping of hair follicles with prominent follicular plugs (Fig. 4-24). The lesions are usually hypopigmented and demonstrate fine scale on the intrafollicular skin.

Follicular mucinosis, also called *alopecia mucinosis,* presents with lesions that appear to be lichen spinulosus but have absent hairs (Fig 4-25).[34] The intrafollicular skin demonstrates scale and may be

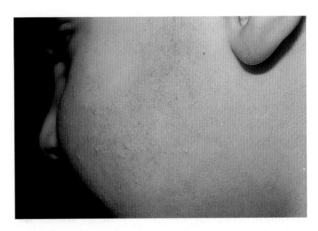

Fig. 4-23 Keratotic papules and telangiectatic erythema on face of child with keratosis pilaris.

Fig. 4-22 Dry pinpoint red and white discrete papules on the extensor surface of the arm and keratosis pilaris.

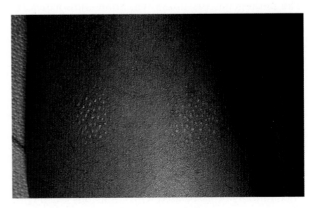

Fig. 4-24 Two areas of lichen spinulosus associated with prominent white follicular plugs.

Fig. 4-25 Hypopigmented plaque of follicular mucinosis with associated follicular plugging and absence of hairs.

indurated, giving the appearance of hairless plaques with follicular prominence.

Differential Diagnosis

Keratosis pilaris may be confused with microcomedones of acne, molluscum contagiosum, warts, milia, psoriasis, or occasionally folliculitis. Inflamed keratosis pilaris is often erroneously diagnosed as dermatitis. Because it is not seen at birth, it should be easily distinguished from neonatal acne and erythema toxicum. Lichen spinulosus may resemble lesions of keratosis pilaris, but they group together involving every follicle in one or several skin areas. Follicular mucinosis lesions are more indurated, localized, and have a more plaquelike appearance. Skin biopsy will distinguish between the two.

Pathogenesis

The pathogenesis is unknown. Some authorities regard keratosis pilaris as a disorder of keratinization. They believe that the keratinous plug is produced through abnormal keratinization of the follicular channel. Others believe it is a response to drying of the skin surface, which results in a dry plug of scale lodged in follicular openings. It is more severe in cold, dry climates. Skin biopsy will separate these conditions because follicular mucinosis will demonstrate mucin in sebaceous glands and the outer root sheaths of affected hair follicles. Follicular mucinosis is occasionally associated with lymphoma in adults, and may uncommonly be associated with cutaneous T-cell lymphoma in children.[35]

Treatment

In the very mild forms of keratosis pilaris, the use of lubricants applied to wet skin may be sufficient to improve the condition because total resolution is often not possible. In more extensive keratosis pilaris, topical keratolytics may be required, frequently in combination with lubricants. Lactic acid 12% cream (Lac-Hydrin), a 10% urea cream, or a cream with both lactic acid and urea (Eucerin Plus Creme) applied several times a day is frequently beneficial. All treatment strategies require many weeks of therapy to see improvement. Therapy must be continued after improvement is seen. Topical tretinoin (Retin-A) or other retinoids are also effective but may cause significant irritation to the skin, particularly if the child has ichthyosis or associated atopic dermatitis. Often, when the child moves to a more humid climate the condition spontaneously improves. The facial telangiectasia, often a source of embarrassment to the child, may be treated with the vascular pulsed dye laser.

Lichen spinulosus may require low-potency topical steroid ointments in addition to lubrication for improvement. The plaques of follicular mucinosis require more potent topical steroid ointments and lubrication. Both conditions are difficult to resolve completely.

Patient Education

The patient and family should be informed of the nature of this disease and its likelihood of becoming chronic if untreated and even if treated (see patient education handouts for Keratosis Pilaris, p. 339 and Creams and Ointments, p. 335) They should also be advised of the slow response to therapy, the necessity of long-term treatment, and the usual eventual improvement or resolution of these conditions.

Follow-up Visits

A follow-up visit in 4 to 8 weeks to determine response to therapy is usually indicated. Thereafter, follow-up during routine evaluations is sufficient.

REFERENCES

1. Foley P et al: The frequency of common skin conditions in preschool-age children in Australia, *Arch Dermatol* 137:293, 2001.
2. McNally NJ et al: Is there a geographical variation in eczema prevalence in the U.K.? Evidence from the 1958 British Birth Cohort Study, *Br J Dermatol* 142:712, 2000.
3. Williams HC, Burney PGJ, Hay RJ: The U.K. working party's diagnostic criteria for atopic dermatitis. I. Derivation of a minimum set of discriminators for atopic dermatitis, *Br J Dermatol* 131:383, 1994.

4. Su JC et al: Atopic eczema: its impact on the family and financial cost, *Arch Dis Child* 76:159, 1997.

5. Emerson RM, Williams HC, Allen BR: What is the cost of atopic dermatitis in preschool children? *Br J Dermatol* 144:514, 2001.

6. Halbert A, Morelli JG, Weston WL: Atopic dermatitis: Is it an allergic disease? *J Am Acad Dermatol* 33:1008, 1995.

7. Weston WL: Allergy in atopic dermatitis: more harm than good? *J Cutan Med Surg* 3:199, 1999.

8. Hara J et al: High-expression of syphingomyelin deacyclase is an important determinant of ceramide deficiency leading to barrier disruption in atopic dermatitis, *J Invest Dermatol* 115:406, 2000.

9. Dupre D, Audrezet M-P, Ferec C: Atopy and a mutation in the interleukin-4 receptor gene, *N Engl J Med* 343:69, 2000.

10. Chavanas S et al: Mutations in SPINK 5, encoding a serine protease inhibitor, cause Netherton syndrome, *Nat Gen* 25:141, 2000.

11. Ellison JA et al: Hypothalamic-pituitary-adrenal function and glucocorticoid sensitivity in atopic dermatitis, *Pediatrics* 105:794, 2000.

12. Hoeger PH, Ganschow R, Finger G: Staphylococcal septicemia in children with atopic dermatitis, *Pediatr Dermatol* 17:111, 2000.

13. Loden M, Andersson AC, Lindberg M: Improvement in skin barrier function in patients with atopic dermatitis after treatment with a moisturizing cream (Canoderm), *Br J Dermatol* 140:264, 1999.

14. Orchard D, Weston WL: The importance of the vehicle in topical therapy, *Pediatr Ann* 30:207, 2001.

15. Fleischer AB Jr: Treatment of atopic dermatitis: role of tacrolimus ointment as a topical noncorticosteroid therapy, *J Allergy Clin Immunol* 104:S126, 1999.

16. Harper JI et al: Cyclosporin for severe childhood atopic dermatitis: short course versus continuous therapy, *Br J Dermatol* 142:52, 2000.

17. Liu T et al: Why children get Kwashiorkor in the United States: fad diets, perceived and true milk allergies and nutritional ignorance, *Arch Dermatol* in press, 2001.

18. Ward DB et al: Characterization of diaper dermatitis in the United States, *Arch Pediatr Adolesc Med* 154:943, 2000.

19. Visscher MO et al: Development of diaper rash in the newborn, *Pediatr Dermatol* 17:52, 2000.

20. Darmstadt GL, Dinulos JG: Neonatal skin care, *Pediatr Clin North Am* 47:757, 2000.

21. Boiko S: Treatment of diaper dermatitis, *Dermatol Clin* 17:235, 1999.

22. De Zeeuw R, van Praag MC, Oranje AP: Granuloma gluteale infantum: a case report, *Pediatr Dermatol* 17:141, 2000.

23. Bruckner A, Weston WL: Contact dermatitis, *Pediatr Ann*, 30:203, 2001.

24. Mortz CG, Andersen KE: Allergic contact dermatitis in children and adolescents, *Contact Dermatitis* 41:121, 1999.

25. Weston WL, Bruckner A: Allergic contact dermatitis, *Pediatr Clin North Am* 47:897, 2000.

26. Sasseville D: Phytodermatitis, *J Cutan Med Surg* 3:263, 1999.

27. Bruckner A, Morelli JG, Weston WL: Does sensitization to contact allergens begin in infancy? *Pediatrics* 105:1 e3, 2000.

28. Cetta F, Lambert GH, Ros SP: Newborn chemical exposure from over-the-counter skin care products, *Clin Pediatr* 30:286, 1991.

29. Gawkroger DJ, Lewis FM, Shah M: Contact sensitivity to nickel and other metals in jewelry, *J Am Acad Dermatol* 43:31, 2000.

30. Katsarou A et al: Contact reactions to fragrances, *Ann Allergy Asthma Immunol* 82:449, 1999.

31. Adachi A et al: Mercury-induced nummular dermatitis, *J Am Acad Dermatol* 43:383, 2000.

32. Lateef A, Schwartz RA: Keratosis pilaris, *Cutis* 63:205, 1999.

33. Popescu R et al: The prevalence of skin conditions among Romanian school children, *Br J Dermatol* 140:891, 1999.

34. Gibson LE, Muller SA, Peters MS: Follicular mucinosis of childhood and adolescence, *Pediatr Dermatol* 5:231, 1988.

35. Hodak E et al: Follicular cutaneous T cell lymphoma: a clinicopathological study of nine cases, *Br J Dermatol* 141:315, 1999.

Bacterial Infections (Pyodermas) and Spirochetal Infections of the Skin

Bacteria constantly colonize the skin surface and occasionally invade the epidermal barrier to replicate within the skin. The majority of skin microorganisms in healthy children are nonpathogenic. The two major pathogens found on children's skin are *Staphylococcus aureus* and *Streptococcus pyogenes*.[1,2] The former is found in 5% of children and the latter in 1%. However, during epidemics and in endemic areas, either of these organisms may be recovered from the skin of 50% to 80% of children. In warm, humid climates, and in those with poor skin hygiene, pyodermas are common in childhood.[1,3] Bacterial toxin–induced syndromes, such as scarlet fever, scalded skin syndrome, and toxic shock syndrome (TSS), are uncommon in childhood and result from skin injury by circulating toxins rather than direct bacterial invasion of skin.

IMPETIGO AND ECTHYMA
Clinical Features

Erosions covered by moist, honey-colored crusts are suggestive of impetigo (Figs. 5-1, 5-2, and 5-3).[1-5] Impetigo begins as small (1 to 2 mm) vesicles with fragile roofs that are quickly lost. Multiple lesions are often present, and exposed areas, such as the face, nares, and extremities, are the most common sites of involvement. The term *bullous impetigo* has been used to describe lesions with a central moist crust and an outer zone of blister formation (Figs. 5-3 and 5-4).[2] The blister is translucent, with a flaccid roof that is easily shed (Fig. 5-4), such that bullous impetigo may be seen as shallow erosions with an outer rim of desquamation.[2] Whether blisters are small or large, *impetigo* is the preferred term. Impetigo has a high attack rate, and its spread is enhanced by crowding and poor socioeconomic conditions.[1,4] In contrast, ecthyma is characterized by a firm, dry, dark crust with surrounding erythema and induration (Fig. 5-5).[2]

Direct pressure on the crust results in the extrusion of purulent material from beneath the crust.

Both ecthyma and impetigo may occur simultaneously in the same patient. The clinical features are so characteristic that bacterial culture is not routinely performed.

Differential Diagnosis

Subacute dermatitis, such as nummular dermatitis, herpes simplex infections, and a kerion resulting from dermatophyte infections, may have moist crusts and mimic impetigo. Nummular dermatitis has dozens of symmetrically distributed lesions, as opposed to impetigo, which has a few asymmetric lesions. Herpes simplex is usually a distinct group of lesions that even when crusted demonstrate a group of individual papules or vesicles beneath. Viral culture, fluorescent antibody testing of smears, or examination of Tzanck smear may be required to differentiate. A potassium hydroxide (KOH) examination or fungal culture may be required to distinguish a kerion from impetigo. Bullous impetigo must be differentiated from second-degree burns, fixed drug eruption, or the uncommon immunobullous diseases seen in childhood, such as linear immunoglobulin A (IgA) dermatosis, bullous pemphigoid, and bullous forms of erythema multiforme. A crusted second-degree burn, cutaneous diphtheria, or cutaneous anthrax may be confused with a solitary lesion of ecthyma. Bacterial culture of the purulent material beneath the crust may be required.

Pathogenesis

Invasion of the epidermis by pathogenic *S. aureus* or group A streptococci occurs in impetigo and ecthyma.[1,4] The depth of invasion in impetigo is superficial (into the upper epidermis), whereas the entire epidermis is involved in ecthyma (Fig. 5-6).

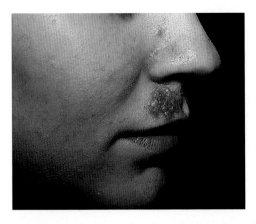

Fig. 5-1 Impetigo. Honey-colored, moist crust just above the upper lip.

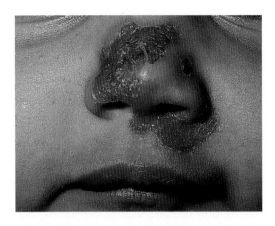

Fig. 5-2 Impetigo. Spread of infection to top of nose from beneath the nose in an infant with impetigo.

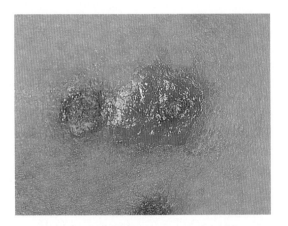

Fig. 5-3 Bullous impetigo. Flaccid blister with thin border of desquamation on the abdomen of an infant.

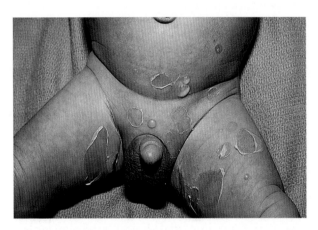

Fig. 5-4 Bullous impetigo in a newborn. Multiple areas of flaccid blisters and shallow erosions on a red base.

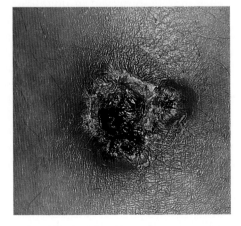

Fig. 5-5 Dry crust with indurated border in a child with ecthyma.

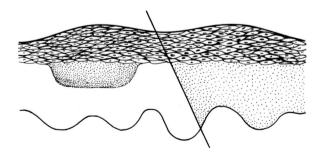

Fig. 5-6 Difference between impetigo and ecthyma. Superficial neutrophilic collection in middermis (shaded area on left) in impetigo in contrast to full-thickness involvement (shaded area on right) in ecthyma.

Microscopic breaks in the epidermal barrier, such as the trauma of scratching dermatitic skin, predispose to impetigo, whereas staphylococci or streptococci penetrate the lower epidermis in ecthyma after injury to the mid and upper epidermis. Often, colonization of the skin surface with the two major pathogens occurs several days to a month before the appearance of clinical lesions.[1] It is now recognized that in many areas of North America, methicillin-resistant staphylococci are more likely to be responsible for impetigo than streptococci and account for 70% to 80% of childhood impetigo.[2,4-6] For impetigo secondary to an underlying skin disease, such as dermatitis, scabies, psoriasis, or varicella, staphylococci are virtually always responsible.[2,5] Poststreptococcal glomerulonephritis may follow such infections of the skin if nephritogenic strains of streptococci are involved.[6]

Treatment

Systemic antibiotics to eradicate staphylococci and streptococci are the treatment of choice.[2,5] To treat both pathogens, dicloxacillin, 15 to 50 mg/kg/day; cephalexin, 40 to 50 mg/kg/day; or cloxacillin, 50 to 100 mg/kg/day orally for a total of 10 days, may be used. Erythromycin, 40 mg/kg/day orally for 10 days, is an alternative, but in many areas of North America, strains of staphylococci resistant to erythromycin have been encountered.[2,5,6] If streptococci are cultured, penicillin V, 125 to 250 mg two times daily for 10 days, may be used.[4-8] Use of most topical antibiotics may result in partial clinical improvement but may also prolong the carriage state of the pathogen on the skin.[1,2,5] Topical mupirocin ointment is as efficacious as oral cephalexin.[7] Removal of crusts and scrubbing the impetigo skin lesions with antibacterial soaps has not been shown to be effective.[2] Hand washing with a surgical soap and simple measures of good hygiene may reduce the likelihood of spread.

The risk of nephritogenic strains of streptococci varies considerably throughout North America, but an active program in which both patients and contacts are treated will significantly reduce the incidence of acute glomerulonephritis in endemic areas.[2,6]

Patient Education

Good hand-washing techniques for the caregivers and the infected child, and good general personal hygiene, are useful in preventing further infection of contacts and reducing the chances for future infections. The child should begin treatment with antibiotic therapy at least 24 hours before returning to school or day care.[4] The highly contagious nature of these infections should be strongly emphasized, and contacts should be examined if feasible.

Follow-up Visits

A visit 10 days to 2 weeks after therapy has begun is useful to determine the therapeutic response and possible spread of the organism to contacts. In recurrent or persistent infections, bacterial culture should be performed to determine if an unusual or antibiotic-resistant organism is present.

CELLULITIS
Clinical Features

Tender, warm, erythematous plaques with ill-defined borders are seen in cellulitis.[4,9-11] Occasionally, linear red macules proximal to the large plaque are seen. Regional lymphadenopathy and fever are common findings. A preceding puncture wound or other penetrating trauma to the skin is often noted (Figs. 5-7 and 5-8). Cellulitis of the fingertips in infants is called *blistering dactylitis* (Fig. 5-9), and several fingers may be involved. Perianal cellulitis in infants is increasingly recognized in North America and is characterized by tender perirectal erythema and pain on defecation (Figs. 5-10 and 5-11).[13] Superficial erosions of the perianal skin may be seen (Fig. 5-11). Lesions may extend beyond perianal skin and involve perivaginal skin (Fig. 5-12). Infants and toddlers with perianal streptococcal cellulitis often present with constipation. Perianal cellulitis in infants is virtually always caused by streptococci.

Cellulitis over large joints such as the hip, shoulder, or knee may be observed in infants and toddlers.[9,10] Extension into the joint cavity and bone is seen with cellulitis overlying a joint, particularly in infants. A bluish hue within the lesion in infants is particularly seen with *Haemophilus influenzae* cellulitis, but is also observed in cellulitis caused by other bacteria. Cellulitis of the cheeks (buccal cellulitis) or over joints in children ages 3 months to 3 years is predominantly caused by *H. influenzae* infection, whereas in older children it may result from streptococci or staphylococci.[4,9-11] *Haemophilus influenza* is now less common in North America since the introduction of the vaccine.[4] Streptococcal cellulitis spreads rapidly, within hours, in contrast to staphylococcal cellulitis. Septicemia may follow cellulitis in untreated patients.[4] Periorbital cellulitis is of great concern because of its potential for spread to the brain.[10,11]

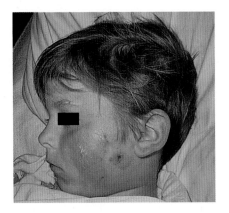

Fig. 5-7 Puncture wound with surrounding cellulitis of the cheek.

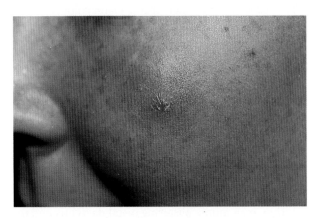

Fig. 5-8 Cellulitis following self-manipulation of acne pustule.

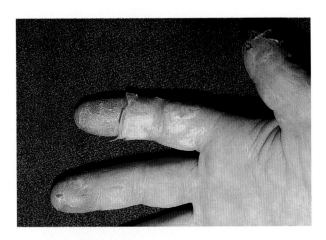

Fig. 5-9 Blistering distal dactylitis.

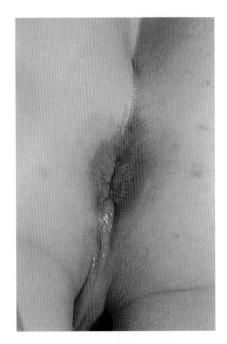

Fig. 5-10 Streptococcal perianal cellulitis. Acutely tender red perianal skin.

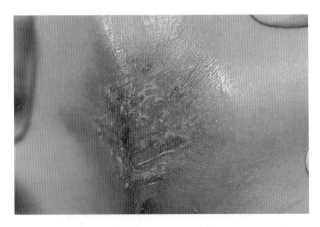

Fig. 5-11 Streptococcal perianal cellulitis. Superficial erosions and erythema of perianal skin.

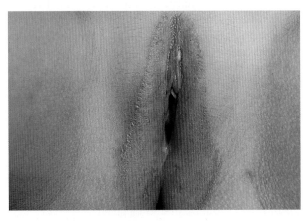

Fig. 5-12 Streptococcal perianal and perivaginal cellulitis.

Differential Diagnosis

Erythematous swellings overlying an unrecognized bony fracture may mimic cellulitis, although they may not feel warm. Similarly, pressure erythema, giant urticaria, and contact dermatitis in the early stages may be difficult to distinguish from cellulitis, but they do not produce tenderness. The redness and swelling over a septic joint may also mimic cellulitis. Acute cold injury to the fat of the cheeks of infants (popsicle panniculitis) may mimic facial cellulitis. Herpetic whitlow may mimic blistering distal dactylitis and diaper dermatitis, or painful rectal fissures may mimic perianal cellulitis.

Pathogenesis

Invasion of bacteria into the deep dermis and subcutaneous fat, with subsequent spread via the lymphatics, is responsible for the clinical features of cellulitis. Pathogenic streptococci account for most cases of cellulitis; *H. influenzae* and *S. aureus* may also be responsible.[9-11] Blood cultures are most likely to reveal the responsible bacteria.[14] Aspiration of the center or advancing edge of the cellulitis is rarely positive.[14]

Treatment

In an acutely ill child or a child with periorbital cellulitis, hospitalization should be considered. Prompt administration of antibiotics is essential. If a streptococcal infection is suspected, systemic penicillin is given, either as benzathine penicillin, 600,000 to 1,200,000 U intramuscularly, or oral penicillin V, 30 to 60 mg/kg/day for 10 days.[4] In an acutely ill febrile infant or child, hospitalization and intravenous penicillin, up to 2 million U/day, is recommended. If staphylococcal cellulitis is suspected, oral dicloxacillin, 50 to 100 mg/kg/day, is recommended. With blue cellulitis suggestive of infection with *H. influenzae*, a blood culture should be obtained before starting antibiotics. Common treatment regimens include cefotaxime, 75 to 100 mg/kg day or ceftriaxone, 50 to 75 mg/kg/day intramuscularly or intravenously, or ampicillin, 100 to 200 mg/kg/day given intravenously in combination with chloramphenicol, 50 to 85 mg/kg/day.[4]

Patient Education

The serious and potentially life-threatening nature of cellulitis should be explained to the patient and family. A thorough understanding of the portal of entry of bacteria is required. Instructions on the prompt cleansing of wounds should be given.

Follow-up Visits

If it is decided not to admit the child to a hospital, a visit within 24 hours is mandatory to assess the response to therapy and observe for signs of toxicity. Daily visits may be required until the child is recovering.

NECROTIZING FASCIITIS (STREPTOCOCCAL GANGRENE)
Clinical Features

Diabetic children with ketoacidosis and immunosuppressed children are susceptible to streptococcal gangrene.[15-19] This condition is rare, but public awareness is increasing in North America as stories about the "flesh-eating bacteria syndrome" make headlines. Prompt recognition of necrotizing fasciitis may be lifesaving. The lesion begins as cellulitis, with tender erythematous plaques, usually on the leg. Within 2 hours bullae appear on the erythematous surface, accompanied by severe pain. A purulent center develops, followed by the appearance of a black eschar and the subsidence of the acute pain (Fig. 5-13). The decrease in pain correlates well with destruction of the cutaneous nerves as they course through the fascia and subcutaneous tissue. Shock may develop. Over the next 2 days frank gangrene may be observed. Usually a clinical diagnosis is sufficient, but when difficulty distinguishing between cellulitis and necrotizing fasciitis occurs, magnetic resonance imaging (MRI) may be helpful.[17-19] In newborns the most common location for necrotizing fasciitis is on the abdominal wall,

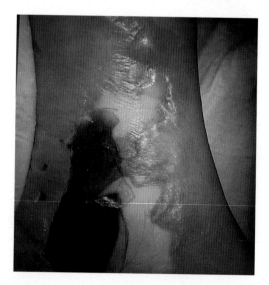

Fig. 5-13 Central black, painless necrosis; painful, yellow, purulent lake and surrounding erythema in necrotizing fasciitis in the leg of a diabetic adolescent.

where the first sign is redness and swelling of the peri-umbilical skin, and the diagnosis of omphalitis is considered. Culture of the deep tissues or blood yields group A streptococci.

Pathogenesis

Invasion by group A streptococci through the dermis and subcutaneous fat into the deep fascial compartments occurs because of the faulty host defenses of the immunosuppressed or diabetic patient.[18-20] Often, trauma to the skin precedes the appearance of these lesions. Rapid spread and destruction of tissue occur. Compromise of blood flow occurs in deep fascial or muscular compartments, and infarction of large areas of skin and subcutaneous tissue occurs.[18-20]

Differential Diagnosis

Cellulitis may mimic necrotizing fasciitis early in the disease, but the rapid evolution of necrotizing fasciitis to form necrotic areas within hours after the onset helps distinguish the two. With the development of gangrene, arterial embolism or thrombosis should be considered. Metastatic calcification with occlusion of major skin vessels may also mimic necrotizing fasciitis, but its slow onset and lack of acute pain are important differentiating features.

Treatment

Prompt surgical debridement down to the fascia is essential and is the most important aspect of therapy.[4,16-19] Fluid management to maintain adequate venous return is essential, along with intravenous antimicrobial therapy at maximal doses for age, with a β-lactamase resistant bactericidal cell-wall inhibitor plus a bacterial protein synthesis inhibitor such as clindamycin.[4] Correction of the metabolic abnormalities of diabetic ketoacidosis is important. For infection refractory to several hours of aggressive therapy, intravenous immunoglobulin may be considered.[4] Even with prompt surgical intervention, mortality is high.

Patient Education

The clinician should emphasize to the patient and family that good control of diabetes and proper personal hygiene are essential to prevent such episodes. Prompt cleansing of cuts or skin abrasions and application of topical antibiotics are suggested, and the patient should be strongly advised to seek prompt medical attention when the early signs of infection appear. Persons that have close contact with the affected child should contact their physician regarding prophylaxis with antibiotics.[4]

Follow-up Visits

After the patient is discharged from the hospital, a follow-up visit a week later is most helpful to evaluate the patient's progress. Weekly visits may be required to assess healing of the devitalized skin and deeper tissues.

SCARLET FEVER
Clinical Features

Scarlet fever occurs most often in children between 2 and 10 years of age.[4,20] The portal of entry of the streptococci may be either the pharynx or a skin wound. The exanthem appears 24 to 48 hours after infection and consists of erythematous macules and papules, beginning on the neck and spreading downward over the trunk to the extremities (Fig. 5-14).[4,20] In severe cases the exanthem may be petechial, and a positive tourniquet test is common. Petechiae in a linear pattern are seen along the major skin folds in the axillae and antecubital fossa (Pastia's sign). The palms and soles in scarlet fever are characteristically uninvolved, and a facial flush with circumoral pallor is common. Tongue involvement (a thick white coat with hypertrophied red papillae) is helpful in the differential diagnosis because a strawberry tongue is seen

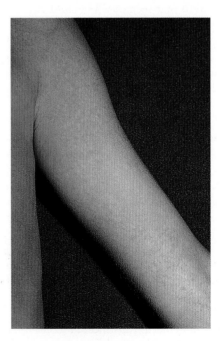

Fig. 5-14 Red, rough eruption of trunk and arm in streptococcal scarlet fever.

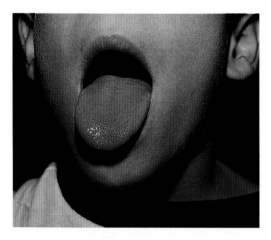

Fig. 5-15 Bright red erythema and strawberry tongue in streptococcal scarlet fever.

with streptococcal but not staphylococcal scarlet fever (Fig. 5-15). Generalized lymphadenopathy is common, with the inguinal lymph nodes particularly enlarged. Desquamation occurs as the eruption fades, progressing in the same manner as it began. In black skin, tiny, slightly erythematous papules resembling gooseflesh are found. Although it is difficult to observe the erythema and the papular nature of the eruption in dark-skinned children, scarlet fever in these children is identical to that seen in white children.

Recent outbreaks of severe septicemic scarlet fever in North America have been noted. Hypotension and a toxic shock–like syndrome are reported. This severe disease is less likely in children than in adults.[4,19,20]

Differential Diagnosis

The scarlatiniform eruption is seen in other infectious diseases, such as that appearing in the early stages of viral hepatitis, infectious mononucleosis, Kawasaki disease, TSS, measles, and rubella. Drug-associated eruptions may also mimic scarlet fever. Drugs that result in scarlatiniform eruptions include the sulfonamides, penicillin, streptomycin, quinine, and atropine. Drug eruptions are more likely to produce mucosal erosions and crusts, which may be a helpful distinguishing sign.

Pathogenesis

Three immunologically distinct scarlet fever–producing toxins have been identified from cultures of Streptococcus.[4,20] Toxin release from streptococci is mediated

by viral infection of the streptococci. The mechanism of action by the toxin on the skin is believed to depend on receptor-mediated activation of skin cells. Severe scarlet fever has been associated with the appearance of M protein type 1 and 3 strains of Streptococcus of an increased virulence.

Treatment

Penicillin, in the same doses as used for impetigo and streptococcal pharyngitis, is the treatment of choice for scarlet fever.[4,8,20] Erythromycin is used in penicillin-allergic patients. If staphylococcal scarlet fever is suspected, dicloxacillin, 15 to 50 mg/kg/day orally for 10 days, is recommended. Prompt treatment virtually eliminates the complications of scarlet fever, such as bacteremia, rheumatic fever, pneumonia, and meningitis.

During the later stages of desquamation, bland ointments applied to wet skin will restore the skin surface integrity and reduce cutaneous pain.

Patient Education

The association of scarlet fever with rheumatic fever is of great concern to patients and their families. It is important to reassure them that prompt treatment has virtually eliminated this association. Identification and cultures of patient contacts are essential.

Follow-up Visits

Approximately 7 to 10 days after the first visit, another visit is helpful to observe the response to therapy and to assess further any other sources of streptococcal infection in the household.

FOLLICULITIS, FURUNCULOSIS, AND CUTANEOUS ABSCESSES
Clinical Features

The manifestations of infection of the hair follicle vary clinically with the depth of bacterial invasion. Infection at the follicular orifice (superficial folliculitis) appears as tiny pustules, 1 to 2 mm in diameter (Fig. 5-16).[4] Folliculitis may be accompanied by impetigo (Fig 5-17).[21] Furunculosis (deep folliculitis) appears as tender erythematous nodules (Fig. 5-18). Confluence of several adjacent areas of furunculosis produces a tender, erythematous tumor that becomes soft and fluctuant after several days. Abscesses are commonly found on the buttocks and trunk but may appear in any location (Fig. 5-19). Other household members may be affected. *S. aureus* is regularly cultured from furuncles and abscesses, although gram-

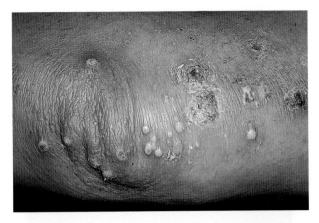

Fig. 5-16 Staphylococcal superficial folliculitis and ecthyma.

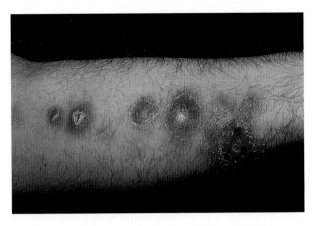

Fig. 5-18 Deep bacterial folliculitis (furunculosis) on arm.

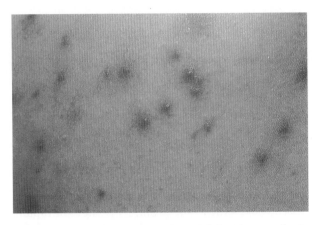

Fig. 5-17 Staphylococcal superficial folliculitis. Multiple pustules on a red base.

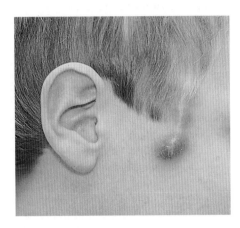

Fig. 5-19 Bacterial abscess. Staphylococcal infection of the cheek of a child.

negative organisms may occasionally be found, such as in Pseudomonas folliculitis, associated with the use of hot tubs.[22] Superficial folliculitis is often found to contain the normal skin flora. Bacteremia from furunculosis or abscess may occur in an unpredictable fashion, particularly after manipulation of the lesion.

Differential Diagnosis

Acne pustules and chemical folliculitis from tars and other compounds contacting the skin may mimic superficial folliculitis. Occasionally, dermatophyte infections caused by animal ringworm or *Candida albicans* infections will produce follicular pustules.

Pathogenesis

Invasion of the follicular wall by bacteria is the usual cause of the disease (Fig. 5-20). Obstruction of the follicular orifice is an important factor in the development of the bacterial infection, particularly with staphylococcal folliculitis. Transmission of staphylococci among household members may occur. Occlusion of the skin or prolonged submersion in water contaminated with bacteria also predisposes to folliculitis.[22]

Treatment

Superficial folliculitis may be treated by topical antibiotics, applied twice daily for 10 to 14 days, and

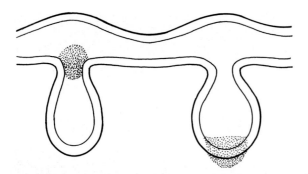

Fig. 5-20 Superficial folliculitis (left) with inflammation of the follicular mouth compared with deep folliculitis (right) with involvement of the base of the follicle and adjacent deep dermis.

good skin hygiene. Furunculosis and abscesses are best treated by incision and drainage.[21] Systemic antistaphylococcal antibiotics, such as dicloxacillin, 15 to 50 mg/kg/day orally, or cephalexin, 40 to 50 mg/kg/day for 7 to 10 days, may be required in more severe cases. In chronic recurrent furunculosis, attention to nasal and skin carriers of staphylococci is required. Mupirocin 1% nasal ointment, with half of the prescribed amount applied to each naris daily for 5 days, and chronic antibiotic treatment with antistaphylococcal drugs or rifampin may be necessary if good personal hygiene fails.

Patient Education

Good personal hygiene is important in preventing follicular skin infections. Thorough hand washing and daily skin cleansing with an antibacterial soap are most useful. It is advisable to instruct all household members in good hand-washing techniques. Avoiding chemicals that have resulted in follicular obstruction is beneficial. In Pseudomonas or gram-negative folliculitis resulting from contaminated tubs or pools, proper chlorination or other treatment of the water should be emphasized.

Follow-up Visits

Poor personal hygiene is the most likely cause in children with recurrent episodes of furunculosis. Reemphasizing good hygiene for the entire household at the follow-up visit is most important.[21] Evaluation for diabetes mellitus and immunodeficiency is not warranted without recurrent or systemic infection of other organ systems such as the lungs (e.g., pneumonia), central nervous system (CNS) (e.g., encephalitis), or bone.

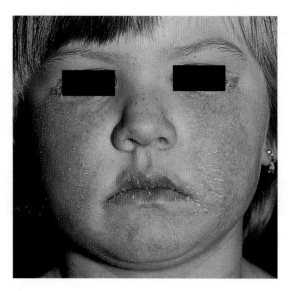

Fig. 5-21 Early SSSS in a toddler, with erythema of cheeks.

STAPHYLOCOCCAL SCALDED SKIN SYNDROME
Clinical Features

A spectrum of clinical presentations of staphylococcal scalded skin syndrome (SSSS) is now recognized, ranging from purely localized forms (bullous impetigo) to generalized involvement. In the generalized form, after an upper respiratory tract infection, a faint erythematous eruption begins on the central face (Fig. 5-21), neck, axillae, and groin.[4,20,23] The skin rapidly becomes acutely tender, with crusting around the mouth, eyes, and neck (Fig. 5-22). Mild rubbing of the skin results in epidermal separation, leaving a shiny, moist, red surface (Figs. 5-23 and 5-24).[23] In infants and preschool children the lesions are usually limited to the upper body, but in the newborn the entire cutaneous surface may be involved (Ritter's disease) (Fig. 5-25).[23] SSSS is uncommon over 5 years of age.

Differential Diagnosis

Toxic epidermal necrolysis, which is often drug induced, may be differentiated from SSSS by skin biopsy and by a preceding history of urticarial or target lesions occurring 2 to 3 days before the appearance of bullae.[23] Pathologic examination of tissue from a patient with toxic epidermal necrolysis shows full epidermal necrosis, with a prominent perivascular dermal infiltrate of inflammatory cells. SSSS shows no epidermal necrosis or inflammatory cells on micro-

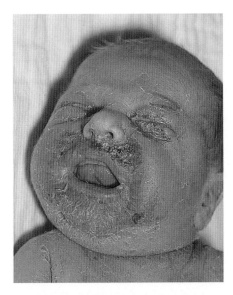

Fig. 5-22 SSSS, with periorbital and perioral crusting.

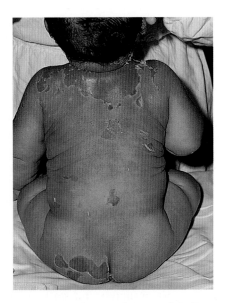

Fig. 5-24 SSSS in an infant. Erythema and shallow erosions, with desquamation of the back.

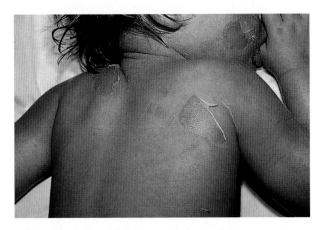

Fig. 5-23 SSSS in a toddler. Erosion, with skin separated during examination by pushing on the skin surface.

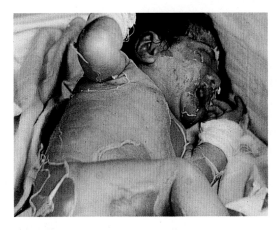

Fig. 5-25 Diffuse erythema and extensive peeling in a newborn with Ritter's disease.

scopic examination. In the newborn, diffuse cutaneous mastocytosis may mimic Ritter's disease.[24] Occasionally SSSS may resemble exfoliative erythroderma, sunburn, thermal burn, TSS, or streptococcal scarlet fever.

Pathogenesis

S. aureus of phage group II[23,25-27] elaborates a toxin (Staphylococcus exfoliatin A), a serine protease that is carried via the circulation to the skin, where it acts on the cell surface of the epidermal granular cells and activates serine proteinases.[26,27] Injury to these kera-

tinocytes results in intraepidermal separation of the cells within the granular layer and subsequent shedding of the entire granular layer and stratum corneum when a minor trauma occurs.

Treatment

Oral dicloxacillin, 15 to 50 mg/kg/day, is the treatment of choice. Newborns require intravenous antistaphylococcal antibiotics.[24] The skin should be handled minimally, especially during the first 24 hours. Newborns may require burn-therapy protocols, with careful attention to fluid and electrolyte losses and prevention of secondary infection of affected skin.[23,27] During the desquamation stage, bland ointments used twice a day may be helpful in restoring the skin surface and reducing cutaneous pain.

Patient Education

It is important that clinicians emphasize to patients and family that such lesions are not like a burn and that they heal without scarring. In children with normal host defenses, neutralizing antitoxins to the staphylococcal exfoliatin are rapidly formed, and the child recovers promptly. It should also be stressed that only certain staphylococci are capable of producing this condition, and that household carriers should be investigated.[23] Asymptomatic carriers may transmit the organism.[27] Nursery outbreaks require prompt investigation and culturing of all those entering the nursery, cohorting of infants and staff, emphasis on hand washing with an antibacterial soap, and alleviating overcrowding and understaffing.[4]

Follow-up Visits

Routine follow-up care in regular pediatric visits is recommended.

TOXIC SHOCK SYNDROME
Clinical Features

A typical presentation of TSS would involve a menstruating adolescent female who presents with a high fever, a scarlatiniform rash, and hypotension, with systolic blood pressure less than 90 mm Hg or orthostatic syncope.[20,28] Prominent desquamation of the palms and soles follows the acute onset of the eruption by 1 to 2 weeks. These four features are the major diagnostic criteria for diagnosis of TSS (Box 5-1).[4,28,29]

Vomiting and diarrhea frequently precede the hypotensive state, and laboratory signs of liver, kidney, or muscle injury may be present. Diffuse redness of the conjunctival, oral, and vaginal mucosa may be present.[28,29] Swelling of the hands and feet may be prominent. Severe myalgias or arthralgias and disorientation, meningismus, seizure, or coma may appear.[28,29] Although the majority of cases have been described in adolescent females, TSS was first noted in infants and children of either sex. In nonmenstrual TSS, pharyngitis or conjunctivitis lasting more than 5 days is observed, and the onset of fever and scarlatiniform rash is early in the course of disease. Nonmenstrual TSS has less frequent CNS manifestations, more frequent musculoskeletal involvement, and less anemia than that reported for menstrual TSS.[28,29] The

circulatory collapse may be mild or severe, and a fatality rate of 10% has been reported.[28,29]

Differential Diagnosis

Rocky Mountain spotted fever, meningococcemia, and leptospirosis may each present with high fever, dizziness, and a rash. In each, the eruption is acral and purpuric and not scarlet fever–like. Blood cultures and specific serologic tests will help to distinguish these conditions. SSSS and TSS have considerable overlapping cutaneous features. The presence of skin tenderness and a positive Nikolsky sign favor SSSS. Streptococcal TSS and streptococcal scarlet fever may mimic SSSS and can be distinguished by pharyngeal and blood cultures. Kawasaki disease is more likely to occur in patients under age 5, lacks hy-

---

Box 5-1 Case Definition of Toxic Shock Syndrome

Fever (temperature greater than 39.9° C)
Rash (diffuse macular erythroderma)
Desquamation 1 to 2 weeks after the onset of illness, particularly of the palms and soles
Hypotension (systolic blood pressure less than 90 mm Hg for adults or below the fifth percentile for children, or orthostatic syncope)
Involvement of three or more of the following organ systems:
  Gastrointestinal (vomiting or diarrhea at onset of illness)
  Muscular (severe myalgia or creatine phosphokinase level greater than two times normal)
  Mucous membrane (hyperemia)
  Hepatic (total bilirubin, serum glutamate oxaloacetate transaminase [SGOT], serum glutamate pyruvate transaminase [SGPT] two times normal)
  Hematologic (platelets less than 100,000/mm³)
  Renal (BUN or creatinine greater than two times normal)
  CNS (disorientation or alterations in consciousness without focal neurologic signs when fever and hypotension are absent)
Negative results:
  Blood, throat, and CSF cultures
  Serologic tests for Rocky Mountain spotted fever, leptospirosis, or measles
  Blood urea nitrogen (BUN), SGOT, SGPT

potension, and has prominent mucous membrane involvement. The fever in Kawasaki disease lasts for a week or more rather than the 2 or 3 days in TSS. The scarlatiniform skin eruption and desquamation may be the same in both TSS and Kawasaki syndrome.

Pathogenesis

S. aureus infection of the vagina or other tissues, such as the upper respiratory tract and sinuses, initiates the disease.[23,28,29] Prolonged tampon use, with positive cultures obtained from tampons, in adolescent females is very frequent.[23,28] Blood cultures positive for *S. aureus* may be obtained. Most authorities consider the staphylococcal toxin designated TSS-1 or enterotoxin C as responsible for the skin eruption and the systemic symptoms.[23,28] Both of these distinct exotoxins have been implicated.

Treatment

Prompt replacement of fluids to correct the hypotension is recommended, as are other general supportive measures for shock.[23] Treatment with an antistaphylococcal antibiotic, usually given intravenously, is recommended. Bland lubricants may be used on the desquamating skin.

Patient Education

It is important for the clinician to emphasize the conditions that might favor the growth of the pathogenic organism. In adolescent females, discontinuing the use of tampons is advisable. It is unknown whether other antibacterial measures to reduce skin or mucous membrane colonization of staphylococci are useful.

Follow-up Visits

The hypotension and acute illness at the onset usually result in hospitalization. Daily examination, with documentation of the sequence of events, is often necessary to confirm the diagnosis. A follow-up visit at 1 week after discharge is advisable, as is a visit during the next anticipated menses for follow-up bacterial cultures.

CAT-SCRATCH DISEASE
Clinical Features

A primary inoculation papule on skin or mucous membrane 3 to 10 days after the scratch of a cat is found in 58% of patients (Fig. 5-26).[29,30] Inoculation of the ocular conjunctivae occurs in 5% of children, which will produce conjunctival granuloma. Persistent tender regional lymphadenitis of the lymph nodes draining

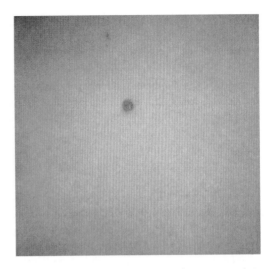

Fig. 5-26 Solitary papule at the site of a cat scratch in cat-scratch disease.

the site of the cat scratch is observed in virtually all patients.[30] The lymph nodes become swollen 14 to 50 days after the scratch and remain enlarged for about 3 months, but may be enlarged for up to 1 year later. Spontaneous suppuration of lymph nodes occurs in 30% of cases.[4] About one third of patients will experience a few days of fever, but occasionally fever persists for several weeks. Fatigue, headache, anorexia, vomiting, splenomegaly, sore throat, morbilliform exanthem, purulent conjunctivitis, and parotid swelling are uncommon findings in children with cat-scratch disease.[30] Quite rare are Parinaud's oculoglandular syndrome, encephalitis, and erythema nodosum.

Differential Diagnosis

Bacterial lymphadenitis caused by *S. aureus, S. pyogenes,* atypical mycobacteria, *Francisella tularensis,* or Brucella species may mimic cat-scratch disease. Biopsy of a papule or lymph node with Warthin-Starry silver impregnation stain will reveal the cat-scratch bacillus within areas of necrosis or granulomas. Molecular diagnosis by amplifying deoxyribonucleic acid (DNA) obtained from a papule or lymph node by the use of the polymerase chain reaction (PCR) is available in a few centers. Other causes of persistent lymphadenopathy in children include lymphomas, cytomegalovirus (CMV), Epstein-Barr virus (EBV), mycobacterial infection, human immunodeficiency virus (HIV), toxoplasmosis, and deep fungus infection. Kerion caused by dermatophyte infection will produce local lymphadenopathy, but the kerion is much larger than an inoculation papule of cat-scratch disease.

Pathogenesis

The domestic cat is the primary reservoir of cat-scratch disease. A cat scratch (found in 80% of children with cat-scratch disease), bite, or other contact may inoculate the bacteria into the skin.[30] In 4% of cases the contact is a dog. The gram-negative pleomorphic bacillus responsible for cat-scratch disease is *Bartonella henselae,* and may be detected in the dermis of inoculation papules or the microabscesses of enlarged lymph nodes if obtained within 1 month of the onset of symptoms. The host response may obscure the bacillus in long-standing disease. Skin test antigen for cat-scratch disease also contains the organism.[29] This organism is also believed to be responsible for bacillary angiomatosis.[30]

Treatment

In most patients spontaneous resolution of the disease occurs in 2 to 4 months.[4,30] Antibacterial therapy with rifampin, ciprofloxacin, azithromycin, gentamicin, or trimethoprim-sulfamethoxazole has been reported to be effective.[4,30,31] Needle aspiration of a tender lymph-node abscess is preferable to incision and drainage. Surgical excision of the lymph node is often done, especially when the diagnosis is in doubt.

Patient Education

Disposal of the healthy cat suspected of being the vector is not recommended.[30] About 5% of household contacts may develop cat-scratch disease, usually within 3 weeks of the first case. There is no evidence that the infection can be transmitted from human to human. Children should avoid rough play with a cat, and children with immune deficiencies should avoid contact with cats that scratch or bite.[4]

Follow-up Visits

Follow-up 1 week after the first visit is useful to ascertain the growth rate of enlarged nodes or to discuss biopsy results. Further visits are dictated by the child's recovery.

SPIROCHETAL DISEASES
Lyme Disease
Clinical features

The earliest feature of Lyme disease is the unique skin eruption called *erythema chronicum migrans* (ECM). ECM begins 4 to 20 days after the bite of a tick, although only one third of patients distinctly recall a tick bite.[32-34] A red papule begins at the site of the tick bite, then slowly enlarges over several weeks to form an annular ring with a flat red border that clears in the center (Fig. 5-27). Sometimes the center remains a red, edematous plaque that feels hot. Fifty percent of patients will develop multiple secondary annular rings, which begin 1 to 6 days after the primary lesion appears.[33,34] Untreated ECM lasts about 3 weeks, then spontaneously resolves but may recur for up to 1 year or more, accompanied by arthritis or other symptoms. Skin lesions are associated with headaches, fatigue, myalgias, and low-grade fever.[33,34] Sometimes nausea, vomiting, sore throat, and lymphadenopathy will accompany ECM. A red nodule may appear on the ear, chest, or axillary fold, which represents borrelial lymphocytoma. Joint, CNS, and cardiac abnormalities begin about 4 weeks after the tick bite, after the ECM has resolved.[33,34] Fifty percent of untreated Lyme disease patients will develop arthritis.[33,34] The onset of arthritis is abrupt and usually monarticular (knee, shoulder, elbow, temporomandibular, ankle, wrist, or hip), and the affected joint is warm, swollen, and tender, but not red. The first episode lasts 1 week, but up to three recurrences are common. CNS disease occurs in 10% to 15% of untreated patients, with the classic triad of meningitis, cranial nerve palsies, and peripheral radiculoneuropathy. The meningitis is characterized by an excruciating headache and stiff neck and may include changes in behavior. The seventh nerve is most frequently involved, with recurrent episodes of facial palsy. Neuritic pain or focal weakness is seen with the peripheral radiculoneuropathy of Lyme disease. Less than 10% of patients experience cardiac in-

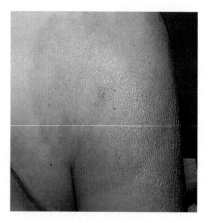

Fig. 5-27 Lyme disease. Annular erythema and central tick-bite papule.

volvement, with atrioventricular block or myoperi-carditis reported. A great variety of additional neurologic and other organ symptoms are occasionally reported. The erythrocyte sedimentation rate (ESR) is usually elevated, but other routine laboratory studies are variable.

Differential diagnosis

ECM may mimic ringworm or be diagnosed as erythema multiforme or erythema marginatum. Tinea infections demonstrate disruption of the epidermis, but ECM does not. ECM evolves slowly, over days; erythema marginatum is transient, often changing hourly. A negative KOH examination and a skin biopsy will help distinguish. In ECM, a dense mononuclear cell accumulation around blood vessels and adnexal structures without epidermal changes is seen. A two-test approach using serologic tests for Lyme disease, with an enzyme immunoassay for immunoglobulin M (IgM) and a Western immunoblot test, is recommended when noncutaneous symptoms develop.[4,33,34] Ordering serologic tests for Lyme disease for patients with nonspecific symptoms such as fatigue or arthralgia is not recommended.[4] Diagnosis using the PCR amplification of spirochetal DNA is not widely available. The organism can be cultured on modified Kelly's medium, but yields are too low for practical use.

Pathogenesis

The spirochete *Borrelia burgdorferi* is carried by a variety of ticks, predominantly the deer tick, *Ixodes dammini*. The ticks may be carried by rodents or house pets, or they may attach themselves to grasses or bushes. Humans are incidental hosts. The spirochete has irregular coils, is 10 to 30 μm long, and is found worldwide, although most cases come from northern Europe or the eastern, mid-Atlantic, or upper midwest regions of the United States.[32] Subtypes of *B. burgdorferi* differ in North America and Europe by molecular typing, and this may account for the differences in prevalence. Within a few days after a tick bite, the spirochete migrates within the skin or enters the bloodstream. The incubation period is usually 7 to 14 days.[4] It appears that all symptoms and signs are directly related to the presence of the spirochete in affected tissues or the immune response to the organism.

Treatment

Some authorities advocate antibiotic treatment at the time of a deer-tick bite rather than observation, but this recommendation remains controversial and is not endorsed by the Committee on Infectious Diseases of the American Academy of Pediatrics.[4] For children over 8 years of age, oral tetracycline or doxycycline, 100 mg twice a day for 3 weeks, is the treatment of choice.[4,34] Younger children are treated with oral amoxicillin, 25 to 50 mg/kg/day divided in two doses for 14 to 21 days.[4] The ECM will disappear within 3 days with successful treatment, and secondary complications are almost always prevented. For mild secondary complications without heart block, the same oral regimens for early disease are recommended. If cerebrospinal fluid (CSF) pleocytosis or complete heart block is present, intravenous therapy with ceftriaxone, 75 to 100 mg/kg daily for 14 to 21 days, or penicillin G, 300,000 U/kg/day for 2 to 4 weeks, may be required.[4]

Patient education

Avoidance of the tick vector is the basis of prevention.[35] Avoiding high-risk areas, such as wooded, grassy areas during tick season; wearing protective light-colored clothing with long sleeves and caps; using insect repellent; and periodic examination for ticks are required.[35] For children with ECM, parents should be advised about the possibility of secondary complications of arthritis or neurologic disease. The importance of completing the 3 weeks of therapy to avoid complications should be emphasized.

For children living in endemic areas that are 15 years of age or older, Lyme disease vaccine may be considered.[4,35,36]

Follow-up visits

After successful treatment, monthly visits for 3 months are useful to observe for late complications. A second antibiotic course may be required should secondary symptoms occur.

Syphilis
Clinical features

Acquired syphilis and congenital syphilis are uncommon, yet increasing, in industrialized countries, and common in Third World countries.[37,38] Acquired syphilis has three distinct stages.[4,37] Primary acquired syphilis is characterized by the chancre, a painless, shallow ulcer surrounded by a red indurated border that appears about 3 weeks after exposure (Fig. 5-28). If untreated, the chancre heals spontaneously in 1 to 2 months. Secondary syphilis is usually seen as a morbilliform generalized eruption accompanied by

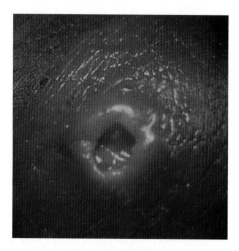

Fig. 5-28 Syphilitic chancre. Painless scrotal ulcer with indurated borders in an 11-year-old boy.

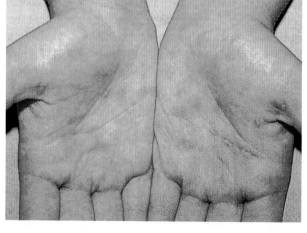

Fig. 5-29 Secondary syphilis. Ham-colored palmar macules on an adolescent with secondary syphilis.

lymphadenopathy, fatigue, headache, and, sometimes, low-grade fever.[4,37] Involvement of the palms and soles is frequently observed (Fig. 5-29). Nodular, pustular, annular, and papulosquamous lesions are occasionally seen. Mucous patches are seen as weeping erosive areas on oral or genital mucosa. Tertiary stages are rare in childhood.

Congenital syphilis is usually asymptomatic in the newborn period, but may be observed as a persistent rhinorrhea that develops during the newborn period, or in severe cases, as hydrops fetalis or stillbirth.[4,39] The newborn with syphilis is usually small for gestational age and has mild hepatosplenomegaly.[4,39] Serologic testing of the mother is critical to the diagnosis because usually the newborn's symptoms are so mild they are overlooked.[4,39,40] Signs of late congenital syphilis may be the first clue to maternofetal transmission of syphilis. Late signs begin around 6 years of age and include cloudy corneas (interstitial keratitis) accompanied by photophobia and pain, bilateral eighth nerve deafness, notching of small central and lateral incisors (Hutchinson's teeth), painless swelling of the knees (Clutton's joint), perforation of the nasal septum leading to a saddle-nose deformity and perforated palate, saber tibia, and radial scarring about the mouth (rhagades).

Differential diagnosis

Syphilis is known as the great mimic, and a high index of suspicion for syphilis should be maintained. The primary chancre of acquired syphilis must be distinguished from bacterial ulcers, herpes simplex infec-

tions, chancroid, or lymphogranuloma venereum. The absence of pain is a useful distinguishing feature, and identification of *Treponema pallidum* by dark-field microscopic examination of smears of the ulcer base is definitive. Secondary acquired syphilis must be distinguished from pityriasis rosea, infectious mononucleosis, many other viral exanthems, and a number of papulosquamous diseases. Biopsy of a secondary syphilis lesion will reveal numerous plasma cells within a perivascular dermal infiltrate and swelling of the vascular endothelium.[41]

Both a nontreponemal and a treponemal serologic test for syphilis or PCR testing are required to make a presumptive diagnosis.[4,37,39] Nontreponemal tests include the Venereal Disease Research Laboratory (VDRL) test, the rapid plasma reagin (RPR) test, and the automated reagin test (ART). Treponemal tests include the fluorescent treponemal antibody absorption (FTA-ABS) test, the microhemagglutinin for *T. pallidum*, Western immunoblotting for *T. pallidum* antigen, and the *T. pallidum* immobilization test. In congenital syphilis the newborn presents a particularly difficult diagnostic problem because of maternally transferred immunoglobulin G (IgG).[39] In congenital syphilis the maternal syphilis serology should be positive, and the Western IgM immunoblotting test to *T. pallidum* antigen should be positive in the affected infant. The IgM enzyme-linked immunosorbent assay (ELISA) test and the FTA-ABS should be positive in 80% of the affected babies.[39] HIV testing of the mother should be considered in babies with congenital syphilis.

Hydrops fetalis caused by congenital syphilis must be differentiated from blood group incompatibility and the rhinorrhea from upper respiratory tract bacterial and viral infections. Hepatosplenomegaly and intrauterine growth failure in newborns must be distinguished from other congenital infections, such as herpes simplex, CMV, rubella, and toxoplasmosis.

Pathogenesis

T. pallidum is the spirochete responsible for syphilis. It is spread primarily through sexual contact and invades the bloodstream in the early phase of infection.[37] The incubation period is 10 to 90 days.[4] The chancre of primary syphilis develops at the time the blood-borne infection is maximal; the morbilliform rash of secondary syphilis represents spirochetes that have left the bloodstream and entered the skin. Congenital syphilis represents a more massive infection than acquired syphilis, being blood borne in the fetus from the fourth month of pregnancy onward.[4,37,39,40] Rhinorrhea represents tissue infection of the nasopharynx, and late signs of congenital syphilis represent effects on developing tissues or osteomyelitis caused by *T. pallidum*.[41]

Treatment

Penicillin is the treatment of choice. Parenteral penicillin given intramuscularly weekly in the form of benzathine penicillin, in doses of 50,000 U/kg/day up to a total of 2.4 million U in a 3-week period, is recommended for children and adolescents with primary or secondary syphilis.[4] If the patient is allergic to penicillin, tetracycline, 500 mg four times a day for 14 days, or doxycycline, 100 mg twice daily for 4 weeks, is recommended. Aqueous crystalline penicillin G, 100,000 to 150,000 U/kg/day given intravenously every 8 to 12 hours for 10 to 14 days, is recommended for neonates with congenital syphilis.[4] If more than 1 day of therapy is missed, the entire course should be repeated. Retreatment is indicated if the clinical signs persist or recur, or if a sustained fourfold increase in a serologic test titer occurs, or if an initial high-titer serologic test fails to show a fourfold decrease within 6 months.

Patient education

Children and adolescents with primary or secondary syphilis should be thoroughly educated on transmission of the disease as recommended by the National Syphilis Elimination Program of the Centers for Disease Control and Prevention.[42] All recent sexual contacts of a child or adolescent with acquired syphilis should be identified, examined, serologically tested, and receive treatment if appropriate. Sexual abuse must be suspected in any young child with acquired syphilis. Routine serologic testing for syphilis in early pregnancy, and the importance of prenatal care for prevention, should be emphasized for congenital syphilis. It should also be emphasized that untreated syphilis in pregnancy results in death of the affected babies in 40% of cases.[4] Pregnant women at high risk for syphilis should also have serologic testing at 28 weeks of gestation. The clinician should emphasize to the pregnant woman that in congenital syphilis the long-term prognosis for the infant is good with prompt treatment, but delayed treatment may result in developmental delays and the complications of late congenital syphilis.[40,42]

Follow-up visits

After treatment, children should be seen monthly for 6 months to observe for recurrence and to monitor serologically. In congenital syphilis, serology tests should be obtained at 3, 6, and 12 months of age. Otherwise, follow-up during routine well-child care will suffice.

MYCOBACTERIAL DISEASE

Mycobacterial infections of the skin in children are uncommon. Of the mycobacterial infections, the one most likely encountered is *Mycobacterium marinum* infection, although *Mycobacterium chelonei* and *Mycobacterium avium-intracellulare* are increasingly identified as causes of lymphocutaneous syndromes.[43-47] Most Mycobacterial infections cause cervical lymphadenitis in children, but cutaneous granulomas and necrotizing granulomas resulting in skin ulcers are increasingly seen.[43-48]

Mycobacterial Granulomas
Clinical features

Atypical mycobacteria, particularly *M. marinum*, produce a chronic granulomatous infection of the skin after direct inoculation through injured skin.[43-48] Contaminated fresh or salt water of warm temperatures (30° to 32° C), such as tropical fish tanks or hot swimming pools, is the usual source of infection in children. The first appearance of red papules occurs at the site of abrasion or skin injury within 3 or 4 weeks (Fig. 5-30). The papules may ulcerate, or more likely coalesce to form a red-brown plaque or nodule (Fig. 5-31).[48] The surface of the plaque may become

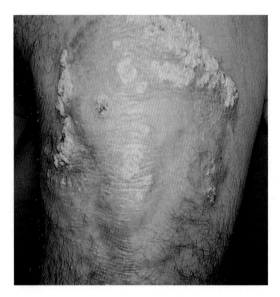

Fig. 5-30 Scaly plaques on the knee of an adolescent male with *M. marinum* infection (swimming pool granuloma).

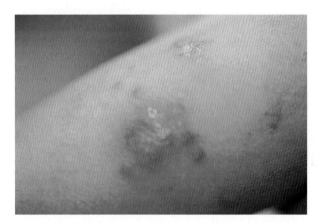

Fig. 5-31 Multiple red nodules in *M. marinum* infection.

verrucous (Fig. 5-30). The plaque may persist for months to years if untreated. The arm and dorsum of the hand account for 80% of lesions, with the remainder on the knee. Usually the lesions are solitary, although a pattern of ascending skin nodules on an extremity has been described (sporotrichoid pattern). No lymphadenopathy is found. Adolescents are most commonly infected, but toddlers may also be infected.

Differential diagnosis

Verrucous plaques need to be distinguished from warts, psoriasis, or other granulomatous diseases such as sarcoidosis, tuberculosis, or foreign-body granulomas. The sporotrichoid pattern must be distinguished from sporotrichosis, and the ulcerative lesions must be distinguished from Langerhans cell histiocytosis, Leishmaniasis, and bacterial or fungal ulcers. A skin biopsy stained for acid-fast organisms will help, but culture of the biopsy for atypical mycobacteria and deep fungal organisms will be definitive. History of exposure to a tropical fish tank or swimming in warm waters is helpful.

Pathogenesis

Abrasion or disruption of the skin, plus exposure to warm water containing the organism, is required for infection by the slender, aerobic, acid-fast rod *M. marinum*.[45] The organism induces a granuloma with a mixture of lymphocytes, macrophages, and epithelioid giant cells. The verrucous lesions also feature epithelial hyperplasia. Other mycobacteria may be found in soil.

Treatment

Spontaneous resolution has been reported, but it may require 1 or 2 years, and most authorities recommend antibiotic therapy. There are no blinded trials of therapy for *M. marinum* cutaneous granulomas. Treatment with rifampin, clarithromycin, doxycycline, trimethoprim-sulfamethoxazole, or ciprofloxacin has been most successful.[4,47-51] If *Mycobacterium chelonei* is isolated, then two drugs are required. Surgical excision of the area, if feasible, is also recommended. Adjunctive therapy with recombinant cytokines such as interleukin-2 (IL-2), interferon-γ (IFN-γ), and granulocyte-macrophage colony–stimulating factor (GM-CSF) is now under study.[52]

Patient education

The clinician should emphasize that the skin abrasion is vulnerable to infection, and the child should not swim or immerse his or her skin in a tropical fish tank when a cut or abrasion is present. Cleaning the fish tank and changing the water may help, but the organism is difficult to remove from contaminated fish tanks.

Follow-up visits

After initiating antibiotic therapy, a follow-up visit at 2 weeks to monitor side effects of the therapy is indicated. If tolerated well, monthly visits are indicated until antibiotics are discontinued. Most authorities recommend continuing treatment for 1 month after the lesion has cleared.

REFERENCES

1. Ferrieri P: The natural history of impetigo, *J Clin Invest* 51:2851, 1972.
2. Brook I, Frazier EH, Yeager JK: Microbiology of nonbullous impetigo, *Pediatr Dermatol* 14:192, 1997.
3. Taplin D: Prevalence of streptococcal pyoderma in relation to climate and hygiene, *Lancet* i:501, 1973.
4. Report of the Committee on Infectious Disease: *Red book 2000,* Elk Grove Village, Ill, 2000, American Academy of Pediatrics.
5. Hogan P: Pediatric dermatology: impetigo, *Aust Fam Physician* 27:735, 1998.
6. Savoia D et al: Macrolide resistance in group A Streptococci, *J Antimicrob Chemother* 45:41, 2000.
7. Bass JW et al: Comparison of oral cephalexin, topical mupirocin and topical bacitracin for the treatment of impetigo, *Pediatr Infect Dis J* 16:708, 1997.
8. Bass JW, Person DA, Chan DS: Twice-daily oral penicillin for treatment of streptococcal pharyngitis: less is best, *Pediatrics* 105:423, 2000.
9. Williams SR, Carruth JA: Orbital infection secondary to sinusitis in children: diagnosis and management, *Clin Otolaryngol* 17:550, 1992.
10. Baddour LM: Cellulitis syndromes: an update, *Int J Antimicrob Agents* 14:113, 2000.
11. Danik SB, Schwartz RA, Oleske JM: Cellulitis, *Cutis* 64:157, 1999.
12. McCray MK, Esterly NB: Blistering distal dactylitis, *J Am Acad Dermatol* 5:592, 1981.
13. Mogielnicki NP, Schwartzman JD, Elliott JA: Perineal group A streptococcal disease in a pediatric practice, *Pediatrics* 10:276, 2000.
14. Howe PM: Etiologic diagnosis of cellulitis: comparison of the aspirates obtained from the leading edge and the point of maximal inflammation, *Pediatr Infect Dis J* 6:685, 1987.
15. Ahmed S, Ayoub EM: Severe, invasive group A streptococcal disease and toxic shock, *Pediatr Ann* 27:287, 1998.
16. Zoger S, Harrison MR: Necrotizing fasciitis in two children with acute lymphoblastic leukemia, *J Pediatr Surg* 27:668, 1992.
17. File TM Jr, Tan JS, DiPersio JR: Group A streptococcal necrotizing fasciitis: diagnosing and treating the "flesh eating bacteria syndrome," *Cleve Clin J Med* 65:241, 1998.
18. Stevens DL: Streptococcal toxic shock syndrome associated with necrotizing fasciitis, *Ann Rev Med* 51:271, 2000.
19. Davies HD et al: Apparent lower rates of streptococcal toxic shock syndrome and lower mortality in children with invasive group A streptococcal infections compared with adults, *Pediatr Infect Dis J* 13:49, 1994.
20. Manders DM: Toxin-mediated streptococcal and staphylococcal disease, *J Am Acad Dermatol* 39:383, 1998.
21. Zimakoff J et al: Recurrent staphylococcal furunculosis in families, *Scand J Infect Dis* 20:403, 1988.
22. Trueb RM, Gloor M, Wuthrich B: Recurrent Pseudomonas folliculitis, *Pediatr Dermatol* 11:35, 1994.
23. Ladhani D, Evans RW: Staphylococcal scalded skin syndrome, *Arch Dis Child* 78:85, 1998.
24. Farrell AM: Staphylococcal scalded-skin syndrome, *Lancet* 354:880, 1999.
25. Murono K, Fujita K, Yoshioka H: Microbiologic characteristics of exfoliative toxin-producing *Staphylococcus aureus, Pediatr Infect Dis J* 7:313, 1988.
26. Lina G et al: Toxin involvement in staphylococcal scalded skin syndrome, *Clin Infect Dis* 25:1369, 1997.
27. Saiman L et al: Molecular epidemiology of staphylococcal scalded skin syndrome in premature infants, *Pediatr Infect Dis J* 17:329, 1998.
28. Kain KC, Schulzer M, Chow AW: Clinical spectrum of nonmenstrual toxic shock syndrome (TSS): comparison with menstrual TSS by multivariate discriminant analysis, *Clin Infect Dis* 16:100, 1993.
29. Margileth AM: Cat scratch disease, *Adv Pediatr Infect Dis* 8:1, 1993.
30. Koehler JE: Rochalimaea henselae infection: a new zoonoses with domestic cat as reservoir, *JAMA* 271:531, 1994.
31. Zangwill K: Therapeutic options for cat-scratch disease, *Pediatr Infect Dis J* 17:1059, 1998.
32. Orloski KA at al: Surveillance for Lyme disease—United States, 1992-1998, *MMWR Morb Mortal Wkly Rep* CDC surveillance summaries 49:1, 2000.
33. Seltzer EG et al: Long-term outcomes of persons with Lyme disease, *JAMA* 283:609, 2000.
34. Gardner P: Long-term outcomes and management of patients with Lyme disease, *JAMA* 283:658, 2000.
35. Committee on Infectious Diseases, American Academy of Pediatrics: Prevention of Lyme disease, *Pediatrics* 105:142, 2000.
36. Lutwick LI, Abramson JM: Pediatric immunization for the future: Lyme disease vaccine and beyond, *Pediatr Clin North Am* 47:465, 2000.
37. Brown TJ, Yen-Moore A, Tyring SK: An overview of sexually transmitted diseases. Part I, *J Am Acad Dermatol* 41:511, 1999.
38. Primary and secondary syphilis—United States, 1998, *MMWR Morb Mortal Wkly Rep* 48:873, 1999.
39. Wicher K, Horowitz HW, Wicher V: Laboratory methods of diagnosis of syphilis for the beginning of the third millenium, *Microbes Infect* 1:1035, 1999.
40. Reyes MP et al: Maternal/congenital syphilis in a large tertiary care urban hospital, *Clin Infect Dis* 17:1041, 1993.
41. Godschalk JC, van der Sluis JJ, Stolz E: The localization of treponemes and characterization of the inflammatory infiltrate in skin biopsies from patients with primary or secondary syphilis or early infectious yaws, *Genitourinary Med* 69:102, 1993.
42. Koplan J: Syphilis elimination: history in the making, *Sex Transm Dis* 27:63, 2000.
43. Hazra R et al: Lymphadenitis due to nontuberculous mycobacteria in children: presentation and response to therapy, *Clin Infect Dis* 28:123, 1999.
44. Pzniak A, Bull T: Recently recognized mycobacteria of clinical significance, *J Infect* 38:157, 1999.
45. Edelestein H: Mycobacterium marinum skin infections, *Arch Intern Med* 134:1359, 1994.

46. Smego RA Jr, Castiglia M, Asperilla MO: Lymphocutaneous syndrome: a review of non-sporothrix causes, *Medicine* 78:38, 1999.

47. Maltezou HC, Spyridis P, Kafetzis DA: Nontuberculous mycobacterial lymphadenitis in children, *Pediatr Infect Dis J* 18:968, 1999.

48. Dobos KM et al: Emergence of a unique group of necrotizing mycobacterial diseases, *Emerg Infect Dis* 5:367, 1999.

49. Jacobs MR: Activity of quinolones against mycobacteria, *Drugs* 58:19, 1999.

50. Evans MJ et al: Atypical mycobacterial lymphadenitis in childhood: a clinicopathologic study of 17 cases, *J Clin Pathol* 51:925, 1998.

51. Bartralot R et al: Cutaneous infections due to nontuberculous mycobacteria: histopathological review of 28 cases. Comparative study between lesions observed in immunosuppressed patients and normal hosts, *J Cutan Pathol* 27:124, 2000.

52. Holland SM: Cytokine therapy of mycobacterial infections, *Adv Intern Med* 45:431, 2000.

| # Fungal and Yeast Infections of the Skin

DERMATOPHYTES

Dermatophytes are fungi that invade and proliferate in the outer layer of the epidermis (stratum corneum). In addition to invading the stratum corneum, some species may also invade the hair and nails. Dermatophyte infections are common and increase in frequency with increasing age; in hot, humid climates; and in crowded living conditions. For example, tinea capitis is quite prevalent in North America, especially in urban areas.[1-3] In one area of the United States, 4% of asymptomatic children had a positive fungal culture for scalp dermatophytes,[1] and 50% of children with tinea capitis had a household member who was culture positive.[2,3]

HAIR INFECTIONS (TINEA CAPITIS)
Clinical Features

Scalp hair involvement is usually seen in prepubertal children and is largely due to infections with either *Trichophyton tonsurans* or *Microsporum canis*.[1,4-7] Each infection has a noninflammatory stage lasting 2 to 8 weeks, followed by an inflammatory stage. Hair loss is a regular feature of tinea capitis. *M. canis* infections are characterized by one or several patches of broken-off hairs that appear thickened and white (Fig. 6-1). The hairs fluoresce yellow-green under Wood's light examination. In contrast, *T. tonsurans* produces several distinct clinical presentations: a noninflammatory stage in which hairs break off at the follicular orifice in a circumscribed area of the scalp, which leaves small, dark hairs in the follicles, or so-called *black-dot ringworm* (Fig. 6-2); and three inflammatory stages, including (1) diffuse fine scaling of the scalp without obvious broken-off hairs (Fig. 6-3); (2) multiple scaly, pustular bald areas with indistinct margins (Fig. 6-4); or (3) multiple kerions. The widespread inflammatory stages are more commonly seen than the black-dot form and usually are associated with regional lymphadenopathy. The presence of enlarged suboccipital or posterior cervical lymph nodes in association with hair loss should make one consider first the diagnosis of tinea capitis.[7] *T. tonsurans* infections account for 95% of tinea capitis in North America.[1,3-7]

The diagnosis in the noninflammatory stage should be confirmed by the following three steps: (1) Wood's light examination, (2) potassium hydroxide (KOH) examination, and (3) fungal culture.[1,4,7-9]

Wood's light examination

Wood's light examination is best performed with a hand-held ultraviolet black lamp with two fluorescent bulbs. The lamp should be held within 6 inches of the scalp to observe for yellow-green fluorescence of the thickened scalp hairs. Lint from clothing fluoresces white from the addition of optical brighteners, and scale entrapped in sebum appears a dull yellow. These may be confused with fungal fluorescence. *M. canis* fluoresces, but the epidemic form of tinea capitis caused by *T. tonsurans* does not. The Wood's light examination cannot be used to exclude the diagnosis of tinea capitis or for screening children during epidemics.

KOH examination

KOH examination should be performed in every case of hair loss associated with broken hairs and in children with diffuse scaling of the scalp. If the hair fluoresces, the clinician should hold the Wood's lamp in one hand and a curette in the other and gently remove the fluorescent hairs for KOH examination and culture by scraping the scalp with the curette. The involved hairs are loosened in the follicles and will be included in the scrapings. Scrapings should not be painful to the child. If the hair does not fluoresce, the clinician should use the curette or a cotton swab to scrape the follicular openings in the involved area of the scalp hair loss. If a kerion is present, scrape the border of the lesion, not the inflammatory center. The scrapings that include infected hair are placed on a glass microscope slide, partially dissolved in KOH 20%, and placed under a coverslip. After 20 to 40

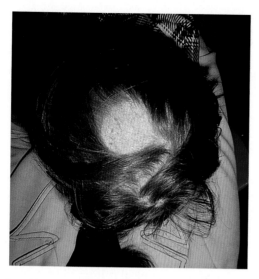

Fig. 6-1 Circumscribed patch of scalp hair loss with thick scales caused by *M. canis* infection.

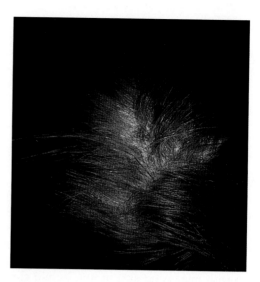

Fig. 6-3 Diffuse scaling in a dandruff-like pattern in *T. tonsurans* infection.

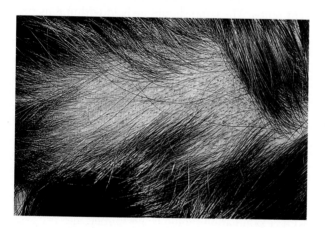

Fig. 6-2 Circumscribed area of hair loss without scalp change and with hairs broken off at the follicular orifice. This is the black-dot pattern of *T. tonsurans* infection.

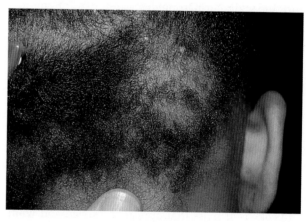

Fig. 6-4 Numerous triangle-shaped patches of hair loss accompanied by pustular kerion formation and enlarged lymph node in *T. tonsurans* infection.

minutes, the clinician should examine the specimen under the 10× and 40× lenses. In fluorescent hairs the outer surface of the hair is coated with mats containing thousands of tiny spores (Fig. 6-5), and hyphae may be seen within the hair shaft. In nonfluorescent hairs, hyphae and spores are seen within the hair shaft (Fig. 6-6). KOH examinations for dermatophytes are simple procedures that can be performed in the office or clinic, but interpretation may be difficult for the inexperienced clinician.[1,3,8]

Fungal culture

Fungal culture is the most reliable test in the diagnosis of tinea capitis and should be routinely performed in children with suspected tinea capitis. Fungal culture also should be considered for household contacts because 50% of children have a culture-positive household member, including adults.[2,3] A modified Sabouraud dextrose agar (dermatophyte test medium [DTM]) makes this procedure simple. Broken hairs or scrapings obtained by a sterile curette or cotton

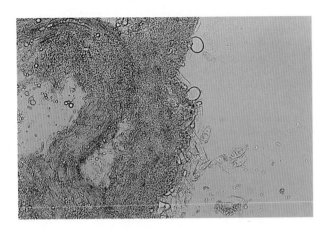

Fig. 6-5 Photomicrograph of hair dissolved in KOH. Mats containing billions of small spores coat the outside of hair, with hyphae seen within the hair shaft in *M. canis* infection.

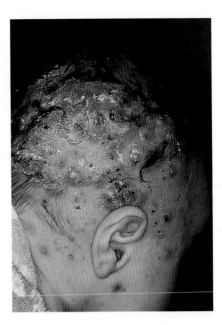

Fig. 6-7 Multiple boggy, red scalp nodules with multiple pustules in newborn with kerion.

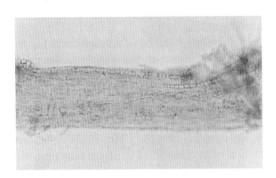

Fig. 6-6 Photomicrograph of hair dissolved in KOH. Hyphae and spores of *T. tonsurans* appear as chains within the hair shaft. There are no spores coating the hair.

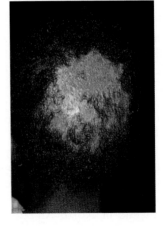

Fig. 6-8 Scarring hair loss in child with previously undiagnosed tinea capitis and kerion.

swab are inoculated so as to break the agar surface. The bottle cap is loosely applied and the culture bottles are left at room temperature.[4,9] If a dermatophyte is present, the agar medium turns from yellow to red in 4 to 5 days, and a fuzzy white or tan growth appears on the agar surface. A positive culture can be subcultured on Sabouraud dextrose agar for precise identification.

Inflammatory lesions produce a kerion, which is an erythematous boggy nodule with multiple superficial pustules (Fig. 6-7).[1,4,5,7] These lesions are almost completely devoid of hair and will lead to scarring and permanent hair loss if untreated (Fig. 6-8). A kerion will appear 2 to 8 weeks after infection begins and represents an exaggerated host response to the invading fungus. Approximately 40% of untreated tinea capitis caused by *M. canis or T. tonsurans* may eventuate in a kerion. Scrapings for KOH examination and fungal culture should be obtained from the edge of lesions, not the inflammatory center.

Differential Diagnosis

Alopecia areata and trichotillomania are the major considerations in the differential diagnosis of tinea capitis in children. Alopecia areata may be distinguished by the total absence of hair in a circumscribed patch, without any associated scalp change. In trichotillomania, odd patterns of hair loss, scalp excoriations, perifollicular petechiae, and hairs broken off at differing lengths are the distinguishing features. Seborrheic dermatitis may mimic the diffuse forms of *T. tonsurans* scalp infection.

In inflammatory tinea capitis (kerion), bacterial pyodermas are often mistaken for kerion. The pustules in kerion are sterile, however, and incision produces only serosanguineous fluid. Bacterial culture of the skin surface may yield *Staphylococcus aureus* and lead to the incorrect diagnosis of pyoderma, but one should recall that *S. aureus* frequently colonizes the skin surface, and such cultures would not detect bacterial invasion. Less commonly, traction alopecia, scleroderma, lichen planus, psoriasis, lupus erythematosus, dandruff, or porokeratosis of Mibelli may be confused with tinea capitis.

Pathogenesis

M. canis is harbored by cats, dogs, and certain rodents, and children handling such animals are susceptible to infection. Humans appear to be a terminal host for *M. canis,* and human-to-human transmission does not occur. When there is delayed hypersensitivity to the organism, a kerion may develop. Histologic study of this lesion shows a mononuclear cell infiltrate consistent with that seen in delayed hypersensitivity reactions. *M. canis* accounts for much of the tinea capitis in suburban and rural areas (Table 6-1). *T. tonsurans* is transmitted from human to human and is currently epidemic in North America. It is most prevalent in areas of crowding and accounts for virtually all tinea capitis in inner-city children in North America.[1-7] Transmission is predominantly from sharing hats, caps, scarves, combs, or brushes with infected individuals.[1-7]

Treatment

In suspected *T. tonsurans* infection, griseofulvin in a micronized form, 20 mg/kg/day for a minimum of 6 weeks, or terbinafine 3 mg/kg/day for 2 to 4 weeks is the treatment of choice.[4,5,10-13] Often, treatment for 2 to 3 months is required with griseofulvin. Itraconazole and ketoconazole are far less effective against *T. tonusrans* than griseofulvin or terbinafine. Topical

Table 6-1	Organisms Responsible for Tinea Capitis	
Feature	*M. canis*	*T. tonsurans*
Source	Cats and dogs	Other children
Fluorescence	Yellow-green	None
Human-to-human spread	No	Yes
Hair loss	Yes	Yes
Kerion	Yes	Yes
Children infected	Rural and suburban	Urban
Clinical patterns	Thickened hairs	Black-dot, dandruff-like, or multiple areas of alopecia

antifungal agents cannot reach the hyphae within the hair shaft and are ineffective. In *M. canis,* with successful treatment the lesions become nonfluorescent within 2 weeks after the administration of griseofulvin is begun. Although griseofulvin has many rare, severe side effects, including agranulocytosis and aplastic anemia, it is a relatively safe drug in children. Absorption is enhanced by a fatty meal; taking griseofulvin once or twice a day with ice cream or whole milk is a popular prescription. In addition to oral griseofulvin, many authorities advocate an antifungal shampoo such as selenium sulfide 2.5% shampoo or ketoconazole 2% shampoo, applied twice weekly to the scalp, to reduce infectivity and to hasten the child's return to school or child-care setting. Kerion responds well to griseofulvin alone. The addition of antibiotics or steroids is not required.[14,15]

If *M. canis* infection is suspected (and a Wood's light examination is positive), either griseofulvin, 10 to 20 mg/kg/day for 4 weeks, or itraconazole, 5 mg/kg/day for 2 weeks is recommended.[5,10-13] Terbinafine is less efficacious against *M. canis*.[10,11,13]

Patient Education

If *M. canis* is found, animal sources should be identified and the animal treated by a veterinarian to prevent infection of other children. In *T. tonsurans,* identification of the likely contacts is necessary. Household contacts should be cultured if possible. Children should not share combs, brushes, or head wear. School and day-care contacts should be referred for evaluation if scaling hair loss is present. Screening of contacts with a Wood's lamp is of no value because the epidemic strains in North America are not fluorescent. Patients should be instructed that hair regrowth is slow, often taking 3 to 6 months. If a kerion is present, some scarring and permanent hair loss may result. For a patient handout on Scalp Ringworm (Tinea Capitis), see p. 347.

Follow-up Visits

A visit in 2 to 4 weeks is helpful to ascertain the effectiveness of the griseofulvin or terbinafine therapy. Reexamination for fluorescence, a KOH examination, and a repeat culture will serve as guidelines for increasing the therapeutic dosage. If the lesions are fluorescence negative, KOH negative, and culture negative at 2 weeks, a total of 6 weeks therapy with griseofulvin or 2 weeks with terbinafine may be all that is required. With griseofulvin therapy, treatment 4 to 6 weeks after the lesions are culture negative is a useful rule of thumb. Once treatment is initiated with antifungal shampoos plus griseofulvin or terbinafine, the child can return to school.[5,13,16] Shaving the head, short hair cuts, or wearing a cap to school is unnecessary.[5,16] A follow-up visit every 2 to 4 weeks until hair growth begins is advised to assess for treatment failures. Asymptomatic carriers may be treated with sporicidal shampoos, such as ketoconazole or selenium sulfide, used twice weekly for 4 weeks. Asymptomatic carriers may be more likely to spread tinea capitis in school or day care than overtly infected children.[2,16]

FUNGAL INFECTION INVOLVING THE SKIN ONLY
Tinea Corporis
Clinical features

Dermatophyte infections on the body often consist of one or several circular erythematous patches (Fig. 6-9). The patches may have a papular, scaly, annular border and a clear center (Fig. 6-10), or they may be inflammatory throughout, with superficial pustules (Fig. 6-11). A most common pattern is a red, scaly patch with partial clearing and follicular pustules (Fig. 6-12). Multiple annular lesions may be seen (Fig. 6-13). In immunosuppressed children, including those with cancer, or those who use potent topical steroids, invasion of the follicular orifice by the dermatophytes may predominate. This produces a folliculitis pattern known as *Majocchi's granulomas* (Fig. 6-14). *M. canis, T. mentagrophytes,*

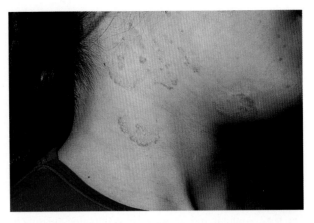

Fig. 6-9 Annular, red, scaly borders with clear center in tinea corporis.

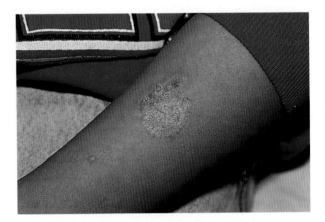

Fig. 6-10 Red, scaly plaque with partial clearing in center in tinea corporis caused by *M. canis.*

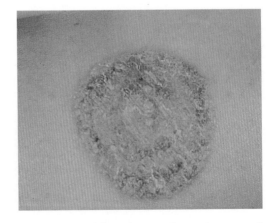

Fig. 6-11 Plaque, red throughout, with prominent pustules, in tinea corporis caused by the cattle ringworm, *T. verrucosum.*

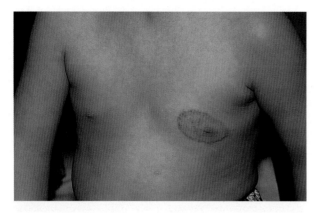

Fig. 6-12 Annular, red, scaly patch, with partial clearing in the center and red follicular papules.

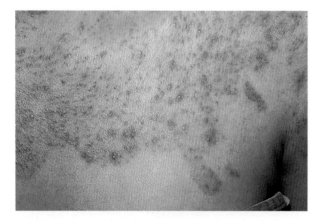

Fig. 6-13 Tinea incognito. Multiple follicular pustules with partial loss of annular border in adolescent mistreated with potent topical steroids.

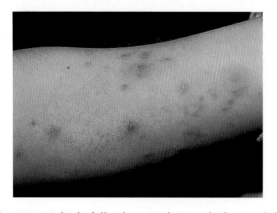

Fig. 6-14 Multiple follicular pustules in a leukemic child with Majocchi's granulomas caused by *T. rubrum*.

T. tonsurans, T. verrucosum, and *T. rubrum* are the most common dermatophytes responsible for tinea corporis. Epidemics of tinea corporis have occurred in wrestlers (tinea gladiatorum) as a result of contaminated wrestling mats.[17] Misdiagnosed tinea corporis treated with potent or superpotent topical steroids will not display scaling, and the annular border may be obscured (tinea incognito).[18] Diagnosis is confirmed by KOH examination of scrapings of thin scales obtained from the border of the lesion. Cultures are not usually done routinely.

Differential diagnosis

Any skin eruption that produces an annular configuration can mimic tinea corporis. The herald patch of pityriasis rosea may mimic tinea corporis, as may any of the forms of dermatitis. The herald patch clears in the center but has central scale rather than scale at the edge. It is not unusual to confuse the annular nodules of granuloma annulare for tinea corporis. In granuloma annulare, there is no scale or surface disruption. Psoriasis, parapsoriasis, figurate erythemas, sarcoidosis, secondary syphilis, and lupus erythematosus can also mimic tinea corporis.

Tinea Pedis (Athlete's Foot)
Clinical features

There are three clinical forms of tinea pedis. All are found predominantly in the postpubertal adolescent and are uncommon in early childhood.[19] The most common form consists of vesicles and erosions on the instep of one or both feet (Figs. 6-15 and 6-16).[20] The dermatophyte may be identified by removing the vesicle roof, scraping the underside of the roof, and examining the scrapings under the microscope for hyphae. Occasionally, fissuring between the toes, with scaling and erythema in the surrounding skin, is seen. Rarely, diffuse scaling of the weight-bearing surface of one or both feet, with exaggerated scaling in the skin creases, the so-called moccasin foot tinea pedis, is seen. The most common organisms responsible for tinea pedis are *T. rubrum* and *T. mentagrophytes*.

Differential diagnosis

Atopic dermatitis mimics tinea pedis in prepubertal children. Contact dermatitis and other forms of dermatitis may also mimic tinea pedis. Contact dermatitis usually involves the tops of the feet, whereas tinea pedis involves the weight-bearing surface. Juvenile plantar dermatosis (JPD) is characterized by redness,

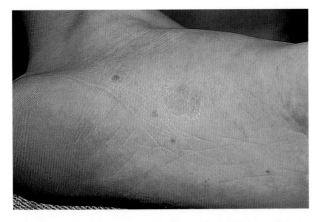

Fig. 6-15 Annular erythema with vesicles on instep of large adolescent male foot. Tinea pedis caused by *T. rubrum.*

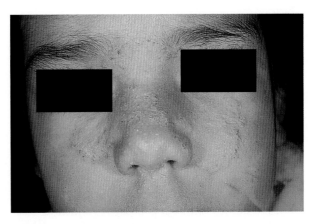

Fig. 6-17 Annular, red, scaly lesions of the nose and malar skin of a girl misdiagnosed as having lupus erythematosus. Tinea faciei caused by *M. canis.*

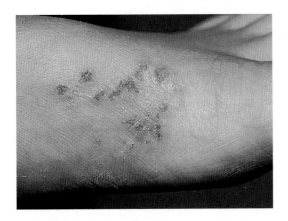

Fig. 6-16 Erosions and blisters on the instep of an adolescent's foot in bullous tinea pedis.

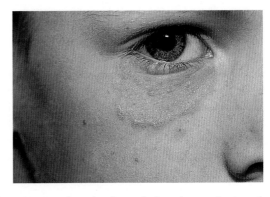

Fig. 6-18 A red, scaly plaque below the eye in tinea faciei caused by *M. canis.*

dryness, and fissures of the weight-bearing surface of the foot and may be easily confused with tinea pedis. Fungal scrapings and culture are needed to distinguish tinea pedis from JPD. Scabies, granuloma annulare, and psoriasis may also mimic tinea pedis.

Tinea Faciei
Clinical features

Dermatophyte infections on the face occur commonly in children. They are erythematous, scaly, and may have a "butterfly" distribution (Fig. 6-17). In other children the lesions may be unilateral (Fig. 6-18). KOH examination of the scaly border will confirm the diagnosis. *M. canis* and the cattle ringworm, *T. verrucosum,* are the most commonly involved fungi of tinea faciei in children.

Differential diagnosis

Tinea faciei may mimic lupus erythematosus and other collagen vascular diseases. A KOH examination for hyphae should always be performed in children in whom the butterfly rash of lupus is considered. Atopic dermatitis, contact dermatitis, and seborrheic dermatitis should also be considered.

Tinea Cruris
Clinical features

An erythematous, scaly eruption on the inner thighs and inguinal creases characterizes tinea cruris.[5] Sometimes an elevated, papular, scaly border is present to suggest the diagnosis. KOH examination of the border for hyphae will confirm the diagnosis. Tinea cruris is unusual before adolescence. *T. mentagrophytes* and

Epidermophyton floccosum are the organisms most often responsible.

Differential diagnosis

Diaper dermatitis and candidiasis may mimic tinea cruris, but these usually occur in infants. Yeast infection in the perineal area may be distinguished by involvement of the scrotum. Several forms of dermatitis also occur in this area. Rarely, erythrasma, a superficial bacterial infection caused by *Corynebacterium minutissimum,* will be confused with tinea cruris. Wood's light examination in erythrasma produces a coral-red fluorescence but is negative in tinea cruris.

Pathogenesis

Dermatophyte invasion of the stratum corneum, but not the remainder of the epidermis or dermis, is responsible for superficial dermatophyte infections. The exact mechanism of the inflammation is not known, but toxins released by the dermatophyte are thought to be important in initiating the inflammatory response.

Treatment

Topical therapy is the treatment of choice (Table 6-2).[17-22] The fungicidal and fungistatic preparations are all efficacious against 90% of dermatophyte species. The allylamines are more efficacious and more expensive than the imidazoles.[22] They are applied twice daily, either as a cream or solution, to the entire area until the lesions have cleared. This often takes 2 to 4 weeks of therapy. Topical terbinafine may produce clinical and mycologic clearing within 1 week.[5,17] Rarely are oral terbinafine, griseofulvin, itraconazole, fluconazole, or other systemic antifungal agents required.

Patient Education

Knowledge that these fungi are found in soil or animals may help identify the source and prevent other family members from being infected. The clinician should be certain to instruct the patient to treat the entire lesion plus about a 1-cm border beyond it. Efforts to keep the affected skin area dry after successful treatment, and changing habits regarding family pets, such as keeping the pets out of the child's room and not allowing the child to carry the pet, may be useful in preventing reinfection until the pet is cured. When epidemic dermatophytes are involved, examination of contacts and fungal culture of suspicious lesions is recommended.

Follow-up Visits

A visit 2 weeks after therapy is started is helpful to ascertain its efficacy. If no response has occurred, either the diagnosis is incorrect or a resistant dermatophyte has been encountered. At this point it is useful to culture the lesion and perhaps change to a different class of topical antifungal agent. Further follow-up visits may be needed.

Table 6-2 Topical Antifungal Agents

Class	Agent	Brand Name	Action
Allylamines	Terbinafine	Lamisil	Fungicidal
	Butenafine	Mentax	Fungicidal
	Naftifine	Naftin	Fungicidal
Hydroxypyridones	Ciclopirox	Loprox	Fungicidal
Imidazoles	Clotrimazole	Lotrimin, Fungoid, Mycelex	Fungistatic
	Econazole	Spectazole	Fungistatic
	Ketoconazole	Nizoral	Fungistatic
	Miconazole	Micatin, Desenex	Fungistatic
	Monistat-Derm		
	Oxiconazole	Oxistat	Fungistatic
	Sulconazole	Exelderm	Fungistatic
Polyenes	Nystatin	Mycostatin, Nilstat	Fungistatic*
Thiocarbamates	Tolnaftate	Tinactin, Aftate, Ting Tolnaftate	Fungistatic†

*No activity against dermatophytes.
†No activity against yeast.

FUNGAL INFECTION OF THE NAILS (ONYCHOMYCOSIS, TINEA UNGUIUM)

Clinical Features

Distal thickening and yellowing of the nail plate are regular features of onychomycosis (tinea unguium) (Fig. 6-19).[5,22] The yellowing represents separation of the distal nail plate from the nail bed, and entrapment of air between these two structures. Usually only one or two nails, most often the toenails, are involved. It is uncommon to find onychomycosis in childhood; it is almost exclusively limited to adolescence. Usually there is a family member with untreated or recurrent athlete's foot. With toenail involvement, a concurrent tinea pedis is usually present.[5,19,21,22]

Differential Diagnosis

Psoriasis also causes distal yellowing and thickening of the nail, but eventually all 20 nails are involved, and superficial nail pitting is also present. Lichen planus and trachyonychia (20-nail dystrophy) also usually involve all 20 nails. Hereditary nail disorders associated with ectodermal defects, such as pachyonychia congenita, are sometimes confused with onychomycosis. Bacterial and candidal nail involvement characteristically result in proximal rather than distal nail plate disease.

Pathogenesis

Some dermatophytes may invade nails and the stratum corneum as well. They proliferate within the nail plate, destroying its integrity.

Treatment

Successful therapy of onychomycosis is difficult. Clinical and mycologic cures have been obtained with oral treatment.[23,24] Itraconazole pulse therapy at 5 mg/kg/day orally for 1 week each month for 3 to 5 months has resulted in long-term clinical and mycological cures

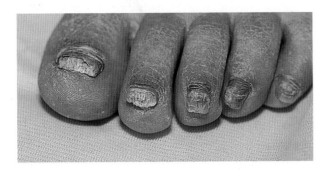

Fig. 6-19 Onychomycosis. Distal thickening and yellowing of four toenails in an adolescent.

(up to 4 years) and is the recommended treatment if there are no contraindications.[24] Itraconazole and other azoles have significant hepatic side-effects, and liver function tests should be monitored monthly. In contrast, only 17.5% of treated patients responded after 6 to 12 months of daily griseofulvin therapy. The clinician should weigh the consequences of prolonged therapy with griseofulvin against the poor success rate. Oral terbinafine (95%), ketoconazole (80%), and itraconazole (71%) used daily for 4 to 8 weeks have somewhat higher reported success rates, but there are little data for long-term relapse rates. Topical agents, with the possible exception of 1% terbinafine, generally are not successful in long-term cures unless used in combination with systemic antifungal agents.[22]

Patient Education

The difficulty in obtaining a cure with this disease should be thoroughly explained to the patient and the parents. The hepatic and other side-effects of the oral antifungal agents and drug interactions should be explained. They may not desire oral antifungal therapy simply to achieve temporary improvement.

Follow-up Visits

Visits at 6-month intervals are useful to follow the course of the illness and observe for the possible involvement of other nails. If oral antifungal agents are used, then evaluation for side effects, including laboratory tests at 1-month intervals, is recommended.

YEAST SKIN INFECTIONS

Tinea Versicolor

Clinical features

In tinea versicolor, multiple oval macules with a fine scale are found on the neck, chest, upper back, shoulders, and upper arms of children and adolescents (Fig. 6-20).[25] Occasionally, the lesions are confluent and present as a continuous sheet. Their color depends on the state of pigmentation. In well-tanned or darkly pigmented adolescents, the lesions appear as discrete hypopigmented macules. In the winter months, as normal pigment fades, the lesions may appear as tan or dark-brown macules, hence the term *versicolor* (Fig. 6-21). The infection tends to be persistent. KOH examination of scrapings reveals numerous short, curved hyphae and circular spores—the so-called *spaghetti and meatballs* appearance (Fig. 6-22). Some authorities recommend application of clear tape to the skin to pull off skin surface cells followed by microscopic examination.[26] Occasionally, Wood's light examination reveals an orange fluorescence of the

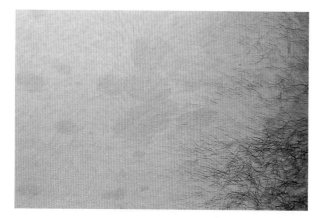

Fig. 6-20 Multiple tan macules with a fine scale over the chest of an adolescent with tinea versicolor.

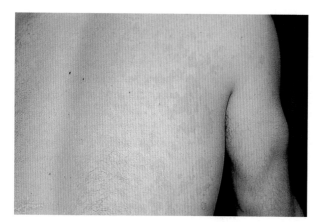

Fig. 6-21 Tan macules of tinea versicolor on a light-skinned child.

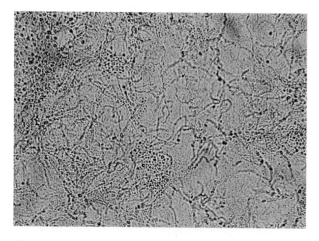

Fig. 6-22 Photomicrograph of KOH examination of tinea versicolor. Multiple short hyphae and spores are seen.

lesions if the patient has not cleansed the affected area recently.[25] Biopsy of these lesions will show periodic acid-Schiff (PAS)–positive hyphae and spores within the stratum corneum.

Differential diagnosis

Seborrheic dermatitis, contact dermatitis, and tinea corporis can mimic tinea versicolor. Vitiligo, pityriasis alba, and other hypopigmented states are also sometimes confused with it. Direct microscopic examination of scales will distinguish tinea versicolor from other possible causes.

Pathogenesis

The yeastlike organism *Malassezia furfur,* which in its culture phase is called *Pityrosporum orbiculare* or *Pityrosporum ovale,* invades the stratum corneum to produce the lesions of tinea versicolor.[25] The organism thrives in hot, humid climates and commonly colonizes the skin by adolescence. It may colonize the skin of neonates as well.

Treatment

Miconazole, ciclopirox, clotrimazole, terbinafine solutions, or fluconazole shampoos applied twice daily for 2 or 3 weeks may be efficacious but are costly when one considers the amount required to cover the trunk of a child or adolescent.[27,28] Applying ketoconazole shampoo or selenium sulfide 2.5% for 30 minutes daily for 1 week followed by monthly applications for 3 months is considered the treatment of choice by many.[5,28] Application of sodium hypochlorite 15% once weekly for 2 months will result in temporary clearing, but the recurrence rate is high.[2] After initial clearing, prevention of recurrence by monthly treatment may be considered. In tropical and subtropical climates, oral ketoconazole, fluconazole, or itraconazole given in a single dose once daily for 2 weeks may be considered in difficult cases.[5,29] A single oral dose of fluconazole may produce acceptable results.[29]

Patient education

Patients should be instructed that repigmentation of the hypopigmented areas will not occur until they are exposed to the sun, and that a recurrence is likely.

Follow-up visits

A follow-up visit at 1 month to evaluate therapy should be considered. If oral therapy is considered, monthly visits to monitor side effects should be instituted.

Candidiasis
Clinical features

In regions of the body in which warmth and moisture lead to maceration of the skin or mucous membranes, the tissue is predisposed to invasion by the pathogenic yeast *Candida albicans.* Candidiasis in different body sites has distinct clinical features.[5,30,31] In neonates and infants, white plaques on an erythematous base (thrush) are commonly seen on the buccal mucosa and other sites in the oral cavity.[5,31] In this same age group, intertriginous involvement of the body folds is also common, such as in the diaper area. The use of pacifiers in infants may be permissive for oral candidiasis, including involvement of the angles of the lips (angular cheilitis).[5,31]

Fully established diaper candidiasis demonstrates beefy erythema with elevated margins and satellite red plaques (Fig. 6-23).[33] However, erosions, pustules, erythematous papules, and vesicles may also be features of candidiasis of the diaper area. *C. albicans* colonizes the diaper area within 3 days of the development of diaper dermatitis and should always be considered as a secondary infection in long-standing diaper dermatitis.

Intertriginous candidiasis involving the inframammary, axillary, neck, and inguinal body folds may also be seen in obese infants, children, and adolescents.

A rare form of candidiasis (congenital candidiasis) acquired in utero results in generalized erythema of the newborn, with scaling and pustule formation (Fig. 6-24). It is particularly observed in very-low-birth-weight infants and is acquired from maternal *C. albicans* vulvovaginitis.

Paronychia caused by candidiasis is a common result of thumb sucking. The erythema and swelling around the base of the nail are usually not tender (Fig. 6-25).

Vulvovaginal candidiasis appears as a cheesy vaginal discharge, with whitish plaques on erythematous mucous membranes.[34] It is most common in adolescent females.

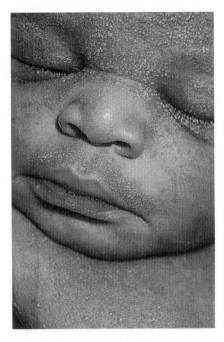

Fig. 6-24 Hundreds of pinpoint pustules with an erythematous base on the face of a newborn with congenital candidiasis.

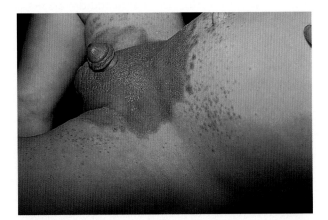

Fig. 6-23 Beefy-red central erythema with satellite pustules in candidiasis of diaper area. Positive cultures can be obtained only from satellite lesions, not from central erythema.

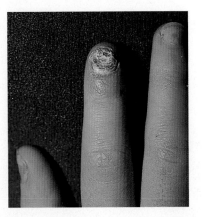

Fig. 6-25 Cuticular nontender swelling and erythema with thickened, disrupted nail surface in paronychia caused by *C. albicans.*

The rare candidal granulomas are oval, red plaques with a thick yellow crust. They are found on the head and neck and other areas of skin in children with defective host defenses.[5] In the syndrome of chronic mucocutaneous candidiasis (Fig. 6-26), seen in patients with defective host defenses, persistent thrush with extensive involvement of the tongue and lips and chronic paronychia are present. Severe thrush may be observed in immunodeficient children infected with the human immunodeficiency virus (HIV). Patients on long-term glucocorticosteroid, antibiotic, or oral contraceptive therapy (in adolescent females) appear unusually susceptible to candidiasis. Similarly, children with diabetes mellitus and reticuloendothelial neoplasms are also predisposed to candidiasis.

The diagnosis can be established by scraping the skin or mucosal lesion and observing the single budding yeast in a KOH preparation under the microscope. *C. albicans* is readily cultured on Sabouraud dextrose agar or cornmeal agar. Interpretation of a positive culture must be made with caution because *C. albicans* may reflect simple colonization.

Differential diagnosis

Herpes simplex, aphthous stomatitis, epidermolysis bullosa, geographic tongue, burns, and erythema multiforme of the oral cavity may mimic thrush. Diaper dermatitis, bacterial infection of intertriginous areas, Letterer-Siwe disease, linear immunoglobulin A (IgA) dermatosis, and maceration may mimic the intertriginous forms of candidiasis.

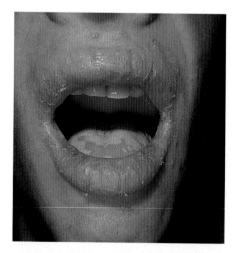

Fig. 6-26 Thick white coating of tongue with scaling and fissuring of lips in chronic mucocutaneous candidiasis.

Congenital candidiasis may be confused with severe erythema toxicum, ichthyosiform erythrodermas, immunodeficiencies, miliaria, transient neonatal pustular melanosis, infantile acropustulosis, and congenital syphilis or other intrauterine infections.

Paronychia caused by *S. aureus* may mimic candidal paronychia, but it usually has an acute onset, and the affected nail is tender and fluctuant. Psoriasis, lichen planus, and pachyonychia congenita should also be considered. Gonorrhea, Trichomonas infections, and chemical vaginitis may mimic vaginal candidiasis. Psoriasis, impetigo, and deep fungal infections such as sporotrichosis may be similar to candidal granulomas.

Acrodermatitis enteropathica, acquired zinc deficiency, and vitamin deficiency states may be confused with chronic mucocutaneous candidiasis.

Pathogenesis

C. albicans may be considered a part of the normal flora of the skin and mucous surfaces in certain body areas. Colonization of the oral cavity, intestinal tract, and vagina of healthy individuals is common. Moisture, warmth, and breaks in the epidermal barrier permit overgrowth and invasion of the epidermis by the organism. It has been demonstrated that *C. albicans* generates inflammation by activation of the complement system within the skin and attraction of neutrophils to skin sites of Candida invasion. Keratolytic proteases and other enzymes in *C. albicans* species allow them to penetrate the epidermal barrier more easily than other organisms.

Treatment

Topical therapy with several anticandidal agents is usually efficacious.[30-32] For infantile thrush the use of nystatin oral suspension four times daily for 5 days is efficacious.[5] In older children with thrush or angular cheilitis, clotrimazole troches may be useful.[5] For cutaneous candidosis, nystatin, oxiconazole, ketoconazole, ciclopirox, econazole, haloprogin, miconazole, or clotrimazole in a cream vehicle applied four times daily will result in prompt clearing of the lesions in 3 to 5 days.* In the diaper area, application with each diaper change for 2 to 3 days is useful. The antifungal creams may sting or burn if there are breaks in the skin surface. Antiyeast ointments may be substituted.

Correction of the predisposing factors, such as good care of the diaper area, drying of intertrigi-

*References 5, 30, 32, 33, 35, 36.

nous areas, and withdrawal of broad-spectrum antibiotics or glucocorticosteroids is also important in the management of candidiasis. Treatment of candidal vulvovaginitis or candidal infections of the nipples in nursing mothers is valuable in the therapy of thrush.

Oral therapy with fluconazole or itraconazole 5 mg/kg/day for 21 days may be required for oral candidosis in immunosuppressed children.[5,30,34-36] Vaginitis in the adolescent may be treated with a single 150-mg dose of fluconazole.[5,34]

The following specific treatment protocols may be utilized:
1. **Thrush:** Apply nystatin solution topically to the area four times daily for 5 days. With recurrence, a second course of this therapy may be helpful. Simultaneous therapy of Candida vulvovaginitis or nipple infection in the mother is most helpful in reducing surface colonization with *C. albicans*. Discarding the infant's pacifier may help.
2. **Diaper candidiasis:** Application of nystatin (or one of the other agents listed) in a cream form with each diaper change for 2 to 3 days is most useful if combined with the usual measures to keep the diaper area dry and cool. Mupirocin applied 4 or 5 times a day for 5 days may also be effective.[32]
3. **Paronychia:** Nystatin cream applied nightly under occlusion (a plastic glove covered by a cotton stocking) for 3 to 4 weeks will often clear candidal paronychia. This should be done with caution in infants to be certain they do not aspirate the plastic into their airways.

Patient education

The patient or parents should understand that *C. albicans* is part of the normal skin flora in certain individuals and will reinvade susceptible tissue sites if the predisposing factors favoring overgrowth are not eliminated. Thus careful attention to the treatment of intertrigo and good diaper-area care are essential to achieve long-term satisfactory results. Recurrences should be retreated.

Follow-up visits

An examination 5 to 7 days after initiating therapy is useful to evaluate the therapeutic response and reinforce the measures to diminish warmth and moisture in intertriginous areas. Most therapy failures are due to poor compliance, not host defense defects. Widespread involvement of oral cavity, nails, and skin should trigger a suspicion of immunodeficiency.

REFERENCES

1. Aly R: Ecology, epidemiology and diagnosis of tinea capitis, *Pediatr Infect Dis J* 18:180, 1999.
2. Pomeranz AJ et al: Asymptomatic dermatophyte carriers in the households of children with tinea capitis, *Arch Pediatr Adolesc Med* 153:483, 1999.
3. Frieden IJ: Tinea capitis: asymptomatic carriage of infection, *Pediatr Infect Dis J* 18:186, 1999.
4. Friedlander SF: Tinea capitis: past, present and future, *Curr Probl Dermatol* 12:126, 2000.
5. Committee on Infectious Diseases: *2000 Red book,* Elk Grove Village, Ill, 2000, American Academy of Pediatrics.
6. Tack DA et al: The epidemic of tinea capitis disproportionately affects school-aged African Americans, *Pediatr Dermatol* 16:75, 1999.
7. Hubbard TW: The predictive value of symptoms in diagnosing childhood tinea capitis, *Arch Pediatr Adolesc Med* 153:1150, 1999.
8. Miller MA, Hodgson Y: Sensitivity and specificity of potassium hydroxide smears of skin scrapings for the diagnosis of tinea pedis, *Arch Dermatol* 129:510, 1993.
9. Friedlander SF et al: Cotton swab method for the diagnosis of tinea capitis, *Pediatrics* 104:276, 1999.
10. Friedlander SF: The evolving role of itraconazole, fluconazole and terbinafine in the treatment of tinea capitis, *Pediatr Infect Dis J* 18:205, 1999.
11. Bennett ML et al: Oral griseofulvin remains the treatment of choice for tinea capitis in children, *Pediatr Dermatol* 17:304, 2000.
12. Gupta AK et al: Tinea capitis: an overview with emphasis on management, *Pediatr Dermatol* 16:171, 1999.
13. Krafchik B, Pelletier J: An open study of tinea capitis in 50 children treated with a two week course of oral terbinafine, *J Am Acad Dermatol* 41:60, 1999.
14. Honig PJ, Caputo GL, Leyden JJ: Microbiology of kerions, *J Pediatr* 123:422, 1993.
15. Honig PJ, Caputo GL, Leyden JJ: Treatment of kerions, *Pediatr Dermatol* 11:69, 1994.
16. Honig PJ: Tinea capitis: recommendations for school attendance, *Pediatr Infect Dis J* 18:211, 1999.
17. Kohl TD, Martin DC, Berger MS: Comparison of topical and oral treatments for tinea gladiatorum, *Clin J Sport Med* 9:161, 1999.
18. Romano C, Asta F, Massai L: Tinea incognito due to *Microsporum gypseum* in three children, *Pediatr Dermatol* 17:41, 2000.
19. Merlin K et al: The prevalence of common skin conditions in Australian school students: 4 tinea pedis, *Br J Dermatol* 140:897, 1999.
20. Geary RJ, Lucky AW: Tinea pedis in children presenting as unilateral inflammatory lesions of the sole, *Pediatr Dermatol* 16:255, 1999.
21. Rebell G, Zaias N: Tinea pedis: the child and the family, *Pediatr Dermatol* 16:157, 1999.
22. Hart R, Bell-Syer SEM, Crawford F: Systematic review of topical treatments for fungal infections of skin and nails of the feet, *Br Med J* 319:79, 1999.
23. Haneke E, Roseeuw D: The scope of onychomycosis: epidemiology and clinical features, *Int J Dermatol* 38(suppl): S27, 1999.

24. Huang P-H, Paller AS: Itraconazole pulse therapy for dermatophyte onychomycosis in children, *Arch Pediatr Adolesc Med* 154:614, 2000.

25. Geis PA: Epidemiology, etiology, clinical aspects and diagnosis of tinea versicolor, *Int J Dermatol* 38:558, 1999.

26. Rogers CJ, Cook TF, Glaser DA: Diagnosing tinea versicolor: don't scrape, just tape, *Pediatr Dermatol* 17:68, 2000.

27. Savin R et al: Tinea versicolor treated with terbinafine 1% solution, *Int J Dermatol* 38:863, 1999.

28. Lange DS et al: Ketoconazole 2% shampoo in the treatment of tinea versicolor: a multicenter, randomized, double-blind, placebo-controlled trial, *J Am Acad Dermatol* 39:944, 1998.

29. Montero-Gei F, Robles ME, Suchil P: Fluconazole vs. itraconazole in the treatment of tinea versicolor, *Int J Dermatol* 38:601, 1999.

30. Hay RJ: The management of superficial candidiasis, *J Am Acad Dermatol* 40:S35, 1999.

31. Khoory BJ et al: Candida infections in newborns: a review, *J Chemother* 11:367, 1999.

32. de Wet PM et al: Perianal candidosis: a comparative study of mupirocin and nystatin, *Int J Dermatol* 38: 618, 1999.

33. Hogan P: Nappy rashes, *Austr J Dermatol* 1999.

34. Nyirjesy P: Vaginitis in the adolescent patient, *Pediatr Clin North Am* 46:733, 1999.

35. Hoppe JE: Treatment of oropharyngeal candidiasis and candidal diaper dermatitis in neonates and infants: review and reappraisal, *Pediatr Infect Dis J* 16:885, 1997.

36. Schwarze R, Penk A, Pittrow L: Treatment of candidal infections with fluconazole in neonates and infants, *Eur J Med Res* 5:203, 2000.

CHAPTER SEVEN | Infestations

Arthropods are constantly present in the human environment, and hundreds of species are known to cause skin disease.[1,2] Arthropods may be divided into arachnids, which have eight legs (e.g., mites, ticks, spiders), and hexapods, with six legs (e.g., lice, mosquitoes, fleas, bedbugs, ants, bees, and other insects). Biting and stinging insects may produce wheals, erythema, and even bullae from contact with the skin.[1,2] The erythematous papule with a central punctum is a common feature of insect bites. In this chapter, scabies, pediculoses, and papular urticaria are discussed in detail because they are the most common forms of infestations and often require therapeutic intervention. Cutaneous eruptions related to ticks, spiders, mites, and parasitic worms (helminths) are also considered.

HUMAN MITE INFESTATION
Scabies
Clinical features

Pruritic papules on the abdomen, dorsa of the hands, flexural surface of the wrist, elbows, periaxillary skin, genitalia, ankles, feet, and interdigital webs of the hands are seen in scabies (Figs. 7-1 and 7-2).[1-4] In infants eczematous eruptions of the face and trunk are also seen (Fig. 7-3). In contrast, the head and neck regions are almost never involved in older children, adolescents, or adults. Most infants have acute dermatitis that is characterized by excoriations, erythematous papules, honey-colored crusts, and pustules. Infants have hundreds of lesions, older children and adults have few. In all children with widespread scabies, secondary impetigo is common.

Crusted nodules that may become brown with time may be apparent on the trunk of the infant with scabies (Fig. 7-4).[1] When present, S-shaped burrows are diagnostic (Fig. 7-5).[1,4] They are usually found on the wrist, palm, feet, ankles, interdigital webs, or genitalia. Nocturnal pruritus is severe. Within one household the disease may vary in severity from asymptomatic infested children to a child with a few nonpruritic papules to hundreds of lesions. Infants are likely to have dozens of lesions (Fig. 7-6), whereas older children and adults may have less than 10. A high index of suspicion should be maintained in any patient with pruritic skin disease.

Children who are severely retarded and unable to scratch effectively may be infested with thousands of scabies mites, which produce a diffuse hyperkeratosis of the skin and lichenification that may be confused with ichthyosis.[1,4,5] Hyperkeratosis and scaling may be particularly prominent on the hands, feet, and genitalia.[4,5] This form of scabies is called *Norwegian scabies* (Fig. 7-7). Children with malignancies or immunodeficiencies, or those who are on immunosuppressive drugs or who suffer local immunosuppression from the use of superpotent topical steroids may similarly suffer widespread scabies infestation, with extensive scalp involvement.[1,5,6]

Differential diagnosis

The diagnosis of scabies is confirmed by scraping an unscratched burrow that is covered with a drop of microscope immersion oil and placing the scrapings on a glass slide with a coverslip. Under the $10\times$ objective of the microscope, the female mite (Figure 7-8) and/or her eggs or feces should be visible (Fig. 7-9). Examination of skin scrapings obtained from the finger webs, wrists, or ankles is most likely to be positive.[1] Excoriated and crusted lesions are often negative. In children with Norwegian scabies, scraping of the thick scales will often yield several viable mites.[1,4-6] Atopic dermatitis, lichen planus, dermatitis herpetiformis, and other severely pruritic skin conditions mimic scabies. Scabies should be suspected in any infant with a sudden onset of severely itchy dermatitis. A careful inspection for burrows and identification of household members who may have a history of itchy bumps are necessary. Seborrheic dermatitis of the scalp may mimic scabies in children with malignancy or immunosuppression.

Pathogenesis

Scabies is caused by the eight-legged human mite *Sarcoptes scabiei*, which may be up to 4 mm in length.[1,3,4] The female mite remains in the stratum corneum, which she traverses at a rate of 0.5 to 5 mm/day. She deposits her eggs during her journey

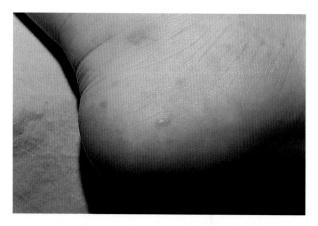

Fig. 7-1 Scabies. Papules and burrows on the foot of an infant.

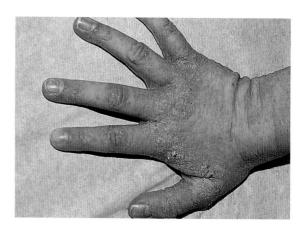

Fig. 7-2 Scabies. Involvement of the dorsa of the hands and interdigital webs in a child.

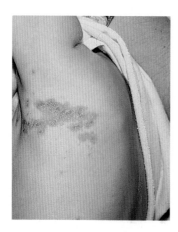

Fig. 7-3 Scabies. Nonspecific eczematous lesions in a child's axilla.

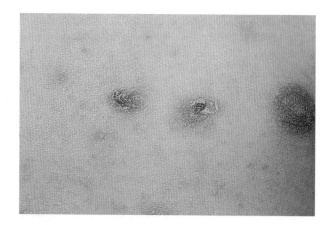

Fig. 7-4 Scabies. Crusted nodules on the trunk of an infant.

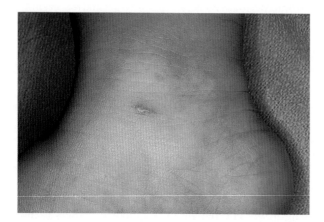

Fig. 7-5 S-shaped burrow diagnostic of scabies. This is the preferred lesion from which to obtain a scraping.

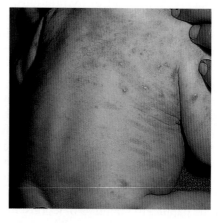

Fig. 7-6 Scabies in an infant. Hundreds of lesions are present.

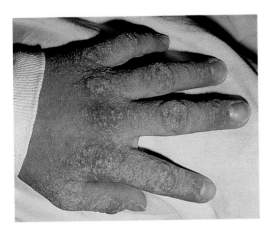

Fig. 7-7 Norwegian scabies. Diffuse scaling of the dorsum of the hand. Scraping of the scales revealed dozens of motile mites.

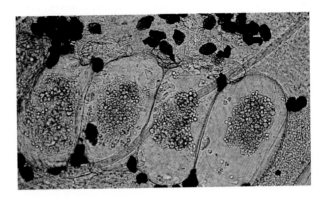

Fig. 7-9 Photomicrograph of oval eggs and dark brown scybala in skin scraping from an infant with scabies.

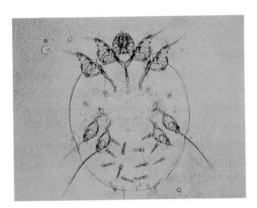

Fig. 7-8 Photomicrograph of female scabies mite recovered from scrapings of burrow.

and dies after 30 or 40 days. Her eggs reach maturity in 10 to 14 days, and a new cycle begins. Transmission of scabies requires human contact, although female mites can survive 2 to 3 days off the human body. A pandemic of scabies has followed each major war of the twentieth century. Human scabies is quite contagious because newly infested individuals may not experience itching for the first 3 weeks of infestation, and only casual contact is required for spread of mites to others.[3,4] Humans are the reservoir for scabies, and infestation of children with animal mites (e.g., dog, cat, chicken) is rare.

Treatment

Application of a scabicide, such as 5% permethrin creme or 1% gamma benzene hexachloride lotion, is curative.[1,2,5-8] The lotion or cream should be dispensed

as the calculated dose needed for therapy. In children and adolescents, application of 5% permethrin creme for 8 to 14 hours produces a 98% cure rate.[1,4,7,8] One 2-hour application of lindane lotion followed by a bath is curative in approximately 82% of cases; one 6-hour application cures 96% of cases. Prolonged contact with the skin may result in significant percutaneous absorption. Gamma benzene hexachloride is concentrated in the central nervous system if absorbed; percutaneous absorption with central nervous system symptoms has been reported in a few infants. Some instances of lindane-resistant scabies in North America have been reported. Ivermectin at 200 µg/kg in a single oral dose has also been demonstrated to be curative.[1,4,7] Topical permethrin may be superior to single-dose ivermectin.[4,7,8] In children under 5 years of age and in pregnant or lactating women, gamma benzene hexachloride lotion and ivermectin are not recommended.[1,2,4,7] Permethrin creme is approved for use for infants 2 months of age or older. In any infant or toddler, covering the hands with clothing to prevent licking the scabicide from the skin is recommended. For children with only a few lesions, routine retreatment is not necessary. In infants with extensive involvement, several retreatments 7 or 8 days apart may occasionally be required. Simultaneous treatment of all household contacts is required.[1,2,4,7]

Even with the elimination of all viable scabies mites and eggs, itching may persist for 7 to 10 days after successful therapy. Despite the persistence of pruritus, no new lesions should be detected. Treatment failures are often the result of poor compliance or failure to treat an infested household member. In treatment failures with topical scabicides, in immunosuppressed children, or others with Norwegian scabies, single-dose ivermectin should be considered.[1,4-8]

Patient education

The clinician should emphasize to the patient and family the mode of transmission of scabies and identify all household contacts. Instructions on the treatment schedule should be specific; the persistence of itching even after scabicidal therapy and the importance of treating all household contacts should be emphasized (see p. 346 for a patient education handout on Scabies).

Follow-up visits

A follow-up visit in 2 weeks is important to ascertain success or failure of therapy. Any new lesions that may have appeared should be scraped to determine whether infestation has persisted or the child is reinfested. If the mite or her products are found, retreatment is suggested. Infants, who tend to have hundreds of lesions, may require several retreatments.

Other Mite Infestations
Clinical features

Mites from nonhuman sources occasionally infest the skin of children. The canine scabies mite, usually carried on the fur of puppies with mange, may be temporarily transferred to the child.[1] The puppy will have fur loss and crusted lesions. Similarly, harvest mites or chiggers, found in grasses, grains, or overgrowth of bushes, may similarly infest children. Grain mites found in stored seeds and grains, and fowl mites found on chickens or domesticated birds such as canaries, pigeons, or swallows may also infest children. In each instance the clinical lesions are characterized by urticarial papules, sometimes with hemorrhagic puncta, and, in intense responses, blister formation. Burrows are absent. The distribution on the child's skin depends on the location of the exposed skin. Characteristically, canine scabies produces lesions on the forearms, abdomen, and thighs. Harvest mites characteristically produce lesions on the legs and around the beltline. Grain-mite lesions occur on the exposed areas of the arms and legs but may be quite

Table 7-1 Insect Repellents for Children

Brand	Manufacturer	% DEET
DEET-CONTAINING		
Skedaddle for Children	Minnetonka	6.5
Skeddadle for Children with sunscreen SPF 15		6.5
Off! Skintastic for Kids spray	Johnson Wax	5.0
Cutter Just for Kids	United Industries	5.0
Cutter Pleasant Protection with sunscreen SPF 15		7.0
Repel Camp Lotion for Kids	Wisconsin Pharmacal	10.0
Repel Soft Unscented gel		7.0
PLANT-BASED REPELLANTS		
Bite Blocker (geranium oil)	Consep, Inc	
Avon Skin So Soft Bug Guard spray (citronella 0.10%)	Avon	
PERMETHRIN INSECTICIDE SPRAYS		
NOTE: For clothing only! Not to be applied on skin.		
Cutter Outdoorsman Gear Guard spray (Permethrin 0.5%)	Cutter	
(Permethrin 0.5%)	Wisconsin Pharmacal	

generalized. Fowl mites produce lesions on exposed areas of skin.

Differential diagnosis

Scabies and papular urticaria are the most important considerations in the differential diagnosis. A history of exposure to the appropriate source is most significant in the diagnosis of mite infestation. Important historical information includes the new puppy with hair loss and crusts on his skin, exposure to deep grasses and grain or stored grain, and association with birds. Exposed skin infested with fowl mites may mimic a photoeruption.

Pathogenesis

In each case the mites attach themselves to the skin to inject an irritating secretion and then fall off in a few days. Identifying the mites within skin lesions is very difficult. They do not persist on skin, however.

Treatment

Symptomatic relief with topical steroids or oral antihistamines, or both, is useful. Specific scabicides are not required.

Patient education

Prophylaxis is an important part of patient education. Treatment of the infested puppy, use of good insect repellents (Table 7-1), and staying away from those areas containing sources that are likely to produce the infestation should be emphasized. Parents and children should know that they cannot pass this eruption to others, and that itching can be quite severe, lasting for several weeks after the initial exposure.

Follow-up visits

A follow-up visit in 2 weeks to ascertain the institution of prophylaxis and the response to therapy is useful.

TICKS
Clinical Features

Tick bites are usually painless and inapparent to the child. Usually the tick is noted several days after contact with the skin when pruritus begins. Localized urticarial reactions can be found. A diagnosis is usually made by identifying the presence of the tick in particular cutaneous locations. The most common sites for tick attachment are the occipital scalp (Fig. 7-10), ear canal, axilla, groin, and vulva.[1,2,9,10] Rarely, a systemic reaction to a tick bite, characterized by fever, nausea, abdominal cramping, and headache, may occur, as may paralysis similar to Guillain-Barré syndrome, with ascending symmetric paralysis. A persistent, pruritic nodule, sometimes surrounded by hair loss, may be the result of an incompletely removed tick in which mouth parts remain in the skin. Because ticks in certain areas of North America and Europe may carry *Borrelia burgdorferi,* the spirochete responsible for Lyme disease, observation for expanding rings of erythema about the site of the bite is advised for 3 weeks after the bite (see Chapter 5). The potentially severe nature of Lyme disease, and its prominence in the news media, has prompted excessive concern regarding tick bites.[2,9,10]

Differential Diagnosis

Most tick-bite reactions are obvious because the tick is found attached to the skin. If the mouth parts are left in the skin and a pruritic nodule remains, the diagnosis may be quite difficult to distinguish from scabies, lichen simplex chronicus, or other infestations. The expanding annular red rings of erythema chronicum migrans (ECM) may be confused with ringworm, urticaria, or other annular conditions.

Pathogenesis

Tick bites may occur when children play in the woods and when ticks are transferred from dogs or other incidental hosts to children. The tick attaches itself to the skin by its head in an effort to suck blood. The tick cuts the skin surface with chelicerae, introduces its proboscis, and secretes saliva into the wound. The saliva contains a cement substance, anesthetic, and anticoagulant, and may include the neurotoxin responsible for tick paralysis or the spirochete responsible for Lyme disease. After 24 to 48 hours, the tick engorges with blood from the child, which allows Borrelia to proliferate in the tick gut and then reenter

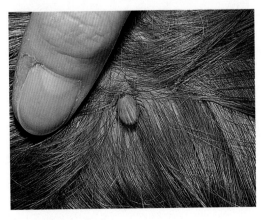

Fig. 7-10 Tick embedded in the occipital scalp of a child.

the child from the tick saliva. A foreign body granuloma is seen in persistent nodules in the skin where tick head parts remain.

Treatment

Removal of the tick is the treatment of choice. The preferred method of removal is the insertion of a blunt instrument, such as a forceps or tweezers, between the tick head and the child's skin (Fig. 7-11). Gentle outward pressure will cause the tick to back out. This method prevents any injury to the skin and the retention of tick parts within the skin. All methods that may injure the skin, such as burning the tick or using noxious substances on the skin, should be avoided. The body of the tick should not be squeezed, and if there is a remnant in the skin, the clinician should consider simple surgical removal. If the child acquired the tick in an area endemic for Lyme disease, it should be saved in a glass jar for analysis if the child becomes ill later. Routine prophylactic administration of oral antibiotics after tick removal is not recommended.[2]

Patient Education

Prevention is the best method for tick bites. As much as possible, children should try to avoid tick habitats, such as dense brush or tall grass, and stay in the center of the path on wooded trails.[2] Children should wear protective clothing, such as long sleeves and caps, preferably of light color so the ticks can be easily seen. They should wear a shirt with a collar to prevent migration and tuck their pants into boots or socks. In endemic areas the regular and careful use of insect repellents (see Table 7-1) during tick season is recommended. Children and their dogs should be routinely inspected for ticks if they have been in wooded areas, and parents should be advised of the most common locations of tick bites and the preferred method of removal.[2,9,10] Clinicians should emphasize that most ticks do not carry Lyme disease. In endemic areas, Lyme vaccine may be considered for adolescents over age 15.[2,10] For a patient information handout on Insect Repellents for Children, see p. 338.

Follow-up Visits

A follow-up visit 2 weeks after a bite to observe for signs of ECM should be considered in areas endemic for Lyme disease.

SPIDERS
Clinical Features

Spider bites may produce local or systemic reactions. The most common is the urticarial papule from nonvenomous spiders. After a bite from a venemous spider, such as a brown recluse, hemorrhagic, painful blisters may appear on the skin and evolve over the next few days into a cutaneous infarct with skin necrosis and dry, gangrenous eschar (Fig. 7-12). This reaction usually occurs on exposed areas of skin in a single lesion around the site of a spider bite.[11] The area of skin loss may be large. With black widow spider bites, systemic reactions, including headache, nausea, vomiting, chills, malaise, syncope, and coma, may develop. Thrombocytopenia, hemolysis, and hemoglobinuria, which might result in renal failure, have been reported.[11]

Differential Diagnosis

Venemous spider bites must be differentiated from other forms of vascular infarction, such as vasculitis.

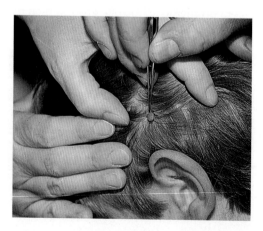

Fig. 7-11 Removal of tick by placing a forceps between the tick and the skin.

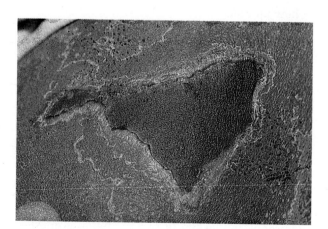

Fig. 7-12 Spider bite. Central necrosis with eschar and surrounding giant erythema.

In vasculitis, numerous lesions are present, whereas in spider bites, a single lesion is seen. Other necrotizing infections, such as ecthyma gangrenosum, caused by Pseudomonas infection, and streptococcal gangrene syndrome should be considered in the differential diagnosis. Lesions of herpes zoster, herpes simplex, cutaneous diphtheria, or anthrax may occasionally be confused with spider bite. In children who do not give a definite history of a spider bite, viral and bacterial cultures may be required.

Pathogenesis

Spiders with venom jaws powerful enough to penetrate human skin, such as the Loxosceles species, produce necrotic skin reactions. In North America, the brown recluse spider *(Loxosceles reclusa)* is usually responsible for the lesion.[11] This spider is very prevalent in the midwestern United States but has occasionally been reported over many other areas of North America. The spider is small, 8 to 10 mm in diameter, and bears a violin-shaped band over the dorsal thorax. It is often found in old buildings. A number of toxins have been found in the venom. Neurotoxins are carried by Latrodectus spiders, including black widow spiders.[11] These spiders are responsible for systemic symptoms after a spider bite.

Treatment

With venemous spider bites, high doses of oral corticosteroids may be useful in reducing or preventing the extent of tissue damage in necrotic spider bites. Doses of 2 mg/kg/day of prednisone are usually recommended for a period of 5 days.[11] Surgical removal of the necrotic area has been performed in some instances to prevent spread of the toxin. Hospitalization may be required in severe systemic toxic reactions caused by black widow spider bites.

Patient Education

The clinician should emphasize that venomous spiders may hide in basements and that recognition of the small, thin-legged spider is important. Children should be kept from abandoned buildings, woodpiles, or other sites favored by spiders.

Follow-up Visits

A daily follow-up visit after initiation of treatment for the spider bite is necessary to evaluate for the development of systemic symptoms and progression of the individual lesion. The child should be seen until healing is observed.

PEDICULOSES (LOUSE INFESTATIONS)
Clinical Features

In human body-louse infestations, excoriated papules and pustules on the trunk and perineum are found in children and adolescents with body-louse infestations.[1,4,12,13] Often only excoriations or their resultant hyperpigmented or hypopigmented scars are seen on the skin. The louse may be discovered by closely examining the seams of the patient's underwear or the scalp hair.

In human head-louse infestations, the gelatinous nits of the head louse appear as white, ovoid bodies tightly adherent to the hair shaft (Figs. 7-13 and 7-14). Nocturnal pruritus is often severe with all hu-

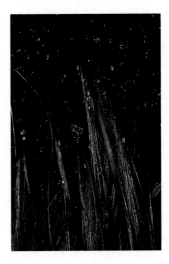

Fig. 7-13 Head lice. Numerous white nits attached to hairs.

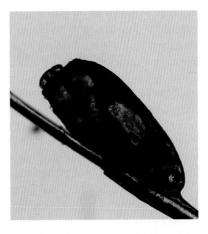

Fig. 7-14 Head lice. Photomicrograph of nit tightly adherent to one side of a hair shaft.

man louse infestations.[1,4] The prevalence of louse infestations is 34 times higher in whites than in blacks.

In human pubic-louse infestations, the pubic (crab) louse may be seen crawling among the pubic hairs, or infestation with the pubic louse may present as blue-black crusted macules (maculae ceruleae) in the pubic area. Nits may also be seen attached to pubic hairs.[1,4] The pubic louse may be seen in the eyelashes or the scalp of newborns.[1,4] Any "bug" seen crawling from the newborn's eye should be considered a pubic louse unless proved otherwise.

Differential Diagnosis

Scabies, dermatitis herpetiformis, neurotic excoriations, and other highly pruritic dermatoses may be confused with pediculoses. Parents with delusions of parasitosis may transfer their delusion to their children. In certain children the retained external hair-root sheath may resemble head louse nits in the scalp. Retained hair root sheaths completely surround the hair, but the nit is attached to one side of the hair. Retained hair root sheaths may be easily removed by sliding them distally down the hair shaft, whereas the nit is tightly adherent to it. The blue-black, crusted macules caused by pubic lice may be confused with vasculitis, folliculitis, or impetigo.

Pathogenesis

The human louse, a six-legged insect, attaches itself to the skin, ingests blood, and produces skin lesions by mechanical puncture and perhaps by injecting toxic secretions.[1,4] There are two species of human lice, *Pediculus humanus,* the body louse, which has subspecies *capitis* (head lice) and *humanus* (body lice), and *Pthirus pubis,* the crab louse.[4] The body louse, which is 2 to 4 mm in length, is the longest of the lice that infest humans; the pubic louse is 1 to 2 mm in length. The female produces new offspring every 2 weeks, and each female may produce over 80 offspring during her lifetime. The body louse produces more eggs during her lifetime than the pubic louse. Newly hatched lice mate with old, and hundreds of nits result every 2 weeks. The female body or head louse attaches herself to a hair and slides along it, laying eggs. If hair is not available, clothing fibers are used. Nits are firmly attached to one side of the hair.[1,4,12,13] Crowded living conditions are most conducive to the spread of lice, which can be transmitted either by person-to-person contact or by fomites, such as hairbrushes, caps, scarves, coats, or carpets.[1,4,12] Sharing of clothing is a common source of transmission.

Treatment

The application of 1% gamma benzene hexachloride lotion to the affected skin area for 12 to 24 hours is effective in body-lice infestation.[1,4,14-16] For head-lice or crab-lice infestations, 1% gamma benzene hexachloride shampoo, 1% permethrin shampoo, or 0.3% pyrethrin shampoo applied for 10 minutes and then rinsed out results in an 80% cure rate. Malathion 0.5% lotion left on for 8 to 12 hours is also effective.[1,2] Resistance of head lice to permethrins, pyrethrins, and malathion has been reported.[16,17] Shampoo treatments will not, however, remove the gelatinous nits. The use of a warm damp towel for 30 minutes on the scalp will loosen the nits and allow their mechanical removal with a fine-toothed comb (nit comb). Most pediculocide shampoos are supplied with a nit comb. Retreatment in 7 days is recommended. Measuring the distance of the nit closest to the scalp surface will provide a baseline measurement to help determine adequacy of treatment on follow-up. Boiling of clothing, bedding, and other possible fomites is ovicidal and lousicidal, and it is necessary because nits may be attached to clothing.

Patient Education

It is tempting for parents to use pediculicides repeatedly in children with lice infestations. The clinician should emphasize the hazards of central nervous system and other toxicities posed by such usage. All contacts should be identified and treated simultaneously. Students should be readmitted to school the morning after the first treatment. "No-nit" policies for return to school cannot be justified. Cutting the child's hair short should be discouraged. Parents should be advised that mechanical removal of nits is required. Schoolmates should be examined by the school nurse to determine if other children are infested. For a patient information handout on Head Lice, see p. 337.

Follow-up Visits

An office or visiting nurse follow-up to evaluate therapy 1 week after the initial visit is most helpful. If new eggs or nits are seen on the proximal hair shafts, as close or closer to the scalp than the original measurement, then retreatment is necessary. Nits will grow out with the hair shaft and by 7 days after successful treatment should be at least 6 to 7 mm from the scalp margin.

PAPULAR URTICARIA
Clinical Features

Pruritic erythematous papules, with or without an erythematous, urticarial flare, are characteristically arranged in clusters in papular urticaria (Fig. 7-15). Such clusters are usually seen over the shoulders, upper arms, and buttocks. Papular urticaria occurs predominantly between the ages of 18 months and 7 years.[18] In intense hypersensitivity, vesicles and bullae may be seen (Figs. 7-15 and 7-16). Recurrent crops of these papules are the rule, with each crop

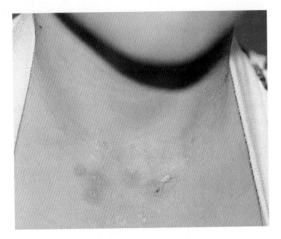

Fig. 7-15 Papular urticaria. Grouped lesions on the lower neck where a puppy was carried by the child.

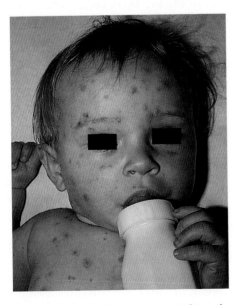

Fig. 7-16 Papular urticaria. Numerous central papules or edematous papules surrounded by an outer zone of urticaria.

lasting 2 to 10 days. Characteristically the affected child is the only household member involved. The problem may persist from 3 to 9 months and most often begins in spring or summer.

Differential Diagnosis

Insect bites, viral exanthems, photoeruptions, acute parapsoriasis, and the early stages of other papulosquamous diseases (see Chapter 9) may be confused with papular urticaria.

Pathogenesis

The lesions represent delayed hypersensitivity reactions to a variety of biting or stinging arthropods.[17,18] Dog and cat fleas are the usual offenders. Less commonly, mosquitoes, lice, scabies, fowl mites, and grain or grass mites are responsible.[1,18] Epicutaneous testing with homogenized arthropods has reproduced the urticarial papule within 4 to 8 hours. The pathologic features of naturally occurring lesions are similar to those of a delayed-type (tuberculin) skin test.

Treatment

The logical therapy is to remove the offending insect. Dogs or cats should be treated for fleas or mites by a veterinarian. The child should be kept away from the pet. Protective clothing, such as long sleeves, may be useful. The prophylactic use of an oral antihistamine, such as cetirizine, may reduce the reactions. Use of insect repellents may make the child less attractive to the insect (see Table 7-1). See p. 338 for a patient information handout on Insect Repellents for Children. The most successful repellent for mosquitoes is Bite Blocker, with DEET-containing insect repellents almost as efficaceous.[2] Caution should be exercised to not use DEET on large areas of skin or in concentrations greater than 10%.[19] DEET preparations that are 6.5 %, listed in Table 7-1, may be used cautiously on the child's skin. Fleas or mites living in carpets or furniture may be eliminated by treatment with a commercial insecticide. Window casings should be treated in the case of bird mites. Symptomatic relief may sometimes be obtained with topical mid-potency glucocorticosteroid creams or ointments applied three times daily.

Patient Education

When only one member of the household is affected, it is difficult to convince some parents of the cause. The extreme sensitivity of the affected person to the offending arthropod should be explained. Often an

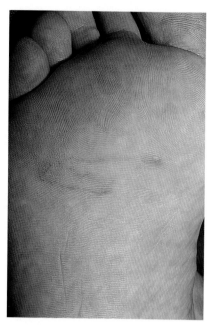

Fig. 7-17 Creeping eruption. Serpiginous red track on the plantar surface of a child with *A. braziliensis* infestation.

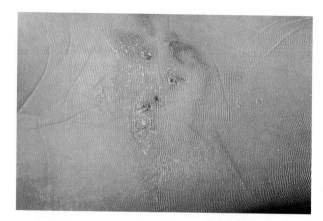

Fig. 7-18 Creeping eruption. Serpiginous tract accompanied by crusted and excoriated lesions from the child's scratching.

obvious source is not evident from the initial history, and a thorough search should be made for the source, including inquiries into day care, preschool, and visits to neighbors, friends, and relatives. It is a great relief to both the parents and the child to learn that the sensitivity is limited to 3 to 6 months. For a patient information handout on Papular Urticaria, see p. 341.

Follow-up Visits

A visit within 2 weeks is most useful in reviewing the possible sources and evaluating the response to therapeutic measures. At the follow-up visit it is often easier to convince parents of the cause of the eruption.

HELMINTHS (PARASITIC WORMS)
Cutaneous Larva Migrans (Creeping Eruption)
Clinical features

Pruritic, serpiginous, erythematous, linear lesions of the skin that advance at the rate of 1 cm/day represent the classic pattern seen in cutaneous larva migrans (Fig. 7-17).[1,21] Lesions are usually on the feet (Fig. 7-18) and occasionally the arms or legs. Vesicles and bullae may be present along the tract, and pulsatile edema within the erythematous, serpiginous tract may be observed. Some children complain of pain at the site, and edema of the area is noted in about 25% of cases. A history of a child having

played along the shorelines of the southeastern or eastern United States is usually obtained. A second clinical form involves strictly the perianal area, buttocks, and thighs, with serpiginous tracts that spread 5 to 10 cm/hr.[1,21] The child may have peripheral blood eosinophilia, with 10% to 35% eosinophils present.

Differential diagnosis

The annular erythemas, including ECM, urticaria, and even tinea infections, may be confused with cutaneous larva migrans. The rapid progression and advancement of the border in cutaneous larva migrans and the presence of pulsations within the serpiginous tract are useful differentiating features.

Pathogenesis

Two larvae are primarily responsible for the cutaneous lesions in cutaneous larva migrans found in North America. *Ancylostoma braziliensis* is the most common of these larvae and produces the clinical pattern involving the feet.[1,21] Children playing along the shore of the southern United States are at the greatest risk. *A. braziliensis* is the dog and cat hookworm, and ova of this organism are deposited in the soil or in the sandy beaches from dog and cat excretions and hatch into larvae that will penetrate bare skin. The larvae migrate 1 to 2 cm/day and produce the serpiginous lesions of the skin. Stools are negative for parasite eggs, and identification of the larvae within the tract is quite difficult because they are often found beyond the area of obvious inflammation. This parasite cannot complete its life cycle in humans, and the larvae disappear within 4 to 6 weeks of their onset.

The second form of cutaneous larva migrans is due to the larvae of *Strongyloides stercoralis*. These larvae usually penetrate the skin near the anus and spread onto the buttocks. They are able to leave the skin and may settle in the gastrointestinal tract, and a stool sample examined for ova and parasites will identify the Strongyloides larvae or eggs. Larvae from fish or squid nematodes may also produce a creeping eruption, particularly among travelers to the Caribbean.[1,20]

Treatment

Topical thiabendazole 15% cream, applied three times a day for 5 to 7 days, is the treatment of choice for creeping eruption caused by *A. braziliensis*. Parents should be instructed to treat well beyond the area of obvious skin redness. Oral thiabendazole is also quite effective in a dose of 25 mg/kg two times a day for 2 days and should be used for creeping eruption caused by *S. stercoralis*.[1,20] Oral albendazole, 400 mg/day for 7 days,[22] and ivermectin, 200 μg/kg as a single dose have also been shown to be efficacious.[1,20]

Patient education

Parents should understand that these infestations may be acquired from sandy beaches or sandboxes, and only in certain regions of North America. Further, they should know that the lesions are not contagious to other children, and that usually one treatment protocol is curative.

Follow-up visits

A visit at 4 to 5 days after initiation of therapy is useful to evaluate the response.

Swimmers' Itch, Seabather's Eruption, and Jellyfish Stings
Clinical features

Pruritic papules appearing in areas not protected by the swimsuit are characteristic of swimmers' eruption, which has occurred in those who have swum in freshwater lakes of the upper Great Lakes region of North America.

In seabather's eruption, the pruritic 2- to 5-mm papules occur under the swimsuit-covered areas after swimming in salt waters of the southern United States.[1,24] Jellyfish stings may be linear when the jellyfish tentacles strike the skin (Fig. 7-19). The papules or linear lesions are persistent and may last for at least 2 weeks.

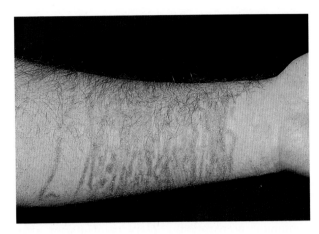

Fig. 7-19 Jellyfish eruption. Multiple linear erythematous areas where jellyfish tentacles contacted the skin.

Differential diagnosis

Papular urticaria, insect bite reactions, and infestations caused by scabies or other mites should be considered in the differential diagnosis. The strong historical and temporal association with swimming is a very useful differentiating point. Linear lesions of jellyfish stings may mimic phytophotodermatitis, in which plants such as tall grasses contact the skin and produce linear erythema or vesicles.

Pathogenesis

Parasitic flatworms have been implicated in swimmers' itch. Cercariae are released into the water from infected snails in freshwater lakes of the upper Great Lakes region. The parasites finish their cycle by penetrating the skin of warm-blooded hosts, but do not survive after penetration. The schistosomes usually come from the droppings of infested mammals and waterfowl and are then involved with the snail as intermediate host.

Seabather's eruption is due to cercariae of the *Linuche ungauiculata* jellyfish. When the seawater containing jellyfish larvae flows through the bathing suit, the larvae contact the skin and discharge nematocysts. Linear lesions of jellyfish stings are the direct result of contact with jellyfish tentacles.

Treatment

Because this is a self-limited disease, no specific anticercarial treatment need be introduced.[25] Symptomatic treatment, such as the use of topical steroid preparations, oral antihistamines, or both, is usually recommended. In severe eruptions, oral prednisone for 5 days may be considered.

Patient education

Parents and patients should be given an explanation of the source of the itchy eruption and should know that it cannot be transmitted from the infested individual to other humans. They should also be told to recognize that this disease is self-limited and will disappear.

Seabather's eruption can be prevented or minimized by showering immediately after removal of swimwear.[22] Immediate application of ice to a jellyfish sting will provide relief, as will topical papain-containing preparations.[23] Hyperpigmentation after jellyfish stings may require months to resolve.

Follow-up visits

Follow-up visits are usually unnecessary.

REFERENCES

1. Angel TA, Nigro J, Levy ML: Infestations in the pediatric patient, *Pediatr Clin North Am* 47:921, 2000.
2. Report of the Committee on Infectious Diseases: *2000 Red book*, Elk Grove Village, Ill, 2000, American Academy of Pediatrics, pp 474, 506.
3. Downs AM, Harvey I, Kennedy CT: The epidemiology of head lice and scabies in the UK, *Epidemiol Infect* 122:471, 1999.
4. Chosidow O: Scabies and pediculosis, *Lancet* 355:819, 2000.
5. Gladstone HB, Darmstadt GL: Crusted scabies in an immunocompetent child: treatment with ivermectin, *Pediatr Dermatol* 17:144, 2000.
6. Jaramillo-Ayerbe F, Berrio-Munoz J: Ivermectin for crusted Norwegian scabies induced by the use of topical steroids, *Arch Dermatol* 134:143, 1998.
7. Meinking TL, Elgart GW: Scabies therapy for the millennium, *Pediatr Dermatol* 17:154, 2000.
8. Usha V, Gopalakrishnan Nair TV: A comparative study of oral ivermectin and topical permethrin cream in the treatment of scabies, *J Am Acad Dermatol* 42:236, 2000.
9. Gardner P: Long-term outcomes and management of patients with Lyme disease, *JAMA* 283:658, 2000.
10. Committee on Infectious Diseases, American Academy of Pediatrics: Prevention of Lyme disease, *Pediatrics* 105:142, 2000.
11. Bond GR: Snake, spider and scorpion envenomation in North America, *Pediatr Rev* 20:147, 1999.
12. Speare R, Buettner PG: Head lice in pupils of a primary school in Australia and implications for control, *Int J Dermatol* 38:285, 1999.
13. Burkhart CN et al: The adherent cylindrical nit structure and its chemical denaturation in vitro: an assessment with therapeutic implications for head lice, *Arch Pediatr Adolesc Med* 152:711, 1998.
14. Pollack RJ, Kisnewski A, Armstrong P: Differential permethrin susceptibility of head lice sampled in the United States and Borneo, *Arch Pediatr Adolesc Med* 153:969, 1999.
15. Burkhart C, Burkhart C, Burkhart K: An assessment of topical and oral prescription and over-the-counter treatments for head lice, *J Am Acad Dermatol* 38:979, 1998.
16. Dawes M, Hicks NR, Fleminger M: Treatment for head lice, *Br Med J* 318:385, 1999.
17. Howard R, Frieden IJ: Papular urticaria in children, *Pediatr Dermatol* 13:246, 1996.
18. Hansen RC: Guidelines for the treatment of resistant pediculosis, *Contemp Pediatrics* 8(suppl):4-10, 2000.
19. Greaves MW: Chronic urticaria in childhood, *Allergy* 55:309, 2000.
20. Fradin MG: Mosquitoes and mosquito repellents: a clinician's guide, *Ann Int Med* 128:931, 1998.
21. Tremblay A et al: Outbreak of cutaneous larval migrans in a group of travelers, *Trop Med Int Health* 5:330, 2000.
22. Grassi A et al: Perianal cutaneous larval migrans in a child, *Pediatr Dermatol* 15:367, 1998.
23. Veraldi S, Rizzitelli G: Effectiveness of a new therapeutic regimen with albendazole in cutaneous larval migrans, *Eur J Dermatol* 9:352, 1999.
24. Kumar S, Hlady WG, Malecki JM: Risk factors for seabather's eruption: a prospective cohort, *Pub Health Rep* 112:59, 1997.
25. Landow K: Best treatment of jellyfish stings? *Postgrad Med* 107:27, 2000.

CHAPTER EIGHT | Viral Infections

Viruses may involve the skin by either dissemination to skin during a systemic viral infection accompanied by viral replication in skin (viral exanthem) or by producing a virus-induced skin tumor. A number of viruses are epidermotropic and replicate within keratinocytes.

VIRAL EXANTHEMS

Any cutaneous eruption associated with an acute viral syndrome has been termed a *viral exanthem*. If mucosa is involved, it is termed an *enanthem*. The exact incidence of viral exanthems is unknown, but herpes simplex alone accounts for a yearly incidence of 5.1 children affected per 1000. Most clinicians who care for children report that viral exanthems are common. Enteroviral and adenoviral exanthems are the most frequently encountered in the United States and account for the majority of viral exanthems seen.[1] It should be emphasized that all viruses may cause an exanthem, including those that are rarely associated with one.[1]

Viral exanthems are seen frequently in general pediatric settings and are considered in the differential diagnosis of drug eruptions. Frequently the clinician will see a child with a generalized eruption who received a medication for the illness. There is no current method to reliably distinguish a viral exanthem from a drug eruption. A variety of different patterns of viral exanthem are seen: a generalized maculopapular eruption that mimics measles (morbilliform), petechial eruptions, vesiculobullous eruptions, scarlet fever–like (scarlatiniform) eruptions, papulonodular eruptions, and oral erosions.[1] Morbilliform eruptions are the most common. It is important to recall that any viral exanthem, including morbilliform eruptions, may have a photodistribution or be exaggerated in areas of prior skin inflammation.[1-4] Some exanthems may also be photoactivated by ultraviolet injury.[4] Skin injury by factors other than ultraviolet light may also result in localization of the viral exanthem to the site of injury.[3] Exanthems may also be unilateral, as reported in the asymmetric periflexural exanthem (Fig. 8-1).[5,6]

VIRAL EXANTHEMS: THE MORBILLIFORM ERUPTIONS

Eruptions that mimic measles (morbilli) are called *morbilliform eruptions.*[1,7] They are seen as generalized, discrete, red to pink macules. The morbilliform eruptions include measles, rubella, enteroviral and adenoviral exanthems, roseola, the mononucleosis syndromes, and erythema infectiosum (EI).[1,7] In immunized children, other viruses may mimic measles and rubella. Parvovirus B19, enteroviruses, and adenoviruses are the most likely causes of morbilliform eruptions in immunized children.[1,7-10] Many other viruses may occasionally produce a morbilliform eruption (Box 8-1).[10]

Measles (Rubeola)
Clinical features

Classic measles. The features of classic measles include a severe prodrome followed by an exanthematous phase. During the entire course of the illness, the child appears quite ill. After an incubation period of 9 to 14 days, a prodrome of high fever, cough, rhinitis, and conjunctivitis appears.[1,7] The cough is described as barking, and a diagnosis of bronchitis or croup is usually considered. The prodrome typically includes cervical lymphadenopathy and lasts 3 to 5 days.[7] The preauricular lymph nodes are enlarged. The prodrome is then followed by a cutaneous eruption.

The exanthem begins on the forehead as blotchy erythema and progresses to involve the face, trunk, and extremities, with multiple discrete macules and papules (Fig. 8-2). The eruption is preceded by intense erythema of the mucous membranes with focal 1 mm white areas, the so-called *Koplik's spots* (Fig. 8-3).[7,12] Bacterial otitis media, bacterial pneumonia, and encephalitis may complicate measles.[1,7] Their exact incidence in measles is unknown. Severe pneumonia and encephalitis are primary causes of death in measles and are more likely to complicate measles in young infants and the malnourished or immunodeficient child. Mortality related to measles in the United States is estimated at 1 per 1000.[1,7,11] Low vitamin-A levels, in particular, have been implicated

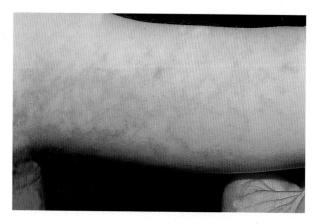

Fig. 8-1 Asymmetric periflexural exanthem. Annular erythema on the inner arm and adjacent axilla in an 8-year-old child.

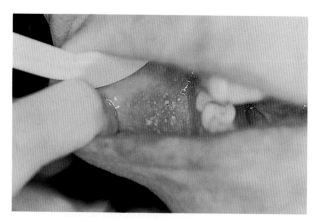

Fig. 8-2 Red macules and conjunctival erythema in a child with rubeola (measles).

Box 8-1 Differential Diagnosis of Morbilliform Eruptions Caused By Viruses

Measles (rubeola)
Rubella
Roseola
Boston exanthem
Erythema infectiosum
Infectious mononucleosis
Pityriasis rosea (presumed viral)
Hepatitis
Mumps
Echoviruses 1, 2, 4, 5, 7, 9, 13, 14, 22, 25, 30
Reoviruses 2, 3
Coxsackieviruses A1, 2, 3, 4, 5, 7
Respiratory syncytial virus
Cytomegalovirus
Adenoviruses 1, 2, 3, 4, 5, 7
Colorado tick fever
Dengue
Herpesvirus 6
Echovirus 16
Parvovirus B19
Epstein-Barr virus

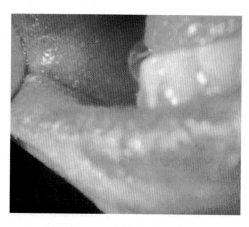

Fig. 8-3 Koplik's spots. Bright erythema of buccal mucosa with pinpoint white macules in rubeola.

cination has failed, a syndrome of high fever, abdominal pain, pulmonary consolidation, and an acral eruption consisting of vesicular, vesiculopustular, or purpuric lesions may occur (atypical measles) (Fig. 8-4). This is rarely observed in the United States.

Differential diagnosis

Classic measles. The severity of the prodrome, a high fever, and Koplik's spots in an acutely ill child are the most distinctive features differentiating measles from the other morbilliform eruptions (Boxes 8-1 and 8-2). Viral isolation from mucosa, although difficult, will distinguish measles from other exanthems. Acute and convalescent sera, obtained 1 week and 3 weeks after the onset of the illness, will assist with a retrospective diagnosis.[14]

in the severity of measles.[7,13] Other complications of measles include myocarditis, pericarditis, thrombocytopenia, hepatitis, acute glomerulonephritis, and Stevens-Johnson syndrome.

Atypical measles. In patients who have received killed measles vaccine, or in whom live measles vac-

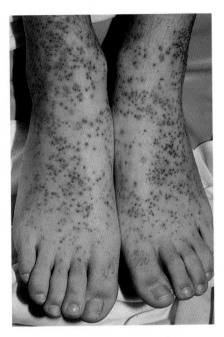

Fig. 8-4 Petechiae and palpable purpura on the feet of an adolescent with atypical measles.

Atypical measles. Atypical measles may mimic meningococcemia and Rocky Mountain spotted fever, which are the main considerations in the differential diagnosis. Primarily acral petechiae may be the presenting symptom in echovirus 9 and other enterovirus infections. Other conditions to be considered in the differential diagnosis are listed in Box 8-3.

Pathogenesis

Despite the very active measles immunization program in the United States, outbreaks of measles continue to occur.[11] Measles has not been eradicated but is at the lowest incidence reported in the United States.[11] The cutaneous eruption is related to the presence of the measles virus within keratinocytes and endothelial cells of the superficial dermal vessels.[7,15] The clinical lesions are believed to be due to the host response to the virus within the skin. The measles virus, a paramyxovirus, replicates within keratinocytes and induces increased nuclear volume within the epidermal cells, producing multinucleated giant cells (Warthin-Finkeldy cells).[15]

The purpuric cutaneous eruption of atypical measles is thought to be the result of immune complex formation.[16]

Treatment

No specific treatment is available for classic or atypical measles. For children 1 year of age and older a

---

Box 8-2 Differential Diagnosis of Morbilliform Eruptions

COMMON VIRUSES
Measles
Rubella
Roseola
Erythema infectiosum
Infectious mononucleosis
Pityriasis rosea

COMMON BACTERIA
Scarlet fever

DRUG ERUPTIONS
Ampicillin
Penicillin
Nonsteroidal antiinflammatory drugs
Salicylic acid
Barbiturates
Phenytoins
Phenothiazines
Thiazide diuretics
Isoniazid

PAPULOSQUAMOUS DISORDERS
Guttate psoriasis
Graft-vs.-host disease

REACTIVE ERYTHEMAS
Urticaria
Papular urticaria
Erythema multiforme

Box 8-3 Differential Diagnosis of the STAR* Complex

Rubella
Human parvovirus B19
Hepatitis B
Adenovirus
Echoviruses
Coxsackieviruses
Epstein-Barr virus

*STAR, Sore throat, arthritis, rash.

single oral dose of 200,000 IU of vitamin A is recommended.[7] For children with evidence of vitamin-A deficiency, the dose should be repeated in 1 day and at 4 weeks. Symptoms should be treated and children should be closely monitored for complications. If secondary bacterial otitis media or bacterial pneumonia occurs, antibiotic therapy should be instituted.

Patient education

The high attack rate of measles should be emphasized, and the patient should be isolated during the contagious period (from the onset of respiratory symptoms through the third day of the cutaneous eruption). Unimmunized normal infants under 1 year of age and immunosuppressed children should receive a preventive dose of immune serum globulin, 0.25 ml/kg intramuscularly, as soon as possible after exposure.[7] Unvaccinated infants and children with malignancies or immunodeficiencies, or those receiving immunosuppressive therapy, should be given 0.5 ml/kg of immune serum globulin intramuscularly to a maximum dose of 15 ml. Exposure to measles is not a contraindication to vaccination if given within 72 hours of exposure. Outbreaks should be reported to local public health authorities.

Follow-up visits

Close contact should be maintained with the patient with rubeola to watch for bacterial superinfection, the development of severe pneumonia with pulmonary compromise, or encephalitis. A prompt revisit should be scheduled if fever recurs, headache or change in the level of consciousness is observed, or seizures or motor defects are noted. Frequent visits may be required during the course of the illness.

Rubella
Clinical features

Classic rubella. Classic rubella is a mild illness in most children.[3,7,10,17-20] Rubella acquired postnatally in infants and children usually is accompanied by few or no prodromal symptoms. Up to 50% of rubella infections may be entirely asymptomatic.[7,10,17-20] Mild lymphadenopathy may precede the cutaneous eruption by several days. The suboccipital and posterior auricular lymph nodes are usually prominently enlarged. A faint pink, macular eruption appears first on the face and spreads to the trunk and proximal extremities. Within 48 hours, the face and trunk have cleared and the eruption involves the distal extremi-

ties. The child usually appears well. Rarely, petechiae or purpura may be seen. A monarthric arthritis may accompany the syndrome, particularly in adolescent girls.[17-20] It may present as the so-called *STAR* (*s*ore *t*hroat, *a*rthritis, *r*ash) *complex*.[21] In the STAR complex, rubella and human parvovirus B19 are the most likely viruses responsible.[21] The arthritis may persist for several months. Fever is usually absent or low-grade in young children with rubella, but may be present in older children and adolescents, particularly when arthritis is present.[3,7,17-19]

Congenital rubella. Rubella acquired during the first trimester of pregnancy may result in rubella embryopathy.[18-20] This may be manifested by neonatal purpura and petechiae caused by thrombocytopenia. Of cases of congenital thrombocytopenia, rubella is responsible for 10%.[19-20] Occasionally, jaundice caused by rubella hepatitis occurs. Accompanying features include deafness, congenital heart defects, cataract, retinopathy, glaucoma, growth retardation, behavioral disorders, meningoencephalitis, and psychomotor retardation.[18-20] Any or all of these features may accompany the typical rubella exanthem. Rubella embryopathy can even be found during reinfection of the mother with rubella.[20] The exanthem may recur any time during the first 5 years. In infants with congenital rubella, rubella virus may be recovered from peripheral blood leukocytes, stool, or urine for months to years after birth.

Differential diagnosis

Classic rubella. In distinguishing classic rubella from rubeola, the absence of fever is helpful. Rubella may be difficult to distinguish from enteroviral exanthems, infectious mononucleosis syndromes, parvovirus B19 infections, or drug eruptions.[19] In the STAR complex, rubella may be indistinguishable from human parvovirus B19 infections or from other viral causes of the exanthem (see Box 8-3).[21] Culture of the virus from nasal mucosa will distinguish rubella from other exanthems.

Congenital rubella. Other congenital infections may produce the thrombocytopenia and hepatitis seen with rubella.[18,20] These include toxoplasmosis, syphilis, cytomegalovirus (CMV), and herpes simplex virus (HSV). Rarely, neonatal lupus, Wiskott-Aldrich syndrome, and hereditary platelet disorders may mimic congenital rubella. The presence of cataracts and congenital heart defects should suggest congenital rubella. Viral cultures of urine and throat will distinguish rubella from other congenital infections.

Pathogenesis

Rubella virus, a rubrivirus, is a ribonucleic acid (RNA) virus that enters the bloodstream via the respiratory mucosa.[7] The mechanism of the exanthem is unknown but is believed to be the result of viral dissemination to skin. Rubella virus has been cultured from the synovia in rubella arthritis. Rubella embryopathy is still seen because young women are vaccine failures or have not received the vaccine. The exact mechanism of the embryopathy is unknown.[20]

Treatment

There is no specific treatment for rubella. If the patient is febrile, fever-control measures will suffice. Nonsteroidal antiinflammatory agents may be required for the arthritis. The management of rubella embryopathy requires a multidisciplinary team to include ophthalmologists, cardiologists, neurologists, and developmental specialists.

Patient education

Exposure or potential exposure of susceptible women in the first trimester of pregnancy should be determined. If possible, the rubella patient should be kept isolated from pregnant women for 7 days after the rash has appeared.[7] In patients who acquire rubella postnatally, it is contagious from 2 days before the onset of the cutaneous eruption to 7 days after the onset. In congenital rubella, virus shedding usually ends by age 6 months but may continue up to 5 or 6 years.[7] The incubation period ranges from 14 to 21 days.[7]

When a pregnant woman is exposed to rubella, a serum specimen should be obtained and tested for rubella antibody.[7] If antibody is present, there is no risk of infection. If no rubella antibody is detectable, a second blood specimen should be obtained 2 or 3 weeks later. If antibody is present in the second specimen and not the first, infection is presumed to have occurred, and termination of pregnancy may be considered. If termination of pregnancy is not an option, immune serum globulin should be given, 0.55 ml/kg intramuscularly.[7]

Follow-up visits

Follow-up visits are usually unnecessary in postnatally acquired rubella. In congenital rubella a multidisciplinary approach, such as that offered by a birth defects clinic, is advisable.

Roseola (Exanthem Subitum, Human Herpesvirus 6 Infection)
Clinical features

Roseola occurs predominantly in infants under 2 years of age.[7,22,23] It is characterized by 2 or 3 days of sustained fever in an infant who otherwise appears well, following which the temperature falls (often to a subnormal level), and a pink, morbilliform, cutaneous eruption appears transiently and fades within 24 hours (Fig. 8-5). A convulsion at the onset of fever is noted occasionally, but the exact incidence of febrile convulsions is unknown.[23] Mild edema of the eyelids and posterior cervical lymphadenopathy are occasionally seen. More frequently, human herpesvirus type 6 (HHV-6) infection produces an illness with cough, fever, and otitis media or a febrile convulsion.[22-24] An infantile infectious mononucleosis syndrome has also been described.[22,23] HHV-6 infections are predominantly acute febrile illnesses in infants under 24 months of age.[7,22,23]

Differential diagnosis

Roseola can be distinguished from most other morbilliform eruptions (see Boxes 8-1 and 8-2) by the distinctive history of 3 days of sustained fever in an infant followed by the appearance of a morbilliform eruption after the fever ends. It may be indistinguishable from echovirus 16 infections. Eruptions resulting from treatment with drugs may easily be confused with roseola in infants who received antibiotics for the febrile portion of the illness. The HHV-6 infections that cause otitis media may be difficult to distinguish from bacterial otitis media, and the infectious mononucleosis syndrome mimics illness induced by

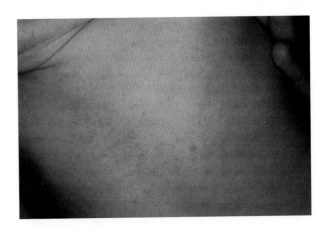

Fig. 8-5 Roseola. Faint pink papules on the trunk of an infant with HHV-6 infection.

the Epstein-Barr virus (EBV), CMV, or HHV-7. The febrile convulsion may mimic bacterial or viral meningitis. HHV-6 can be identified by culture of peripheral blood leukocytes, by serodiagnosis, or from skin lesions by molecular diagnosis.[7,22-24]

Pathogenesis

HHV-6 infection is thought to be the major causative agent for roseola worldwide, whereas in North America, children with echovirus 16 infections probably account for some cases of roseola.[22,23] HHV-6 is a herpes-group virus that preferentially involves circulating leukocytes. It produces predominantly acute febrile illnesses in infants, and it may be associated with a few cases of infectious mononucleosis, leukemias, or histiocytic syndromes.[23]

Treatment

In roseola, fever can be controlled with wet dressings or tepid-water sponge baths, supplemental fluids, and antipyretics. HHV-6 is insensitive to current antiviral agents, but in immunocompromised children with severe disease some authorities recommend treatment with ganciclovir.[7]

Patient education

Parents should be informed of the viral nature of this disorder and told that there is no necessity for antibiotics. If the child is seen during the febrile state, it is worthwhile to document the morbilliform eruption by personally observing it. Parents should be told that the virus responsible for roseola predominantly infects children under 24 months of age, and most older children and adults are immune.

Follow-up visits

To be certain to exclude other infections that may mimic roseola, a follow-up visit 2 days later to ascertain the course of the illness is recommended.

Human Parvovirus B19 Infection (Erythema Infectiosum)
Clinical features

The eruptions of EI (fifth disease) classically begin with an intense, confluent redness of both cheeks, the so-called *slapped-cheek appearance* (Fig. 8-6), seen in 75% of patients.[7,25-28] It may then spread to involve the arms (86%), legs (75%), chest (47%), and abdomen (45%), with a lacy, pink to dull-red macular eruption (Figs. 8-7 and 8-8); 25% of patients will have only the lacy eruption on their extremities. The original eruption lasts from 3 to 5 days. Stimulation

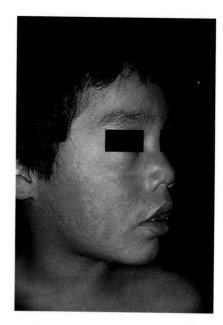

Fig. 8-6 Slapped-cheek appearance of a child with parvovirus B19 infection (erythema infectiosum).

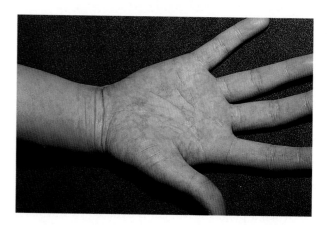

Fig. 8-7 Lacy pink eruption over the palms in erythema infectiosum.

of cutaneous vasodilation, however, will cause the eruption to reappear up to 4 months later.[26,27] This may result from vigorous exercise, overheating of the skin, or sun exposure. Only 20% of affected children will have mild fever. Occasionally, morbilliform, vesicular, or purpuric skin eruptions are seen. A purpuric hand and foot eruption (purpuric gloves-and-socks syndrome) may develop.[7,25,27] About 20% of infected children and adults are asymptomatic. During some outbreaks of EI, symmetric arthritis of hands, wrists, or knees will be observed.[7,21,26] The STAR complex is caused by parvovirus B19 equally

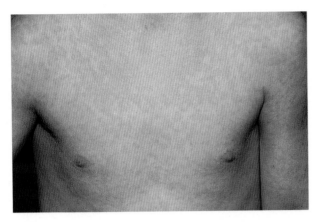

Fig. 8-8 Lacy pink eruption on chest and upper abdomen.

Box 8-4   Morbilliform Viral Exanthems With Petechiae

Echovirus 9
EBV
Hepatitis
Atypical measles
Echoviruses 4, 7
Coxsackievirus A9
Respiratory syncytial virus
Rubella
Dengue
Parvovirus B19 (petechial gloves-and-socks syndrome)

---

as often as by rubella.[21] Joint symptoms usually resolve in 1 to 2 months. In patients with chronic hemolytic anemias, EI may be the cause of transient aplastic crises, and in immunosuppressed children it may be responsible for red-cell aplasia and severe anemia.[7,26,28] Immunosuppressed children may be susceptible to persistent infection.[7] Conjunctivitis may occasionally be a presenting symptom, and chronic infection has resulted in a picture of systemic necrotizing vasculitis.[7,26] EI in pregnant women may result in fetal death.[7,26,28]

Differential diagnosis

Drug eruptions and the other morbilliform eruptions may be considered in the differential diagnosis, but the lacy, mottled appearance of the EI eruption is characteristic. Occasionally the more violaceous livedo reticularis pattern of skin mottling associated with collagen vascular disease (periarteritis nodosa or lupus erythematosus) may be confused with EI, especially if associated with arthropathy. The STAR complex can also be caused by rubella and other viruses (see Box 8-3).[21] The petechial or purpuric gloves-and-socks syndrome[25] should be differentiated from other petechial exanthems, such as enteroviral infections (Box 8-4). Diagnosis can be confirmed by analysis of serum obtained within 30 days of the onset of illness for the presence of immunoglobulin M (IgM) B19 antibodies.[29]

Pathogenesis

Human parvovirus B19 is the causative agent of EI.[7,25-29] The virus has been identified within EI skin lesions. The organism replicates in erythroid bone marrow cells, accounting for its role in red-cell aplasia of immunodeficiency and transient aplastic crises in children with chronic hemolytic anemias.[7,26] Suscep-

tibility to infection has been linked to the presence of the erythrocyte P antigen, which serves as the receptor for parvovirus B19.[26,30] It is thought that hereditary lack of the receptor is protective against infection.[30] Among other viruses, Parvovirus B19 has been implicated in the etiology of Kawasaki disease (see Chapter 11), although the association is controversial.[31-34]

Treatment

There is no specific treatment for EI, nor are there any specific control measures, although isolation of patients at risk for complications (pregnant women, immunosuppressed patients, patients with chronic hemolytic anemia) is recommended.[7] Administration of intravenous immunoglobulins may be effective in immunosuppressed children.[7] The disease may no longer be contagious once the skin eruption occurs.

Patient education

The patient or family should be informed of the dangers of parvovirus B19 virus to pregnant women, immunosuppressed patients, and patients with chronic hemolytic anemia (e.g., sickle cell disease). They should be advised to keep the infected child away from these individuals for 2 weeks, and good hand-washing techniques in the affected family should be emphasized. Pregnant women should be offered serologic testing for IgG antibody, and fetal ultrasonography may be useful. Children with EI may return to school or day care because they are no longer infectious.[7] They should also be told of the likely reappearance of the cutaneous eruption for up to 4 months. In children with the STAR complex, the likelihood of persistence of the arthritis should be emphasized.

Follow-up visits

Follow-up visits are unnecessary for the child with normal immunity unless arthritis or exposure of persons at risk is involved.

Echovirus Exanthems
Clinical features

Echovirus exanthems result in morbilliform eruptions associated with two predominant clinical patterns: a roseola-like pattern and the petechial pattern. Infants and toddlers are more likely to have a viral rash with echovirus infections than are older children.[35,36] Echovirus 16 infection in children is usually seen in epidemic form and may mimic roseola in that the cutaneous eruption may appear after the end of 2 or 3 days of fever.[7,8] Since its first report, it has been known as the *Boston exanthem,* although it is found worldwide. The eruption is characteristically morbilliform, but vesicles or punched-out erosions have occasionally been described. The morbilliform eruption lasts 1 to 5 days. Cervical, suboccipital, and postauricular lymphadenopathy are seen. Aseptic meningitis may occasionally occur, but it is usually seen in children without the cutaneous eruption.

Echovirus 9 results in a morbilliform eruption with acral petechiae (Fig. 8-9). Although a great number of viral infections may present with petechial eruptions (see Box 8-4), echovirus 9 accounts for most epidemics of petechial eruptions.[35,36] Echovirus 9 infects preschool children primarily, and they present with a syndrome of fever, sore throat, abdominal pain, and vomiting. Echoviruses 2, 4, 6, 11, 25, and 30 produce similar morbilliform exanthems, often without gastrointestinal symptoms (Fig. 8-10). Aseptic meningitis is common.[7,35,36] The petechial eruption lasts 2 to 7 days. Some coxsackieviruses produce similar clinical patterns. Complete recovery follows.

Differential diagnosis

Roseola caused by HHV-6 should be considered in the differential diagnosis of echovirus morbilliform eruptions (see Boxes 8-1 and 8-2). Roseola may mimic the Boston exanthem, but the fever and eruption in the latter often overlap. The identification of echovirus 16 in stools or throat washings helps to distinguish between these two disorders.[35,36] Atypical measles, Rocky Mountain spotted fever, and meningococcemia are the major considerations of serious diseases in the differential diagnosis of echovirus 9 infections (see Box 8-4). Other echoviruses, streptococcal infections, EBV, hepatitis, rubella, coxsackieviruses, dengue, and typhus may also be considered.

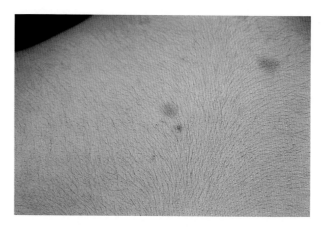

Fig. 8-9 Discrete red macules and a petechia in a child with echovirus infection.

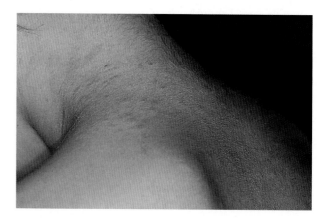

Fig. 8-10 Enterovirus exanthem. Pink papules over the back.

Pathogenesis

Echoviruses are small RNA viruses of the picornavirus group, which have been found worldwide.[7] There are 31 known types. The viruses are characteristically "summer" viruses and produce epidemics, particularly in crowded living conditions. The incubation period is 3 to 5 days when the virus is spread by the enteric route.[7,35,36] The viruses use decay-accelerating factor (CD55) as a receptor.[35,36] Despite enteric replication of the echovirus, gastrointestinal symptoms are uncommon, except for ECHO 9. It is not known whether the virus appears within the cutaneous eruption. The mechanism that produces the cutaneous eruption is also unknown.

Treatment

There is no specific treatment. Symptomatic fever control is useful.

Patient education

The contagious nature of the disease should be emphasized.

Follow-up visits

Follow-up visits are unnecessary.

Infectious Mononucleosis (Human Herpesvirus 4, 5, 6, and 7 Infections)
Clinical features

The annual incidence of infectious mononucleosis is estimated at 50 per 100,000 children, with the highest incidence found among adolescents and young adults.[7,37] As opposed to acute viral infections, the onset is often insidious. The usual presenting symptoms and signs are fatigue (100%), fever (in 85%), generalized lymphadenopathy (85%), sore throat with exudative tonsillitis (70%), headache (45%), and splenomegaly (45%).[37-41] Jaundice and hepatomegaly occur in up to 30% of patients. A pink, fleeting morbilliform eruption occurs in 15% of patients and may last 1 to 5 days.[7,37,41] Treatment of children with infectious mononucleosis with ampicillin, penicillin, or azithromycin for the sore throat results in an increase in incidence of morbilliform eruption in up to 80% of patients.[7,39] With antibiotic use, the eruption becomes bright red and more papular and may persist for 7 to 10 days (Fig. 8-11). The morbilliform eruption is the most characteristic seen with infectious mononucleosis, but occasionally other cutaneous eruptions may occur. Urticaria has been described as a prominent presenting feature, and petechial eruptions associated with thrombocytopenia may be seen occasionally.[7,37,41] Palmar erythema has also been reported as a presenting symptom of infectious mononucleosis. Neurologic symptoms, such as spatial and visual distortion or signs of encephalitis, meningitis, neuritis, or Guillain-Barré syndrome, may accompany the cutaneous eruption.

The acute phase with fever and sore throat lasts 2 to 3 weeks. Extreme fatigue and lethargy may persist for 3 months, however.[7,37,41] Rare complications include splenic rupture, thrombocytopenia, agranulocytosis, hemolytic anemia, orchitis, and cardiac involvement.[41] Blood transfusions may occasionally precede the onset of mononucleosis because the viral agents are carried in leukocytes.[7,37-41] In children infected with the human immunodeficiency virus (HIV), EBV infections are commonly seen.[7,41]

Differential diagnosis

Laboratory studies are most useful in aiding with the diagnosis, with the detection of heterophil antibodies

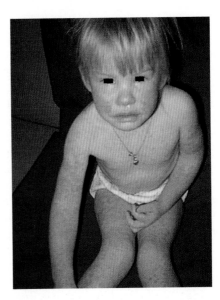

Fig. 8-11 Child with bright red morbilliform eruption caused by infectious mononucleosis plus ampicillin.

Table 8-1 Frequency of Laboratory Findings in Infectious Mononucleosis	
Finding	**Patients (%)**
Epstein-Barr virus antibody IgG or IgM	85
Lymphocytosis	92
Atypical mononuclear cells in peripheral blood film	92
Liver enzyme abnormalities	80
Hypergammaglobulinemia	80
Heterophil antibodies	75
Indirect Coombs' test	50
Thrombocytopenia	50
Hyperbilirubinemia	40

by Paul-Bunnell test as the most important diagnostic criterion.[7,40,41] The laboratory findings most often encountered and their frequencies are shown in Table 8-1. During the early phase of infectious mononucleosis, the possibility of streptococcal pharyngitis is usually considered, as are other causes of pharyngitis. Infectious mononucleosis can be distinguished from the other morbilliform eruptions (see Boxes 8-1 and 8-2) by its prolonged course, the prominent symptom of excessive fatigue, and the laboratory findings. If arthritis occurs, it must be differentiated from rubella or parvovirus B19 as causes of the STAR complex (see Box 8-3).[21] The petechial eruption must be differentiated from other causes of thrombocytopenic purpura in children, such as idiopathic thrombocytopenic purpura, lupus erythematosus, and malignancies. A similar syndrome may be produced by CMV, HHV-6 and HHV-7, rubella, and parvovirus B19, but exudative tonsillitis and heterophil antibodies are not present (see Table 8-1).[1,19,21,22] EBV mononucleosis is most prevalent in the adolescent, whereas CMV and others are most prevalent in infantile and childhood mononucleosis. Tests of serum for IgM anti-EBV viral capsid antigen or isolation of EBV from oropharyngeal secretions will distinguish.[7,40,41]

Pathogenesis

It is now accepted that EBV (HHV-4) is responsible for most cases (85%) of infectious mononucleosis.[7,37-39,41] The incubation period is 4 to 8 weeks in adolescents but is usually shorter in prepubertal children. The period of communicability is uncertain because most patients with infectious mononucleosis excrete small amounts of virus for months after the onset of symptoms, and there are asymptomatic carriers of EBV. In crowded conditions, intrafamilial spread of EBV is common, and infants may be infected. HHV-5 (CMV), HHV-6 and HHV-7, and parvovirus B19 may be responsible for the infectious mononucleosis syndrome, particularly in infants and toddlers.[37,41]

Treatment

In mild cases no treatment is required. In hemolytic anemia, thrombocytopenic purpura, airway interference, neurologic involvement, or in selected patients with toxemia and prolonged fever, systemic glucocorticosteroids may be given. Prednisone, 2 or 3 mg/kg/day for 3 days, is recommended for adolescents. Ampicillin or penicillin should not be administered in routine cases because of the high frequency of drug rashes. Acyclovir has yet to be convincingly demonstrated to be efficacious in infectious mononucleosis, but the drug is active against EBV in vitro.[42]

Patient education

Concern that the spleen may rupture, which occurs in 0.5% of patients, should prompt avoidance of contact sports or other vigorous activity in which abdominal injury is likely.[7,37,41] Neurologic complications occur in 1.5% of cases, and patients should be warned about mental symptoms such as hallucinations and mood changes. They should also be ap-

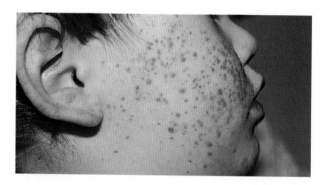

Fig. 8-12 Gianotti-Crosti syndrome. Multiple discrete papules on the cheek.

prised of the prolonged convalescence from this disorder and of the need to increase activities in a stepwise fashion.

Follow-up visits

Weekly visits should be scheduled in patients with mild to moderate disease to ascertain the course of the disease and observe for complications. In severe disease daily visits or hospitalization may be necessary.

Papular Acrodermatitis (Gianotti-Crosti Syndrome)
Clinical features

A distinct eruption called *papular acrodermatitis* (Gianotti-Crosti disease) is characterized by groups of large, flat-topped, nonpruritic papules that appear in acral areas.[43] Involvement of the cheeks (Fig. 8-12), buttocks, and limbs is characteristic. Papules are particularly prominent over the hands (Fig. 8-13), elbows, and knees (Fig. 8-14), although with some outbreaks the distribution is more widespread.[43,44] The skin lesions may be preceded by low-grade fever and mild upper respiratory tract symptoms. Of children described as having this syndrome, 85% are less than 3 years of age, although it may occur in school-age children. The eruption persists unchanged for 2 to 8 weeks and may be recurrent.[43,44] Generalized lymph-adenopathy and hepatosplenomegaly develop in some children along with the cutaneous eruption. In such children, atypical lymphocytes are seen in peripheral blood films, and liver enzyme levels, especially serum aminotransferases, are elevated. EBV has been associated with outbreaks of papular acrodermatitis in North America,[44,45] and other viruses such as CMV and coxsackievirus A16 may be involved (Box 8-5).

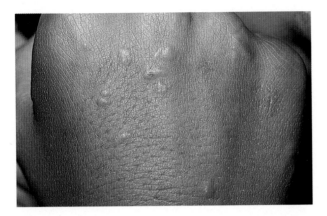

Fig. 8-13 Gianotti-Crosti syndrome. Skin-colored papules on top of the hand.

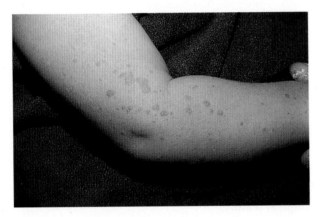

Fig. 8-14 Gianotti-Crosti syndrome. Grouped papules on the proximal extremities.

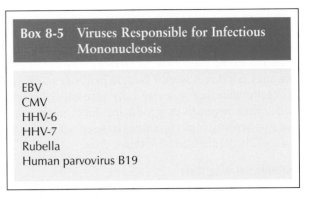

Box 8-5	Viruses Responsible for Infectious Mononucleosis

EBV
CMV
HHV-6
HHV-7
Rubella
Human parvovirus B19

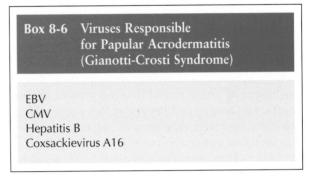

Box 8-6	Viruses Responsible for Papular Acrodermatitis (Gianotti-Crosti Syndrome)

EBV
CMV
Hepatitis B
Coxsackievirus A16

In Europe 30% of patients with papular acrodermatitis have mild viral hepatitis B; hepatitis B surface antigen (HBsAg) has been demonstrated in the lymph nodes in such children, with liver biopsy findings consistent with acute viral hepatitis.[43]

Differential diagnosis

In irritant contact dermatitis, atopic dermatitis, and lichen planus, flat-topped acral papules that mimic papular acrodermatitis may be seen, but they are usually associated with severe pruritus and disruption of the skin surface.

Pathogenesis

In infants with papular acrodermatitis in the United States, EBV has been identified, but in a few CMV or coxsackievirus A16 has been associated (Box 8-6).

Treatment

No treatment is needed for Gianotti-Crosti syndrome. Individual lesions are not responsive to topical steroids.

Patient education

The prolonged nature of the Gianotti-Crosti syndrome eruption should be emphasized. It should also be emphasized that several virus agents may be responsible for papular acrodermatitis, and its significance is the prolonged course.

Follow-up visits

Follow-up visits are unnecessary unless hepatosplenomegaly is present.

Hepatitis Viruses
Clinical features

Although viral hepatitis is usually not associated with exanthems, it is a disease that should not be overlooked when searching for the cause of a viral exanthem. Exanthems associated with hepatitis viruses A, B, C, and E are primarily morbilliform, but urticarial and scarlatiniform eruptions have been described.[7,46-49] Children infected with hepatitis A often have nonspecific symptoms of low-grade fever, irritability, and upper respiratory tract symptoms without cutaneous involvement or mild jaundice.[7] Subclinical hepatitis is more likely to occur in a 10 to 1 ratio. The morbilliform eruption of hepatitis A, B, and E (Fig. 8-15) characteristically precedes the icteric stage by 1 to 10 days. The entire disease may last 3 to 4 weeks. Both hepatitis A and E are primarily waterborne, enterically transmitted infections, with hepatitis A producing local outbreaks, whereas hepatitis E has produced large epidemics in the Indian subcontinent and Southeast Asia.[7]

Differential diagnosis

The other viral exanthems, particularly rubella and parvovirus B19, should be considered during the prodromal phase of morbilliform and urticarial eruptions (see Boxes 8-1 and 8-2). Urticaria resulting from other causes may be impossible to distinguish. The serum aminotransferase levels will be markedly elevated early in hepatitis, and will be an important distinguishing test. The eventual development of icterus, hepatic tenderness, and hepatic enlargement will allow a retrospective diagnosis of hepatitis. Pruritus may be severe during the icteric phase, particularly in hepatitis E. Diagnosis is usually made by the serologic test for IgM antihepatitis A or IgM antihepatitis E by enzyme-linked immunosorbent assay (ELISA) or radioimmunoassay.[7]

Pathogenesis

Both hepatitis A and E are single-stranded RNA viruses that replicate in the liver but not the bowel. Virus shedding into the bowel occurs during the prodromal phase and may last throughout the remainder of the illness. A viremic phase may occur that is believed to be responsible for the cutaneous eruptions. The usual source of infection is human feces through contaminated water supplies and food, particularly shellfish.

Treatment

Only symptomatic treatment is usually given. Bed rest and adequate diet are supportive measures. For exposed individuals, human immune serum globulin, 0.02 ml/kg, is given as soon as possible after exposure.[50] It is not known whether hepatitis A vaccines given after exposure are preventive.[7,50]

Patient education

It should be emphasized that both hepatitis A and E are transmitted by the enteric route and possibly the oral route. Contaminated food or water sources should be sought. The importance of personal hygienic measures, such as hand washing, in preventing spread should be emphasized.[7,50] Vaccination for hepatitis A is recommended for children living in high-risk areas.[7,50]

Follow-up visits

Patients should be seen weekly until the jaundice has disappeared. Although the course is benign in 95% of children, hepatitis is variable and may progress to liver failure.

Hepatitis B, C, and D Infections
Clinical features

Urticarial and serum-sickness–like eruptions are the most common skin eruptions seen with hepatitis B, and hepatitis-associated antigen may be detected in these children 10 days after the eruption appears. Icterus usually does not develop.

If a child is infected with both hepatitis B and D, a fulminant picture of severe jaundice, with encephalopathy, bleeding, and fluid and electrolyte imbalance may ensue.

The urticarial or serum-sickness–like eruption of hepatitis B and C is characterized by joint swelling and fixed urticaria.[48] It lasts 7 to 10 days and resolves with the onset of hepatic symptoms. Anaphylactoid purpura with purpuric papules on the distal extremities and a periarteritis nodosa pattern are rarely associated with hepatitis B infection.[7]

Differential diagnosis

A serum-sickness reaction resulting from drugs or serum products, or from rubella or parvovirus B19 in-

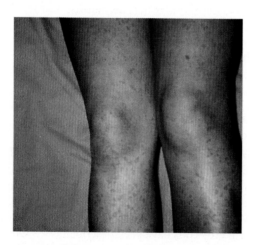

Fig. 8-15 Morbilliform eruption of the legs in an adolescent with preicteric hepatitis.

fections, may mimic the prodrome of hepatitis. In hepatitis, however, the joint swelling is usually symmetric, in contrast to rubella, in which it is often monarthritic.

Pathogenesis

HBsAg antigenemia persists for 2 months in affected children and may last for several years. Hepatitis B virus has been identified as a double-stranded DNA virus that replicates via reverse transcriptase. It produces complete virus particles and capsids that circulate in the blood and can be detected ultrastructurally or by antibody testing.[7,50] Hepatitis C is a single-stranded RNA virus. Hepatitis D is a unique single-stranded RNA virus that cannot enter the hepatocytes unless accompanied by the hepatitis B virus. The morbilliform eruption is associated with HBsAg-positive hepatitis. Hepatitis antigen-antibody immune complexes have been identified in the sera and skin of patients with eruptions of the urticarial, anaphylactoid purpura, and periarteritis nodosa types.

Treatment

If children are hepatitis B positive, it is important to prevent them from donating blood or blood products and to protect laboratory personnel. Enteric transmission of hepatitis can occur, and contact with patients' blood should be avoided. Isolating the patients from contact with persons at risk for severe hepatitis may be important. Exposed persons may be given large doses of hepatitis B immunoglobulin (HBIG), 0.06 ml/kg, within 24 hours of exposure, and 1.0 ml of hepatitis B vaccine given intramuscularly within 7 days of exposure.[7,50] The vaccine should be repeated 1 and 6 months later. For perinatal exposure, 0.5 ml of HBIG should be administered within 12 hours of birth, with 0.5 ml of vaccine given within 7 days and at 1 and 6 months. The incubation period for hepatitis B and C is 6 weeks to 6 months.[50]

Patient education

The importance of evaluating contacts if hepatitis B is found should be emphasized.

Follow-up visits

A visit 2 weeks after the initial visit to determine whether the signs and symptoms of hepatitis B have developed is recommended. If the child is hepatitis B positive, sera should be retested for HBsAg and antibodies to HBsAg 3 months later to detect possible chronic carriers.[50]

VIRAL EXANTHEMS: VESICULOBULLOUS ERUPTIONS

After dissemination to skin during a viremic phase, there may be productive viral infection of keratinocytes, with ballooning degeneration of cells resulting in vesicle formation. This is particularly characteristic of the herpes group of viruses.

Herpes Simplex (Human Herpesvirus 1 and 2 Infections)
Clinical features

Grouped vesicles on an erythematous base are the characteristic lesions of herpes simplex in the skin, regardless of the location.[7,51] On mucous membranes the blister roof is easily shed and the blister base (erosion) is seen. HHV infections may be primary or recurrent.[7,51] Recurrent infections represent reactivation of latent HSV. In the immunosuppressed child the erythematous base may be lost, or large erosions may be seen. Several distinct clinical patterns are seen.

Primary infections

Gingivostomatitis. In infants and children, 60% of herpes simplex infections appear as a gingivostomatitis (Figs. 8-16 and 8-17) and are almost always caused by HSV type 1 (HSV-1). It primarily appears in infants less than 6 months of age, with pain in the mouth and throat on attempted swallowing, accompanied by fever and irritability. Erosions are extensive throughout the oral cavity, with moist crusts and foul breath. The child often is unable to eat. It lasts 7 to 14 days. Many infants are asymptomatic or suffer a mild pharyngitis on their first encounter with HSV-1.

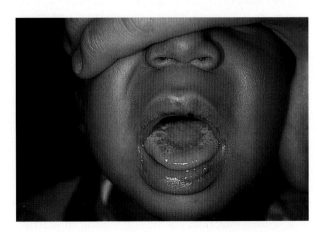

Fig. 8-16 Infant with primary herpes gingivostomatitis.

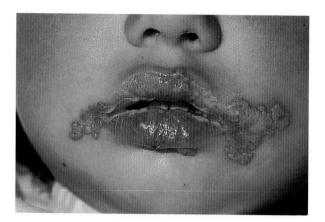

Fig. 8-17 Primary HSV-1 gingivostomatitis in an infant.

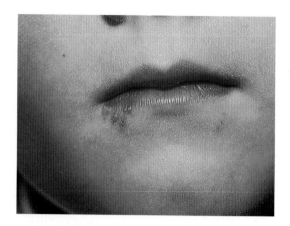

Fig. 8-18 Recurrent herpes labialis of the lower lip and adjacent skin in a child.

Recurrent herpes simplex virus infections. HSV after initial exposure may persist in nerve ganglia and be reactivated by a number of factors, including fever, ultraviolet light, trauma, and the menses.[7,51-53] The mechanisms of this reactivation of latent virus and its subsequent replication within epidermal cells are unknown. Nonetheless, once recurrent skin involvement appears, the disease is contagious and can be transmitted to other areas of skin or to other persons.

Sites of involvement vary, but the most common are the lips, eyes, cheeks, and hands.[7,51,52] When different skin locations are involved, the clinical appearance may vary, and all may be photoactivated.[52] In all forms, however, grouped vesicles on a red base are present. Regional lymphadenopathy may occur in all forms of herpes simplex.

Herpes labialis. Recurrent HSV infection of the lip occurs in 20% of all infants and children previously infected and accounts for the majority of all recurrent infections.[51] It appears as grouped vesicles on one portion of the lip, usually the lower lip, and typically follows an acute febrile illness or intense sun exposure (Fig. 8-18).[7,51] The period from the appearance of the vesicles until complete healing averages 8 days. HSV-1 can be recovered from the vesicles during the first 24 hours after onset. A prodrome of severe pain accompanies the lesions in 85% of patients.

Herpes keratitis. Although the cornea is involved in only 8% to 10% of children infected with HSV-1, this is a serious infection, potentially leading to scarring and loss of vision.[7,51] Any HSV infection on the skin around the eye, whether accompanied by a red eye,

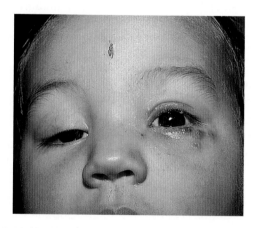

Fig. 8-19 Herpetic keratitis. Involvement of eyelid and conjunctiva in a child.

should prompt a search for herpes keratitis (Fig. 8-19). Dendritic ulceration of the cornea may be present and is an important characteristic. Ophthalmologic consultation should be obtained.

Herpes hand and finger infections. HSV-1 infection of the hand and finger occurs in 10% of infants and children, with perhaps a predilection for thumb suckers (Fig. 8-20).

Because it causes severe pain and erythema, it is often initially considered a pyoderma or cellulitis. A careful history will elicit the prodrome of pain, and careful examination will reveal thick-roofed blisters. Because the stratum corneum is thick on the palms and fingers, the vesicles appear deceptively deeper in the skin than in their epidermal location.[54]

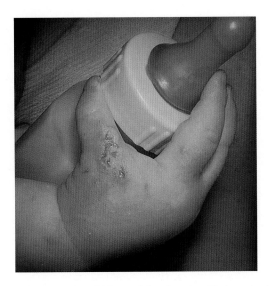

Fig. 8-20 Herpetic whitlow of the thumb of baby who is a thumb sucker.

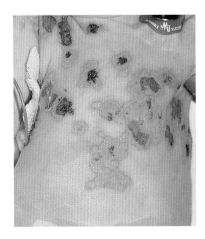

Fig. 8-22 Widespread blisters on the trunk in neonatal herpes.

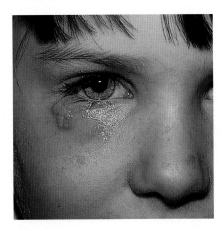

Fig. 8-21 Recurrent eruption of cheek in a child with herpes facialis.

Herpes facialis. Recurrent episodes of grouped vesicles on the cheek or forehead are less common than other forms of HSV of the head and neck, but frequently they are confused with impetigo (Fig. 8-21).

Herpes progenitalis. Herpes progenitalis, predominantly caused by HSV type 2 (HSV-2) infection, occurs almost exclusively in adolescents and young adults.[7,51,53] Just as in HSV-1 gingivostomatitis, the symptoms may vary from none to severe widespread erosions, accompanied by fever, lymphadenopathy, severe pain, and lassitude. Recurrent herpes progenitalis characteristically presents with a prodrome of pain followed by the appearance of grouped vesicles on an erythematous base in a localized area of the genitalia. It is important to bear in mind that recurrent genital herpes is contagious and sexually transmitted. It is a common venereal disease among adolescents and young adults.

Neonatal herpes simplex. Neonatal herpes simplex may develop in approximately 10% of infants born of parents with active HSV-2 infection.[7,53] In natally acquired herpes simplex, 67% of cases are caused by HHV-2 and 33% by HHV-1. Signs may be present at birth, but grouped vesicles on an erythematous base may appear up to 7 days after birth (Figs. 8-22 and 8-23). The disease may be mild, with primarily cutaneous manifestations, but central nervous system function may ultimately be impaired.[53,55] More usual is a systemic illness with jaundice, progressive hepatosplenomegaly, dyspnea, hypothermia, and central nervous system symptoms. A severe encephalitis ensues, and death occurs in 48 to 96 hours.[7,55]

Herpes simplex virus infections in immunodeficiency states. In infants or children with genetic immunodeficiency, those receiving immunosuppressive drugs, and those with severe protein-calorie malnutrition or cancer-associated immunodeficiency, atypical forms of HSV infection occur. Grouped vesicles often become large bullae and may lack an erythematous border. Deep erosions may occur even in the absence of

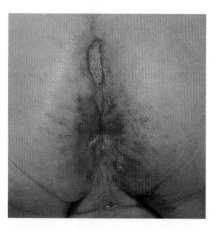

Fig. 8-23 Perianal erosions in a newborn with HHV-2 infection.

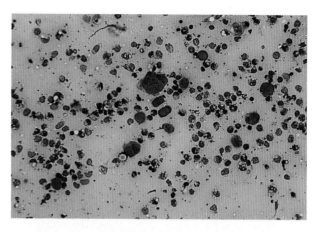

Fig. 8-25 Photomicrograph of smear of blister contents shows giant cells in herpes simplex infection (Tzanck smear).

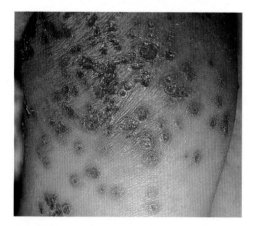

Fig. 8-24 Discrete ulcers and hundreds of erosions associated with dermatitis in an infant with atopic dermatitis and widespread herpes simplex infection (Kaposi's varicelliform eruption, eczema herpeticum).

Box 8-7 Vesiculobullous Virus Infections

COMMON
Herpes simplex
Varicella-zoster
Hand-foot-and-mouth disease (coxsackievirus A16)

UNCOMMON
Orf
Influenza
Coxsackieviruses A5, 9, 10
Echoviruses 4, 9, 11, 17, 25
Variola
Vaccinia (cowpox)

---

inflammation. Purpura or hemorrhage appears within the bullous lesions. After 24 to 48 hours of local skin involvement, generalized skin involvement and visceral involvement may ensue. Herpes encephalitis or pneumonia may result in death.

Kaposi's varicelliform eruption (eczema herpeticum).
Infants and children with atopic dermatitis, burns, and other conditions that disrupt the epidermal barrier are susceptible to the development of generalized HSV infection characterized by high fever, lassitude, hundreds of skin vesicles, and sometimes death. Severe infections may develop in these patients, even when their dermatitis is inactive (Fig. 8-24).

Differential diagnosis

A rapid clinical clue to HSV (or varicella-zoster virus [VZV]) infection is the finding of epidermal giant cells on a Tzanck preparation (Fig. 8-25; see Chapter 2 for technique).

Rapid diagnostic tests using fluorescent- or dye-labeled monoclonal antibodies are available to stain smears and are 90% or more reliable.[56] Isolation of HHV-1 or HHV-2 is the diagnostic gold standard but requires at least 24 hours. Molecular diagnosis using the polymerase chain reaction (PCR) techniques can be done in less than 24 hours, but it is not widely available.

Other virus infections to be considered in the differential diagnosis of herpes simplex are listed in Box 8-7.

Gingivostomatitis. Gingivostomatitis must be differentiated from aphthous ulcers, which are shallow, irregular, ragged, recurrent ulcerations on the oral mucosa. In erythema multiforme, in contrast to HSV gingivostomatitis, symmetric iris and target lesions are present on the skin. In herpangina, which is caused by enteroviruses, ulcers are limited to the anterior tonsillar pillars and have a linear arrangement; isolation of coxsackievirus A confirms the diagnosis.

Recurrent herpes simplex virus infection. Recurrent skin infection caused by HSV must be differentiated from herpes zoster. Because both infections demonstrate epidermal giant cells on Tzanck smear, antibody testing or viral culture is the preferred method for differentiating the two on first infection. The history of recurrent lesions in the same skin area suggests HSV rather than varicella-zoster virus. VZV infections often have three or more groups of vesicles, HSV infections have one or two.

Herpes labialis. Impetigo may mimic herpes labialis. Gram's stain and bacterial culture of the lesions will help distinguish the two.

Herpes keratitis. Herpes keratitis should be differentiated from bacterial conjunctivitis and epidemic adenovirus keratoconjunctivitis. The characteristic grouped vesicles on an erythematous base in periocular skin will help distinguish HSV from these infections. Furthermore, HSV is usually unilateral, whereas bacterial and adenovirus infections, although initially unilateral, often become bilateral.

Herpes hand and finger infections. HSV hand and finger infections are often confused with bacterial cellulitis. A Tzanck smear of the vesicle base is a rapid method of distinguishing HSV from bacterial infection.

Herpes facialis. Impetigo may mimic facial herpes on the cheek or forehead. A Tzanck smear, HSV antibody test, or bacterial and viral culture will often distinguish the two.

Herpes progenitalis. Herpes progenitalis may mimic other venereal diseases. Also, it is not unusual to note more than one venereal disease simultaneously in the sexually active person. A smear and culture for gonorrhea and a serologic test for syphilis are most helpful in such cases.

Neonatal herpes simplex. Other congenital infections (e.g., *t*oxoplasmosis, *o*ther [congenital syphilis and viruses], *r*ubella, CMV, and *h*erpes simplex virus, the so-called *TORCH complex*) may mimic neonatal HSV. Vesicular skin lesions are not present in any of these, however. In neonatal bacterial sepsis, isolated vesicular or pustulovesicular lesions may occur. They are not grouped as in HSV infection, and Gram's stain and bacterial culture will distinguish them from herpes simplex.

Pathogenesis

HHV-1 and HHV-2 are complex DNA viruses with an incubation period of 2 to 12 days. They are epidermotropic viruses, and productive viral infection occurs within keratinocytes. Active infection occurs despite high titers of specific antibody. This no doubt reflects the intracellular infection characteristic of these viruses in which antibody cannot interact with the active virus, which is transferred from cell to cell. There are two possible outcomes of epidermal cellular infection: productive and nonproductive infection. Productive infection is characterized by the biosynthesis of infectious progeny and epidermal cell death, producing the intraepidermal vesicle. Nonproductive infection results in the perpetuation of all or part of the viral genome and survival of the epidermal cell, producing epidermal giant cells. It is uncertain whether fusion of several epidermal cells or nuclear division without cytoplasmic division is responsible for the epidermal giant cells seen on Tzanck smear.

Treatment

Oral acyclovir, famciclovir, or valacyclovir are the specific therapy for localized cutaneous herpes simplex infections.[7,51,57] Oral acyclovir has been safe and effective in children. In severe primary HSV infections, such as herpes gingivostomatitis or Kaposi's varicelliform eruption, acyclovir may be very useful, especially if initiated within 72 hours of the onset, in doses of 20 to 40 mg/kg/day. In localized forms of herpes simplex, such as those limited to a certain small area of skin, systemic therapy is usually not required. Neither topical nor systemic antiviral agents, however, will prevent recurrences of herpes simplex, although they may prevent transfection of the virus to adjacent skin sites or to family members or playmates if given prophylactically. In patients experiencing frequent, severe recurrences, 6 months of acyclovir prophylaxis may be considered.

In herpes keratitis, topical 5-iodo-2-deoxyuridine, topical adenine arabinoside (Vira-A), or 1% to 2% trifluridine ophthalmic ointments may be most efficacious. Before initiation of treatment, consultation with an ophthalmologist is recommended.

In neonatal HSV infections and in Kaposi's varicelliform eruption, intravenous acyclovir has proved effective.[7] Supportive measures, such as fever control, maintenance of fluid and electrolyte balance, and thermal regulation, are necessary. Infected patients shed virus and should be isolated.

Patient education

Patients with local cutaneous infection should be informed of the contagious nature of the disease. Avoidance of precipitating factors may be most useful (e.g., avoiding sun exposure or using sunscreens in sun-activated recurrent HSV, and discontinuing sexual activity in herpes progenitalis). In patients with atopic dermatitis or other skin diseases susceptible to disseminated HSV infections, optimal treatment of the underlying skin disease and consistency of care may be useful in preventing future episodes.

Follow-up visits

Careful ophthalmologic follow-up (every 1 to 2 days) is required in herpes keratitis. Disseminated infections often require hospitalization and intensive supportive therapy. Neonatal HSV requires careful developmental and neurologic examinations at 3-month intervals. Cutaneous herpes lesions may recur throughout childhood after neonatal HSV.

Chickenpox and Zoster (Human Herpesvirus 3 Infections)
Clinical features

Varicella (chickenpox). Varicella is characterized by the abrupt onset of crops of skin lesions.[7,58,59] Individual lesions begin as faint erythematous macules that progress to edematous papules and then to vesicles during 24 to 48 hours (Fig. 8-26). The vesicles then develop moist crusts that dry and are shed, leaving a shallow erosion. Successive crops of lesions appear during the next 2 to 5 days, so that at any one time several stages of skin lesions can be observed concomitantly: macules, papules, vesicles, and crusted lesions (Fig. 8-27). Skin lesions may appear in sites of skin injury or be localized to areas of sun exposure. Lesions frequently involve mucous membranes, and isolated erosions may be seen in the conjunctiva, oral cavity, or nasal mucosa.[7,59] Fever is usually low grade,

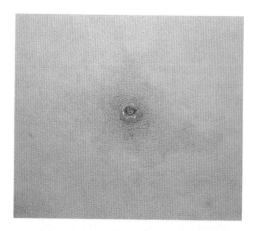

Fig. 8-26 Varicella. Umbilicated vesicles on a red base.

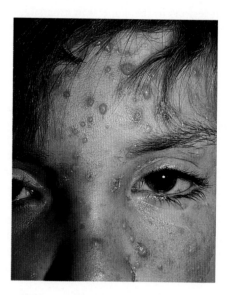

Fig. 8-27 Blisters, papules, and crusted lesion in a child with varicella.

and associated symptoms are mild. In a single family, varicella lesions may vary from fewer than 10 in one child to hundreds in another. The total duration is 7 to 10 days, but frequently children stay home 14 days because of school or other contagion-restriction policy.[7] The disease is highly contagious from 1 to 2 days before the onset of the skin eruption to 5 to 6 days afterward.[7,59]

Secondary bacterial infection of one to three of the many varicella skin lesions is common (1% to 4%), producing the so-called *bullous varicella.* Often this is the result of *Staphylococcus aureus* infection. Pneumonia may complicate varicella in some children, and

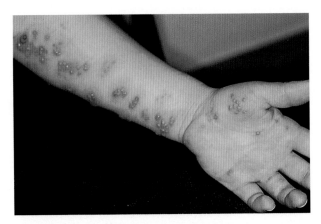

Fig. 8-28 Many groups of blisters occurring over the arm in a child with herpes zoster.

rarely, Reye's syndrome, acute cerebellar ataxia, or encephalitis may ensue.[7] Severe generalized HHV-3 infections may develop in immunosuppressed persons, with high fever, encephalitis, pneumonia, hepatitis, or disseminated intravascular coagulation.[7,59]

Herpes zoster. In children who have previously had varicella, recurrent infection results in herpes zoster.[7,58,59] Two to three groups of lesions appear within several adjacent dermatomes (Fig. 8-28). They begin as macules and edematous papules and progress to grouped vesicles on an erythematous base. Rarely, dermatomal pain may precede the eruption in children, and postzoster neuralgia may also occur, but rarely. Almost all children, however, have a mild illness lasting 7 to 10 days. Pruritus may be severe. The thoracic segments are involved in 60% of children with herpes zoster, with the childhood distribution depicted in Figure 8-29. If the nose is involved, herpes zoster keratitis is likely to occur, and it may be as severe as HSV keratitis. Ophthalmic zoster is also more likely to be associated with severe pain than is zoster of other skin regions in children. Herpes zoster involving skin around the eyes, nose, and forehead requires a careful ophthalmologic examination. Herpes zoster may be the initial finding in acquired immune deficiency syndrome (AIDS), but it is rarely the presenting finding in childhood cancer. In immunosuppressed children, disseminated herpes zoster occurs 1 to 5 days after the dermatome infection begins. Even immunosuppressed children with disseminated herpes zoster recover without sequelae, but visceral involvement can occur. Involvement of the geniculate ganglion results in pain in the ear, vesicles on the pin-

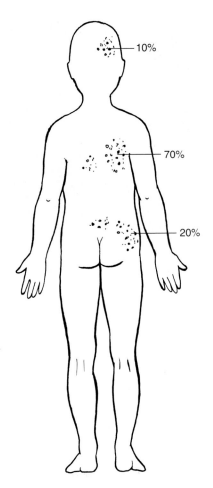

Fig. 8-29 Common distribution of herpes zoster in childhood: 10% cranial nerve involvement, 70% thoracic dermatome, 20% lumbosacral involvement.

nae, and facial palsy (Ramsay Hunt syndrome) (Fig. 8-30). Motor paralysis of other nerves may follow herpes zoster.

Differential diagnosis

Varicella. Typical varicella is seldom confused with other illnesses (Box 8-7). In hand-foot-and-mouth disease, vesicles are limited to acral areas, and vesicular forms of insect-bite reactions (papular urticaria) usually have a typical history of bites. Acute parapsoriasis may mimic varicella in that it produces crops of lesions in different stages. True vesicles are less common in parapsoriasis, and papules with central purpura are more common. Rickettsialpox and dermatitis herpetiformis are rare in children, but may mimic varicella. A Tzanck smear of the vesicle base will differentiate varicella from

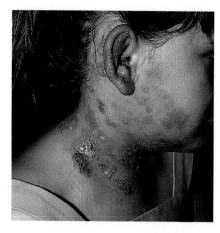

Fig. 8-30 Involvement of the ear and adjacent skin associated with facial palsy in herpes zoster of geniculate ganglion (Hunt syndrome).

these vesicular diseases. Occasionally, disseminated HSV infection will mimic varicella. Viral cultures may be necessary to distinguish between HSV and varicella.

Herpes zoster. Local cutaneous HSV infections may also mimic herpes zoster in children.[52] Usually HSV involves one group of vesicles, and herpes zoster involves three to four clusters of grouped vesicles. Viral culture or fluorescent antibody tests may be required to distinguish the two. Impetigo is sometimes confused with herpes zoster, but honey-colored crusts, Gram's stain of lesions, and bacterial cultures will help distinguish it from herpes zoster.

Pathogenesis

HHV-3 is a complex herpes-group DNA virus that infects in much the same way as herpes simplex (see Herpes Simplex, Pathogenesis, p. 105). The incubation period ranges from 10 to 27 days and averages 14 days.[7,59] Productive infection occurs within keratinocytes, producing ballooning degeneration of cells and an intraepidermal blister. Reactivation is more likely in herpes simplex–seronegative subjects.[60]

Treatment

In the healthy child, varicella does not require specific therapy. Wet dressings, soothing baths, and oral antihistamines will give symptomatic relief of the pruritus in children.[7,61] Salicylates should not be administered.[7] Zoster immune globulin, if given within 72 hours after exposure of an immunosuppressed host (including newborns or hospitalized premature infants), may modify varicella.[7,61] Secondary bacterial infection of varicella lesions should be treated with antistaphylococcal drugs, such as dicloxacillin, 12.5 to 25.0 mg/kg/day in four divided oral doses for 7 to 10 days.

Systemic antiviral agents, such as intravenous or oral acyclovir, valacyclovir, famciclovir, and foscarnet, have been used for childhood HHV-3 infections with success.[7,61,62] It is recommended that antivirals not be given to otherwise healthy children, but their use should be considered in those likely to have complications, such as adolescents and children with chronic pulmonary disease, especially if they are taking inhaled or systemic steroids, or children receiving chronic salicylate therapy. In immunosuppressed children, children with ophthalmic zoster, or children with Ramsay Hunt syndrome, acyclovir, 20 mg/kg/dose in four daily doses for 5 days, may be a valuable therapeutic strategy.[62] If administered within 72 hours of exposure, varicella vaccine is efficacious in preventing or attenuating varicella.[7,61,62]

Patient education

The highly contagious nature of varicella should be emphasized, and the child should be isolated until all lesions are crusted, which usually occurs 5 to 6 days after eruption of the lesions. Contact with the elderly, neonates, and immunocompromised children should be avoided.

Postvaricella scarring is always a concern for parents. What appear to be highly vascular purple-red scars return to normal skin color in 6 to 12 months and often leave little evidence of scarring. Patients should be advised to wait at least 1 year before seeking help for postvaricella scars.

Follow-up visits

A visit in 48 hours to assess the development of secondary bacterial infection is useful in children with varicella. Children with disseminated zoster, ophthalmic zoster, or Ramsay Hunt syndrome should be seen daily until symptoms improve.

Hand-Foot-and-Mouth Disease (Coxsackievirus Infection)

An abrupt onset of scattered papules that progress to oval or linear vesicles in an acral distribution should suggest hand-foot-and-mouth disease.[35,36,63] The individual lesions are seen on the palms, fingertips, interdigital webs, and soles of the feet, and are few in num-

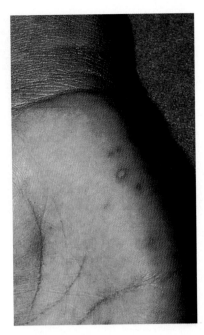

Fig. 8-31 Oval blisters of the palms in child with hand-foot-and-mouth disease (coxsackie virus A16 infection).

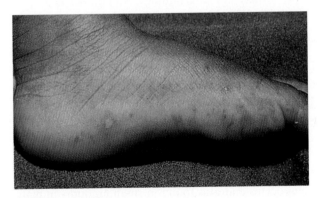

Fig. 8-32 Oval blisters on the feet of a child with hand-foot-and-mouth syndrome.

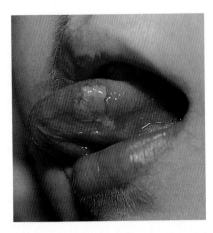

Fig. 8-33 Erosion of the tongue in a child with hand-foot-and-mouth syndrome.

Differential diagnosis

In the early nonvesicular stage, rubella and the other morbilliform lesions must be considered (see Box 8-4), but the sparsity of lesions and the lack of truncal involvement make those diagnoses unlikely. In the vesicular stage, the disease may be confused with varicella, but the acral distribution of the lesions, the lack of pruritus, and the oval to linear nature of the individual vesicles will help differentiate hand-foot-and-mouth disease from varicella. Insect bites may also mimic hand-foot-and-mouth disease, particularly if they occur on exposed acral skin. Isolation of coxsackievirus or enterovirus 71 from throat washings or serologic evidence will distinguish.

Pathogenesis

Several coxsackievirus group A enteroviruses and enterovirus 71 have been found to be responsible for hand-foot-and-mouth disease.[7,35,36,63,64] The epidemic form is almost always caused by coxsackievirus A16 or enterovirus 71, but coxsackieviruses A2, A5, and A10 have also been associated. Molecular analysis reveals homology among coxsackievirus A16, A2, and enterovirus 71. The incubation period is 3 to 5 days, and the virus enters by the enteric route, with the eruption reflecting a viremic phase. The disease is contagious from 2 days before to 2 days after the onset of the eruption, but virus excretion in feces may persist for 2 weeks.

Treatment

No treatment is necessary in mild cases. In severe illness with enterovirus 71 infection, immune globulin

ber (Figs. 8-31 and 8-32). Discrete oral lesions may also be seen (Fig. 8-33). Such children are not ill and characteristically are afebrile. During epidemics, incomplete forms may be seen.[35,36,63] In some epidemics skin lesions may be more numerous and involve both proximal and distal extremities. Oral lesions appear as discrete, shallow, oval erosions. In recent years fatal cases have been described that are predominantly caused by enterovirus 71.[63,64] Fatal cases often present with high fever.[63,64] Nail matrix arrest with shedding of nails may follow the acute infection.[65]

intravenous or the antiviral agent pleconaril may be effective.

Human Immunodeficiency Virus Infections
Clinical features

The cutaneous manifestations of HIV-1 disease in children are predominantly the result of bacterial, fungal, and viral infections.[7,66,67] Clinical findings of perinatally acquired HIV infection are usually noted at about 4 months of age, but may be first manifested as early as 3 months or as late as 21 months.[67] The initial features are usually lymphadenopathy, persistent diarrhea, hepatosplenomegaly, and failure to thrive. As HIV infection progresses to AIDS, more features of opportunistic infections appear. AIDS has many features that mimic hereditary immunodeficiency diseases, such as severe combined immunodeficiency (SCID). Often the first sign of AIDS is persistent thrush, recalcitrant to antiyeast therapy. The failure to clear thrush should be distinguished from the infant who gets thrush, clears with therapy, and then has a recurrence off therapy. Infants with AIDS and thrush also will have failure to thrive, lymphadenopathy, hepatosplenomegaly, and esophageal involvement. Chronic cough, clubbing of the fingers, and hypoxemia are the features of *Pneumocystis carinii* pneumonia, the most common infection of children with AIDS.[66,67]

A dermatitis that mimics seborrheic dermatitis is observed in half of the children who have HIV infection. It is not specific. Severe herpes gingivostomatitis or zoster (Fig. 8-34) may be the presenting finding. Children with HIV infection may exhibit hundreds of molluscum contagiosum lesions, and giant molluscum lesions may be seen. Recurrent pyodermas caused by *S. aureus* are frequent, and cellulitis or septicemia may develop from cutaneous infections that otherwise should be well localized to the epidermis. Unusual dermatophyte infections in children, such as onychomycosis and widespread tinea faciei, may be found. Severe crusted scabies with hundreds of live mites, the so-called *Norwegian scabies,* may occur. Purpura is common and may be the result of thrombocytopenia or severe viral or bacterial infections. A persistent folliculitis called *eosinophilic folliculitis* may be seen.[66,67]

Drug eruptions are far more common than predicted, particularly morbilliform and toxic epidermal necrolysis reactions caused by trimethoprim-sulfamethoxazole.[66,67] A clinical syndrome that mimics acrodermatitis enteropathica may accompany the failure to thrive and result from nutritional zinc defi-

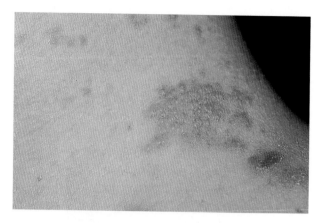

Fig. 8-34 Herpes zoster in a 12-year-old boy who is HIV positive.

ciency. Kaposi's sarcoma of skin has not been reported in children with HIV infection.

Differential diagnosis

Virtually every known skin infection will mimic some infection seen in the infant or child with AIDS. Severe malnutrition states and congenital immunodeficiencies may display the same findings. An HIV serology confirmed by Western immunoblotting techniques are the most sensitive tests utilized to distinguish HIV infection, and they should be done on every infant or child suspected of having HIV.[7] In HIV-1 exposed infants, it may be difficult using serologic tests alone to establish the diagnosis, and HIV DNA PCR may be required.[7]

Pathogenesis

The agent responsible for AIDS is HIV-1, a retrovirus that selectively infects T lymphocytes, including those that are epidermotropic.[7] It can be isolated from blood leukocytes and also found in small amounts in tears, semen, saliva, vaginal secretions, cerebrospinal fluid, and breast milk. Eighty percent of affected infants in the United States are infected by transplacental passage of HIV from the mother. Older children are infected by sexual contact and from blood products administered before 1985. In sexually active adolescents, seroprevalence is 0.2%. If the infant's mother was a prostitute or intravenous drug user, the likelihood of infant infection is quite high.[7] Once T lymphocytes are infected by HIV, it relentlessly destroys the child's cell-mediated immunity, leaving the child at the mercy of a huge variety of opportunistic infectious agents.

Treatment

Children with AIDS are best managed at large medical centers experienced in the care of AIDS patients.

Infectious disease experts should be involved in their care. Treatment is directed at the specific opportunistic infection, and the antimicrobial selected is directed by culture and sensitivities. Combinations of antiretroviral drugs, including nucleoside analog reverse transcriptase inhibitors, protease inhibitors, and nonnucleoside reverse transcriptase inhibitors may effectively suppress the disease.[7,68] Assessment of the viral load by HIV RNA PCR will assist the evaluation of response to therapy.[68]

Patient education

Information about the transmission of HIV and support groups for AIDS families are essential. Preventive measures such as sex education for adolescents and treatment of HIV-positive mothers with antiretroviral agents may reduce the disease.[7,66] It should be emphasized that many unusual infections may be encountered, and vigilance for early signs and symptoms of infection must be encouraged. There is currently no effective vaccine.

Follow-up visits

Frequent visits are required, and establishing a close relationship with an AIDS clinic is advisable.

VIRUS-INDUCED TUMORS

Certain viruses, such as human papillomaviruses and molluscum contagiosum viruses, do not destroy keratinocytes but induce proliferation, resulting in benign tumors of skin.

Warts (Human Papillomavirus Infection)
Clinical features

Human papillomavirus (HPV)–induced epithelial tumors produce a variety of clinical lesions known collectively as *warts*.[7,69] Different HPVs are associated with specific clinical patterns. Table 8-2 lists the clinical types of warts and the HPV type responsible.

Warts are very commonly seen in children. By age 11, 5% of children will have warts.[69]

The common wart *(verruca vulgaris)* appears as a solitary papule, with an irregular, rough surface (Figs. 8-35 and 8-36). They are usually found on the extremities, but they may be found anywhere on skin, including the scalp and genitalia. *Periungual* warts occur around the cuticles of fingers or toes and are spread by trauma (Fig. 8-37). *Filiform* warts appear as spiny projections from the skin surface with a narrow stalk (Fig. 8-38). In children they are usually seen on the lips, nose, or eyelids. *Flat* warts have a flat-topped, smooth surface. They tend to be multiple and

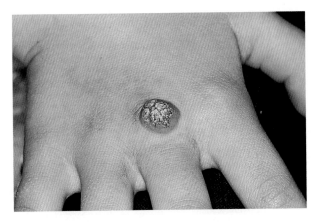

Fig. 8-35 Common wart on the hand.

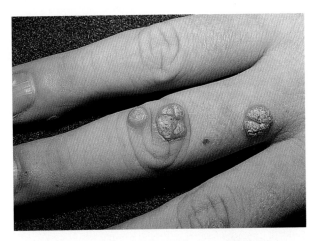

Fig. 8-36 Common warts on a child's fingers.

Table 8-2	Clinical Warts and Associated Human Papillomavirus Type
Clinical Wart Type	**HPV Type**
Common wart	HPV-2a, b, c, d, e; some HPV-4
Plantar wart	HPV-1a, b, c; HPV-4, 60, 63, 65 (weight-bearing)
Flat warts	HPV-3a, b; HPV-10a, b
Condyloma acuminata	HPV-6a, b, c, d, e, f; HPV-11a, b; HPV-16

skin-colored to light tan (Fig. 8-39). They are grouped, will appear within sites of skin trauma, and are usually observed on the face or extremities. *Plantar* (weight-bearing) warts appear as rough papules that disrupt the dermal ridges (Fig. 8-40). They are

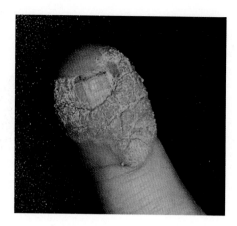

Fig. 8-37 Periungual warts.

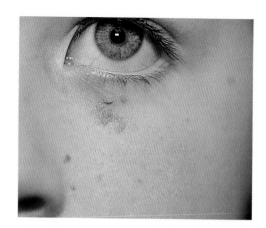

Fig. 8-39 Multiple flat warts (verruca plana) of the eyelid and cheek.

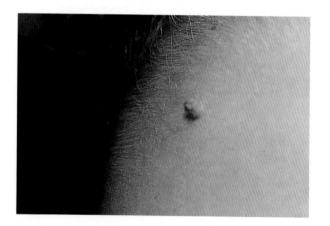

Fig. 8-38 Filiform wart.

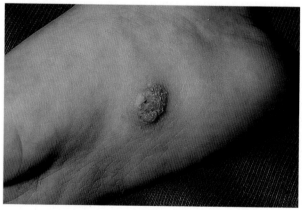

Fig. 8-40 Plantar (weight-bearing) wart.

frequently painful when the child is walking. They may be grouped together to produce mosaic warts.

Venereal warts *(condylomata acuminata)* are multiple discrete or confluent papules with a rough surface that appear on the genital or oral mucosa, adjacent dry skin, or both (Figs. 8-41 and 8-42).[69-71] Common warts also appear on genital or perigenital skin, particularly in toddlers.[71]

The natural history of warts is variable, and the incubation period is unknown, but transmission from child to child, adult to child, and mother to newborn is well documented.[71] Most warts spontaneously resolve in 12 to 24 months but may persist for longer periods in some children. Warts in the immunosuppressed child are very persistent. Most

warts are asymptomatic, except weight-bearing warts, although large warts anywhere may develop painful fissures.

Differential diagnosis

Common warts and filiform warts are so characteristic that they present no diagnostic problem. Plantar warts must be differentiated from calluses, which have a smooth, rather than irregular, surface and preserve the dermal ridges. Condylomata acuminata must be distinguished from the moist, smooth papules of secondary syphilis (condylomata lata), which appear as moist papules in genital areas. A serologic test for syphilis will readily distinguish the two. Flat warts are often overlooked and may be misdiagnosed as

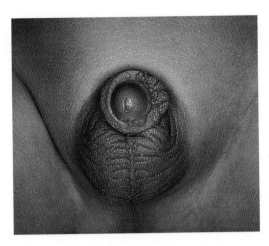

Fig. 8-41 Venereal warts (condyloma acuminata) of the foreskin in a male infant.

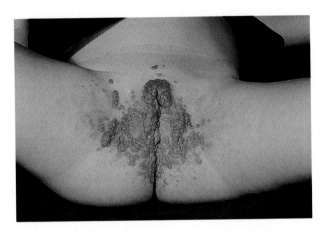

Fig. 8-42 Venereal warts in a female infant.

lichen planus, lichen nitidus, seborrheic keratosis, or birthmarks. The linear or grouped arrangement of flat warts is helpful in diagnosis, as is their occurrence along areas of skin trauma. Diagnosis can be established by biopsy and HPV molecular typing, but these procedures are rarely required, and warts remain a clinical diagnosis.

Pathogenesis

Immunity to warts is not well understood, but inducing inflammation around a single wart may result in regression of all others. The HPV is located within the epidermal cell nucleus, which may be an immunologic privileged site where viral antigen has little opportunity to interact with antibody or white blood cells and may encode receptors that prevent interferon release.[69] HPV induces vacuolated epidermal cells with eosinophilic inclusions. The HPV induces keratinocyte proliferation with relatively normal differentiation, giving rise to a benign epithelial tumor.

Treatment

Wart therapy may be cytodestructive, immunologic, antiproliferative, or psychological.[71-75] Cytodestructive therapy is designed to destroy all of the epidermal cells within the wart tumor and, hopefully, all of the HPV as well. The recurrence rate for all wart treatment strategies is high, and it is unlikely the wart will resolve with a single treatment. Of cytodestructive therapies, cryotherapy usually has the smallest recurrence rate from a single treatment. Table 8-3 summarizes usual treatments for wart types.

Cytodestructive therapies

CRYOTHERAPY. A cryosurgery probe, spray unit, or copper bar cooled in liquid nitrogen may be used for cryotherapy, but a cotton swab with a loose, pointed tip is most commonly used. The cotton swab is dipped in a thermos containing liquid nitrogen (–195° C), and the saturated swab is applied to the center of the wart until a white ice ball extending 1 to 3 mm beyond the margin of the wart is formed. The freeze is maintained 10 to 30 seconds. Warts greater than 7 mm in diameter should not be frozen, because scarring is likely to result. In 1 to 2 days a blister, sometimes hemorrhagic, forms. Removing the blister roof in 1 week and refreezing may be necessary. Cryotherapy spray is best for common warts because it is the coldest but should not generally be used on periungual or plantar warts. Freezing a forceps with cotton wrapped around the ends in liquid nitrogen and grasping the narrow stalk of a filiform wart for 30 to 45 seconds is effective.

SALICYCLIC ACID PLASTERS. Cotton plasters impregnated with 40% salicylic acid can be used on plantar and periungual warts. The plaster is cut to size, the paper backing removed, and the gummed side placed against the wart. It should be secured by trainer's tape so the plaster does not move for 3 to 5 days. Sweating mobilizes the salicylic acid out of the plaster so that it may enter the skin. When the plaster is removed, the patient should soak the wart in water for 45 minutes, then rub off the dead, white skin of the wart. A new plaster is taped in place, and the process is repeated for two more changes.

Table 8-3 Treatment of Viral Warts

	TREATMENT		
Type of Wart	First Choice	Alternative	Response Rate (%)
Common	Cryotherapy	Salicylic acid paint	60–90
Periungual	Imiquimod cream	Cantharidin	60
Flat	Retinoic acid	Imiquimod cream	50
Filiform	Surgery	Cryotherapy with forceps	50
Plantar	Salicylic acid plaster	Imiquimod cream	60
Venereal	Podophyllum or Condylox	Imiquimod cream	90

SALICYCLIC ACID PAINTS. Prescriptions for salicylic acid–containing solutions can be provided for home use. The solutions should be applied with a toothpick by microdrops. They should be applied once or twice a day for 4 to 6 weeks. This method will not work on warts over 5 mm. Redness around the base of the wart and itching may herald the onset of wart regression. These preparations should be used for periungual warts or small common warts.

VASCULAR SELECTIVE LASERS. The pulsed-dye laser will not scar and is equally effective as cryosurgery. Several treatment sessions may be required.

CO_2 LASERS, ELECTRODESICCATION, AND X-RAYS. CO_2 lasers, electrodesiccation, and x-ray therapies always result in scarring and other undesirable side effects, with high recurrence rates. They are not recommended.

VESICANTS (CANTHARIDAN). Currently unavailable in the United States, the vesicant cantharidin can be quite effective in the treatment of periungual warts. It should be applied carefully with a toothpick to cover the size of the wart. It produces a tender blister beneath the wart 2 or 3 days after application, and the wart is eventually sloughed off. It is difficult to regulate the size of the blister, and the response may vary from application to application. Cantharidin should never be used in intertriginous areas.

SURGERY. The recurrence rate after surgical excision of a wart approaches 100%, presumably because of transfection of HPV at the time of surgery. Removing a filiform wart by cutting its narrow base is one exception. Some authorities recommend the use of a sharp curette on the remaining plantar wart after 3 or 4 weeks of salicylic acid plasters.

Immunologic therapies

INTERFERON INDUCERS. Imiquimod cream applied daily for 1 to 2 months is a painless and effective treatment. The drug induces interferon production by keratinocytes. Instructions to discontinue when the warts become red will prevent crusting or oozing from excessive interferon release.

ALPHA INTERFERONS. Alpha interferon preparations must be injected either intralesionally or subcutaneously twice weekly. The injection requirement limits their use in children.

CIMETIDINE. Some authorities have used 3 months of oral cimetidine, an H_2 blocking agent, to nonspecifically improve immunity to HPV. This is usually used in conjunction with another strategy and should be reserved for resistant warts.

VACCINES. There are currently no effective wart vaccines.

Antiproliferative agents

RETINOIC ACID. Retinoic acid in a 0.025% cream or 0.05% cream may be used for flat warts and applied once or twice daily for 4 to 6 weeks. It is ineffective in common, plantar, or periungual warts.

PODOPHYLLUM. Podophyllum, a plant extract, is a microtubule inhibitor that blocks cell division. It can be effective against genital warts and common warts. It is applied by the health care provider in a 25% alcohol solution and applied with a toothpick to the warts. It should be washed off in 4 hours. It is an irritating substance, and application to perianal skin often induces defecation. A purified podophyllotoxin is now available for use by the patient (podofilox [Condylox]). It is applied carefully with a toothpick twice daily for 3 days, then 4 days later reapplied for 3 days if the warts remain. Podophyllum in excessive doses is a neurotoxin and can cause an areflexic coma.

Psychotherapy. Because warts regress without therapy, most studies demonstrate a placebo effect of 30%. Suggestion therapy such as "buying the wart" from the child, or a variety of folk medicines, is expected to have a similar regression rate.

Patient education

It should be emphasized from the initial visit that one treatment is unlikely to cure the wart, and many treatments may be necessary (see the patient education handout on Warts, p. 349). A careful explanation of the poor host immunity to the HPV is helpful. For genital warts in infants and toddlers, the possibility of sexual abuse should be considered. However, it is well established that vertical transmission of genital warts from an infected mother can occur, and many genital warts are of common HPV types, with a parent, sibling, or care giver having common warts of the same type.[71] This makes it impossible to diagnose sexual abuse by the presence of genital warts alone. The clinician should carefully examine the child for other forms of physical or sexual abuse, including examination of the oral cavity and genitalia. A history of unusual behavior in the child, such as withdrawal, sleep disturbances, phobias, or new onset of enuresis or encopresis, should be solicited. If suspicious history or physical findings other than the genital warts are obtained, reporting to the appropriate social agencies is recommended.[71]

Follow-up visits

A visit 2 weeks after initiating therapy is needed to ascertain the need for retreatment.

Molluscum Contagiosum
Clinical features

White or yellow-white 1- to 6-mm discrete papules with a central umbilication are seen in molluscum contagiosum (Figs. 8-43 and 8-44).[7,76] Occasionally, lesions as large as 15 mm will be found. A dermatitis often surrounds larger lesions (Fig. 8-45). Lesions larger than

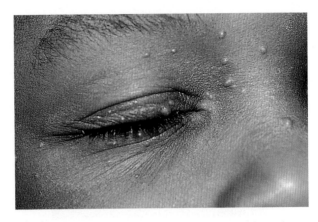

Fig. 8-43 Multiple molluscum papules on an infant's face.

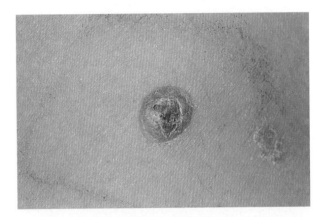

Fig. 8-44 Umbilicated dome-shaped papule characteristic of molluscum contagiosum.

6 mm may occasionally become red and purulent, healing with a slightly depressed scar. Some lesions may extrude keratinous contents from the central umbilication (Fig. 8-46). In infants and toddlers, lesions are usually observed around the eyes, axilla, and proximal extremities, but lesions can be found in other locations. In the child with atopic dermatitis, dozens to hundreds of lesions can be seen. Genital grouped lesions can be found in sexually active adolescents. Hundreds of lesions in the older child or the presence of facial or perioral lesions should raise the suspicion of AIDS.[77]

Differential diagnosis

Warts, closed comedones, and tiny epidermal cysts may mimic molluscum contagiosum. Careful inspection, however, will reveal the central umbilication characteristic of molluscum contagiosum, and microscopic examination will differentiate the disease from

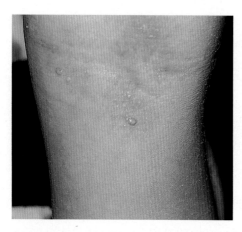

Fig. 8-45 Erythema and scaling surround resolving lesions of molluscum contagiosum (molluscum dermatitis).

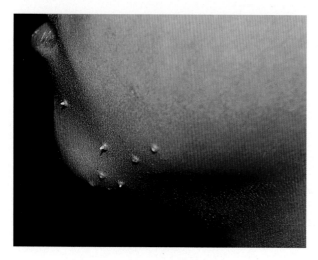

Fig. 8-46 Molluscum extruding their contents.

other skin papules. At first glance, molluscum may appear to be blisters, but palpation and careful inspection will reveal their solid nature. Extrusion of the papule contents onto a glass slide and Wright's stain will reveal the characteristic viral inclusions. Serologic diagnosis is usually not required.[78]

Lesions of molluscum dermatitis may mimic other forms of dermatitis, and pustular lesions may mimic bacterial folliculitis.

Pathogenesis

Molluscum contagiosum is caused by a poxvirus that induces epidermal cell proliferation.[7,76] Three types are recognized by restriction endonuclease analysis of viral DNA. Molluscum type 1 is believed to be re-sponsible for common lesions on the extremities, head, and neck. Types 2 and 3 are most often associated with genital lesions in the adolescent or young adult. The incubation period is 2 to 7 weeks, and the child is contagious as long as active lesions are present. The molluscum contagiosum viruses evade intracellular interferon production by encoding a faulty chemokine receptor.[79] Untreated molluscum may require 1 to 5 years to resolve.

Treatment

Removal of a papule is curative. In older children the use of a sharp dermal curette to remove the entire papule is the treatment of choice. Some clinicians prefer to empty the contents with a needle. In infants and young children this method is frightening and painful. In such children, daily application of imiquimod cream is preferred.[74] Oral cimetidine has been reported to be successful by some.[80] Alternatives include application of a drop of cantharidin, potassium hydroxide, or podophyllum applied to the central umbilication with a wooden toothpick. This is less traumatic than curettage and may avoid scarring.[81,82] Recurrences are common because it is often difficult to detect the pinpoint early lesions of molluscum. Pustular molluscum lesions do not require antibiotics.

Patient education

The highly contagious nature of molluscum contagiosum should be emphasized. The lesions are benign, and patients should not be unduly concerned (see patient education handout on Molluscum Contagiosum, p. 340).

Follow-up visits

A visit 1 to 2 weeks after initial therapy is advisable to determine the need for retreatment.

REFERENCES

1. Mancini AJ: Exanthems in childhood: an update, *Pediatr Ann* 27:398, 1998.
2. Norval M, El-Ghorr A, Garssen J: The effects of ultraviolet light irradiation on viral infections, *Br J Dermatol* 130:693, 1994.
3. Messner J et al: Accentuated viral exanthems in areas of inflammation, *J Am Acad Dermatol* 40:345, 1999.
4. Jones VF, Badgett JT, Marshall GS: Repeated photoreactivation of herpes simplex virus type I in an extrafacial dermatomal distribution, *Pediatr Infect Dis J* 13:238 1994.
5. Coustou D et al: Asymmetric periflexural exanthem of childhood: a clinical pathologic and epidemiologic prospective study, *Arch Dermatol* 135:799, 1999.

6. Gelmetti C, Grimalt R, Cambiaghi S: Asymmetric periflexural exanthem of childhood: report of two new cases, *Pediatr Dermatol* 11:42, 1994.

7. Report of the Committee on Infectious Diseases: *Red book 2000,* Elk Grove Village, Ill, 2000, American Academy of Pediatrics.

8. Weston WL, Morelli JG: Newly recognized infectious exanthems, *Dermatol Nurs* 10:191, 1998.

9. Kaplan SL: Newer pediatric pathogens, *Adv Pediatr* 46:189, 1999.

10. Davidkin I et al: Etiology of measles- and rubella-like illnesses in measles, mumps and rubella-vaccinated children, *J Infect Dis* 178:1567, 1998.

11. Centers for Disease Control and Prevention: Measles—United States 1999, *MMWR Morb Mortal Wkly Rep* 49:557, 2000.

12. Koplik H: The diagnosis of the invasion of measles from a study of the exanthema as it appears on the buccal mucous membrane, *Arch Pediatr* 13:918, 1896.

13. West CE: Vitamin A and measles, *Nutr Rev* 58:S46, 2000.

14. Ratnam S et al: Performance of indirect immunoglobulin M (IgM) serology tests and IgM capture assays for the laboratory diagnosis of measles, *J Clin Microbiol* 38:99, 2000.

15. Schneider-Schaulies S, ter Meulen V: Pathogenic aspects of measles virus infections, *Arch Virol* 15:139, 1999.

16. Fulginiti VA, Eller JJ, Downie AW: Altered reactivity to measles virus: atypical measles in children previously immunized with inactivated measles virus vaccine, *JAMA* 202:1075, 1967.

17. Sullivan EM, Burgess MA, Forrest JM: The epidemiology of rubella and congenital rubella in Australia, 1992 to 1997, *Commun Dis Intell* 23:209, 1999.

18. Rosa C: Rubella and rubeola, *Semin Perinatol* 22:318, 1998.

19. Turner AJ: Surveillance of congenital rubella in Great Britain: rubella can be mistaken for parvovirus B19 infection, *Br Med J* 318:769, 1999.

20. Webster WS: Teratogen update: congenital rubella, *Teratology* 58:13, 1998.

21. Jundt JW, Creager AH: STAR complexes: febrile illness associated with sore throat, arthritis and rash, *South Med J* 86:521, 1993.

22. Kosuge H: HHV-6 & 7 and their related diseases, *J Dermatol Sci* 22:205, 2000.

23. Stoeckle MY: The spectrum of human herpesvirus 6 infection: from roseola infantum to adult disease, *Ann Rev Med* 51:423, 2000.

24. Teach SJ et al: Human herpesviruses types 6 and 7 and febrile seizures, *Pediatr Neurol* 21:699, 1999.

25. Ongradi J et al: Simultaneous infection by human herpesvirus 6 and human parvovirus B19 in papular purpuric gloves-and-socks syndrome, *Arch Dermatol* 136:672, 2000.

26. Barton Rogers B: Parvovirus B19: twenty-five years in perspective, *Pediatr Develop Pathol* 2:296, 1999.

27. Seishima M, Kanoh Izumi T: The spectrum of cutaneous eruptions in 22 patients with isolated serological evidence of infection by parvovirus B19, *Arch Dermatol* 135:1556, 1999.

28. Gilbert GL: Parvovirus B19 infection and its significance in pregnancy, *Commun Dis Intell* 24:69, 2000.

29. Chen MY, Lee KL, Hung CC: Immunoglobulin M and G immunoblots in the diagnosis of parvovirus B19 infection, *J Formos Med Assoc* 99:24, 2000.

30. Brown KE, Hibbs JR, Gallinella G: Resistance to parvovirus B19 infection due to a lack of virus receptor (erythrocyte p antigen), *N Engl J Med* 330:1192, 1994.

31. Han RK et al: Recognition and management of Kawasaki disease, *Can Med Assoc J* 162:807, 2000.

32. Barone SR, Pontrelli LR, Krilov LR: The differentiation of classic Kawasaki disease, atypical Kawasaki disease and acute adenoviral infection: use of clinical features and a rapid direct fluorescent antigen test, *Arch Pediatr Adolesc Med* 154:453, 2000.

33. Chua PK et al: Lack of association between Kawasaki syndrome and infection with parvovirus B19, human herpesvirus 8, TT virus, GB virus C/hepatitis G virus or *Chlamydia Pneumoniae*, *Ped Infect Dis J* 19:477, 2000.

34. Boyd AS et al: Mercury exposure and cutaneous disease, *J Am Acad Dermatol* 43:81, 2000.

35. Sawyer MH: Enterovirus infections: diagnosis and treatment, *Pediatr Infect Dis J* 18:1033, 1999.

36. Zaoutis T, Klein JD: Enterovirus infections, *Pediatr Rev* 19:183, 1998.

37. Godshall SE, Kirchner JT: Infectious mononucleosis: complexities of a common syndrome, *Postgrad Med* 107:175, 183, 2000.

38. Niedobitek G et al: Epstein-Barr virus (EBV) in infectious mononucleosis: detection of the virus in tonsillar B lymphocytes but not in desquamated oropharyngeal epithelial cells, *Mol Pathol* 53:37, 2000.

39. Schissel DJ, Dinger D, David-Bajar K: Azithromycin eruption in infectious mononucleosis: a proposed mechanism of interaction, *Cutis* 65:163, 2000.

40. Brigden ML et al: Infectious mononucleosis in an outpatient population: diagnostic utility of 2 automated hematology analyzers and the sensitivity and specificity of Hoagland's criteria in heterophile-positive patients, *Arch Pathol Lab Med* 123:875, 1999.

41. Peter J, Ray CG: Infectious mononucleosis, *Pediatr Rev* 19:276, 1998.

42. Torre D, Tambini R: Acyclovir for treatment of infectious mononucleosis: a meta-analysis, *Scand J Infect Dis* 31:543, 1999.

43. Caputo R, Gelmetti C, Ermacora E: Gianotti-Crosti syndrome: a retrospective analysis of 308 cases, *J Am Acad Dermatol* 26:207, 1992.

44. Boeck K et al: Gianotti-Crosti syndrome: clinical, serologic and therapeutic data from nine children, *Cutis* 62:271, 1998.

45. Cohen JI: Epstein-Barr virus infection, *N Engl J Med* 343:481, 2000.

46. Muir AJ: The natural history of hepatitis C viral infection, *Semin Gastrointest Dis* 11:54, 2000.

47. Dollberg S, Berkun Y, Gross-Kieselstein E: Urticaria in patients with hepatitis A virus infection, *Pediatr Infect Dis J* 10:702, 1991.

48. Reichel M, Mauro TM: Urticaria and hepatitis C, *Lancet* 336:822, 1990.

49. Sokal EM, Bortolotti F: Update on prevention and treatment of viral hepatitis in children, *Curr Opin Pediatr* 11:384, 1999.

50. National guideline for the management of the viral hepatidides A, B and C: Clinical effectiveness group (Association of Genitourinary Medicine and the Medical Society for the Study of Veneral Diseases, *Sex Transm Dis* 75: S57, 1999.

51. Riley LE: Herpes simplex virus, *Semin Perinatol* 22:284, 1998.

52. Jones VF, Badgett JT, Marshall GS: Repeated photoreactivation of herpes simplex virus type 1 in an extrafacial dermatomal distribution, *Pediatr Infect Dis J* 13:238, 1994.

53. ACOG practice bulletin: management of herpes in pregnancy. Clinical management guidelines for obstetrician-gynecologists, *Int J Gynaecol Obstet* 68:165, 2000.

54. Weeks BS et al: Herpes simplex virus type-1 and -2 pathogenesis is restricted by the epidermal basement membrane, *Arch Virol* 145:385, 2000.

55. Bale JF Jr: Human herpesviruses and neurological disorders of childhood, *Semin Pediatr Neurol* 6:278, 1999.

56. Goodyear HM: Rapid diagnosis of cutaneous herpes simplex infections using specific monoclonal antibodies, *Clin Exper Dermatol* 19:294, 1994.

57. Emmert DH: Treatment of common cutaneous herpes simplex virus infections, *Am Fam Phys* 61:1697, 2000.

58. Takayama N, Takayama M, Takita J: Herpes zoster in healthy children immunized with varicella vaccine, *Pediatr Infect Dis J* 19:169, 2000.

59. Arvin AM: Chickenpox (varicella), *Contrib Microbiol* 3:96, 1999.

60. Furuta Y et al: High prevalence of varicella-zoster virus reactivation in herpes simplex-seronegative patients with acute peripheral nerve palsy, *Clin Infect Dis* 30:529, 2000.

61. Arvin AM: Management of varicella-zoster infections in children, *Adv Exp Med Biol* 458:167, 1999.

62. Lin F, Hadler JL: Epidemiology of primary varicella and herpes zoster hospitalizations: the pre-varicella vaccine era, *J Infect Dis* 181:1897, 2000.

63. Chang LY, Lin TY, Huang YC: Comparison of enterovirus 71 and coxsackievirus-A16 clinical illnesses during the Taiwan enterovirus epidemic, 1998, *Pediatr Infect Dis J* 18:1092, 1999.

64. Shimizu H et al: Enterovirus 71 from fatal and nonfatal cases of hand, foot and mouth disease epidemics in Malaysia, Japan and Taiwan in 1997-98, *Jap J Infect Dis* 52:12, 1999.

65. Clementz GC, Mancini AJ: Nail matrix arrest following hand, foot and mouth disease: a report of five children, *Pediatr Dermatol* 17:7, 2000.

66. Raj R, Verghese A: Human immunodeficiency virus infections in adolescents, *Adolesc Med* 11:359, 2000.

67. Smith KJ, Skelton HG, Yeager J: Cutaneous findings in HIV-1 positive patients: a 42 month prospective study, *J Am Acad Dermatol* 31:746, 1994.

68. Johnson SC, Gerber JG: Advances in HIV/AIDS therapy, *Adv Intern Med* 45:1, 2000.

69. Tyring SK: Human papillomavirus infections: epidemiology, pathogenesis and host immune response, *J Am Acad Dermatol* 43:S18, 2000

70. Squires J et al: Oral condylomata in children, *Arch Pediatr Adolesc Med* 153:651, 1999.

71. Atabaki S, Paradise J: The medical evaluation of the sexually abused child: lessons from a decade of research, *Pediatrics* 104:178, 1999.

72. Raimer S: New and emerging therapies in pediatric dermatology, *Dermatol Clin* 18:73, 2000.

73. Hobbs CJ, Wyunne J: How to manage warts, *Arch Dis Child* 81:460, 1999.

74. Edwards L: Imiquimod in clinical practice, *J Am Acad Dermatol* 43:S12, 2000.

75. Orlow SJ, Paller A: Cimetidine therapy for multiple viral warts in children, *J Am Acad Dermatol* 28:794, 1993.

76. Smith KJ, Yeager J, Skelton H: Molluscum contagiosum: its clinical, histopathologic and immunohistochemical spectrum, *Int J Dermatol* 38:664, 1999.

77. Kolokotronis A et al: Facial and perioral molluscum contagiosum as a manifestation of HIV infection, *Aust Dent J* 45:49, 2000.

78. Konya J, Thompson CH: Molluscum contagiosum virus: antibody responses in persons with clinical lesions and seroepidemiology in a representative Australian population, *J Infect Dis* 179:701, 1999.

79. Luttichau HR et al: A highly selective CC chemokine receptor (CCR) 8 antagonist encoded by the poxvirus molluscum contagiosum, *J Exp Med* 191:171, 2000.

80. Yashar SS, Shamiri B: Oral cimetidine treatment of molluscum contagiosum, *Pediatr Dermatol* 16:493, 1999.

81. Romiti R et al: Treatment of molluscum contagiosum with potassium hydroxide: a clinical approach to 35 children, *Pediatr Dermatol* 16:228, 1999.

82. Weller R, O'Callaghan CJ, MacSween RM: Scarring in molluscum contagiosum: comparison of physical expression and phenol ablation, *Br Med J* 319:154, 1999.

CHAPTER NINE

Papulosquamous Disorders

Children affected with papulosquamous disorders have skin lesions characterized by red or violaceous macules that progress to papules and develop scales. The exact prevalence of this group of diseases is unknown.[1] However, psoriasis alone has a yearly prevalence of 3.1 per 1000 U.S. children. Pityriasis rosea accounts for a further increase in the prevalence of papulosquamous eruptions in childhood. Thus papulosquamous disorders are common in children and should be readily recognized by those caring for them. The clinician should recognize that this group of diseases is chronic, lasting months to years. It is important for the clinician to distinguish these diseases with raised lesions from flat, scaly conditions, such as the ichthyoses or the various forms of desquamation.

PSORIASIS
Clinical Features

Psoriasis is thought to be a hereditary disorder that requires an interplay of genetic and environmental factors for full clinical expression.[2,3] Childhood-onset psoriasis is more likely to demonstrate an affected family member than late-onset psoriasis.[2,4] Psoriasis is a clinical diagnosis based on the presence of thick, silvery scales on at least some lesions, the characteristic distribution, nail involvement, and the presence of the isomorphic phenomenon. The eruption consists of erythematous macular or papular lesions that develop a thick, silvery scale (Fig. 9-1).

Discrete scaly papules (guttate lesions) may be seen, or groups of papules may coalesce to form raised, sharply marginated, erythematous plaques. The sites of predilection for psoriasis include the scalp, ears, eyebrows, elbows, knees, gluteal crease, genitalia, and nails (Fig. 9-2). Complete examination of the entire cutaneous surface is necessary because lesions may be few in number. The most common clinical picture of psoriasis in childhood is involvement of the elbows, knees, and scalp by a few plaques (Figs. 9-3 and 9-4).

Guttate psoriasis, the term given to the form of psoriasis with multiple discrete papules, begins on the trunk as multiple erythematous macules that mimic a viral exanthem (Fig. 9-5). Guttate psoriasis is more common in children than adults. As noted, the lesions progress to papules that develop a silvery scale (Fig. 9-6). These droplike papules (*guttata* is the Latin word for "drop") are seen predominantly on the trunk and proximal extremities. Guttate psoriasis may follow a sore throat, particularly streptococcal pharyngitis, by 2 to 3 weeks.[6] Follicular accentuation of the skin lesions may be seen. Children with guttate psoriasis should be evaluated for pharyngeal[6] or rectal[7,8] streptococcal infection. Children with an episode of guttate psoriasis are likely to develop psoriasis vulgaris within 5 years.[1]

The isomorphic (Koebner) phenomenon, in which psoriatic lesions develop in sites of skin trauma several days after the traumatic event, is a useful diagnostic feature of psoriasis.[1] It occurs in a linear fashion along a scratch, but may also be precipitated by lacerations, abrasions, sunburn, insect bites, or pressure (Fig. 9-7). In some children it may appear in a nevoid distribution and mimic epidermal nevi.[9]

Scalp involvement with psoriasis results in accumulation of thick scales throughout the scalp, with thickened scales along the frontal hairline and behind the ears (Fig. 9-8). The scalp is involved in the majority of children with psoriasis. Hair loss does not occur.

Involvement of the palms and soles is uncommon in children, but psoriasis may appear as fissured, painful, symmetric plaques (Fig. 9-9) or as multiple small, sterile pustules.[10] Pustular lesions on the palms and soles may be associated with common plaques of psoriasis elsewhere.[10] Children may also have involvement of the distal segment of one or more digits.[11]

Genital involvement (e.g., perineal area, penis, inguinal folds, labia) occurs in 44% of children with psoriasis.[4] Gluteal cleft involvement is common (see Fig. 9-2), as is involvement of the penis (Fig. 9-10).

Nail signs in psoriasis (Box 9-1) include the following: multiple tiny pits on the surface of the nails (pitting); yellowing of the distal nail caused by

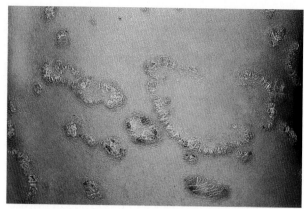

Fig. 9-1 Papules and plaques, some of which are covered with thick, silvery scales over the back of a child with psoriasis.

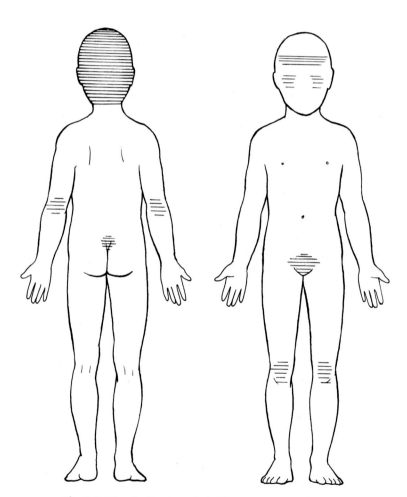

Fig. 9-2 The distribution of childhood psoriasis vulgaris.

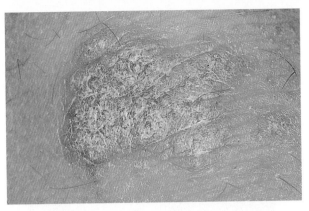

Fig. 9-3 Plaque of psoriasis with silvery scale on the leg of a child.

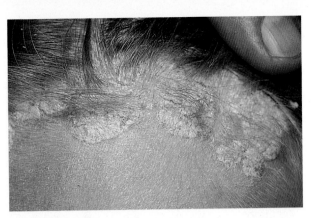

Fig. 9-4 Scaly plaques of the scalp in psoriasis.

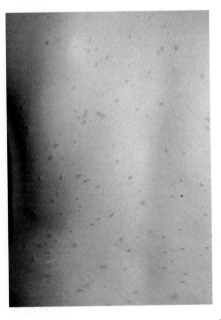

Fig. 9-5 Dozens of discrete, red papules scattered on the back of a child with acute guttate psoriasis after a streptococcal throat infection.

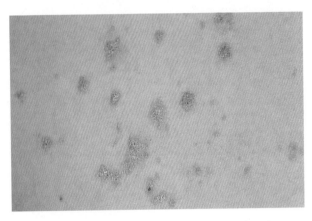

Fig. 9-6 Guttate papules on the back of a child with streptococcal perianal cellulitis.

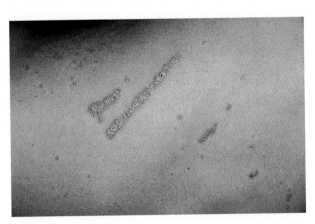

Fig. 9-7 Psoriasis appearing within the line of a previous scratch demonstrating the isomorphic (Koebner) phenomenon.

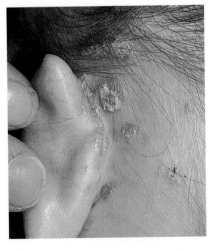

Fig. 9-8 Scaly papules behind the ear and in the scalp.

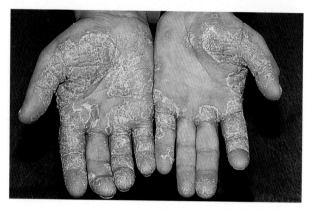

Fig. 9-9 Scaly fissured psoriasis plaques on a child's palms.

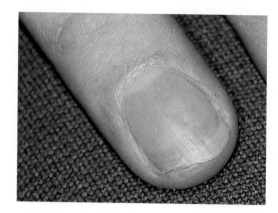

Fig. 9-11 Nail pitting in a child with psoriasis.

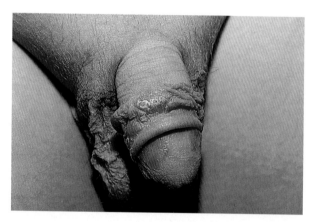

Fig. 9-10 Scaly plaque on foreskin and red plaque on glans penis in child with psoriasis.

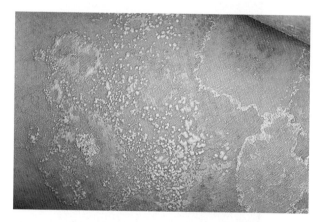

Fig. 9-12 Pinpoint pustules, erythema, and sheets of desquamation in a child with pustular psoriasis.

Box 9-1 Nail Signs in Psoriasis

Pitting of the nail surface
Distal onycholysis
Distal hyperkeratosis
Hyperkeratosis and crumbling of the entire nail

---

separation of the nail plate from the nail bed (onycholysis); thickening of the distal nail (distal hyperkeratosis); or thickening, crumbling, and destruction of the entire nail (Fig. 9-11). All 20 nails may be involved, and rarely, nail changes may be the presenting feature of psoriasis in children. Nail changes are seen in 15% of children with psoriasis, but absence of nail involvement does not exclude the diagnosis of psoriasis. [1,4,12]

Erythroderma with thousands of pinpoint pustules, which eventuates in sheets of desquamation, is called *pustular psoriasis* and is quite rare in childhood but may result from treatment of psoriasis with systemic steroids (Figs. 9-12 and 9-13). [13,14] Pustular psoriasis may be accompanied by lytic bone lesions. [15]

Itching is a variable feature in psoriasis; most children do not complain of it. Scratching of lesions or picking off the scales may induce the isomorphic phenomenon and make individual lesions worse.

Arthritis is seldom seen. It develops in only 1% of children with psoriasis. [16] Arthritis may precede or follow psoriasis and usually begins as oligoarticular disease involving the metacarpophalangeal (MCP) joints, proximal interphalangeal (PIP) joints, or the axial skeleton (Fig. 9-14). [16,17]

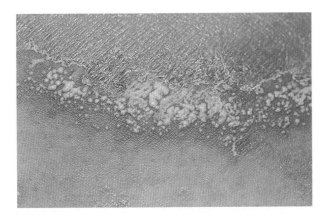

Fig. 9-13 Pinpoint pustules at border of childhood pustular psoriasis.

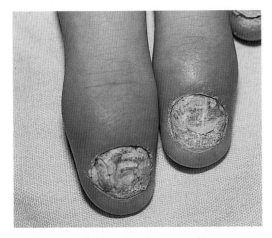

Fig. 9-14 Childhood psoriatic arthritis. Erythema and swelling of the distal interphalangeal joints with total nail dystrophy.

Differential Diagnosis

Conditions to be considered in the differential diagnosis of papulosquamous disorders are listed in Box 9-2. Lichen planus with involvement of the elbows and knees can mimic psoriasis. However, the silvery scale and red color of psoriatic plaques distinguish them from the purple papules of lichen planus. Whitish plaques of the oral mucosa are seen in lichen planus, but not in psoriasis. The isomorphic phenomenon is also seen in lichen planus, but the papules are purple.

In contrast to psoriasis, linear epidermal nevi are present from birth. Flat warts occurring along a line of skin trauma do not have a scaly surface. Lichen striatus appears as a solitary lesion progressing down

---

Box 9-2 Differential Diagnosis of Papulosquamous Disorders

Lichen planus
Lupus erythematosus
Lues (secondary syphilis)
Lichen striatus
Lichen nitidus
Psoriasis
Pityriasis rosea
Parapsoriasis
Pityriasis rubra pilaris
Dermatophyte infections
Dermatomyositis
Nummular eczema

---

an extremity. Scaly macules on the elbows and knees seen in childhood dermatomyositis may be confused with psoriasis. The presence of a malar photoeruption and muscle weakness and pain will help distinguish dermatomyositis. Hypertrophic cutaneous lupus lesions may mimic psoriasis, but the scale is thin, not thick, and central atrophy is present. Guttate psoriasis is most often confused with pityriasis rosea. The large "herald patch" of pityriasis rosea is lacking in guttate psoriasis, and the overlying scale in pityriasis rosea is thin and central, rather than thick and diffuse, as in psoriasis. Early guttate lesions are not scaly and may be confused with a morbilliform viral exanthem, urticaria, drug eruption, or secondary syphilis.

Scaling in the scalp in psoriasis is nongreasy, in contrast to the seborrheic dermatitis of adolescents. Diffuse scaling of the scalp in African-Americans should make one consider tinea capitis. In atopic dermatitis of the scalp, the scales are mild, thin, and dry in contrast to the thick scales of psoriasis.

Nail pitting occurs in alopecia areata, but the pits are broader, more shallow, and fewer in number than in psoriasis. Onycholysis and hyperkeratosis of the nails occur in lichen planus, but synechiae from the cuticle to the fingertip and narrowing of the nail are seen. Fungal involvement of the nail is seen rarely in childhood, and usually only one or two nails are involved in contrast to psoriasis. Trachyonychia may be difficult to distinguish from psoriasis, although onycholysis and "oil spots" found in psoriasis are usually not seen in trachyonychia. In the absence of classical psoriasis skin lesions elsewhere, it requires following the child over many months to finally distinguish the two. All 20 nails are affected in ectodermal dysplasia and its variants, but alopecia, dental disorders, and other features are usually present to distinguish them from psoriasis.

Genital psoriasis must be differentiated from candidal intertriginous infections by potassium hydroxide (KOH) examination and fungal culture.

Pathogenesis

In most families with juvenile-onset (type 1) psoriasis, inheritance is apparently autosomal dominant, but environmental factors influence the expression of psoriasis significantly.[1,3] The histocompatibility antigens HLA-Cw6 and HLA-DR7 are increased in psoriasis, but are not required for the development of psoriasis.[1,3] Preliminary studies indicate psoriasis susceptibility genes on chromosome 17q25, 4q, and 20p.[3]

The classic pathologic features of psoriasis seen on skin biopsy denote inflammation associated with features of epidermal proliferation. The epidermis is thickened, with elongation of the rete ridges to the same level (regular acanthosis), increased epidermal mitosis, parakeratosis (nuclei retained in the stratum corneum), thinning of the granular layer, and microabscesses of neutrophils within the epidermis and stratum corneum. In the dermis the dermal papillae are clubbed, and there is vasodilation of dermal blood vessels with an infiltration of activated T lymphocytes.[18] Increased numbers of epidermal cells enter the mitotic cellular pool; the epidermal turnover time in psoriasis is three to four times faster than that of normal skin.[19]

The factors responsible for increased epidermal turnover are unknown. In many ways the psoriatic epidermis mimics skin healing from a wound. In children the association with streptococcal infection is intriguing, and there is some experimental evidence to suggest that psoriasis patients, particularly children with guttate psoriasis, have greater lymphocyte activation by specific streptococcal antigens than do children without psoriasis.[6,7,19,20] Infection of the throat or perianal skin with streptococci may precipitate acute guttate psoriasis.[6-8] Studies on the inflammatory events before epidermal stimulation, and the regulation of epidermal growth, may help elucidate the mechanism of psoriasis.

Treatment

Most therapies are designed to retard epidermal proliferation but have some antiinflammatory effects as well. It is not certain which of these effects produces the most successful therapeutic results. The treatment of psoriasis can be divided into three levels—topical, ultraviolet light, and systemic therapy—with the choice of treatment dependent on the severity of the disease. In most children psoriasis can be controlled with topical therapy alone.[21]

Steroids are still the mainstay of topical therapy for children. Topical steroids improve psoriasis temporarily, with the most benefit obtained from moderate- to high-potency glucocorticosteroids. Low-potency topical steroids, such as 1% hydrocortisone, are ineffective in childhood psoriasis.[1,21] The maximal benefit is obtained with 2 to 4 weeks of daily therapy, and remissions are shorter than with phototherapy.

Topical calcipotriene (1,25-hydroxyvitamin D3 analog) may be equally effective as potent topical steroids in the management of childhood psoriasis, requiring 4 weeks to clearing.[22] The efficacy of topical calcipotriene is enhanced by alternating with potent topical steroids.[23] Topical calcipotriene is more irritating to the skin than topical steroids.[22]

Anthralin is a tricyclic hydrocarbon that is efficacious in the management of psoriasis by inhibiting epidermal proliferation through downregulation of the epidermal growth factor TGF-alpha and its receptor, the epidermal growth factor receptor. The so-called "short-contact" protocols are particularly useful. Anthralin 1% ointment is applied once daily to the psoriatic lesions for 20 minutes, then neutralized with a pH 7.0 soap, such as Dove soap, thoroughly washing off all of the anthralin. If not washed off, it produces considerable skin irritation. Anthralin stains the skin and clothing brown. Most patients require 4 to 8 weeks of daily anthralin therapy to clear. There is no benefit from adding topical steroids to anthralin.[21] Short-contact anthralin therapy is not quite as effective as topical calcipotriene.[24] Tazarotene is a topically applied retinoid. It is similar in efficacy to mid-potent topical steroids, but it is much more irritating.[25] It may also be used in combination with topical steroids.[26]

For the scalp, softening the scales with salicylic acid 3% in mineral oil or olive oil, or use of a phenol and saline scalp solution massaged in and left in overnight is useful. Then the scalp can be shampooed with a tar shampoo, and the scales can be mechanically removed with a comb and brush. This is repeated daily until the scales are gone. The tar shampoo may be drying, and conditioners applied after shampooing may be helpful. The use of steroid or calcipotriene lotions after shampooing may be necessary in resistant cases.[27,28]

Ultraviolet light (UVL) with artificial ultraviolet (UV) sources (phototherapy) is effective in the management of psoriasis. In general, psoriatic children have better therapeutic response to UVL if it is received in a structured phototherapy protocol rather than during sunbathing. Lubrication of the skin surface with mineral oil or petrolatum before UVL produces uniform penetration of UVL by reducing the reflection of light from the disrupted skin surface.[29] UVL (290 to 320 nm ultraviolet B [UVB]) three times weekly for 18 to 24 treatments) may be quite successful. Photochemotherapy with methoxsalen and long-wave UVL (320 to 400 nm ultraviolet A [UVA]), so-called *PUVA* (psoralen ultraviolet A-range) *therapy,* is reserved for children who have failed on standard therapies. Because of potential mutagenicity, PUVA should be administered only by experienced dermatologists.[30] In the future, narrow band UVB (311 nm) alone or in combination with other therapies may become the treatment of choice for those who fail topical therapy.[31-34]

Children with guttate psoriasis and evidence of streptococcal infection should be treated with antibiotics to eliminate the infection.[6-8]

Systemic steroids are contraindicated in childhood psoriasis because psoriatic erythroderma may follow withdrawal, resulting in fever, hypoalbuminuria, and other metabolic changes associated with generalized skin involvement.[10] Oral retinoids are efficacious in severe forms of childhood psoriasis, such as generalized pustular psoriasis and psoriatic erythroderma.[35] Retinoids should never be considered the drug of first choice in the management of childhood psoriasis. Cyclosporin has been demonstrated to be efficacious in childhood psoriasis, but renal toxicity restricts its use to only the most recalcitrant cases.[36] Antimetabolites, such as methotrexate, inhibit the formation of epidermal deoxyribonucleic acid (DNA), but their use is reserved for the most severe, disabling forms of psoriasis because of significant side effects. The use of antimetabolites in children should generally be avoided, with the exception of those with psoriatic arthritis.[37]

Patient Education

Children with psoriasis have a chronic disease, and education is a crucial aspect of overall care. Patients and parents should understand that the disease is the result of both a genetic susceptibility and environmental factors (see patient handouts on Psoriasis,

p. 343 and Psoriasis Scalp Care, p. 345). Childhood-onset psoriasis tends to increase in severity in adult life.[1,2,5,38] One should emphasize that good remission and good control of psoriasis can be achieved, but that sometimes childhood psoriasis is difficult to treat. One should explain that good treatments require 4 to 8 weeks to obtain significant improvement. It should also be stated that even if psoriasis clears, there is a hereditary susceptibility for psoriasis, and it can reappear in the future. Adolescents, in particular, need considerable emotional support. The occurrence of exacerbations at times of emotional stress is well recognized.

Patients should understand that trauma to the skin induces psoriasis, but severe restriction of activities is unwarranted. Not scratching psoriasis lesions should be stressed. In childhood guttate psoriasis, prompt administration of antibiotics with each sore throat or respiratory illness should be stressed, and children who have multiple episodes of poststreptococcal guttate psoriasis in a year might require prophylactic antibiotics.

Staphylococcus aureus can be cultured in large numbers from the skin surface in psoriasis. Occlusive dressings should be avoided because they enhance the overgrowth of skin bacteria. Hospitalized children with psoriasis will shed bacteria continually into the room air.

Follow-up Visits

Patients should be seen every 2 weeks during therapy to evaluate their response and to provide supportive care. Dermatology nurse specialists or psoriatic day-care centers are ideal for this type of specialized care. An advantage of phototherapy protocols is that emotional support for the patient can be provided with each treatment, and the parents and patient can develop a better understanding of the condition and the care required to successfully control psoriasis.

PITYRIASIS ROSEA
Clinical Features

Pityriasis rosea is most commonly seen in adolescents and children but has been described at all ages, including infancy.[39] It may be preceded by a prodrome of pharyngitis, lymphadenopathy, headache, and malaise, but in most children no history of constitutional symptoms is given. An annular, scaly, erythematous lesion (the herald patch) precedes the appearance of the remainder of the lesions by 1 to 30 days (Fig. 9-15).[39] The herald patch is present in 20% to

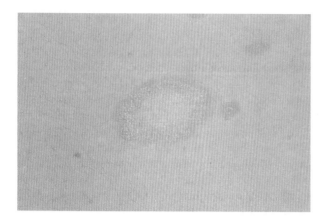

Fig. 9-15 Pityriasis rosea. Herald patch, which is larger than other papules, is seen on the child's chest.

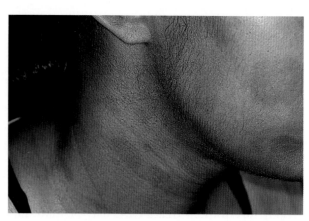

Fig. 9-17 Inverse pityriasis rosea with lesions seen on the neck and face.

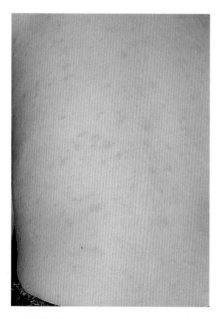

Fig. 9-16 Lesions of pityriasis rosea following a "Christmas tree" distribution.

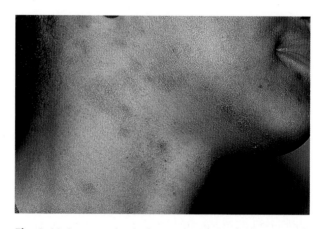

Fig. 9-18 Inverse pityriasis rosea with oval plaques with central scale on the neck of a black child.

80% of children.[40] It is usually on the trunk but may appear on the face or extremities. The herald patch, unlike the other lesions, shows central clearing and may mimic tinea corporis.[39]

The cutaneous lesions consist of multiple erythematous macules progressing to small, red papules that appear over the trunk (Fig. 9-16). The papules enlarge, becoming oval. The long axes of the oval lesions tend to be parallel to each other and follow the lines of skin stress (Fig. 9-17). A thin scale develops in the center of the oval lesions.[39] Individual lesions may be atypical in appearance, including vesicular, crusted, and purpuric types.[39] Asymptomatic oral lesions may be noted in 16% of cases.[39] In black skin, lesions over the proximal extremities, inguinal and axillary areas, and neck often predominate, with few lesions on the trunk (Fig. 9-18).[39] Despite the different distribution, the course is similar. The lesions last 4 to 8 weeks. Mild itching is common during the first week of the generalized eruption, but the lesions are asymptomatic thereafter.

Differential Diagnosis

The herald patch is often confused with tinea corporis before the appearance of the generalized eruption. If an antifungal agent is used, the generalized papular eruption may be mistaken for a drug reaction to the antifungal. The herald patch may also be confused with a lesion of nummular eczema. Nummular eczema usually is crusted, in contrast to the dry, scaly herald patch. The generalized papular eruption may mimic urticaria, the viral exanthems, morbilliform drug eruptions, post–bone marrow transplantation eruption, or guttate psoriasis (see Box 9-2), but the presence of the herald patch is a useful distinguishing feature. As the lesions become more oval, secondary syphilis should be considered. Although secondary syphilis is usually characterized by lesions of the oral and genital mucosa and ham-colored macules on the palms and soles, the adolescent with "pityriasis rosea" accompanied by palmar lesions, fever, or lymphadenopathy should have a Venereal Disease Research Laboratories (VDRL) test to exclude secondary syphilis. The oval lesions may also be confused with pityriasis lichenoides chronica.

Pathogenesis

Because epidemics occur in a susceptible age group, pityriasis rosea has long been considered to be an infectious process. There is debate regarding the role of human herpesvirus (HHV) 7 as the causative agent.[41-44] Pathologic changes consist only of mild inflammation, with edema of the epidermis and dermis, and a mild perivascular accumulation of lymphocytes. Focal areas of parakeratosis are seen.

Treatment

Most children and adolescents require no therapy. A single dose of UVL, either natural sunlight exposure to redness or one minimal erythema dose of sunlamp exposure, will stop itching and hasten the disappearance of the lesions (Fig. 9-19).[45] Oral antihistamines are rarely necessary. Topical steroids do not influence the lesions.

Patient Education

The long duration of the lesions should be explained, with assurance that they will disappear, leaving normal-appearing skin.

A repeat episode of pityriasis rosea may cause concern for the patient and parents, but multiple episodes occasionally occur and there is no need for concern.

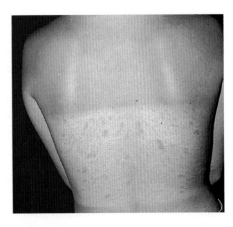

Fig. 9-19 The effect of sunlight on pityriasis rosea. Lesions present only in untanned areas of a child's back.

Box 9-3   Cutaneous Signs of Secondary Syphilis

MAJOR
Papular lesions
Condylomata lata
Mucous patches

MINOR
Annular
Nodular
Pustular crusted lesions
Alopecia
Keratotic macules of palms and soles
Usually associated with generalized lymphadenopathy

Follow-up Visits

Follow-up visits are usually unnecessary except for follow-up on syphilis serology.

LUES (SECONDARY SYPHILIS)
Clinical Features

Secondary syphilis is characterized by discrete pink macules or pink papules with a fine scale distributed over the trunk and is associated with lymphadenopathy (see Chapter 5). Skin lesions erupt 4 to 8 weeks after the appearance of the chancre. Serologic tests for syphilis are always positive at the time of the secondary cutaneous eruption. A list of the cutaneous signs of secondary syphilis is presented in Box 9-3.

The major signs include maculopapular lesions, condylomata lata, and mucous patches.[46]

Condylomata lata are moist, warty papules seen in the perineum and other intertriginous areas, such as under the breast and in the interdigital webs and axillae. The mucous patch is a papular lesion seen most often on the tongue as a red papule lacking tongue papillae. On the buccal mucosa, palate, tonsils, vaginal mucosa, glans penis, and coronal sulcus, it appears as a papule with a central erosion.

The maculopapular lesions, condylomata lata, and mucous patches contain hundreds of spirochetes and are infectious. Generalized lymphadenopathy accompanies these features in 85% of cases; low-grade fever, lethargy, and arthralgias accompany the eruptions in 50% of cases.

Minor variants of secondary syphilis include the following: annular lesions of the face, neck, and genitalia, most commonly seen in blacks; acral nodules that are few in number; sterile pustules and crusted lesions that mimic ecthyma; a "moth-eaten" alopecia of the eyebrows and scalp hair; and keratotic, ham-colored macules of the palms and soles.

Untreated secondary syphilis may progress to nephrotic syndrome, cranial nerve palsies, meningismus, osteolytic lesions, syphilitic hepatitis, or neurosyphilis.

Differential Diagnosis

Syphilis is well known to mimic a wide variety of cutaneous conditions (see Box 9-2), most commonly pityriasis rosea.

The generalized eruptions may be differentiated from pityriasis rosea by the involvement of the palms and soles, lymphadenopathy, mucous patches, and a positive VDRL flocculation test.

Condylomata lata must be distinguished from venereal warts by the VDRL flocculation test or dark-field microscopic examination.

Mucous patches may be confused with geographic tongue, aphthous stomatitis, angular cheilitis, or other mucocutaneous syndromes.

For pathogenesis, treatment, patient education, follow-up visits, and references, see Chapter 5.

PITYRIASIS LICHENOIDES (PARAPSORIASIS)
Clinical Features

Pityriasis lichenoides, an uncommon disorder, may be seen in two distinct childhood forms: pityriasis lichenoides (Mucha-Habermann disease) (pityriasis lichenoides et varioliformis acuta [PLEVA]) and pityriasis lichenoides chronica.[47] Both forms may occur in the same patient, or one form may progress to the other. Thus they are considered two forms of the same disease.[47] The diseases usually have their onset between ages 3 and 15.[47] In pityriasis lichenoides acuta, the eruption consists of recurrent crops of red papules 2 to 4 mm in diameter (Fig. 9-20). The papules have central petechiae and progress to crusting (Fig. 9-21). Lesions in different stages are seen, particularly on the trunk. They heal with depressed scars. The eruption lasts approximately 9 to 12 months and is occasionally associated with low-grade fever. A very rare form of the condition includes acute high fever associated with ulcerative nodules.[48]

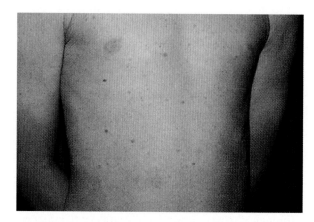

Fig. 9-20 Acute parapsoriasis. Red papules with central purpura or crusts and vesicles scattered over a 10-year-old child's trunk.

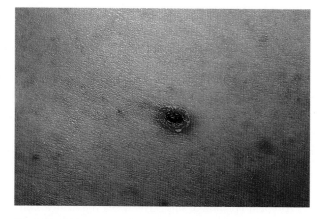

Fig. 9-21 Characteristic red papule with central crust in acute parapsoriasis.

In pityriasis lichenoides chronica, salmon-colored, oval papules with central thin scales are seen primarily in the perineal area, thighs, and trunk (Figs. 9-22 and 9-23).[47] They are few in number, but may persist for 2 to 3 years.[47] Both forms are seldom associated with itching.

Differential Diagnosis

Pityriasis lichenoides acuta mimics varicella, and a child with "prolonged varicella" should bring pityriasis lichenoides acuta to mind. Occasionally insect bites or necrotizing vasculitis are confused with acute parapsoriasis. In pityriasis lichenoides acuta at least some lesions have a purpuric center, which is helpful to distinguish it from varicella or insect bites. The presence of lesions in many different stages is useful in separating pityriasis lichenoides acuta from vasculitis. In a few children lesions appear similar to those of pityriasis lichenoides acuta, but the infiltrating cells will demonstrate abnormal nuclear shapes and size. This condition is called *lymphomatoid papulosis*. A few children with lymphomatoid papulosis may develop a cutaneous T cell lymphoma, mycosis fungoides.[49] A skin biopsy will distinguish.[49]

The chronic form mimics pityriasis rosea, and thus "prolonged pityriasis rosea" should alert one to the diagnosis of pityriasis lichenoides chronica. Dry skin dermatitis, nummular eczema, secondary syphilis, guttate psoriasis, and tinea corporis sometimes confuse the diagnosis (see Box 9-2). The long duration and sparse number of lesions help distinguish.

Pathogenesis

Pityriasis lichenoides acuta is a vascular injury, with extravasation of erythrocytes, a superficial perivascular lymphohistiocytic infiltrate, and necrosis of the overlying epidermis. Focal parakeratosis is also seen. In contrast to necrotizing vasculitis, no fibrinoid necrosis of the vessel walls is seen, neutrophils are not present, and nuclear fragments are not found around vessels. The mechanism of the disease remains unknown.

The histologic findings in pityriasis lichenoides chronica are similar to those of pityriasis rosea. The mechanism of the disease is unknown.

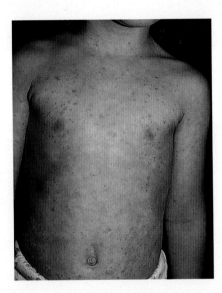

Fig. 9-22 Chronic parapsoriasis. Discrete, oval salmon-colored papules with a thin scale seen on a child's trunk.

Treatment

Treatment with oral erythromycin, 40 mg/kg/day for 1 to 2 months, may benefit some children.[50] For children who fail erythromycin therapy, a conservative approach is recommended. UVB phototherapy may control the disease and some authorities believe it is the treatment of choice for parapsoriasis.[51] Topical steroids do not influence the disease, and claims for efficacy from high-dose tetracycline or low-dose methotrexate cannot be substantiated.

Patient Education

The prolonged course of these disorders should be emphasized.

Follow-up Visits

A visit in 1 month is useful to reevaluate the child's disease state and determine response to therapy. In

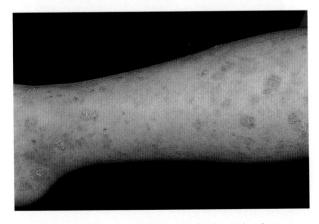

Fig. 9-23 Chronic parapsoriasis. Multiple scaly plaques on child's leg.

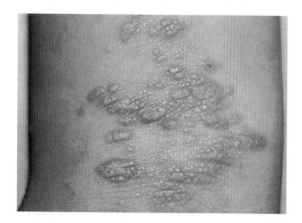

Fig. 9-24 Childhood lichen planus. Purple papules on wrist and forearm.

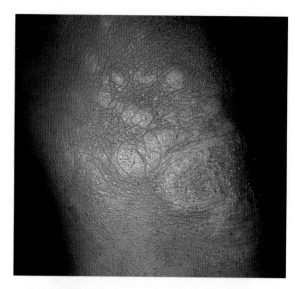

Fig. 9-25 Thick, scaly, purple plaques over the knee in a child with lichen planus.

Box 9-4   The "Ps" of Lichen Planus

Planar (flat-topped)
Pruritic (itchy)
Purple
Polygonal (angulated borders)
Papules
Penile

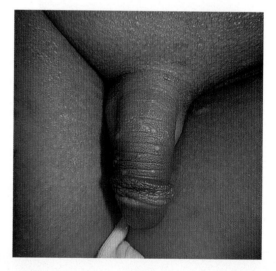

Fig. 9-26 Linear purple papules on the penis in a child with lichen planus.

the child with lesions that persist for over 2 years, reevaluation every 6 to 12 months is suggested, and additional biopsies should be considered because of the possibility of development of a cutaneous T cell lymphoma.[49]

LICHEN PLANUS
Clinical Features

Lichen planus is a chronic papular skin disorder characterized by the appearance of purple, flat-topped papules.[52] The list in Box 9-4 is helpful in recalling the major features. The classic polygonal purple papules occur on the wrist and extensor surfaces of the forearm (Fig. 9-24). On the knees, feet, and lower legs, thick scaling is found over thickened, purple plaques (hypertrophic lichen planus) (Fig. 9-25). Bullae or erosions may be seen on the feet or head and neck.[53] The shaft of the penis is commonly involved (Fig. 9-26). Lichen planus may be inherited in an autosomal dominant manner.[52] The isomorphic phenomenon may be prominent (Fig. 9-27).

Oral lesions are seen most commonly on the buccal mucosa as white, thickened papules in a lacy pattern (Fig. 9-28).[52] Erosions or thickening of the tongue or gingivae may be seen.

In the scalp a circumscribed area of hair loss with replacement of follicles by scarring rarely occurs.[54]

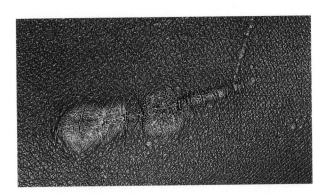

Fig. 9-27 Isomorphic phenomenon in childhood lichen planus. Linear extension of lichen planus along the line of a scratch.

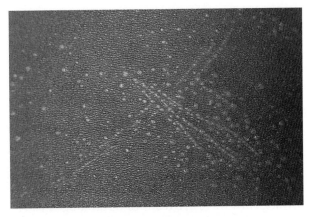

Fig. 9-29 Hundreds of discrete, pinpoint, white, flat-topped papules on a child with lichen nitidus.

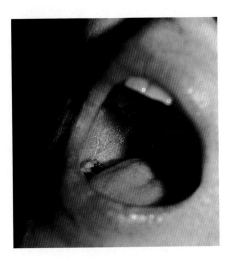

Fig. 9-28 Lacy white thickening of the buccal mucosa in an adolescent demonstrating mucosal involvement in lichen planus.

The nail changes of lichen planus are rare in children, but a roughening of the nail surface (trachyonychia) may be seen.[55] Total destruction of all 20 nails with synechiae formation may precede, accompany, or follow the onset of skin lesions.[55] The nail is narrowed, with an overgrowth of fibrous tissue from the proximal nail fold across the nail plate to the tip of the digit. A few children with lichen planus will present with only nail involvement, which is often labeled trachyonychia until a nail biopsy is done or other mucocutaneous lesions of lichen planus develop.[56]

Itching is severe in lichen planus, and the isomorphic phenomenon occurs commonly, with the appearance of lichen planus papules along an area of skin trauma.[52] Localized forms also occur in children. The natural history of lichen planus is to resolve in 9 to 18 months, leaving hyperpigmented areas in sites where lesions occurred.

A variant of lichen planus, called *lichen nitidus*, has histologic features identical to those of lichen planus yet is more focal in nature.[56] It demonstrates tiny (1 to 2 mm), hypopigmented, flat-topped papules occurring in clusters, usually over the trunk (Fig. 9-29). Lesions may demonstrate the isomorphic phenomenon.[56] They do not itch. Lesions of lichen nitidus have been found in 25% of children with lichen planus.

Differential Diagnosis

The characteristic purple color, with flat-topped papules with angulated borders, distinguishes lichen planus from other papulosquamous disorders (see Box 9-2). The hypertrophic lesions on the lower legs mimic psoriasis. Erosive lesions in the mouth mimic aphthous stomatitis and herpes simplex, and the white, lacy appearance of the buccal mucosa may be confused with premalignant leukoplakia or a white sponge nevus. A skin biopsy may be required to confirm the diagnosis of lichen planus.[52]

A variety of drugs can produce an eruption identical to lichen planus, including thiazide diuretics, quinacrine, chloroquine, quinine, quinidine, and gold, but these agents are rarely used in children.

Lichen nitidus may mimic keratosis pilaris, but the inspissated, dry, scaly, follicular plugs of keratosis pilaris are not seen, and lichen nitidus lesions are smooth-topped.[56]

Pathogenesis

Lichen planus results from an acute injury to the basal cells of the epidermis such that liquefaction degeneration of basal cells occurs and the dermal-epidermal junction is obscured. In bullous lichen planus the epidermis separates from the dermis. Amorphous colloid bodies representing degenerating basal cells combined with immunoreactants such as immunoglobulin A (IgA), immunoglobulin G (IgG), immunoglobulin M (IgM), complement, and fibrin are seen in the basal layer or just beneath it. The damaged basal cells have decreased ability to divide. Thus there are features of prolonged retention of cells in the epidermis, with acanthosis, hyperkeratosis, and a thickened granular layer. The exact mechanism of the epidermal basal cell injury is unknown, but it is thought to be due to inflammatory injury by mononuclear cells that interact with the basement membrane. Hepatitis C has been associated with lichen planus.[57] The actual percentage of lichen planus patients with hepatitis C ranges from 3% to 60% and varies depending on geographic location.[57]

In lichen nitidus the same pathologic changes occur, but they are limited to a single dermal papilla.

Treatment

Topical glucocorticosteroids are effective in controlling the itching and resolution of the lesions.[52] They are used twice daily, and 4 to 8 weeks of therapy are often required for remission. In children with severe generalized lichen planus, prompt relief from prednisone, 1 to 2 mg/kg/day in a single morning dose, can be expected in 2 weeks, although the lichen planus may return as the steroids are reduced. Oral lesions are usually asymptomatic, but when painful they will respond to topical steroid or topical isotretinoin gels applied to the mucosa. Lichen nitidus need not be treated.

Patient Education

Patients should be informed of the prolonged nature of lichen planus and the tendency for dyspigmentation to occur on healing. It should be emphasized that topical steroids are the most effective method to relieve the itching, but that the clearing of individual lesions will be slow.

Follow-up Visits

Follow-up visits every 2 to 4 weeks are needed to monitor the course of the disease and the response to therapy.

LUPUS ERYTHEMATOSUS
Clinical Features

Lupus erythematosus (LE) occurs more often in females than in males.[58] The prevalence may be three times higher in black, Asian, or Hispanic children than in whites.[58] In approximately 15% of all patients with LE, the onset is between the ages of 9 and 15 years, and the incidence is estimated at 1 to 6 per 100,000.[59]

A cutaneous eruption is present in 80% of adolescents with LE, and in 25% it is the presenting sign. The most frequent cutaneous sign is the erythematous maculopapular eruption over the cheeks and nose with a "butterfly" distribution (Fig. 9-30).[59] It is covered by a fine scale and occurs in one third to one half of the patients. Next most common is the discoid lesion, a chronic, persistent skin change that progresses to scarring and pigmentary changes; in black patients, severe hypopigmentation may be seen (Fig. 9-31).[60] Discoid lesions are seen most frequently over the face, hands, ears, and scalp, where scarring hair loss results (Fig. 9-32).[61]

More transient annular papulosquamous lesions limited to sun-exposed areas of skin are observed in subacute cutaneous lupus (Fig. 9-33).[62] Subacute cutaneous lupus is more likely to occur in early childhood and be associated with genetic complement deficiencies and the presence of anti-Ro and anti-La autoantibodies.[63]

Other kinds of skin involvement may occur in adolescents with LE, including telangiectatic erythema on the thenar and hypothenar eminences of the palms and the pulps of the fingers and diffuse erythema and telangiectasia of the cuticle, with erythematous, scaly macules occurring over the dorsa of the fingers between the knuckles (Fig. 9-34).[60] Bullous lesions may occasionally occur. A mottling of the extensor surface of the extremities, the so-called *livedo reticularis*, occasionally occurs.[60] Features of cutaneous vasculitis, such as subcutaneous nodules, splinter nail hemorrhages, purpuric acral infarcts, palpable purpura, and distal gangrene, may be seen. Raynaud's phenomenon, a two-phase color change of the digit after cold exposure, with pallor and cyanosis, occurs in 35% of adolescents. Rarely, persistent, tender, red-purple nodules on the cheeks, proximal extremities, or trunk—which represent lupus panniculitis—will be seen in children (Fig. 9-35).[59] A distinct history of sun sensitivity may not be obtained in children with lupus, and careful questioning may be required to uncover photosensitivity.

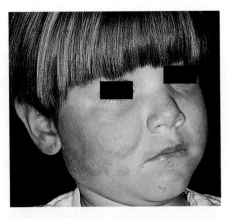

Fig. 9-30 Bright red, scaly plaques on cheeks of a girl with acute systemic lupus erythematosus.

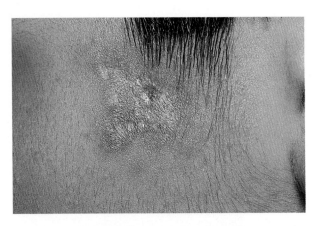

Fig. 9-31 Atrophy, erythema, and scaling of preauricular skin of a child with discoid lupus erythematosus.

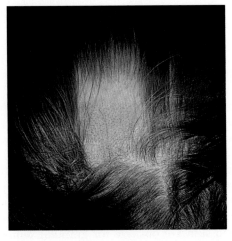

Fig. 9-32 Scarring hair loss with redness and scaling of the underlying scalp in an 8-year-old girl with discoid lupus erythematosus.

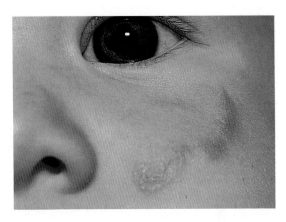

Fig. 9-33 Subacute cutaneous lupus erythematosus. Annular, scaly red plaque of a child's cheek.

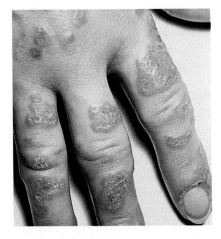

Fig. 9-34 Scaly plaques between the knuckles in systemic lupus erythematosus. Compare with Figs. 9-40 and 9-41.

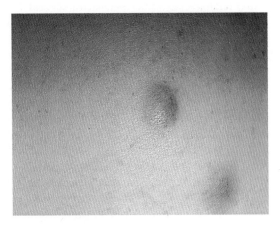

Fig. 9-35 Red-purple nodules on the upper arm of a girl with lupus profundus (panniculitis).

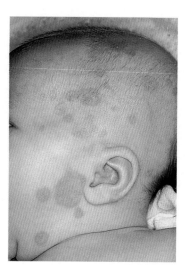

Fig. 9-36 Neonatal lupus syndrome. Four-week-old female with dozens of scaly, annular red macules on the forehead and cheeks.

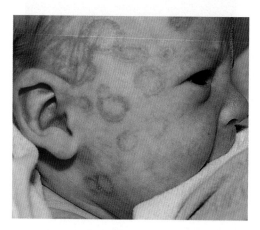

Fig. 9-37 Neonatal lupus syndrome. Five-week-old baby with annular papulosquamous lesions of the head.

Diagnosis depends on a constellation of clinical, pathologic, and serologic findings. Use of American Rheumatism Association (ARA) criteria for LE is recommended.[59]

The neonatal lupus syndrome is characterized by congenital heart block or annular papulosquamous skin lesions or both (Figs. 9-36 and 9-37).[64,65] Although affected infants do not meet ARA criteria for lupus, the association with maternal lupus or Sjögren's syndrome and the clinical skin lesions, skin pathology, and distinctive pattern of autoantibodies similar to those found in subacute cutaneous lupus permit the use of lupus in the diagnosis of this neonatal lupus syndrome. The skin lesions fade by 6 to 7 months of age, but the heart block will persist. Residual telangiectasia may persist for several years. In infants selected by cutaneous involvement, thrombocytopenia and hepatic disease were as frequent as cardiac disease and were more common in males with crusted skin lesions.[65]

The most useful serologic test in the diagnosis of lupus is the fluorescent antinuclear antibody (ANA) test, which is positive in over 90% of children with LE.[59] Autoantibodies in LE are directed against a variety of nuclear components. The most specific is that directed against the nuclear acidic chromosomal proteins, such as the Sm antigen. It is very specific but is found in only 30% of patients. In addition to screening with a fluorescent ANA test, in some children in whom lupus is suspected, an ANA profile in which immunodiffusion tests are done against soluble nuclear antigens may be performed. This is especially useful in detecting antibodies to Sjögren's syndrome A (SS-A) (Ro), which is a diagnostic marker for neonatal lupus syndrome and is found in 98% of reported babies.[64,65] A few babies will have autoantibodies to UI-RNP rather than anti-Ro.[64]

Depressed complement levels, especially the C4 level, are useful for detecting active vasculitis, particularly in the central nervous system and kidney. Direct immunofluorescence of skin biopsy specimens of involved skin are positive for granular deposits of IgG or C3 at the dermal-epidermal junction in 90% of patients. IgG deposits over basal keratinocytes are observed in subacute cutaneous lupus and neonatal lupus.[66]

The initial evaluation of patients with suspected LE should include the tests listed in Box 9-5.

In general, patients with discoid cutaneous lesions, subacute cutaneous lupus, or lupus panniculitis have a low incidence of disease in other organs, whereas those with the butterfly maculopapular eruption or vasculitis lesions are likely to have renal, central nervous system, or other vital organ involvement.

Differential Diagnosis

Childhood dermatomyositis and lupus may present with similar cutaneous features. The photosensitive butterfly eruption may be seen in children with dermatomyositis or drug-induced photosensitivity, such as is seen with the phenothiazines, naproxen, or thiazide diuretics. A butterfly eruption may also be seen

---

Box 9-5   Initial Laboratory Evaluation of Lupus

Skin biopsy, formalin fixed for routine histologic study
Skin biopsy, frozen section, for immunofluorescence
Serum for antinuclear antibody and ANA profile
Serum for total hemolytic complement and complement components
Urinalysis
Complete blood cell count with differential and platelet count

---

Box 9-6   Drugs Responsible for Inducing Lupuslike Syndromes

HIGH RISK
Hydralazine
Procainamide
D-Penicillamine
Practolol

MODERATE RISK
Isoniazid
Phenytoin
Ethosuximide
Propylthiouracil
Trimethadione

---

in polymorphous light eruption. Skin biopsy and immunofluorescence will be useful in distinguishing lupus erythematosus from these processes. The eruption may be scaly enough to consider psoriasis, lichen planus, or other papulosquamous disorders (see Box 9-2). Dermatophyte facial infection (tinea faciei) must be excluded by KOH examination of the scales.

Biopsy is necessary to differentiate discoid lesions of the face from psoriasis and lichen planus, and the discoid lesions of the scalp from other causes of circumscribed alopecia.

Drug-induced LE syndromes rarely cause cutaneous eruptions, but sometimes they may mimic LE. The drugs likely to produce LE syndromes are listed in Box 9-6. The livedo reticularis pattern is seen in dermatomyositis, scleroderma, and other collagen vascular diseases, as is Raynaud's phenomenon, palmar erythema, and cuticular telangiectasia.

Careful examination of the dorsa of the hands may help distinguish LE from dermatomyositis. In LE, scaly erythematous macules are seen between the knuckles on the dorsum of the hand, whereas in dermatomyositis, scaly macules or papules are seen over the knuckle pads. Compare Fig. 9-34 with Fig. 9-40.

The annular papulosquamous lesions of subacute cutaneous LE may mimic tinea corporis, erythema infectiosum, or pityriasis rosea, but a skin biopsy will distinguish.

The red-purple nodules of lupus panniculitis may be confused with vascular tumors or cutaneous lymphomas or leukemias.

Pathogenesis

LE is associated with circulating immune complexes, which may account for many of the vasculitis features in the joints, kidneys, and central nervous system. In the skin there is an injury to epidermal basal cells with liquefaction degeneration, which may lead to dermal-epidermal separation.[66] A patchy accumulation of lymphocytes around dermal blood vessels and hair follicles is seen. These findings are found in acute, subacute, chronic (discoid), and neonatal skin lesions. In addition, discoid lupus shows epidermal atrophy and follicular plugs of scale.[66] Usually no evidence of necrotizing vasculitis is found in the skin, although antigen-antibody complexes have been eluted from the skin. In lupus panniculitis, there is usually a dense lymphocytic infiltrate around subcutaneous vessels between fat lobules, without the superficial skin injury observed in other forms of cutaneous lupus.

The exact mechanism of skin injury and photosensitivity is unknown. A possible association with viruses or virus-induced tissue injury is suggested from animal models of LE-like diseases.

Treatment

It is beyond the scope of this book to discuss the treatment of systemic LE. The chronic cutaneous lesions respond to potent topical fluorinated glucocorticosteroids applied twice daily. In the discoid lupus form, response is slow, over many months. Hydroxychloroquine, 5 mg/kg/day, may be used if topical steroids alone are ineffective.[59] Prior vision screening should be obtained by ophthalmologic consultation. Routine ophthalmologic and hematologic examination should be done throughout the treatment course.[59]

In children and adolescents with systemic involvement, skin lesions clear with immunosuppressive agents in the doses used to treat renal disease. Sometimes skin lesions require additional topical therapy with potent or superpotent topical steroids for control.

Photoprotection should be a mainstay of therapy for cutaneous LE, even when photosensitivity is uncertain. Protective clothing and regular use of sunscreens are recommended.

Patient Education

Sun sensitivity should be discussed and the use of photoprotective agents strongly emphasized. Daily use of a sunscreen of at least SPF-30 is advised. In addition, it is advisable for the patient to avoid sun exposure between the hours of 10 AM and 4 PM, during which time the majority of UVL reaches the earth's surface. The patient should be advised to wear a hat to protect the face. Severe sunburn has resulted in systemic exacerbations of LE. Cosmetic coverings are helpful, both as sunscreens and for disguising unsightly skin lesions.

Follow-up Visits

After the initial visit, a visit in 2 weeks is useful for the evaluation of laboratory evidence, which may indicate potential systemic involvement. Often, adolescents presenting with acute symptoms such as fever, acute arthralgias, or renal disease must be hospitalized. It is important to remember that in 5% to 10% of those presenting with cutaneous lesions only, the disease may progress to involvement of internal organs. Thus reevaluation every 3 months is recommended.

DERMATOMYOSITIS
Clinical Features

The onset of most cases of childhood dermatomyositis is between 4 and 10 years.[59] The incidence is estimated as 0.3 per 100,000.[59] Childhood dermatomyositis often presents with a photosensitive facial rash involving the malar areas and the upper eyelids.[56] Photosensitivity in juvenile dermatomyositis is more frequent than in LE.[59] Periorbital edema and a violaceous hue to the eyelids are seen (Fig. 9-38). Over the elbows and knees, erythematous plaques with a fine scale are observed (Fig. 9-39), and flat-topped red papules over the knuckles (Gottron's papules) are found (Figs. 9-40 and 9-41).[59] Cuticular or eyelid margin telangiectasia is seen. A livedo reticularis pattern on the extremities may be prominent. The skin changes may precede, occur simultaneously with, or

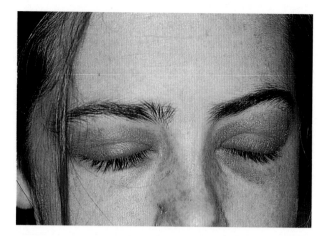

Fig. 9-38 Dermatomyositis. Purple-red discoloration of the eyelids.

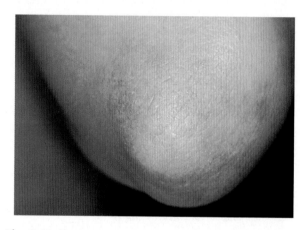

Fig. 9-39 Dermatomyositis. Scaly, rosy-colored plaques over an elbow.

follow signs of muscle disease. Occasionally the cutaneous features are present for months before muscle symptoms are noted.[59] Children with dermatomyositis appear ill, with low-grade fever, malaise, and anorexia noted.

Weakness, with or without pain in the proximal muscles, is the most frequent symptom. Inability to run and climb stairs, easy fatigability during play, and inability to comb hair or reach upward may be presenting symptoms.[59] Difficulty swallowing secondary to pharyngeal muscle weakness may be seen.

As the disease slowly progresses, muscle weakness may be so profound as to make the child bedridden. Calcinosis of skin and muscle eventually develops in 40% to 70% of children and becomes a major problem (Fig. 9-42).[59] Skin calcinosis is seen as crusted papules or plaques around joints or as nonhealing

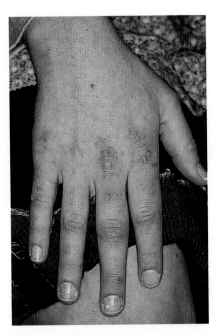

Fig. 9-40 Dermatomyositis. Scaly, red papules over the knuckles (Gottron's papules) in childhood dermatomyositis. Compare with Fig. 9-34.

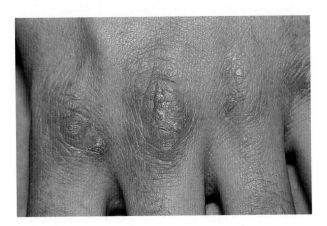

Fig. 9-41 Gottron's papules over the knuckles in juvenile dermatomyositis.

sores. Muscle calcification may result in contractures or severe muscular pain.

Differential Diagnosis

LE is most often confused with dermatomyositis because of the facial photosensitive eruption. Examination of the dorsa of the hands (see the section on lupus) will help differentiate, as will muscle signs and symptoms. Muscle enzyme levels, particularly creatine phosphokinase (CPK), serum glutamate oxaloacetate

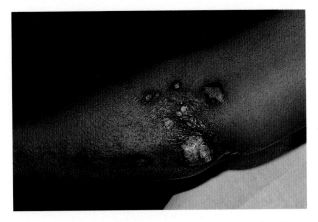

Fig. 9-42 Dermatomyositis. Severe ulceration near the elbow.

transaminase (SGOT), and aldolase may be elevated. Muscle biopsy, electromyography, ultrasonography, or magnetic resonance imaging may assist in the diagnosis.[67] Skin biopsy findings are not diagnostic but are consistent with a diagnosis of collagen vascular disease.

The scaly plaques on elbows and knees are often confused with psoriasis. In dermatomyositis the scale is thin, not thick, and there are associated muscle findings; the child appears ill in contrast to psoriasis.

The livedo reticularis pattern may also be found in periarteritis nodosa and lupus; and the cuticular telangiectasias are found in a number of collagen vascular diseases.

Pathogenesis

The mechanism of cutaneous injury is unknown.[67] Skin biopsies show edema of the upper dermis with a sparse perivascular mononuclear cell infiltrate, and immunofluorescent studies are usually nonspecific. A skin biopsy may be most useful to detect calcification. Children with dermatomyositis may have autoantibodies to muscle proteins such as Jo-1, PM/SCL, or Mi-2 and have positive ANAs.[67]

Treatment

Systemic steroids, either high-dose intravenous pulsing or chronic oral therapy, and steroid-sparing drugs, such as intravenous immunoglobulin and methotrexate, are the primary modes of therapy in dermatomyositis.[55,67] Skin lesions usually are controlled by systemic therapy, but occasionally potent or superpotent topical steroids will be required in addition. Hydroxychloroquine may also be helpful in treating resistant skin disease.[59]

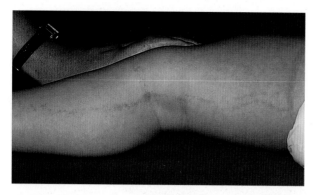

Fig. 9-43 Lichen striatus. Linear, red, scaly papules extending down the flexor surface of a child.

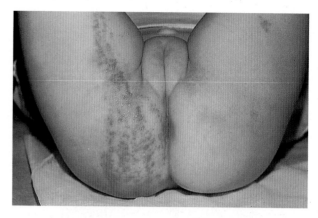

Fig. 9-44 Lichen striatus lesions, which follow the lines of Blaschko.

Patient Education

It should be emphasized that a multidiscipline approach to care for children with dermatomyositis is required. Children should be treated in settings in which muscle disease specialists, dermatologists, and rheumatologists can coordinate the care, and physical therapy and nutritional support are available. Parents must recognize the serious and disabling nature of the condition, be prepared for long-term therapy, and be apprised of the potential complications of the disease and the long-term immunosuppressive therapy.

Follow-up Visits

If not hospitalized, the child should be seen weekly until good control of the disease is achieved.

LICHEN STRIATUS
Clinical Features

Lichen striatus is a disorder peculiar to childhood, characterized by linear, shiny, hypopigmented papules usually limited to one extremity (Fig. 9-43).[68] It does not follow vascular or neural structures, but tends to follow the lines of Blaschko (Fig. 9-44).[68] It is most common in ages 9 months to 5 years, with the majority of children being of preschool age.[68] Although the lesions begin as pink or dull-red papules, they quickly become hypopigmented (Fig. 9-45). Characteristically, the lesions begin on a buttock and spread down the leg, or begin on the shoulder and progress down the arm.[68] They may first be noticed distally, however. The lesion may extend down the digit (Fig. 9-46) and produce a linear nail dystrophy (Fig. 9-47).[68] Occasionally, lesions will be noted on the face. The lesions last 1 week to 3 years, with a mean of 9 months, and

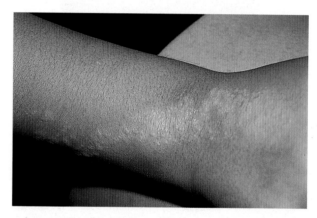

Fig. 9-45 Hypopigmented residual macules in healing lichen striatus.

then spontaneously disappear.[69] Hypopigmented macules occur in 50% of cases and may persist for additional months.[60] Relapses of short duration have been noted after complete clearing.[69]

Differential Diagnosis

The linear lesions of lichen striatus are so characteristic that they are seldom confused with other lesions. The isomorphic phenomenon, seen in lichen planus, lichen nitidus, or psoriasis, may be confused with lichen striatus, but lesions will be present in other areas of the skin in these diseases. Epidermal birthmarks may also be confused for lichen striatus, but they are irregular on the surface rather than shiny and are present from birth, rather than being acquired later in life. Porokeratosis of Mibelli may be confused for lichen striatus, but it does not transcend an entire ex-

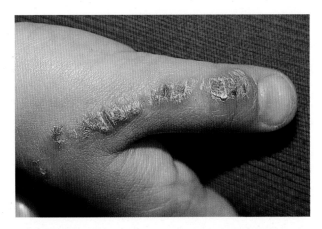

Fig. 9-46 Lichen striatus extending down the digit.

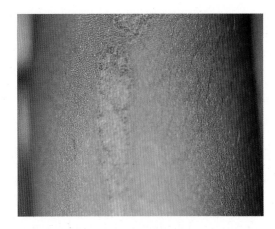

Fig. 9-48 Porokeratosis of Mibelli. Linear, scaly plaque with moatlike border in a 9-year-old child.

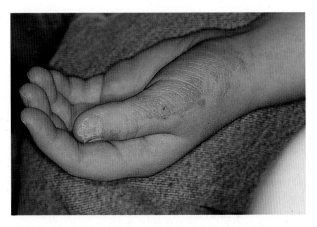

Fig. 9-47 Lichen striatus extending down the thumb and involving the nail.

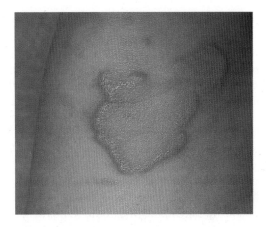

Fig. 9-49 Porokeratosis of the knee of a child.

tremity nor does it follow the lines of Blaschko. A skin biopsy will distinguish it from lichen striatus but is usually not required.

Pathogenesis

A chronic dermatitis is seen on histologic sections, but the mechanism of the disease is unknown.

Treatment

Treatment is unnecessary. Topical steroids may be helpful for the inflammatory component.[68]

Patient Education

The benign nature and complete resolution of these lesions should be emphasized.

Follow-up Visits

A follow-up visit in 4 weeks is useful to examine for skin lesions in other areas to rule out other papulosquamous conditions.

POROKERATOSIS OF MIBELLI
Clinical Features

Porokeratosis of Mibelli may appear as a segmental single lesion or as a group of lesions that may mimic lichen striatus or an epidermal nevus (Fig. 9-48).[70] The condition occurs more frequently in males and has a predilection for the face, neck, forearms, and hands, although the knees (Fig. 9-49), buttocks, and feet may also occasionally be involved. Individual lesions appear as craterlike areas on the skin with a scaly, irregular, oval border.[70] The crateriform area may measure from 5 to 50 mm in diameter, and several craters may be grouped together. The most important diagnostic feature of porokeratosis of Mibelli is the appearance of a scaly border in which a double row of scales surmounted by a furrow is observed. Diagnosis is by biopsy of the border of the lesion.

Differential Diagnosis

Porokeratosis of Mibelli may be confused with lichen striatus or with epidermal nevi. However, in contrast to lichen striatus, lesions are often segmental and do not completely extend down an extremity. In contrast to epidermal nevi, they are never present at birth but develop later in childhood, and do not have as verrucous a surface. Biopsy is often useful in distinguishing among these possibilities.

Pathogenesis

The characteristic biopsy finding demonstrates focal areas of parakeratosis within the epidermis and, if proper sectioning of the double ridge has been obtained, a pair of focal parakeratotic columns with a normal or slightly thinned epidermis sandwiched between them.[67] Sparse or moderate inflammation may be seen beneath the parakeratotic columns. It is believed that this represents hyperplastic clones of keratinocytes, whose phenotypic expression is the result of activation by external trigger factors.[70] This would explain its generalized nature in immunosuppressed patients or in patients with chronic sun damage.[70]

Treatment

The lesions of porokeratosis may produce some concern about cosmetic appearance in the parents, but no satisfactory therapy has been developed. Progressive growth may occur over 2 to 3 years, and some spontaneous resolutions have been reported. Despite numerous case reports and studies, an adequate form of treatment remains elusive.[70]

Patient Education

The parents must be told that the cause is unknown. They must be warned against rushing into cosmetic surgery for improvement because the scarring after surgery may be worse than the lesion itself. The advantages of a conservative approach to such lesions should be emphasized. Malignant degeneration in porokeratosis may occur in less than 10% of patients, with the average time to development being 36 years.[70]

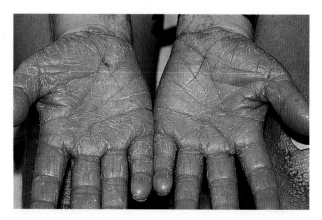

Fig. 9-50 Salmon-colored scaly palms in childhood pityriasis rubra pilaris.

Follow-up Visits

Families should be instructed of the chronic nature of the disease and long-term risk for malignant degeneration.

PITYRIASIS RUBRA PILARIS
Clinical Features

Pityriasis rubra pilaris (PRP) has its onset in the first decade of life.[71] The first sign is commonly salmon-colored diffuse thickening of the palms and soles, with exaggerated scaling in the fissures (Figs. 9-50 and 9-51).[71] The involvement extends beyond the dorsopalmar and dorsoplantar junctions, often involving the knuckle pads (Fig. 9-52).

The condition may remain restricted to the palms and soles, but in the majority of children it will involve other areas of skin, such as circumscribed salmon-colored plaques of elbows and knees with a fine scale. The disease may also produce 2- to 6-mm red follicular papules, particularly over the distal extremities (Fig. 9-53). Widespread involvement of the trunk and progression to exfoliative erythroderma may rarely occur.[71] One feature frequently observed is the presence of an area of uninvolved skin entrapped within a large plaque of involved skin (Fig. 9-54).[71] These so-called "islands of sparing" were once considered a diagnostic feature, but most now believe this can be seen in drug eruptions, psoriasis, and other conditions.[71] Despite widespread involvement, the child with PRP usually has minimal to no itching. Scalp involvement has been reported, as has an asymptomatic white, lacy change of the oral mucosa. Most clinicians appreciate that a wide spectrum

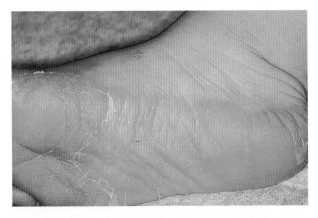

Fig. 9-51 Salmon-colored thickening of the sole in childhood pityriasis rubra pilaris.

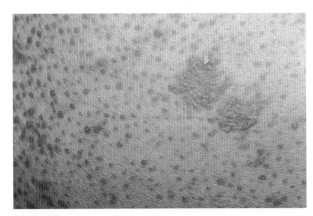

Fig. 9-53 Follicular papules in childhood pityriasis rubra pilaris.

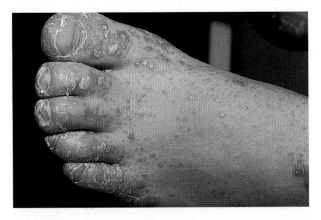

Fig. 9-52 Involvement extending to the dorsa of the foot and toes in childhood pityriasis rubra pilaris.

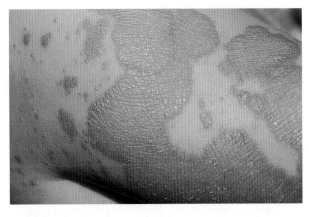

Fig. 9-54 Red plaques on the trunk with "island of sparing" in childhood pityriasis rubra pilaris.

of disease may be observed, and as the condition evolves over many weeks, different skin sites may be affected.[71] The condition tends to be chronic, but most children clear spontaneously within 1 year.[71]

Differential Diagnosis

All of the papulosquamous eruptions may be considered in the differential diagnosis at some point (see Box 9-2). Psoriasis and guttate parapsoriasis are the most likely to be confused. Drug eruptions may mimic PRP, and the involvement of the palms and soles may mimic poststreptococcal desquamation. However, the prolonged duration of PRP and the characteristic salmon-colored thickenings should lead to a suspicion of PRP. Skin biopsies are not diagnostic, but may suggest the diagnosis because of the "moundlike" para-

keratosis around follicular openings accompanied by hyperkeratosis and irregular acanthosis.[71]

Pathogenesis

The cause of the condition is unknown. A rare early onset form with an autosomal dominant pattern of inheritance has been reported.[71] Thickening of the epidermis, with increased keratinocyte proliferation and differentiation, is found.

Treatment

Childhood PRP is quite difficult to treat. It is unresponsive to topical steroids and phototherapy.[71] Some children may respond to topical calcipotriene.[72] Oral retinoids, such as isotretinoin and etretinate have been successful.[71] Methotrexate has been used for refractory disease, but should be avoided in childhood because spontaneous remission is seen. Children unresponsive to topical calcipotriene or with extensive symptomatic disease should be treated with a 4-month trial of isotretinoin, 1 mg/kg/day. Management should be done by an experienced dermatologist.

Patient Education

Patients and parents should understand that this is a condition that can be quite persistent, and therapeutic responses are slow. One should state that the cause is unknown, and the therapy available treats the epidermal proliferation and not the triggering factors. The side effects of the systemic agent chosen should be carefully explained, and the risks and benefits of each therapy discussed.

Follow-up Visits

Follow-up visits should be at 2-week intervals until the response to therapy and side effects are determined. It is usually not necessary to treat until every skin area is cleared. If using retinoids, the clinician should provide a "drug holiday" after 4 months of treatment.

REFERENCES

1. Krueger GG, Duvic M: Epidemiology of psoriasis: clinical issues, *J Invest Dermatol* 102:14s, 1994.
2. Smith AE et al: Bimodality in age of onset of psoriasis in both patients and their relatives, *Dermatology* 186:181, 1993.
3. Bhalerao J, Bowcock AM: The genetics of psoriasis: a complex disorder of the skin and immune system, *Hum Mol Gen* 7:1537, 1998.
4. Braathen LR, Botten G, Bjerkedal T: Psoriasis in Norway, *Acta Derm Venereol Suppl* (Stockh)142:1, 1989.
5. Farber EM, Nall L: Childhood psoriasis, *Cutis* 64:309, 1999.
6. Telfer NR et al: The role of streptococcal infection in the initiation of guttate psoriasis, *Arch Dermatol* 128:39, 1992.
7. Patrizi A et al: Perianal streptococcal dermatitis associated with guttate psoriasis and/or balanoposthitis: a study of five cases, *Pediatr Dermatol* 11:168, 1994.
8. Herbst RA et al: Guttate psoriasis triggered by perianal streptococcal dermatitis in a four year old boy, *J Am Acad Dermatol* 42:885, 2000.
9. Atherton DI, Kahana M, Russell-Jones R: Naevoid psoriasis, *Br J Dermatol* 120:843, 1989.
10. Matsuoka Y, Okada N, Yoshikawa K: Familial cases of psoriasis vulgaris and pustulosis palmaris et plantaris, *Int J Dermatol* 20:308, 1993.
11. Patrizi A et al: Psoriasiform acral dermatitis: a peculiar clinical presentation of psoriasis in children, *Pediatr Dermatol* 16:439, 1999.
12. Akinduro OM, Venning VA, Burge SM: Psoriatic nail-pitting in infancy, *Br J Dermatol* 130:800, 1994.
13. Judge MR, McDonald A, Black MM: Pustular psoriasis in childhood, *Clin Exp Dermatol* 18:97, 1993.
14. Karamfilov T, Wollina U: Juvenile generalized pustular psoriasis, *Acta Dermato-Venereologica* 78:220, 1998.
15. Ivker RA et al: Infantile generalized pustular psoriasis associated with lytic lesions of bone, *Pediatr Dermatol* 10:277, 1993.
16. Biondi-Oreiente C, Scarpa R, Oriente P: Prevalence and clinical features of juvenile psoriatic arthritis in 425 psoriatic patients, *Acta Derm Venereol Suppl (Stockh)* 186:109, 1994.
17. Roberton DM et al: Juvenile psoriatic arthritis: follow-up and evaluation of diagnostic criteria, *J Rheumatol* 23:166, 1996.
18. Onuma S: Immunohistochemical studies of infiltrating cells in early and chronic lesions of psoriasis, *J Dermatol* 21:223, 1994.
19. Ortonne IP: Recent developments in the understanding of the pathogenesis of psoriasis, *Br J Dermatol* 140(suppl):l, 1999.
20. Valdimarsson H, Sigmundsdottir, Jonsdottir I: Is psoriasis induced by streptococcal superantigens and maintained by M-protein–specific T cells that cross-react with keratin? *Clin Exp Immunol* 107(suppl):21, 1997.
21. Linden KG, Weinstein GD: Psoriasis: current perspectives with an emphasis on treatment, *Am J Med* 107:595, 1999.
22. Ashcroft DM et al: Systematic review of comparative efficacy and tolerability of calcipotriol in treating chronic plaque psoriasis, *BMJ* 320:963, 2000.
23. Singh S, Reddy DC, Pandey SS: Topical therapy for psoriasis with the use of augmented betamethasone and calcipotriene on alternate weeks, *J Am Acad Dermatol* 43:61, 2000.
24. Wall AR, Poyner TF, Menday AP: A comparison of treatment with dithranol and calcipotriol on the clinical severity and quality of life in patients with psoriasis, *Br J Dermatol* 139:1005, 1998.
25. Marks R: The role of tazarotene in the treatment of psoriasis, *Br J Dermatol* 140(suppl):24, 1999.
26. Goilnick H, Menter A: Combination therapy with tazarotene plus a topical corticosteroid for the treatment of plaque psoriasis. *Br J Dermatol* 140(suppl):18, 1999.
27. Van de Kerkhof PC et al: Scalp psoriasis, clinical presentations and therapeutic management, *Dermatology* 197:326, 1998.
28. Barnes L et al: Long-term treatment of psoriasis with calcipotriol scalp solution and cream, *Eur J Dermatol* 10:199, 2000.
29. Hudson-Peacock MI, Diffey BI, Farr PM: Photoprotective action of emollients in ultraviolet therapy of psoriasis, *Br J Dermatol* 130:361, 1994.
30. Lindelof B et al: PUVA and cancer risk: the Swedish follow-up study. *Br J Dermatol* 141:108, 1999.
31. Storbeck K et al: Narrow-band UVB (311 nm) versus conventional broad-band UVB with and without dithranol in phototherapy of psoriasis, *J Am Acad Dermatol* 28:227, 1993.
32. Carrozza P et al: Clinical efficacy of narrow-band UVB (311 nm) combined with dithranol in psoriasis: an open pilot study, *Dermatology* 200:35, 2000.
33. Behrens S et al: Combination phototherapy of psoriasis with narrow-band UVB irradiation and topical tazarotene gel, *J Am Acad Dermatol* 42:493, 2000.
34. Calzavara-Pinton P: Narrow band UVB (311 nm) phototherapy and PUVA photochemotherapy: a combination, *J Am Acad Dermatol* 38:687, 1998.

35. Juanquin G et al: Evaluation of effectiveness of childhood generalized pustular psoriasis treatment in 30 cases, *Pediatr Dermatol* 15:144, 1998.

36. Alli N et al: The use of cyclosporin in a child with generalized pustular psoriasis, *Br J Dermatol* 139:754, 1998.

37. Kumar B et al: Methotrexate in childhood psoriasis, *Pediatr Dermatol* 11:271, 1994.

38. Farber EM: Juvenile psoriasis: early intervention can reduce risks for problems later, *Postgrad Med* 103:89, 1998.

39. Hartley AH: Pityriasis rosea, *Pediatr Review* 20:266, 1999.

40. Tay YK, Goh CL: One-year review of pityriasis at the National Skin Centre, Singapore, *Ann Acad Med Singapore* 28:829, 1999.

41. Drago F, Ranieri E, Rebora A: Is pityriasis rosea skin healthier than healthy skin? *Arch Dermatol* 136:932, 2000.

42. Kempf W et al: Pityriasis is not associated with human herpesvirus 7, *Arch Dermatol* 135:1070, 1999.

43. Watanabe T et al: Human herpesvirus 7 and pityriasis rosea, *J Inv Dermatol* 113:288, 1999.

44. Drago F et al: Human herpesvirus 7 in patients with pityriasis rosea, *Dermatology* 195:374, 1997.

45. Arndt KA et al: Treatment of pityriasis rosea with ultraviolet radiation, *Arch Dermatol* 119:381, 1983.

46. Report of the Committee on Infectious disease 2002: Syphilis. In *Red book 2000*, Elk Grove, Ill, 2000, American Academy of Pediatrics.

47. Romani J et al: Pityriasis lichenoides in children: clinicopathologic review of 22 patients, *Pediatr Dermatol* 15:1, 1998.

48. Tsuji T et al: Mucha-Habermann disease and its febrile ulceronecrotic variant, *Cutis* 58:123, 1996.

49. Ko JW et al: Pityriasis lichenoides-like mycosis fungoides in children, *Br J Dermatol* 142:347, 2000.

50. Truhan AP, Hebert AA, Esterly NB: Pityriasis lichenoides in children: therapeutic response to erythromycin, *J Am Acad Dermatol* 15:66, 1986.

51. Tay YK, Morelli JG, Weston WL: Experience with UVB phototherapy in children, *Pediatr Dermatol* 13:406, 1996.

52. Sharma R, Maheshwari V: Childhood lichen planus: a report of fifty cases, *Pediatr Dermatol* 16:345, 1998.

53. Sanchez-Perez I et al: Lichen planus with lesions on the palms and/or soles: prevalence and clinicopathological study of 36 patients, *Br J Dermatol* 142:310, 2000.

54. Nayar M et al: A clinicopathologic study of scarring alopecia, *Br J Dermatol* 128:533, 1993.

55. Joshi RK et al: Lichen planus of the nails presenting as trachyonychia, *Int J Dermatol* 32:54, 1993.

56. Sorpush V, Gurevitch AW, Peng SK: Generalized lichen nitidus: a case report and literature review, *Cutis* 64:135, 1999.

57. Chuang TY et al: Hepatitis C and lichen planus: a case-control study of 340 patients, *J Am Acad Dermatol* 41:787, 1999.

58. Klippel JH: Systemic lupus erythematosus: demographics, prognosis and outcome, *J Rheumatol* 48:67, 1997.

59. DeSilva TN, Kress DW: Management of collagen vascular diseases in childhood, *Dermatol Clin* 16:579, 1998.

60. Yell IA, Mbuagbaw I, Burge SM: Cutaneous manifestations of systemic lupus erythematosus, *Br J Dermatol* 135:355, 1996.

61. McMullen EA et al: Childhood discoid lupus erythematosus: a report of two cases, *Pediatr Dermatol* 15:439, 1998.

62. Parodi A et al: Clinical, histological and immunopathological features of 58 patients with subacute cutaneous lupus erythematosus: a review by the Italian group of immunodermatology, *Dermatology* 200:6, 2000.

63. Buckley D, Barnes L: Childhood subacute cutaneous lupus erythematosus associated with homozygous complement 2 deficiency, *Pediatr Dermatol* 12:327, 1995.

64. Krafchik BR: Neonatal lupus erythematosus, *Adv Exp Med Biol* 455:23, 1999.

65. Weston WL, Morelli JG, Lee LA: The clinical spectrum of anti-Ro-positive cutaneous neonatal lupus erythematosus, *J Am Acad Dermatol* 40:675, 1999.

66. David-Bajar KM et al: Clinical, histologic and immunofluorescent distinctions between subacute cutaneous lupus erythematosus and discoid lupus erythematosus, *J Invest Dermatol* 99:251, 1992.

67. Callen IP: Dermatomyositis, *Lancet* 355:53, 2000.

68. Kennedy D, Rogers M: Lichen striatus, *Pediatr Dermatol* 13:95, 1996.

69. Taieb A et al: Lichen striatus: a Blaschko linear acquired inflammatory skin eruption, *J Am Acad Dermatol* 25:637, 1991.

70. Schamroth JM, Zlotogorski A, Gilead L: Porokeratosis of Mibelli: overview and review of the literature, *Acta Dermatovenerealogica* 77:207, 1997.

71. Albert MR, Mackool BT: Pityriasis rubra pilaris, *Int J Dermatol* 38:1, 1999.

72. Thiers BH: The use of topical calcipotriene/calcipotriol in conditions other than plaque-type psoriasis, *J Am Acad Dermatol* 37:S69, 1997.

CHAPTER TEN | Sun Sensitivity

Sun exposure in children may result in sunburn or sun-induced dermatoses in the skin. Abnormal reactions occur in the skin areas predominantly exposed to sunlight: the face, ears, back of the neck, "V" of the neck, and extensor surfaces of the arms and hands. Sun sensitivity is suspected when the distribution of the cutaneous eruption is limited to these areas. The majority of children with sun sensitivity will have one of the idiopathic photodermatoses, erythropoietic protoporphyria (EPP), or lupus erythematosus (LE) (see Chapter 9). These conditions should be considered in every child with sun sensitivity.

SUNBURN

The acute result of excessive sun exposure is sunburn. Sunburn readily occurs in fair-skinned children, who have less melanin protection than darker-skinned children. However, intense sun exposure can produce sunburn in children with dark skin as well (Table 10-1). Any child who seeks medical assistance because of sunburn should be questioned about exposure to agents that make individuals sun sensitive.

Clinical Features

Erythema and skin tenderness begin 30 minutes to 4 hours after sun exposure, depending on the intensity of the exposure and the degree of the child's natural protection against the sun. They peak at 24 hours and may last up to 72 hours (Fig. 10-1).[1] On the face, sunburn is usually most prominent on the nose and cheeks, with sun-protected areas under the nose, chin, and upper eyelids uninvolved (Fig. 10-2). On the extremities and trunk, protective clothing may produce sharp borders between burned and nonburned areas (Fig. 10-3; see also Fig. 10-1). After intense sun exposure, edema and blistering occur (see Fig. 10-3). Some 2 to 7 days after intense sun exposure, 5 to 10 cell layers of epidermis are shed in one piece as a white scale (desquamation). With acute sunburn, sleep is often disturbed because of the tenderness of the skin. Extensive sunburn causes a reduction in the sweating rate and may contribute to collapse from heatstroke. Sunburn over large areas of the body in a child may result in fever, headache, and fatigue.

Differential Diagnosis

It is occasionally difficult to determine in children what constitutes overexposure to sunlight (Box 10-1). In such a case one should consider the presence of a photosensitizing agent that would induce a sunburn reaction in an unusually short period (5 to 30 minutes of sun exposure). Agents that cause photosensitivity are listed in Chapter 18. Most have been associated with photosensitivity in adults, but they may also occur in children. Burning pain in the skin after 5 minutes of sun exposure should suggest EPP. In contrast, sunburn alone requires at least 30 minutes to produce symptoms. Rapid onset of sunburn and persistent sunburn reactions may be early clues to xeroderma pigmentosum (XP). In LE the eruption occurs 1 to 7 days after sun exposure and is characterized by scaling and erythema, which is persistent for several weeks. Many viral exanthems appear primarily or are exacerbated in sun-exposed areas (see Chapter 8). The laboratory evaluation of photosensitivity, listed in Box 10-2, should be considered when determining the differential diagnosis of sun sensitivity.

Pathogenesis

The tanning or burning rays from the sun represent ultraviolet radiation. The exact cause of ultraviolet radiation damage to the skin is unknown, but it is thought to be a combination of direct effects, generation of toxic oxygen species, and the production of inflammatory mediators.[1] The skin attempts to protect itself against ultraviolet radiation by tanning. Thus tanning is always a sign of ultraviolet injury to the skin. Ultraviolet radiation effects are cumulative as well, with many types of cutaneous cells retaining the additive effects of years of radiation exposure.[2] Long-term effects are expressed as fine and deep wrinkling; scaly, red patches (actinic keratoses); and, ultimately, skin cancer formation.[2] Basal and squamous cell carcinomas of the skin are associated with chronic exposure to ultraviolet radiation, whereas malignant melanoma is more commonly seen in those patients with a history of multiple severe blistering sunburns.

In acute ultraviolet injury the skin changes noted reflect immediate effects of radiation damage.[1] The

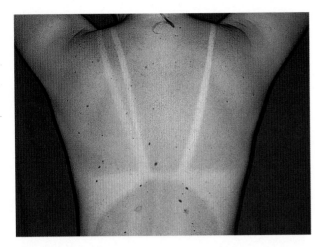

Fig. 10-1 Acute sunburn in an adolescent female. Note the sharp lines of demarcation between uninvolved skin protected by clothing and unprotected skin.

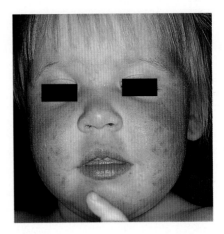

Fig. 10-2 Sunburn of an infant's face. Note protection of the upper eyelids, nasolabial folds, beneath the nose, and under the hair. Note the red papules of sweat duct obstruction.

Table 10-1	Skin Types and Sun Sensitivity

Skin Type	Description
I	Fair skin, always burns, never tans
II	Fair skin, usually burns, sometimes tans
III	Lightly pigmented, usually tans, sometimes burns
IV	Pigmented, always tans, never burns
V	Moderately pigmented, never burns
VI	Heavily pigmented (black) skin

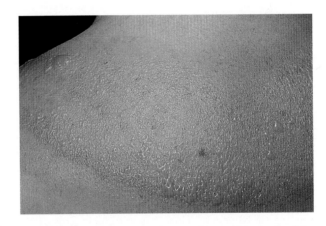

Fig. 10-3 Acute sunburn with vesiculation of the back of the neck. Note sharp demarcation of the area protected by clothing.

first changes noted after prolonged sun exposure are vasodilation of the dermal blood vessels. There is evidence to implicate several prostaglandins as mediators of a portion of the pain and erythema of sunburn, but total inhibition of ultraviolet radiation-induced prostaglandin formation only inhibits sunburn by 30%.[1] Vitamins C and E given together orally for at least 1 week before ultraviolet radiation to the skin also decrease sunburn, presumably by acting as free radical scavengers.[3,4] Metabolic changes then occur within epidermal cells, and individual epidermal cells within the midepidermis demonstrate clumping of tonofilaments and abnormalities of cytoplasmic and nuclear shape, producing the rounded, so-called *sunburn cell*. Such cells lose their epidermal cell attachments; with increased sun exposure, a large number of these cells appear within the epidermis and produce an intraepidermal blister cavity.

Treatment

The pain and erythema of sunburn can be relieved by the use of wet dressings or cool compresses. Inhibitors of prostaglandin synthesis, such as aspirin or indomethacin, may modify sunburn if given within 48 hours of exposure. There is no convincing evidence that vitamins C and E or systemic or topical glucocorticosteroids are beneficial in the treatment of already established sunburn. Topical anesthetics, such as benzocaine, are sensitizing and transient in their relief of pain and thus are not recommended. *Sunburn*

Box 10-1 Differential Diagnosis of Sun Sensitivity

- Sunburn
- Idiopathic photodermatoses
- Erythropoietic protoporphyria
- Lupus erythematosus
- Dermatomyositis
- Photosensitizing drugs
- Viral exanthems
- Xeroderma pigmentosum

Box 10-2 Laboratory Evaluation of Photosensitivity

- Red blood cell fluorescence
- Red blood cell protoporphyrin levels
- Antinuclear antibody and antinuclear antibody profile
- Skin biopsy

Box 10-3 Sunscreen Sun Protection Factor

$$SPF = \frac{MED \text{ of sunscreened skin}}{MED \text{ of unprotected skin}}$$

MED, Minimal erythema dose—that is, the minimal amount of UVB energy required to produce erythema to human skin.

Box 10-4 Recommendations for Sunscreen Use in Children

- Use a broad-spectrum sunscreen with UVB SPF of 30 or greater
- Select a waterproof sunscreen preparation
- Apply at least 30 minutes before sun exposure
- Reapply every 1 to 2 hours

Box 10-5 Types of Available Sunscreens

UVB PROTECTION
- PABA (*p*-aminobenzoic acid) and its derivatives
- Cinnamates
- Salicylates
- Combinations of above ingredients

UVA PROTECTION
- Dibenzoylmethane derivatives

UVB PLUS UVA PROTECTION
- Benzophenones
- Anthranilates
- Physical agents that block light

---

is 100% preventable, and prevention is by far superior to treatment.

Patient Education

Over 80% of lifetime sun exposure is received before the age of 18 years.[3] Thus it is extremely important to protect infants, children, and adolescents against sun exposure. Sun protection habits should be formed at an early age, because adolescents either do not realize or do not admit that they are sun sensitive, and they are likely to be noncompliant.[5] Also, many parents do not recognize the degree of sun sensitivity of their children. Infants younger than 6 months should not be subjected to sun exposure because of the decreased sweating rate and the likelihood of heatstroke.[2] For those older than 6 months, mid-day sun avoidance is still the best method of sun protection. If this cannot be done on a given day, clothing, shade, and umbrellas provide good sun protection. Special sun-protective clothing, such as Solumbra and Frogskin, is available. Sunscreen agents with SPF (sun protection factor) of 30 or greater are recommended as an adjunct to other sun-protective measures (Boxes 10-3, 10-4, and 10-5).[6] Because of the increasing evidence that ultraviolet A (UVA) radiation is also damaging to the skin, many sunscreens now contain agents that block both ultraviolet B (UVB) and UVA (Box 10-5).[7,8] Physical sun blocks, such as zinc oxide pastes and titanium dioxide, have become more cosmetically acceptable and are good sun-protective agents. It must be remembered that sunburn is a gross sign of sun damage, and that cellular damage to the skin can occur even with the use of SPF-15 sunscreens or higher.[6,8] These creams and lotions should be applied to the skin 30 minutes before sun exposure. Sunscreens should be used throughout the spring and summer months and during the winter in sunny cli-

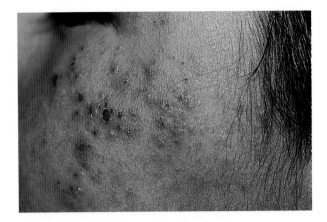

Fig. 10-4 Erythematous papules and plaques in a 9-year-old male with papular polymorphic light eruption.

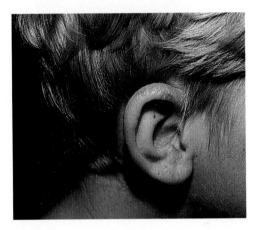

Fig. 10-5 Vesicles and crusts on the tops of the ears in a child with juvenile spring eruption.

Box 10-6 Types of Idiopathic Photodermatoses

- Polymorphous light eruption
- Juvenile spring eruption (hydroa aestivale)
- Actinic prurigo
- Photodermatitis of North American Indians
- Hydroa vacciniforme
- Solar urticaria

mates. Although local reactions to sunscreens are common, these reactions are mostly of the irritant type and not allergic; if allergic reactions occur, they are more frequently caused by the sunscreen vehicle and not the active ingredient.[9] Sun avoidance, such as planning outdoor activities before 10 AM and after 4 PM, is preferable. Sunscreens should not be used to increase the amount of time spent in the mid-day sun. For a patient instructions handout on Sun Protection, see p. 348.

Follow-up Visits

Follow-up visits are unnecessary.

IDIOPATHIC PHOTODERMATOSES
Clinical Features

The idiopathic photodermatoses are a group of related sun-sensitive conditions that are sometimes separated by distinct clinical patterns. Six major types are reported (Box 10-6).[10]

Papular polymorphous light eruption is the most common type.[10] The process begins in the spring and improves throughout the summer. In 75% of patients, onset of the disease is sudden, occurs within the first 3 decades of life, and affects predominantly females. New lesions appear within hours to days of sun exposure, remain 1 to 7 days, and usually heal without scarring. The clinical lesions are discrete erythematous papules and plaques (Fig. 10-4), occurring in sun-exposed areas. For unknown reasons, not all sun-exposed skin is affected. The majority of patients improve with age, and in some patients the disease may totally subside.[11]

Juvenile spring eruption (hydroa aestivale) is described in children of European descent, mainly boys ages 5 to 12 years.[12] Its prevalence in primary school-aged males in Dunedin, New Zealand is 12%.[13] It characteristically begins as 2- to 3-mm discrete papules or vesicles on the ears and cheeks of fair-skinned children. The episode lasts 1 week and reappears the next spring (Fig. 10-5). A small percentage (22%) of patients with juvenile spring eruption will at other times in their lives develop lesions more typical of plaque-type polymorphous light eruption, and some authorities consider it a localized variant of polymorphous light eruption.[12]

Actinic prurigo, Hutchinson's summer prurigo, and photodermatitis of North American Indians have many overlapping features. Females predominate 2:1. Each condition begins as a dermatitis predominantly occurring on the face and extensor surface of the forearms of school-age children. Actinic prurigo has been described in the United Kingdom and northern Europe, and the related form is seen in the Plains Indians of North America.[14,15] Both characteristically start in the early spring, when sufficient sunlight energy reaches the earth's surface. Lesions occur by age 5 years in 35% of children and by 10 years in 70%; the eruption develops during adolescence in the remainder. The initial eruption consists of an itchy, acute facial or forearm dermatitis with edematous papules and vesicles (Fig. 10-6). As the spring progresses, the dermatitis becomes subacute, with crusting on the surface and epidermal thickening or lichenification (Fig. 10-7). Papular lesions may predominate on the face. In the summer the eruption may spontaneously clear, to recur again the next spring. Some very sun-sensitive children will have the eruption throughout the year. It is characteristic that several patches of skin are involved, with uninvolved areas of skin in be-

tween. In North American Indians the disease differs in two respects: (1) a chronic cheilitis of the lower lip is frequently observed (Fig. 10-8), which may be related to living in regions of intense sunlight, and (2) a family history of the disease is often obtained.[15] Overlap with atopic dermatitis that worsens with summer heat is frequent in both actinic prurigo and photodermatitis of North American Indians.

Hydroa vacciniforme is characterized by a few discrete, deep-seated vesicles on the cheeks, ears, or nose that heal with scarring (Fig. 10-9).[16] They are frequently persistent, lasting up to 4 weeks, and more episodes may occur with further sun exposure. Rarely the eye may be affected with conjunctival injection, photophobia, lacrimation, and corneal ulceration.

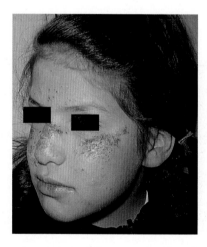

Fig. 10-6 Polymorphous light eruption. Photodermatitis of a North American Indian child, with vesicles and crusting of the face at springtime onset.

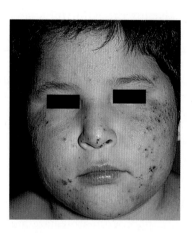

Fig. 10-8 Involvement of the lower lip with redness, edema, and fissures in polymorphous light eruption.

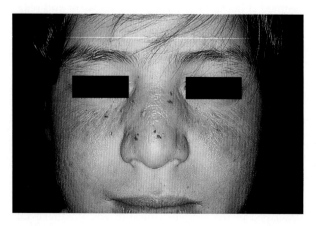

Fig. 10-7 Chronic polymorphous light eruption with lichenification by midsummer.

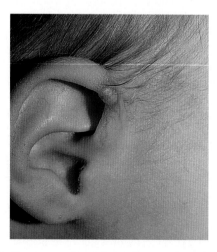

Fig. 10-9 Deep-seated vesicle on the ear of a child with hydroa vacciniforme.

This is the rarest of all forms of polymorphous light eruption. A severe hydroa vacciniforme-like eruption with systemic symptoms is associated with Epstein-Barr virus and lymphoid malignancies.[17]

Solar urticaria is an uncommon idiopathic photodermatosis and an uncommon cause of urticaria. Patients present with urticaria acutely after sun exposure. The disease rarely presents before late adolescence.[18]

It is unclear how these clinical patterns are interrelated, but until pathologic or biochemical tests can distinguish the correct diagnosis they are catalogued under the broad term *idiopathic dermatoses*. Biopsy of early lesions shows an acute dermatitis, whereas biopsy of papular, crusted, and lichenified forms shows a chronic dermatitis.

As in any dermatitis, itching may be severe. Scratching may result in secondary bacterial infection.

Differential Diagnosis

Atopic dermatitis, in addition to other photosensitive states, may mimic idiopathic photodermatoses (see Box 10-1). During hot weather, sweating in children with atopic dermatitis may induce itching and dermatitis on the face and sun-exposed areas. A family history of atopic dermatitis, and the finding of flexural dermatitis in addition to photodermatitis, are useful differentiating features. Acute sensitivity to airborne substances may also lead to the appearance of a contact dermatitis predominantly on sun-exposed areas. In airborne contact dermatitis, the upper eyelids are usually involved, in contrast to polymorphous light eruption. LE, EPP, dermatophyte infections of the face, and sunburn are likely to be confused. Laboratory tests listed in Box 10-2 should be considered. Photodermatitis caused by drugs characteristically produces a diffuse involvement of sun-exposed areas, rather than the patchy areas of dermatitis seen with polymorphous light eruption. Solar urticaria must be differentiated from other causes of urticaria.

EPP and XP have an onset in early infancy rather than childhood, and they may have symptoms out of proportion to skin changes. They usually do not develop dermatitis-like changes.

Pathogenesis

The mechanism of any form of idiopathic photodermatosis is unknown. Patients with idiopathic photodermatosis are generally more likely to be sensitive to both UVA and UVB, but may also be sensitive to either alone.[19] The biochemical change responsible for initiating the dermatitis after sun exposure is unknown.

Treatment

Treatment of polymorphous light eruption involves the use of topical glucocorticosteroids in an ointment base applied twice daily for the dermatitis. In addition, wet dressings in the form of a face mask made of a damp washcloth, with eye, nose, and mouth holes, will serve to enhance the steroid effect on the face. This may be used for 2 to 3 days. Secondary bacterial infection is best treated with systemic antibiotics.

Sun avoidance is crucial in such patients and should be the mainstay of any treatment program. The child should restrict outdoor activities to the hours before 10 AM and after 4 PM. Further photoprotection with a wide-brimmed hat, long-sleeved shirts, and sunscreens with UVB (SPF greater than 30) and UVA protection may be necessary (see Box 10-5).

Children with polymorphous light eruption who are sensitive to the UVA spectrum of light and remain symptomatic despite adequate sun avoidance and UVA sunscreen may be treated with betacarotene capsules, 40 to 120 mg/day, to achieve a serum carotene level of 600 to 800 μg/ml.

In cases of severe polymorphous light eruption, treatment with a UVB or a psoralen and UVA may be considered. Although it appears contradictory to treat a photosensitive disorder with a UVR, UVB or low-dose oral psoralen and UVA will induce melanin pigmentation and epidermal thickening, increasing the natural protection to sunlight.

Patient Education

The concept of sun sensitivity must be understood by patients and their parents. Sun protection methods should be carefully explained and re-explained at each visit. Because of the delayed nature of the eruption, the relationship of the disease to sun exposure is difficult to comprehend. Many parents are reluctant to accept sun avoidance or to restrict their children's activities at school or play.

Follow-up Visits

A visit 1 week after initial therapy is useful to assess the therapeutic response. Visits at 4-week intervals thereafter are advised until the condition has cleared.

ERYTHROPOIETIC PROTOPORPHYRIA
Clinical Features

EPP is an inherited disorder of porphyrin metabolism. In many children EPP shows an autosomal dominant pattern of inheritance, but other modes of inheritance have been described.[20] The preschool child experiences burning, stinging, or itching sensations in the skin. Often this occurs after a sun exposure of only 1 to 10 minutes. Despite the severe discomfort the child suffers, no skin lesions may be found. The child soon learns to stay indoors. Intense sun exposure may result in facial edema, erythema, or urticaria, followed by petechiae, primarily on the face. Less often, vesiculation and crusting of the face appear (Figs. 10-10 and 10-11).

More commonly, however, acute skin changes do not occur, and chronic changes are apparent. Chronic changes usually do not appear until late childhood. Slightly thickened, skin-colored papules appear over the dorsa of the hands (Fig. 10-12), nose, and cheeks. Pitted scars on the face (see Figs. 10-10 and 10-11) and perioral, linear, skin-colored papules may result from previous vesicular injury.

Skin biopsy specimens from sun-exposed skin show thickening of the small blood vessels of the papillary dermis, with a perivascular deposit of periodic acid-Schiff (PAS)–positive material. Direct immunofluorescence of such lesions demonstrates deposits of immunoglobulins, mostly immunoglobulin G (IgG), around superficial dermal blood vessels. Of children with EPP, 5% may suffer cholelithiasis, with porphyrin stones in the gallbladder, and varying degrees of liver injury, which occasionally result in hepatic failure. Mild anemia may also occur.

The diagnosis can be confirmed by laboratory tests. Heparinized blood diluted 1:10 in unpreserved saline solution can be examined with a fluorescence microscope for coral-red fluorescence of red blood cells. It is important that the blood be withdrawn in a light-protected tube because exposure may allow protoporphyrin to be converted to a nonfluorescent metabolite. In unaffected children, less than 1% of red blood cells fluoresce, whereas in those with EPP, from 5% to 30% of the total erythrocytes fluoresce. Quantitative red blood cell protoporphyrins are also useful.

Differential Diagnosis

Most other photosensitive states (see Box 10-1), such as polymorphous light eruption, LE, sunburn, and drug photosensitivity, can be excluded by the striking history of cutaneous burning seen in children with EPP, by a positive family history, and by laboratory studies. Occasionally the family is unable to relate the symptoms to exposure to sunlight, and airborne allergens are suspected. This is particularly true if facial edema or urticaria is a major feature. A careful history, however, will reveal the role of sun exposure.

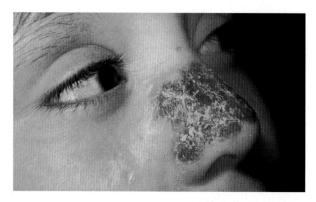

Fig. 10-10 Crusting of the nose after acute sun exposure in erythropoietic protoporphyria. Note depressed scars on the cheek from a prior episode.

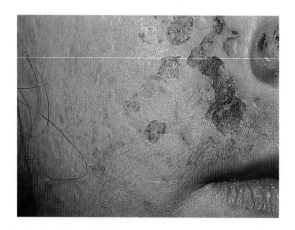

Fig. 10-11 Crusting of the cheek and atrophic scarring in severe erythropoietic protoporphyria.

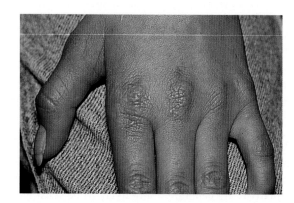

Fig. 10-12 Thickened papules over the dorsa of the left hand of a 12-year-old female with erythropoietic protoporphyria.

Pathogenesis

Abnormally elevated tissue levels of protoporphyrin IX, a normal precursor of heme, are found in EPP. The increased levels of protoporphyrin IX are due to a defect in the enzyme ferrochelatase. Excessive protoporphyrin IX has been found in the circulating erythrocytes, plasma, liver, and bone marrow. Protoporphyrin IX absorbs light at 409 nm and becomes a molecule with an altered energy state. The molecule then transfers energy to molecular oxygen; toxic oxygen products are thought to be responsible for the injury to vascular membranes and perhaps to lysosomal membranes, with subsequent inflammation.

Light-producing 409-nm wavelengths are found in sunlight, reflected sunlight, sunlight traveling through window glass, and fluorescent lighting. Thus a child could develop symptoms indoors or through window glass.

Treatment

Conventional sun protection methods have been uniformly unsuccessful because of the poor ability of sunscreen to protect in the 409-nm range and the small amount of light necessary to induce symptoms.

Oral administration of betacarotene is the treatment of choice.[21] In children, a dosage of 40 to 120 mg/day will raise serum carotene levels to 600 to 800 μg/100 ml, the desired therapeutic range. The child becomes carotenemic, but sun tolerance is greatly increased. Children who previously refused to go outdoors may play for 3 to 4 hours outside without symptoms. Other agents that quench reactive singlet oxygen may also be effective.[21]

Patient Education

The hereditary nature of the disease should be discussed with the patient and the parents, and all family members should be screened by protoporphyrin level determinations. Liver function tests may also be performed on family members. It must be emphasized that photosensitivity can occur with fluorescent lamps, such as those in overhead lighting in school.

Follow-up Visits

During the initiation of therapy, a visit every 2 to 3 weeks is useful to ascertain the response and to adjust the therapeutic dosage of betacarotene. After 4 weeks the serum carotene levels may be used to monitor for the correct dosage. After an effective therapeutic response is achieved, visits every 6 months to examine the patient for possible liver involvement are valuable.

PHYTOPHOTODERMATITIS
Clinical Features

Redness and blisters that occur in bizarre shapes, such as linear streaks, and that leave intense hyperpigmentation are characteristic of phytophotodermatitis (Figs. 10-13 and 10-14).[22] Exposure to plants in the spring and summer months from outdoor activities is the usual history. Some children present with only the hyperpigmented streaks, without a distinct history of erythema or blistering. Exposure to limes or certain perfumes may also produce the syndrome.

Differential Diagnosis

The linear streaks of blisters may be confused with acute allergic contact dermatitis from plants such as poison ivy, whereas the hyperpigmented macules can be confused with incontinentia pigmenti because of the linear arrangement or irregular café-au-lait spots. The bizarre shapes and simultaneous, sudden onset of phytophotodermatitis lesions help differentiate from contact dermatitis.

Pathogenesis

Plants that contain the furocoumarin psoralen are responsible. This includes the celery family and certain grasses and limes. The plants produce the psoralen transiently, usually after a rainy week. The child gets the psoralen onto the skin from the plant touching the skin (the epicutaneous application of a photosensitizer). The psoralen, when exposed to sunlight, produces a photodermatitis with blister formation, followed by intense stimulation of melanin production

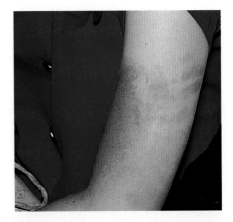

Fig. 10-13 Irregular erythema and hyperpigmentation secondary to contact with riverside grasses followed by sun exposure.

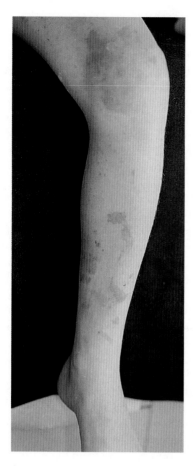

Fig. 10-14 Phytophotodermatitis. Linear and bizarre shapes of hyperpigmentation in an 8-year-old boy from a fight with his brother; they were hitting each other with plants found along a lakeshore.

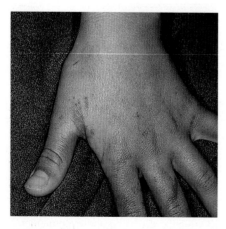

Fig. 10-15 Hyperpigmentation from exposure to celery and sunlight.

(Fig. 10-15). The resultant hyperpigmentation may last for months.

Treatment

The acute dermatitis phase is treated as an acute allergic contact dermatitis with moderate-potency topical steroid ointments twice daily for 2 weeks. The hyperpigmentation is difficult to treat, but bleaching creams may be used if cosmetically important areas are involved.

Patient Education

Patients and parents should be advised that once hyperpigmentation occurs, it may persist for 6 to 12 months. They should be told of the nature of the photosensitizing chemical from plants and should avoid play in the area where the plants were contacted.

Follow-up Visits

A follow-up visit in 4 weeks to evaluate the progress of the condition is recommended.

XERODERMA PIGMENTOSUM
Clinical Features

XP is an autosomal recessive disorder of sun sensitivity in which eight different forms have been recognized.[23] Onset of skin lesions by 18 months of age is characteristic, with early sunburn reactions from minimal sun exposure and numerous freckles as the predominant findings. An important clue is that the sunburn may persist for several weeks rather than resolve within a week. Telangiectasia of the sun-exposed areas and cutaneous atrophy develop within a few years of the other cutaneous findings. Actinic keratoses, which appear as persistent, red, scaly, rough macules in sun-exposed skin, are found next, and the child's skin appears prematurely aged. In dark-skinned children these findings may be difficult to appreciate. Skin cancers may develop by the age of 6 to 8 years, with basal and squamous cell carcinomas and malignant melanomas reported before puberty. Skin-colored or pigmented papules should be regarded as suspicious for skin cancers, and biopsy should be done promptly. The majority of precancerous and cancerous skin lesions occur on the head and neck. Early death from metastatic skin cancers is reported, with 10% of the patients dead before puberty. Ocular disease has a median age of onset of 4 years. Photophobia, eyelid atrophy, ectropion, corneal xerosis and scarring, and ocular neoplasms are seen. Up to 20% of affected patients have neurologic disease. Group A patients have severe early-onset neurologic disease. Groups C and D have milder adult-onset neurologic disease. Immunologic abnormalities, including defective natural killer cell function and a marked deficiency in cellular catalase are seen. Diagnosis and classification of suspected XP are accomplished by examination of abnormal deoxyribonucleic acid (DNA) repair by the patient's cells after ultraviolet light exposure.

Differential Diagnosis

The early freckling should be differentiated from lentigines observed in multiple lentigines syndromes and the LEOPARD (lentigines, electrocardiogram [ECG] abnormalities, ocular hypertelorism, pulmonary stenosis, abnormalities of genitalia, retardation of growth, and deafness) and NAME (nevi, atrial myxoma, myxoid neurofibroma, ephelides) syndromes. Freckling is earlier in onset, macular, and tan, whereas lentigines are slightly raised and brown. Ordinary freckles usually begin between the ages of 3 and 5 years, rather than before 2 years, in children with XP and are not accompanied by skin changes that make the child appear old. Actinic keratoses and skin cancers in prepubertal children may be seen in the basal cell nevus syndrome or in Bazex's syndrome, but not at an age as young as in children who have XP, nor do these children develop the other skin changes associated with XP. Diagnosis is suggested by skin biopsy showing severe actinic skin damage at an early age. Confirmation is made by culture of skin cells with evaluation of DNA repair.

Pathogenesis

Enzymes involved in several steps of DNA repair are abnormal.[15] Thus far at least eight different defects in DNA repair can be found by the fusion of cultured cells from different patient groups with each other to determine if normal DNA repair is restored. Defects have been found in DNA damage recognition, DNA damage binding, DNA helicase and endonucleases. Failure to repair ultraviolet light damage results in carcinogenesis, and XP patients are an important model in the ultimate understanding of sun-induced cancers.

Treatment

Sun avoidance is essential to minimize skin damage and skin cancer formation. Children with XP should avoid sunlight, wear protective clothing, and use sunscreens with maximal SPF each day. Biopsy of any suspect skin lesion is necessary. Referral to a center with experience in management of this condition is recommended. Dermatologic, ophthalmologic, and neurologic consultations should be obtained.

Patient Education

The autosomal recessive inheritance of this disease should be emphasized. A great deal of effort stressing the critical role of sunlight in producing skin cancers is required. The need for frequent evaluations must be emphasized because many skin cancers are preventable or cured if detected early and removed.

Follow-up Visits

A cutaneous examination every 3 months is necessary, preferably at a center with experience in XP. At the follow-up visit, careful examination for skin cancers should be done, with biopsy of any suspect lesions. An evaluation of the child's sun protection program should be performed at each visit.

REFERENCES

1. Hruza LL, Pentland AP: Mechanisms of UV-induced inflammation, *J Invest Dermatol* 100:35S, 1993.
2. American Academy of Pediatrics Committee on Environmental Health: *Pediatrics* 104:328, 1999.
3. Eberlein-Konig B, Placzek M, Pryzbilla B: Protective effect against sunburn of combined systemic ascorbic acid (vitamin C) and D-alpha-tocopherol (vitamin E). *J Am Acad Dermatol* 38:45, 1998.
4. Fuchs J, Kern H: Modulation of UV-light-induced skin inflammation by D-alpha-tocopherol and L-ascorbic acid: a clinical study using solar simulated radiation, *Free Radic Biol Med* 25:1006, 1998.
5. Robinson JK, Rigel DS, Amonette RA: Summertime sun protection used by adults for their children, *J Am Acad Dermatol* 42:746, 2000.
6. Weinstock MA: Updated sunscreen advice: SPF 30, *J Am Acad Dermatol* 43:154, 2000.
7. Roelandts R: Shedding light on sunscreens, *Clin Exp Dermatol* 23:147, 1998.
8. Gasparro FP: Sunscreen, skin photobiology, and skin cancer: the need for UVA protection and evaluation, *Environ Health Perspect* 108:71, 2000.
9. Nixon RL, Frowen KE, Lewis AE: Skin reactions to sunscreens, *Aust J Dermatol* 38:S83, 1997.
10. McGregor JM et al: Genetic modeling of abnormal photosensitivity in families with polymorphic light eruption and actinic prurigo, *J Invest Dermatol* 115:471, 2000.
11. Hasan T et al: Disease associations in polymorphous light eruption: a long-term follow-up of 94 patients, *Arch Dermatol* 134:1081, 1998.
12. Beth-Jones J et al: Juvenile spring eruption of the ears: a probable variant of polymorphic light eruption, *Br J Dermatol* 124:375, 1991.
13. Tan E, Eberhart-Phillips J, Sharples K: Juvenile spring eruption: a prevalence study, *N Z Med J* 109:293, 1966.

14. Grabczynska SA et al: Actinic prurigo and polymorphic light eruption: common pathogenesis and the importance of HLA-DR4/DRB1*0407, *Br J Dermatol* 140:232, 1999.

15. Schnell AH et al: Major gene segregation of actinic prurigo among North American Indians in Saskatchewan, *Am J Med Gen* 92:212, 2000.

16. Gupta J, Man I, Kemmett D: Hydroa vacciniforme: a clinical and follow-up study of 17 cases, *J Am Acad Dermatol* 42:208, 2000.

17. Iwatsuki K et al: The association of latent Epstein-Barr virus infection with hydroa vacciniforme, *Br J Dermatol* 140:715, 1999.

18. Uetsu N et al: The clinical and photobiological characteristics of solar urticaria, *Br J Dermatol* 142:32, 2000.

19. Boonstra HE et al: Polymorphous light eruption: a clinical, photobiologic, and follow-up study of 110 patients, *J Am Acad Dermatol* 42:199, 2000.

20. Murphy GM: The cutaneous porphyrias: a review, *Br J Dermatol* 140:573, 1999.

21. Matthews-Roth MM: Erythropoietic protoporphyria: treatment with antioxidants and potential cure with gene therapy, *Methods Enzymol* 319:479, 2000.

22. Bowers AG: Phytophotodermatitis, *Am J Contact Derm* 10:89, 1999.

23. Cleaver JE et al: A summary of mutations in the UV-sensitive disorders: xeroderma pigmentosum, Cockayne syndrome, and trichothiodystrophy, *Hum Mutat* 14:9, 1999.

Bullous Diseases and Mucocutaneous Syndromes

Blister formation in the skin of children usually brings to mind a viral infection or bullous impetigo. However, a large variety of noninfectious blistering skin diseases may be seen. These may be spontaneously occurring blisters, such as seen in the immunobullous disorders, erythema multiforme (EM), Stevens-Johnson syndrome (SJS), or toxic epidermal necrolysis (TEN), or trauma-produced blisters seen in the hereditary mechanobullous disorders. A history of trauma-induced blisters is important in distinguishing the hereditary mechanobullous disorders from immunobullous disorders. In most of the hereditary mechanobullous disorders the onset of blisters is within the first 3 months of life. Blisters on the palms and soles often have a thick roof of stratum corneum and appear deceptively deep in tissue when they are within the epidermis or at the dermal-epidermal junction. In contrast, blisters on mucous membranes shed their roofs quickly, so that only blister bases (erosions) are seen. Infectious blisters are discussed in detail in Chapters 5 and 8, and mechanobullous diseases are discussed in Chapter 18.

SPONTANEOUS VESICULOBULLOUS ERUPTIONS

Viral blisters (see Chapter 8), bullous impetigo (see Chapter 5), chemical or thermal burns, papular urticaria, and acute dermatitis such as plant allergic contact dermatitis (see Chapter 4) are the most common forms of blisters that appear spontaneously. The injury in thermal burns is similar to that in sunburn. EM is a recurrent blistering disease of the skin. SJS and TEN are uncommon but serious blistering mucocutaneous syndromes in children. Miliaria, aphthous ulcers, and geographic tongue are common, more benign forms of spontaneous vesiculobullous diseases, whereas the immunobullous diseases are quite un-

common to rare. Bullous mastocytosis, an uncommon blistering condition, is discussed in Chapter 14. Kawasaki disease is included in this chapter, although not truly a bullous disease, because it mimics the major mucocutaneous syndromes.

ERYTHEMA MULTIFORME
Clinical Features

EM is a syndrome characterized by the acute onset of oval or round, fixed, erythematous skin lesions appearing symmetrically on the skin.[1-3] Each lesion remains at the same site at least 7 days, and often for 2 or 3 weeks (Fig. 11-1). The lesions progress over several days to form concentric zones of color change in which the central zone of epidermal injury becomes dusky, blistered, or crusted. These lesions are called *target* or *iris* lesions (Fig. 11-2).[1,2,4,5] Prodromal symptoms in EM are conspicuously absent.[1,2] EM lesions are frequently recurrent and preceded by a lesion of herpes labialis (Fig. 11-3).[1-3,6,7] Skin lesions initially involve the dorsal surface of the hands and the extensor aspects of the extremities. The palms and soles are frequently involved, with the flexor aspects of the extremities affected less frequently. The isomorphic (or Koebner) phenomenon has been reported in EM (Fig. 11-4). Systemic symptoms and signs are absent in EM. Usually there are no mucosal lesions, but when present, only the oral mucosa is involved and lesions are few (5 to 10) in contrast to hundreds on the skin (Fig. 11-5). Target lesions may occur on the lips and be mistaken for SJS.[8] EM lasts an average of 3 weeks. It is most common in adolescents but may occur at all ages. Recurrences may occur yearly, but occasionally they happen every 1 or 2 months, particularly if the child has been treated with systemic steroids. Recurrences may be induced by ultraviolet light and mimic polymorphic light eruption.[9] There is no evidence that EM progresses to SJS or TEN.[1,2]

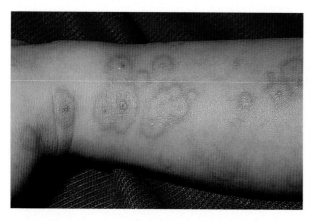

Fig. 11-1 Early fixed papules with a central dusky zone on the dorsum of the forearm of a child with erythema multiforme caused by herpes simplex virus.

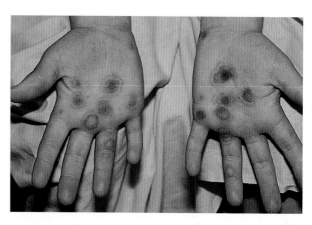

Fig. 11-2 "Target" or "iris" lesions with characteristic central dusky zone on palms of a child with erythema multiforme caused by herpes simplex virus.

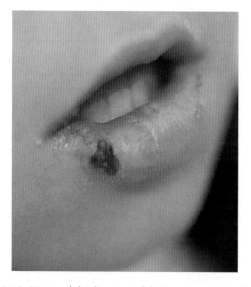

Fig. 11-3 Herpes labialis crusted lesion present on child's lip at the onset of erythema multiforme.

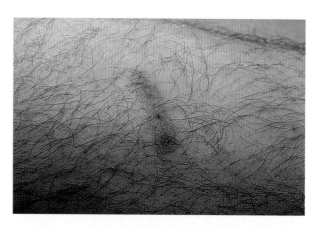

Fig. 11-4 Isomorphic (Koebner) phenomenon in adolescent with erythema multiforme.

Fig. 11-5 Oral involvement in erythema multiforme.

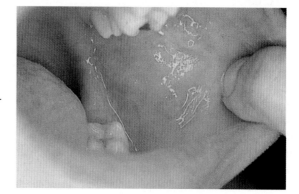

Differential Diagnosis

Acute urticaria is most often confused with EM.[4] This confusion results from the fact that urticaria may frequently have lesions with concentric color changes, with a pale edematous center and an erythematous border. In particular, giant urticaria, with large polycyclic lesions that are often accompanied by angioedema of the hands and feet, may be mistaken for EM. However, urticarial lesions are transient, usually lasting 24 hours or less, whereas EM lesions are fixed and stay at the same site for at least 7 days. Further, the first concentric zone of color change seen in EM minor is not pale in the center, as seen in urticaria, but rather demonstrates epidermal injury with crusting or blister formation.[5] Urticarial lesions will clear with subcutaneous epinephrine, and EM minor will not.[4,5] Skin biopsy will also distinguish EM from urticaria.[5,6]

Oral mucous lesions that are confused with EM include aphthous ulcers, herpes simplex infection, bullous pemphigoid, pemphigus, paraneoplastic pemphigus, and epidermolysis bullosa. Exfoliative cytologic study of the blister base will demonstrate epidermal giant cells of herpes simplex. Immunofluorescent examination of mucosal biopsies will distinguish the immunobullous diseases.

Pathogenesis

In the majority of affected children, EM is thought to be due to a herpes simplex virus (HSV) specific host response to HSV antigens expressed on keratinocytes within the target lesion.[1,3,6,7] There is compelling evidence to show that HSV antigens and deoxyribonucleic acid (DNA) are present within the skin lesions even when a distinctive preceding HSV episode is not observed.[1,3,6,7] Children with recurrent lesions may have recurrent HSV preceding most, but not all, EM episodes. HSV may reside within keratinocytes of previously involved skin and may reactivate at the same sites.[6,7] Children with EM may be unable to effectively clear HSV from keratinocytes. The central necrotic zone of a target lesion shows individual keratinocyte necrosis and inflammatory cells around superficial dermal blood vessels and up into the epidermis.[6] The outer red zone shows dilation of vessels and minimal inflammation. Sheets of necrotic epithelium, as observed in SJS or TEN, are conspicuously absent. In a few children, HSV may not be the precipitating agent. Epstein-Barr virus (EBV), cytomegalovirus (CMV), and other human herpesviruses have been implicated.

Treatment

For EM, symptomatic relief may be obtained from wet compresses or oral antihistamines. There is no evidence to support the use of systemic steroids in EM.[1,2] In children with recurrent episodes of EM, prophylaxis with oral acyclovir may be considered.[10]

Patient Education

Patients should be informed of the role of HSV in EM, and children with recurrent episodes should attempt to reduce sun exposure or other factors that might precipitate the antecedent HSV infection.

Follow-up Visits

A visit in 24 to 48 hours is wise early in the disease to determine the progress of EM.

STEVENS-JOHNSON SYNDROME AND TOXIC EPIDERMAL NECROLYSIS
Clinical Features

Because cutaneous features and etiologies of SJS and TEN may be indistinguishable, they will be considered here together. Both are serious, potentially life-threatening conditions characterized by large areas of epithelial necrosis.[1,11,12] SJS, in contrast to EM, has a distinct prodrome lasting 1 to 14 days and is characterized by fever, headache, sore throat, malaise, and, sometimes, cough, vomiting, and diarrhea. Mucosal involvement is severe, with extensive mucosal necrosis, and it always involves at least two mucosal surfaces (Figs. 11-6 and 11-7). The

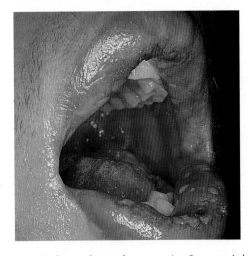

Fig. 11-6 Early oral involvement in Stevens-Johnson syndrome.

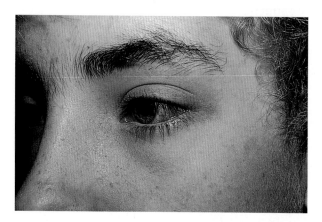

Fig. 11-7 Early eye involvement in Stevens-Johnson syndrome.

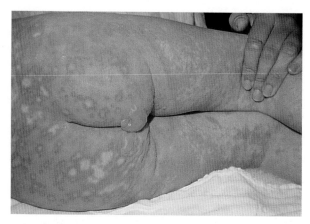

Fig. 11-8 Bullous macules with islands of uninvolved skin in Stevens-Johnson syndrome/toxic epidermal necrolysis.

oral mucosa (Fig. 11-6) and eyes (Fig. 11-7) are the most frequently involved, but vaginal and urethral necrosis and widespread gastrointestinal or lower respiratory tract necrosis may develop. An uncommon variant, sometimes called *recurrent oral erythema multiforme* is limited to the oral mucosa. The initial cutaneous lesions mimic those found in EM but progress rapidly within hours from central blisters to severe epidermal necrosis with loss of the epidermis, leaving a denuded skin. Large sheets of epidermis or mucosa may be lost (Fig. 11-8). The mouth is affected in every case of SJS.[1,11,12] Hemorrhagic crusts often appear on the lips (Fig. 11-9). Mucous membrane involvement often precipitates hospitalization in children because of severe limitation of the ability to eat. Redness, swelling, bullae, or denuded erosions may be seen on the conjunctivae, accompanied by pain and photophobia. Conjunctival scarring may be severe, and ocular complications are the most frequent.[12,13]

TEN has similar cutaneous findings that may occur in the absence of mucosal involvement. Although lesions first begin on the extremities in a pattern similar to that noted in EM, extensive truncal and facial involvement soon follows. A large percentage of the skin may be lost, leading to complications similar to a thermal burn.[1] Healing with scarring and contractures may occur, and loss of hair and nails may ensue.[1,12,13] Permanent areas of depigmentation may develop.[1,12,13]

There may be considerable overlap in the clinical conditions of SJS and TEN. SJS may be mucosal only, but more likely will have mucosal and necrotic skin lesions together. TEN may only involve skin but also

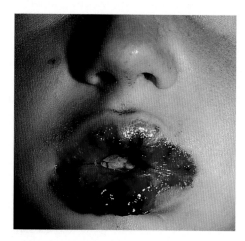

Fig. 11-9 Hemorrhagic crusts on the lips of a child with Stevens-Johnson syndrome.

may exhibit severe necrosis of oral mucosa. Attempts at classification of these two entities have been of help in clarifying the conditions, but the clinician should appreciate that there are overlapping clinical features and that early on it may be difficult to predict areas of involvement.[1,11,12] Most authorities now accept four major types of SJS/TEN.[1] The typical SJS usually has only a few red macules with blisters, which accompany the mucous membrane involvement, and less than 10% of the body surface is involved. The "overlap" SJS/TEN has 10% to 30% of body surface involved. Two types of TEN are recognized: one with "spots" in which many red macules with blisters are seen involving more than 10% of the body surface, and one in which large confluent areas of skin are involved on the face and trunk and more than 30% of the body surface is involved. The course of SJS and TEN disease is more prolonged and accompanied by systemic symptoms of fever, dehydration, cough, and lymphadenopathy. The child is often sick 3 or 4 weeks.[1,11,12,14] SJS and TEN are more likely to occur in children ages 2 to 10 years, which is younger than those with EM. Complications tend to be severe, with pseudomembrane formation of mucosa leading to mucosal scaring and loss of function in SJS.[1,11-13] As in a severe burn, fluid and electrolyte imbalance, renal and respiratory complications, and secondary bacterial infections complicate TEN.[1,11-13] Use of a severity scoring system may help with monitoring and response to therapy.[14]

Differential Diagnosis

SJS may exactly mimic paraneoplastic pemphigus.[15] Immunofluorescent examination of mucosal biopsy will distinguish. SJS and TEN must be distinguished from staphylococcal scalded skin syndrome (SSSS) and acute graft-versus-host disease by skin biopsy. SJS and TEN show full-thickness epidermal necrosis and subepidermal rather than intraepidermal blister formation (Fig. 11-10).[1,6,11] In graft-versus-host disease there is satellite cell necrosis in the epidermis and severe injury to cutaneous vessels not seen in SJS. Early in the course of disease, SJS may be confused with Kawasaki disease. In SJS there is necrosis of mucous membranes, whereas in Kawasaki disease there is redness and edema, but necrotic crusts and severe erosions are not seen. SJS may also be confused with the mucositis produced by chemotherapeutic agents in the child with cancer or with severe herpes stomatitis. Medication history and culture or rapid diagnostic test for herpes will distinguish.

Pathogenesis

In SJS and TEN there is increasing evidence that the toxic injury to keratinocytes and mucosal epithelial cells may be the result of genetic susceptibility to injury. Most cases of SJS and TEN are related to drug ingestion, with nonsteroidal antiinflammatory agents, sulfonamides, and anticonvulsants the most often incriminated.[1,11,16,17] Because the skin is a large organ involved in drug detoxification, toxicity is thought to be related to the accumulation of arene oxides in keratinocytes as the result of cytochrome P-450 action on the parent drug. The detoxification of arene oxides, which bind to keratinocyte ribonucleic acids (RNAs), depends on epoxide hydrolases, which may

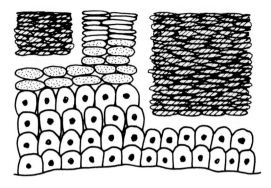

Fig. 11-10 Pathologic differentiation of staphylococcal scalded skin syndrome (left) and toxic epidermal necrolysis (right). Dark areas represent necrosis.

be genetically decreased in children susceptible to SJS or TEN. In some children, infections with *Mycoplasma pneumoniae* or HSV have been associated with SJS. The mechanism of epithelial damage with those infectious agents is not known.

Treatment

Patients with SJS or TEN require treatment as burn patients, preferably in a burn unit or a pediatric intensive care unit.[1,12,17-19] The offending drug must be discontinued.[17] Careful attention to fluid and electrolyte balance, respiratory toilet, fever control, and prevention of secondary bacterial infection of the denuded skin is required.[17-19] Most affected children cannot eat or drink, and parenteral nutrition must be supplied. Ophthalmologic consultation should be obtained, and efforts to prevent conjunctival scarring should be initiated. There is no evidence that systemic steroids are of benefit.[1,12] Intravenous immunoglobulin therapy at 1.5 to 2.0 g/kg/day for 3 days may reduce fever and shorten the hospital stay.[20]

Patient Education

With SJS and TEN, the drugs thought to be associated should be avoided and patients should be informed that they may be genetically susceptible to develop the condition. Each complication should be discussed with the patient and parents, making them aware of potential sequelae.

Follow-up Visits

For hospitalized patients, follow-up should be directed by their complications. Long-term follow-up will be required for those children who develop sequelae of mucosal or skin scarring.

KAWASAKI DISEASE (MUCOCUTANEOUS LYMPH NODE SYNDROME)
Clinical Features

In Kawasaki disease the child presents with a high fever of abrupt onset that lasts longer than 5 days and is accompanied by conjunctival injection (Fig. 11-11).[21,22] One of three oral changes occurs: (1) erythema, fissures, redness, and crusting of the lips (Fig. 11-12); (2) diffuse erythema of the oropharynx; or (3) strawberry tongue.[16-18] One of four changes is seen in the extremities: (1) prominent edema and induration of the hands and feet (Fig. 11-13), (2) erythema of the palms and soles, (3) desquamation beginning at the tips of the digits and spreading proximally in transverse nail grooves (Fig. 11-14), or (4) an erythematous eruption that is polymorphous in character at one point in time but mostly scarlatiniform and gen-

eralized. Lymph node masses greater than 1.5 cm, particularly in the cervical lymph nodes, may be noted. Kawasaki disease is often a diagnosis of exclusion, so that other forms of acute febrile illnesses, including acute adenoviral infection, must be considered first.[22] Laboratory tests related to Kawasaki disease are nonspecific, including an increased sedimentation rate of red blood cells, elevated nonspecific acute-phase reactants, mild anemia, and thrombocytosis that can be quite striking.[21,22]

Aneurysms of the coronary artery occur in 10% to 20% of patients with Kawasaki disease, and 2% will die from thrombosis of the aneurysms of coronary vessels.[21] Echocardiography may detect coronary aneurysms when present, but coronary angiography may be required. Although there is some evidence that coronary aneurysms may heal spontaneously, careful

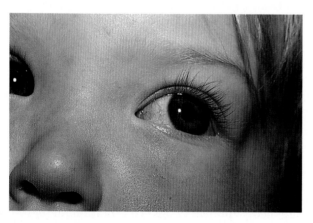

Fig. 11-11 Injected conjunctivae in a child with Kawasaki disease.

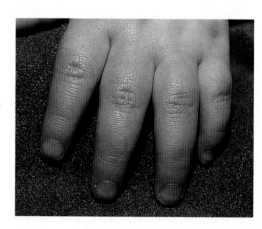

Fig. 11-13 Red, swollen fingers in an infant with Kawasaki disease.

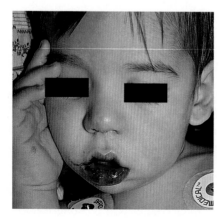

Fig. 11-12 Red, swollen, and slightly crusted lips in a child with Kawasaki disease.

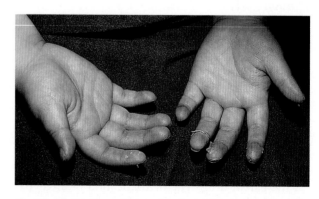

Fig. 11-14 Peeling of fingertips from distal to proximal in Kawasaki disease.

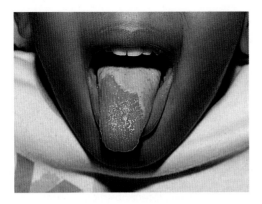

Fig. 11-17 Geographic tongue.

Pathogenesis

Pathologic changes in the annular border of the lesion of the tongue are surprisingly similar to those in psoriasis. There are microabscesses in the epithelium and epithelial thickening, but the pathogenesis is unknown. Although the smooth area looks like an erosion clinically, the epithelium is intact and there is no blister formation.

Treatment

Treatment is usually unnecessary because the lesions are asymptomatic. Oral liquid antacids taken before meals may help if pain occurs when eating.

Patient Education

The benign nature of this condition should be emphasized.

Follow-up Visits

Follow-up visits are unnecessary.

MILIARIA (HEAT RASH)
Clinical Features

There are two forms of miliaria: miliaria crystallina and miliaria rubra.[32] Miliaria crystallina occurs in newborn infants or in areas of sunburn. Miliaria rubra (heat rash) occurs primarily in infants with induced sweating or heat retention. Airtight occlusion predisposes to miliaria. Miliaria crystallina is characterized by clear, thin-walled vesicles that are 1 to 2 mm in diameter, without erythema. The vesicles rupture within 24 to 48 hours and leave a white scale. They are seen on the head and neck and upper trunk in newborn infants and within areas of sunburn in other children.

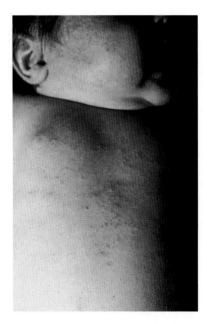

Fig. 11-18 Red pinpoint papules on chest of infant with miliaria rubra.

The characteristic finding in miliaria rubra consists of 2- to 4-mm papules or papulovesicles surrounded by erythema (Fig. 11-18).[32] Lesions are seen in flexural areas, such as the neck, axilla, and groin, after excessive sweating. The face and upper chest may be involved. Miliaria rubra may occur in a localized skin area where airtight occlusion has occurred, for example, in an immobilized or comatose child lying on a plastic bed cover.

Both forms of miliaria may be secondarily infected by *Staphylococcus aureus,* producing pustules in the sweat pores (miliaria pustulosa), which is particularly troublesome in tropical or subtropical areas. If continued sweating occurs, repeated daily episodes of miliaria result. Allowing the skin to cool and dry produces mild desquamation and healing in a few days.

Differential Diagnosis

Box 11-1 presents the conditions to be considered in the differential diagnosis of miliaria crystallina and miliaria rubra. Miliaria crystallina can be distinguished from viral infections of skin or from acute dermatitis by the lack of erythema and the negative exfoliative cytologic findings. On smear of miliaria crystallina lesions, neither giant cells nor inflammatory cells are seen.

Box 11-1 Differential Diagnosis of Spontaneous Vesiculobullous Diseases

COMMONLY SEEN
Viral vesicles (HSV, varicella-zoster virus [VZV])
Bullous impetigo
Thermal or chemical burns
Friction blisters
Acute dermatitis
Miliaria

UNCOMMON DISORDERS
Erythema multiforme
Stevens-Johnson syndrome
Toxic epidermal necrolysis

Autoimmune blistering disorders
Dermatitis herpetiformis, linear IgA dermatosis, pemphigus, pemphigoid epidermolysis bullosa acquisita

Mechanobullous diseases
Epidermolysis bullosa types, especially simplex
Mastocytosis
Bullous insect bite reactions
Lupus erythematosus
Lichen planus
Polymorphous light eruption
Incontinentia pigmenti
Bullous ichthyosis

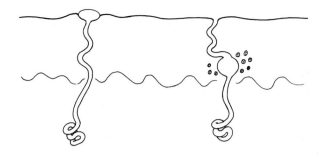

Fig. 11-19 Superficial sweat-duct obstruction in miliaria crystallina (left) does not result in inflammation, in contrast to midepidermal sweat-duct obstruction in miliaria rubra (right).

Miliaria rubra may be confused with neonatal acne, viral exanthems, candidiasis, or drug eruptions, but it is so characteristic that it is seldom misdiagnosed. The febrile child who receives an antibiotic may be mistakenly diagnosed as drug allergic when the eruption with fever was miliaria.

Pathogenesis

Occlusion of sweat ducts after sweating, with rupture of the sweat duct as it spirals through the epidermis, is seen in miliaria (Fig. 11-19). In miliaria crystallina the duct rupture is within the stratum corneum, whereas in miliaria rubra it occurs in the lower epidermis. Induction of sweating, overheating of the skin, and mechanical occlusion of the sweat pores are essential to the production of miliaria. The baby who is overclothed is particularly susceptible to miliaria.

Treatment

The treatment of choice consists of avoidance of further sweating and allowing the skin surface to dry and cool. If pustule formation occurs and secondary staphylococcal infection appears, systemic anti-staphylococcal antibiotics should be administered. Cooling lotions and other agents used for miliaria are not effective unless sweating is reduced. Avoidance of overclothing the baby will be preventive.

Patient Education

The role of overheating the skin and the ease of sweat-duct obstruction should be emphasized. The parent or care giver who overdresses the infant or child should be duly informed. Avoidance of all air-tight dressings, such as plastic occlusion, and the need for cooling the skin must be emphasized.

Follow-up Visits

Follow-up visits are unnecessary.

THE IMMUNOBULLOUS DISEASES

One should suspect an immunobullous disease in the circumstance of a persistent blistering condition, particularly if present for over a month.[33] Immunobullous diseases may present with intraepidermal blister formation, which results in a flaccid, easily eroded blister or a subepidermal blister that is tense (Box 11-2). All are chronic diseases and as a group are quite uncommon to rare.[33] All are characterized by the presence of autoantibodies; the immunobullous diseases are also called the *autoimmune blistering diseases*. In most diseases the autoantibodies are thought to play a role in the pathogenesis of the blister formation. In contrast to the hereditary mechanobullous

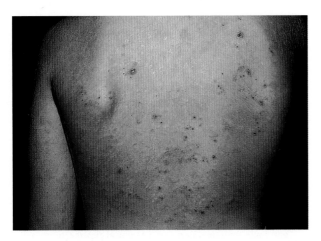

Fig. 11-20 Blisters and excoriated papules on the back of an adolescent with dermatitis herpetiformis.

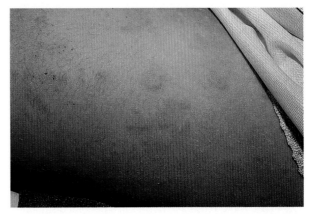

Fig. 11-21 Urticarial papules preceding blister formation on the thigh of an adolescent with dermatitis herpetiformis.

Box 11-2   Childhood Immunobullous Diseases

FLACCID BLISTERS (INTRAEPIDERMAL)
Pemphigus vulgaris
Pemphigus foliaceous
Paraneoplastic pemphigus

TENSE BLISTERS (SUBEPIDERMAL)
Dermatitis herpetiformis
Linear IgA dermatosis
Bullous pemphigoid (including vulvar pemphigoid)
Epidermolysis bullosa acquisita
Systemic lupus erythematosus

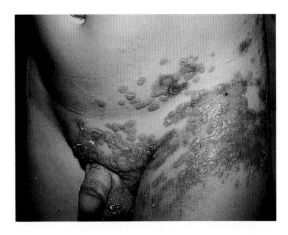

Fig. 11-22 Numerous sausage-shaped tense bullae and crusted lesions in the pelvic area of a toddler with linear IgA dermatosis.

---

diseases (see Chapter 18) in which there are gene mutations resulting in weakening of the epidermal structural proteins, in immunobullous diseases there are autoantibodies to these same structural proteins. The most common of this group of diseases is dermatitis herpetiformis, characterized by severely pruritic vesicles (Figs. 11-20 and 11-21), which usually has its onset in adolescence. The second most common is linear immunoglobulin A (IgA) dermatosis (chronic bullous disease of childhood), which has its onset in infants or toddlers (Figs. 11-22 to 11-24). All of the remaining immunobullous diseases are rare, including the immunobullous disease seen with systemic lupus erythematosus. If mucosa is involved it is usually

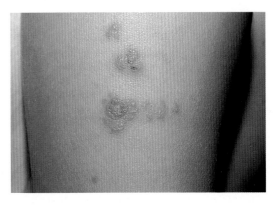

Fig. 11-23 Rosette of blisters on the leg of a child with linear IgA dermatosis.

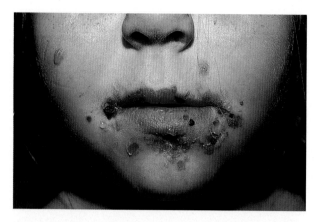

Fig. 11-24 Moist crusts and blisters in a perioral distribution in a child with linear IgA dermatosis.

the oral mucosa in pemphigus and vulvar mucosa in bullous pemphigoid.[33-36]

There are frequent errors made in the diagnosis of this group of diseases, particularly if one relies on clinical features alone. It should be emphasized that the diagnosis of immunobullous diseases is based on a combination of clinical, histologic, and immunofluorescent findings. Immunofluorescence of a skin biopsy is frequently the diagnostic test for these diseases, and one must select noninvolved skin adjacent to a blister for biopsy. One should never biopsy an old blister or a crusted lesion. Obtaining a serum for the examination of circulating autoantibodies is most useful. These diseases are presented in Box 11-2 in order from most common to least common.

Treatment of immunobullous diseases requires long-term immunosuppressive therapy protocols, and the child should be managed by an experienced dermatologist.[33,37]

REFERENCES

1. Leaute-Labreze C et al: Diagnosis, classification and management of erythema multiforme and Stevens-Johnson syndrome, *Arch Dis Child* 83:347, 2000.
2. Weston WL, Morelli JG: Herpes-associated erythema multiforme in prepubertal children, *Arch Pediatr Adolesc Med* 151:1014, 1997.
3. Weston WL, Stockert SS, Jester JD: Herpes simplex virus in childhood erythema multiforme, *Pediatrics* 89:32, 1992.
4. Weston JA, Weston WL: The overdiagnosis of erythema multiforme, *Pediatrics* 89:802, 1992.
5. Weston WL: What is erythema multiforme? *Pediatr Ann* 25:106, 1996.
6. Zaim MT et al: An immunopathological study of herpes-associated erythema multiforme, *J Cutan Pathol* 14:257, 1987.
7. Brice SL, Leahy MA, Ong L: Examination of non-involved skin, previously involved skin and peripheral blood for herpes simplex virus DNA in patients with recurrent herpes-associated erythema multiforme, *J Cutan Pathol* 21:406, 1994.
8. Weston WL, Morelli JG, Rogers M: Target lesions on the lips: childhood herpes simplex–associated erythema multiforme mimics Stevens-Johnson syndrome, *J Am Acad Dermatol* 37:848, 1997.
9. Wolf P et al: Recurrent post-herpetic erythema multiforme mimicking polymorphic light and juvenile spring eruption: two cases in young boys, *Br J Dermatol* 131:364, 1994.
10. Tatnall FM, Schofield JK, Leigh IM: A double-blind, placebo-controlled trial of continuous acyclovir therapy in recurrent erythema multiforme, *Br J Dermatol* 132:267, 1995.
11. Roujeau JC: The spectrum of Stevens-Johnson syndrome and toxic epidermal necrolysis: a clinical classification, *J Invest Dermatol* 102:28s, 1994.
12. Wong KC, Kennedy PJ, Lee S: Clinical manifestations and outcomes of 17 cases of Stevens-Johnson syndrome and toxic epidermal necrolysis, *Aust J Dermatol* 40:131, 1999.
13. Lehman SS: Long-term ocular complications of Stevens-Johnson syndrome, *Clin Pediatr* 38:425, 1999.
14. Bastuji-Garin S et al: SCORTEN: a severity-of-illness score for toxic epidermal necrolysis, *J Invest Dermatol* 115:149, 2000.
15. Lemon MA, Weston WL, Huff JC: Childhood paraneoplastic pemphigus associated with Castleman's tumor, *Br J Dermatol* 136:115, 1997.
16. Rzany B et al: Risk of Stevens-Johnson syndrome and toxic epidermal necrolysis during the first weeks of antiepileptic therapy, *Lancet* 353:2190, 1999.
17. Sullivan JR, Shear NH: The drug hypersensitivity syndrome: what is the pathogenesis? *Arch Dermatol* 137:357, 2001.
18. Roujeau JC: Treatment of severe drug eruptions, *J Dermatol* 26:718, 1999.
19. Sheridan RL et al: Management of severe toxic epidermal necrolysis in children, *J Burn Care Rehab* 20:497, 1999.
20. Morici MV et al: Intravenous immunoglobulin therapy for children with Stevens-Johnson syndrome, *J Rheumatol* 27:2494, 2000.
21. Burns JC et al: Kawasaki disease: a brief history, *Pediatrics* 106:e27, 2000.
22. Barone SR, Pontrelli LR, Krilov LR: The differentiation of classic Kawasaki disease, atypical Kawasaki disease and acute adenoviral infection, *Arch Pediatr Adolesc Med* 154:453, 2000.
23. Michie C et al: Recurrent skin peeling following Kawasaki disease, *Arch Dis Child* 83:353, 2000.
24. Fukunishi M et al: Prediction of the non-responsiveness to intravenous high-dose gamma globulin therapy in patients with Kawasaki disease at onset, *J Pediatr* 137:172, 2000.
25. Verpilleux MP, Bastujin-Garin S, Revuz J: Comparative analysis of severe aphthosis and Behçet's disease: 104 cases, *Dermatology* 198:247, 1999.
26. Ghate JV, Jorizzo JL: Behçet's disease and complex aphthosis, *J Am Acad Dermatol* 40:1, 1999.
27. Thomas KT et al: Periodic fever syndrome in children, *J Pediatr* 135:15, 1999.
28. Feder HM Jr: Periodic fever, aphthous stomatitis, pharyngitis, adenitis: a clinical review of a new syndrome, *Curr Opin Pediatr* 12:253, 2000.

29. McBride DR: Management of aphthous ulcers, *Am Fam Phys* 62:149, 2000.

30. Fridh G, Koch G: Effect of a mouth rinse containing amylo-glucosidase and glucose oxidase on recurrent aphthous ulcers in children and adolescents, *Swed Dental J* 23:49, 1999.

31. Lacour JP, Perrin C: Eruptive familial lingual papillitis: a new clinical entity? *Ped Dermatol* 14:13, 1997.

32. Wenzel FG, Horn TD: Nonneoplastic disorders of the eccrine glands, *J Am Acad Dermatol* 38:1, 1998.

33. Weston WL, Morelli JG, Huff JC: Misdiagnosis, treatments, and outcomes in the immunobullous diseases in children, *Pediatr Dermatol* 14:264, 1997.

34. Farrell AM et al: Childhood vulval pemphigoid: a clinical and immunopathological study of five patients, *Br J Dermatol* 140:308, 1999.

35. Fischer G, Rogers M: Vulvar disease in children: a clinical audit of 130 cases, *Pediatr Dermatol* 17:1, 2000.

36. Edwards S et al: Bullous pemphigoid and epidermolysis bullosa acquisita: presentation, prognosis and immuno-pathology in eleven cases, *Pediatr Dermatol* 15:184, 1998.

37. Harman KE, Black MM: High dose intravenous immune globulin for the treatment of autoimmune blistering diseases: an evaluation of its use in 14 cases, *Br J Dermatol* 140:865, 1999.

CHAPTER TWELVE | Skin Cysts and Nodules

Persistent masses in the skin often result in a child's being brought in for medical examination. Often, parents are concerned that the skin lesion is cancer. Biopsy may be necessary to provide an accurate diagnosis in these conditions, which are rarely symptomatic except in weight-bearing areas. A large number of skin problems can produce nodules. When one observes a skin-colored nodule in an infant or child, an orderly list of possibilities does not easily come to mind. One should first remember that the most common palpable superficial nodule in infants and children is the lymph node. Occipital and cervical nodes are superficial and easily palpated, and sometimes may be mistaken for skin tumors or nodules.

The most common types of superficial skin nodules in infants and children that require skin biopsy are listed in Table 12-1.[1] An estimation of the approximate frequency of each skin nodule in infants and children is provided. Epithelial cysts and pilomatricomas together account for over two thirds of such superficial nodules, and one should particularly remember these two major causes of skin nodules when making a diagnosis.[1] Overall, only 1% of such skin nodules turn out to be malignant growths. The main factors in suspecting whether one of these nodules is malignant are listed in Box 12-1. The most important factor is rapid, progressive growth. Hemangiomas can show rapid growth in infancy (see Chapter 13) and have a benign course. If a clinician is certain that a lesion is not a hemangioma and identifies a skin nodule with rapid, progressive growth, he or she should suspect malignancy and obtain a tissue sample for diagnosis.

SKIN CYSTS

Skin cysts are often solitary in children and produce skin-colored nodules that distort skin contours. They are the most common skin nodule, found predominantly on the lateral border of the eyebrow or under the scalp, both in infants and children (Fig. 12-1).

Clinical Features

Epithelial cysts, dermoid cysts, branchial cleft cysts, and milia

Epithelial cysts are slow-growing, firm, round nodules that reach a maximum size of 1 to 15 cm (Fig. 12-2). Epidermal cysts in the newborn period are found predominantly in the lateral border of the eyebrow or in the scalp.[1] They may also be seen on the palms and soles of newborns. They may not be recognized until childhood when the lesions grow larger. Whether these cysts contain follicular or other adnexal structures and are designated dermoid cysts does not vary their location or clinical features. The presence of midline pits or cysts on the nose poses a special problem related to possible intracranial connection.[2] Papules, cysts, or draining sinus tracts on the lateral aspect of the neck may be associated with branchial cleft cysts or sinus tracts (Fig. 12-3).[3]

In adolescence, solitary cysts appear on the scalp, face, neck, and trunk in the region where acne vulgaris is seen. Multiple cysts in children or adolescents should suggest Gardner's syndrome. Milia are tiny, superficial cysts seen on the faces of newborns and within the scar in scarring conditions such as epidermolysis bullosa (Fig. 12-4).

Steatocystoma multiplex

Steatocystoma multiplex appears as firm, skin-colored or yellowish nodules 1 to 3 cm in diameter in the axillae and on the chest and arms. The condition is inherited as an autosomal dominant mutation of keratin 17. It can be associated with pachyonychia type 2. It begins in late childhood or adolescence and is uncommon.[4]

Eruptive vellus hair cysts

Eruptive vellus hair cysts commonly begin between ages 5 to 10 years as small, skin-colored papules appearing on the lower chest and upper abdomen, areas not usually involved with epithelial or dermoid cysts (Fig. 12-5).[5] Usually five or more lesions are present.

Table 12-1	Skin Nodules and Cysts in Infants and Children	

Type	Approximate Percentage of All Nodules (%)
Epithelial cysts	59
Pilomatricomas	10
Fibromas	4
Neurofibromas	3
Lipomas	3
Lymphangiomas	3
Granuloma annulare	3
Juvenile xantho-granulomas	3
Mastocytomas	2
Miscellaneous lesions	9
Malignant tumors (usually sarcomas)	1

Box 12-1	Factors Associated With Likelihood of Malignancy in Superficial Skin Tumors in Children*	

Rapid, progressive growth
Ulceration
Fixed to deep fascia
Greater than 3 cm and firm
Occurs in first 30 days of life

*Listed in order of importance.

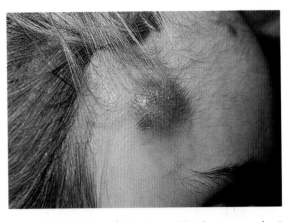

Fig. 12-2 Inflamed epithelial cyst. This lesion may be inflamed secondary to infection or spontaneous rupture and foreign body reaction.

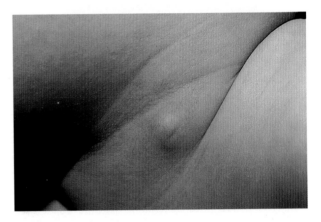

Fig. 12-3 Branchial cleft cyst on the neck of a child.

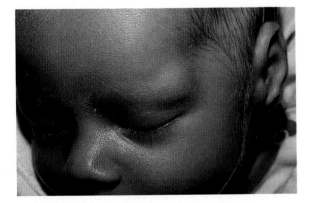

Fig. 12-1 Dermoid cyst. Cystic nodule on lateral aspect of left eyebrow of newborn infant.

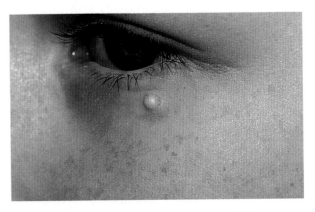

Fig. 12-4 Milia on the cheek of a child.

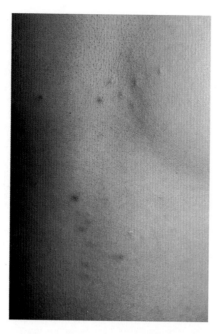

Fig. 12-5 Eruptive vellus hair cyst. Superficial cystic lesions on the midportion of the chest and upper aspect of the abdomen.

Differential Diagnosis

For a list of skin nodules and cysts that should be included in the differential diagnosis, see Table 12-1. Epithelial and dermoid cysts are difficult to distinguish from one another without a biopsy. However, because both conditions are benign, a biopsy is usually not necessary. Midline nasal dermoid lesions are the exception. These appear as a midline pit, fistula, or swelling anywhere from the glabella to the nasal tip. These lesions may have intracranial extensions. Steatocystoma multiplex similarly has a different distribution, with locations around the axilla, neck, and onto the arms. Gardner's syndrome should be considered when multiple epithelial cysts are seen. Branchial cleft cysts are usually on the lateral aspect of the neck and may show inflammation.

Pathogenesis

Epithelial cysts and milia

Although epithelial cysts are commonly called *sebaceous cysts,* they contain neither sebum nor sebaceous glands. Epithelial cysts and milia are filled with keratin in laminated layers and lined by epithelium. When they are ruptured, foreign body reactions occur around the ruptured cyst wall.

Steatocystoma multiplex

Steatocystoma multiplex consists of intricately folded cyst walls of epithelial cells, with flattened sebaceous gland lobules within or close to the cyst wall.

Dermoid cysts

Dermoid cysts represent sequestration of skin along lines of embryonic closure and contain an epithelial lining plus either mature sebaceous glands, eccrine sweat glands, or mature hair.

Branchial cleft cysts

Branchial cleft cysts are defects of embryological closure. They may drain into the pharynx or onto the skin.

Eruptive vellus hair cysts

Most authorities consider eruptive vellus hair cysts a developmental anomaly of body hair follicles. Obstruction at the neck of the follicular channel results in cystic dilation of the follicle, retention of vellus hairs, and atrophy of the hair bulbs.

Treatment

Most cysts require no treatment and may be best left alone. If cosmetic improvement can be obtained, surgical excision is the treatment of choice. Midline nasal dermoid cysts require meticulous surgical excision in an effort to prevent intracranial extension and complications. Before surgery, neuroimaging studies may help to predict intracranial involvement.[2] Branchial cleft cysts and sinus tracts require complete surgical excision to avoid recurrence. No effective therapy for vellus hair cysts is available.

Patient Education

Patients should be aware of the benign nature of these growths despite their prominent size. In children with multiple epithelial cysts, bowel examination for signs of Gardner's syndrome is indicated.

Follow-up Visits

A visit 1 week after surgery to explain the pathologic findings is beneficial.

ADNEXAL TUMORS

A variety of benign growths arise from epithelial adnexal structures (e.g., sebaceous glands, hair follicles, sweat glands) and produce skin nodules or tumors. Some, such as the sebaceous nevus and epidermal nevus, appear at birth and are discussed in the section

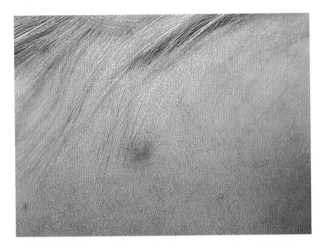

Fig. 12-6 Pilomatricoma. Firm blue papule on the face of a child.

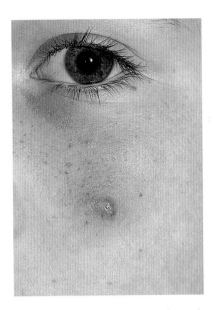

Fig. 12-7 Pilomatricoma. Firm blue papule on the face surrounded by an inflammatory reaction.

on birthmarks (see Chapter 21). Most adnexal tumors do not appear until adult life, but four types—pilomatricomas, syringomas, trichoepitheliomas, and basal cell carcinoma—may be seen in childhood or adolescence.

Clinical Features
Pilomatricoma

Pilomatricomas (calcifying epitheliomas) appear as solitary, hard, multilobular, 2- to 5-mm papules covered by normal skin on the face or extremities (Figs. 12-6 and 12-7).[6] They may have a blue color. Pilomatricomas often begin in infancy or during early school years, but they are not hereditary. Pilomatricomas account for up to 10% of all skin nodules and tumors in children.[1] They may be present in newborns. They are a result of a mutation in hair matrix cells.[7]

Syringomas

Syringomas appear at puberty as small (1 to 2 mm), skin-colored to yellowish, soft nodules (Fig. 12-8). They occur on the eyelids, cheeks, axillae, abdomen, and vulva. They are more common in girls than boys. Most often, lesions are limited to the eyelids.[8]

Trichoepitheliomas

Trichoepitheliomas appear as numerous, round, skin-colored nodules primarily on the midface area of children and adolescents (Fig. 12-9). The nodules are 2 to 8 mm in diameter and also may be seen on the upper trunk, neck, and scalp. A few fine telangiectasias may be observed over the lesions. Multiple lesions are inherited as an autosomal dominant trait,

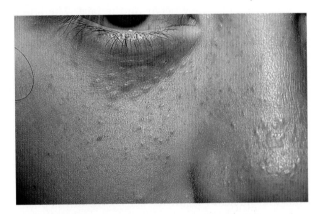

Fig. 12-8 Syringomas. Multiple skin-colored papules on the face and lower eyelid.

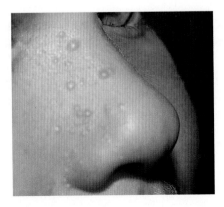

Fig. 12-9 Multiple trichoepitheliomas on the nose of a child.

whereas solitary lesions may appear spontaneously without a family history.

Basal cell carcinoma

Basal cell carcinoma is uncommon in school-age children and adolescents.[9] These lesions appear on the face or upper trunk as a solitary nodule with overlying telangiectasia. They may be seen in otherwise unaffected children, but their presence should suggest three syndromes: the basal cell nevus syndrome,[10,11] xeroderma pigmentosum, and the Bazex's syndrome (Table 12-2). The basal cell carcinoma may progress to ulceration and local invasion of the dermis and deeper tissues. It does not metastasize.

Differential Diagnosis

Pilomatricomas and basal cell carcinoma are characteristically solitary and firm, in contrast to syringomas and trichoepitheliomas. Trichoepitheliomas and syringomas may be confused with acne vulgaris or the multiple angiofibromas of tuberous sclerosis because they occur on the face. The latter are red rather than skin colored, however. A skin biopsy will distinguish between the lesions of tuberous sclerosis, trichoepithelioma, or syringoma. Confirmatory diagnosis of all four adnexal tumors is made by skin biopsy.[12,13]

Pathogenesis
Pilomatricoma

Pilomatricoma is considered a benign hyperplasia of the cells of the hair matrix. It is a tumor located in the deep dermis and is composed of islands of basophilic cells and nuclear "shadow" cells. Calcium deposits appear throughout the tumor.

Syringoma

Syringoma is a benign hyperplasia of the cells of the eccrine sweat ducts. Numerous small ducts are located in the mid to upper dermis with "tennis racquet" shapes and surrounding fibrosis.

Trichoepitheliomas

Trichoepitheliomas consist of multiple horn cysts and basophilic tumor islands in the mid-dermis. They are believed to be derived from the cells of the hair follicle.

Basal cell carcinoma

Basal cell carcinomas are composed of solid masses of cells that contain a large nucleus and little cytoplasm and extend down from the epidermis. Separation from the surrounding fibrous tissue by a clear space is commonly observed. In xeroderma pigmentosum, ultraviolet light–induced DNA damage cannot be repaired because of autosomal recessive inheritance of various enzyme deficiencies.[14] The pathogenesis of basal cell epitheliomas in the basal cell nevus syndrome is associated with mutations in the hedgehog signaling pathway.[15,16] The cause of the Bazex's syndrome is currently unknown.

Treatment

Excision is the treatment of choice for pilomatricomas and basal cell carcinoma. Multiple syringomas and trichoepitheliomas are difficult to treat, and treatment of multiple lesions often has poor cosmetic results.

Patient Education

The benign nature and origin of pilomatricoma, syringoma, and trichoepithelioma should be discussed.

Table 12-2 Syndromes Associated With Basal Cell Carcinoma in Children

Clinical Feature	Basal Cell Nevus Syndrome	Bazex's Syndrome	Xeroderma Pigmentosum
Inheritance	Autosomal dominant	Autosomal dominant	Autosomal recessive
Palmar pits	Present	Present	Absent
Multiple freckles	Absent	Absent	Present
Prominent dilated pores on arms and dorsa of hands	Absent	Present	Absent
Jaw cysts	Present	Absent	Absent
Defective teeth	Present	Absent	Present

Basal cell epitheliomas should be considered to be slowly progressing malignant tumors. In the hereditary syndromes, careful evaluation of family members is necessary.

Follow-up Visits

Children with basal cell carcinoma should be examined every 6 months for the appearance of further skin tumors. The importance of avoiding exposure to the sun and using sunscreens should be emphasized at each visit.

SKIN NODULES
Fibromas
Clinical features

Dermatofibroma. The presenting symptom of dermatofibroma is a small, firm, well-defined, often pigmented nodule on the leg or trunk of children, adolescents or adults (Fig. 12-10). Dermatofibroma may

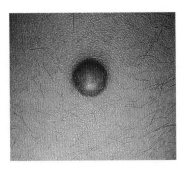

Fig. 12-10 Dermatofibroma. Firm, well-defined pigmented nodule on the leg of an adolescent.

follow minor skin trauma or may appear to occur spontaneously. Multiple lesions can also occur. Lateral pressure on the lesion will produce dimpling of its surface. The lesions may become as large as 1 to 2 cm in diameter, and they persist indefinitely.

Hypertrophic scars. A hypertrophic scar is an overgrowth of fibrous tissue that remains at the site of the original injury (Fig. 12-11). These lesions usually enlarge for several months after the injury along the area of the injury. Eventually the hypertrophic scar will stabilize for several months before regressing in size.

Keloids. Keloids are firm, progressively enlarging nodules with a shiny, hairless surface. They may be painful or itch. They may occur on the extremities but are predominantly located on the earlobes (Fig. 12-12), presternal area, neck (Fig. 12-13), and face after skin trauma. They often have stellate shapes. The tendency to form keloids may be inherited. They may progressively enlarge for 20 to 40 years and form lobulated or pedunculated masses.

Digital fibrous tumor of childhood. Digital fibrous tumor of childhood is a firm nodule occurring around the fingernail or toenail.[17,18] The lesion may be present at birth or will usually arise before 1 year of age. Because excision often results in rapid recurrence, the lesion is also called recurrent digital fibrous tumor. The lesion may initially grow rapidly and require a skin biopsy to confirm that it is not a sarcoma. It will usually spontaneously involute within several years.

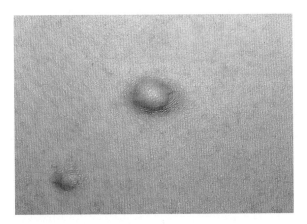

Fig. 12-11 Hypertrophic scar. Site of previous chickenpox lesions.

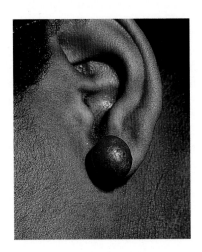

Fig. 12-12 Keloid nodule on ear.

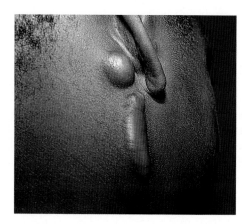

Fig. 12-13 Keloid and epithelial cyst. Superior lesion is an epithelial cyst, and lower lesion is a keloid that formed in an excision scar of a previously excised epithelial cyst.

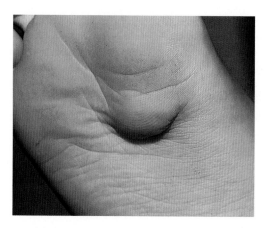

Fig. 12-14 Neurofibroma. Soft, skin-colored papule.

Differential diagnosis

Dermatofibromas. Dermatofibromas may be pigmented and mimic melanoma. They are more likely to be confused with other skin nodules, however (see Table 12-1).

Keloids and hypertrophic scars. Keloids are seldom misdiagnosed, but early keloids mimic ordinary scars. The keloid will extend beyond the bounds of the original injury, whereas the hypertrophic scar will remain within the area of injury.

Digital fibrous tumor of childhood. Digital fibrous tumors may mimic the fibrous thickening overlying a subungual exostosis, a callus, or a corn. A radiograph of the digit should be obtained before biopsy.

Pathogenesis

Dermatofibromas. Dermatofibromas contain numerous fibroblasts with excessive deposition of collagen and proliferation of the overlying epidermis. They are believed to be a reactive proliferation of fibroblasts in response to trauma.

Keloids and hypertrophic scars. Keloids produce nodular patterns of collagen fibers associated with the new blood vessel formation, as expected in healing. However, as the vessels regress, collagen deposition continues and fails to thin as expected. Hypertrophic scars may be a similar process to a lesser degree.

Digital fibrous tumor of childhood. Digital fibrous tumors show proliferating fibroblasts that contain eosinophilic cytoplasmic inclusions thought to represent myofilaments.

Treatment

Dermatofibromas, if symptomatic or worrisome, may be excised. Keloids can be treated by injections of intralesional glucocorticosteroids, which results in softening and flattening of the keloid. Often, triamcinolone acetonide, 5 to 10 mg/ml in saline solution, is injected. Surgery alone will result in rapid reappearance of the keloid, but surgery followed by frequent intralesional injections of glucocorticosteroids may be effective therapy for large keloids. Steroid injections may result in hypopigmentation surrounding the lesion. Applications of silicone occlusive sheeting may also benefit keloids or scars.[19] Months of application may be required. Recurring digital fibrous tumors should be allowed to involute spontaneously if possible because surgical excision may be followed by recurrence.[17,18]

Patient education

The benign nature of these disorders should be emphasized.

Follow-up visits

Keloids may be injected with steroids at 4- to 6-week intervals.

Neurofibromas

Neurofibromas may be present at birth or develop later in life. The neurofibroma is a soft, easily inverted, skin-colored to brown papule that may occur anywhere on the skin (Fig. 12-14). Occasionally, large clustering of neurofibromas will form a plexiform neurofibroma.

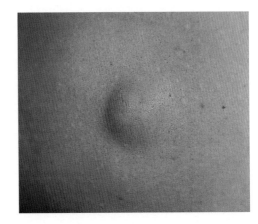

Fig. 12-15 Lipoma. Soft subcutaneous nodule unattached to overlying skin.

Neurofibroma may occur as solitary lesions or may be associated with neurofibromatosis. Neurofibromatosis is discussed in Chapter 17. Solitary lesions may precede the other features of neurofibromatosis.

Differential diagnosis

The differential diagnoses of neurofibromas are listed in Box 12-2. A biopsy may be necessary to confirm the diagnosis.

Pathogenesis

Neurofibromas are benign tumors of nerve sheath cells.

Patient education

The nature of neurofibromas and their association with multiple neurofibromatosis should be carefully explained to the family, and a complete family history and evaluation of family members should be done.

Follow-up visits

Children with a solitary neurofibroma should be followed every 6 to 12 months and examined for the appearance of café-au-lait spots or other signs and symptoms of neurofibromatosis.

Lipomas
Clinical features

Lipomas are soft, subcutaneous nodules unattached to overlying skin (Fig. 12-15). They are usually solitary, begin in adolescence, and are most commonly found on the neck, upper aspect of the chest, and arms. Angiolipomas, variants of lipomas, may present as painful subcutaneous nodules, usually on the upper arms of adolescent females.

Differential diagnosis

Epithelial cysts, neurofibromas, and other skin nodules may mimic lipomas, but the ability to easily slide the overlying skin over the lesion helps to confirm the deep subcutaneous location of lipomas.

Pathogenesis

A lipoma is composed of nodules of normal-appearing fat cells, although unresponsiveness of fat cells to the lipolytic effects of norepinephrine occurs in multiple symmetrical lipomatosis. Capillary proliferation is seen in angiolipoma in addition to an excess of normal fat cells.

Treatment

Lipomas are usually asymptomatic. Angiolipomas may be painful and may require excision for pain relief.

Patient education

The benign nature of these nodules should be emphasized.

Follow-up visits

Follow-up visits are unnecessary.

Lymphangiomas

Lymphangiomas are often present at birth and are discussed in detail in the section on vascular malformations (see Chapter 13). They may, however, be overlooked until later in infancy and childhood, and their presenting symptom is solitary, soft swellings of the face, neck, trunk, or extremities that show progressive growth.

Granuloma Annulare
Clinical features

Small, firm papules or nodules that form a circle or semicircle are characteristic of granuloma annulare.[20] They may be skin-colored, but more often a dusky, violaceous hue is seen. Stretching the skin reveals the ring

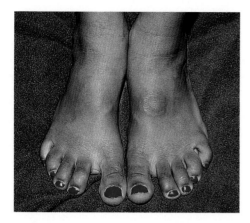

Fig. 12-16 Granuloma annulare. Unilateral oval lesion on dorsum of foot.

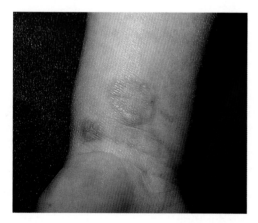

Fig. 12-17 Granuloma annulare. Large and small annular plaques on ventral surface of arm. Central resolution can be seen in larger lesions.

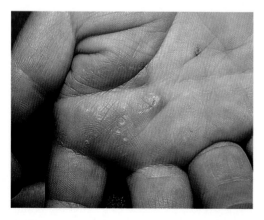

Fig. 12-18 Granuloma annulare. Grouping of firm papules on palm of hand.

of papules or nodules. The lesions occur predominantly in acral areas, on the digits, ankles, and wrists (Figs. 12-16 to 12-18); 50% of affected children have a single ring of lesions. Occasionally, large, firm, subcutaneous nodules may be seen, or multiple small papules are found. Lesions are usually asymptomatic.

Differential diagnosis

Small, annular lesions are often mistaken for dermatophyte infections. The lack of epidermal change or scaling and the deep palpable portion help distinguish granuloma annulare from tinea corporis. Large nodules of granuloma annulare may mimic rheumatoid nodules, and subcutaneous granuloma annulare may be histologically and clinically indistinguishable from rheumatoid nodules. In granuloma annulare, no systemic symptoms are noted. Occasionally, other annulare lesions (e.g., lichen planus, sarcoidosis, syphilis, necrobiosis lipoidica diabeticorum) are confused with granuloma annulare. A biopsy may be necessary to confirm the diagnosis.

Pathogenesis

Focal areas of collagen degeneration surrounded by lymphocytes and epithelioid cells are seen in the mid-dermis and reticular dermis in granuloma annulare. The mechanism of the disease is unknown.

Treatment

Because lesions are asymptomatic, only reassurance is necessary. Although it is tempting to treat such conditions, spontaneous remission in several years is the rule. No effective therapy is available.

Patient education

The benign nature of this disorder and its natural history should be stressed. Its distinct separation from rheumatoid disease states should be explained.

Follow-up visits

Follow-up visits are unnecessary.

Rheumatoid Nodules
Clinical features

True rheumatoid nodules are uncommon in children with rheumatic disease. They are seen in rheumatoid arthritis, rheumatic fever, and systemic lupus erythematosus as 1- to 4-cm subcutaneous nodules not attached to overlying skin. They develop over bony structures such as a joint and are usually associated with severe rheumatoid disease with positive rheumatoid factor. The overlying skin has a normal color.

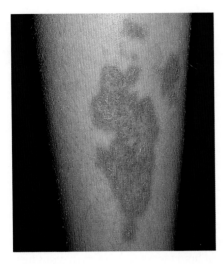

Fig. 12-19 Necrobiosis lipoidica diabeticorum. Large plaque on lower leg of female adolescent. Note elevated border and yellow-red coloration.

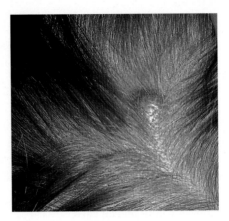

Fig. 12-20 Juvenile xanthogranuloma. Yellow-orange lesion on the scalp.

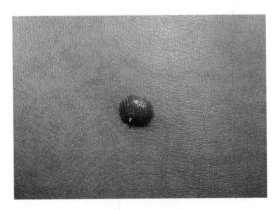

Fig. 12-21 Juvenile xanthogranuloma. Lesion on the abdomen has more of a brown-orange color.

Differential diagnosis

Rheumatoid nodules are most often confused with granuloma annulare (see Table 12-1). However, epithelial cysts, adnexal tumors, lipomas, and other skin nodules may also be confused with rheumatoid nodules.

Pathogenesis

Foci of collagen degeneration surrounded by macrophages are seen in the deep dermis and subcutaneous fat. The mechanism of production of rheumatoid nodules is unknown, but most investigators regard this condition as a form of immune complex disease.

Treatment

If the nodules are symptomatic, excision is the treatment of choice. Therapy used to control other rheumatic symptoms rarely influences rheumatoid nodules.

Patient education

Information about the nature of the associated disease should be given to the patient and family members.

Follow-up visits

The timing of follow-up visits should be based on the severity of the associated systemic illness.

Necrobiosis Lipoidica Diabeticorum

The lesions of necrobiosis lipoidica diabeticorum are irregularly shaped, yellow-red plaques on the lower leg (Fig. 12-19). The lesions may show central atro-phy or sclerosis. Often the lesions are bilateral and symmetric. A skin biopsy specimen of a lesion may have the histologic appearance of granuloma annulare. Children with necrobiosis lipoidica diabeticorum may have associated diabetes mellitus and should be evaluated with a fasting serum glucose test.

Juvenile Xanthogranulomas
Clinical features

In juvenile xanthogranulomas orange to yellow-brown soft nodules appear on the skin of infants and children (Figs. 12-20 and 12-21). The nodules are often multiple, numbering five to ten (Figs. 12-22 and 12-23). They may be present at birth and often involute spontaneously over several years.[21-23] Lesions are seen in the iris and may be mistaken for retino-blastoma, or they may cause glaucoma.[24] Although

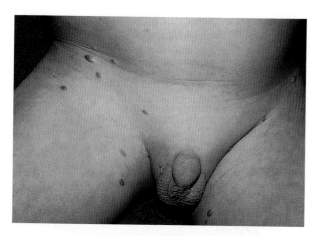

Fig. 12-22 Juvenile xanthogranuloma. Grouping of lesions on lower aspect of trunk and on thigh.

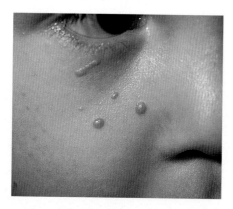

Fig. 12-23 Juvenile xanthogranuloma. Orange-brown coloration is seen on close inspection.

involvement is primarily in the skin, nodules have been described in the testes, lung, liver, spleen, and pericardium.[25]

Differential diagnosis

Xanthomas, spindle and epithelioid melanocytic nevi, histiocytosis, and mastocytomas all may appear as orange or yellow-brown nodules at first presentation (Box 12-3). Skin biopsy is necessary to distinguish juvenile xanthogranuloma from these conditions. Stroking the skin surface covering a mastocytoma will produce urticaria within the nodule (Darier's sign).

Pathogenesis

Within the dermis, large accumulations of macrophages appear. Their cytoplasm gradually fills with lipid, creating a particular type of giant cell called the *Touton giant cell*. Regressing lesions show fibroblas-

---

Box 12-3 Differential Diagnosis of Orange or Yellow-Brown Nodules

Benign cephalic histiocytosis
Langerhans cell histiocytosis
Juvenile xanthogranuloma
Mastocytoma
Spindle and epithelioid cell melanocytic nevus
Xanthoma

---

tic proliferation. There is no apparent relationship between juvenile xanthogranuloma and either abnormalities of lipid metabolism or malignant histiocytosis.

Treatment

Treatment of the individual lesions is usually not necessary. Examination by an ophthalmologist may be necessary to evaluate and possibly treat eye lesions if they occur. Eye lesions appear to be more likely associated with multiple cutaneous lesions and in children younger than 2 years of age.[26] Patients with juvenile xanthogranulomas and multiple café-au-lait spots may have an increased risk of granulocytic leukemia.[27]

Patient education

The natural history of this lesion and the need for careful observation for eye involvement should be emphasized.

Follow-up visits

Ophthalmological follow-up may need to be done to monitor for eye changes. Examination and quantitation of skin lesions can be completed during routine examinations.

Mastocytomas

Mastocytomas are usually present at birth and are discussed in detail in Chapter 14. They may not become apparent until 1 to 2 months of age and appear as macular red or red-brown lesions, usually on the trunk.[28]

Pyogenic Granulomas
Clinical features

Pyogenic granulomas are most common in acral areas, such as the hands and fingers, and on the face (Fig. 12-24). They appear as solitary, dull red, firm nodules that are 5 to 6 mm in diameter. The surface may be

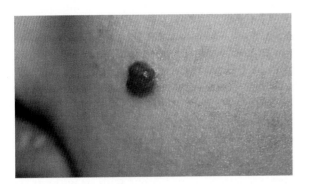

Fig. 12-24 Pyogenic granuloma. Smooth, glistening surface on an erythematous papule.

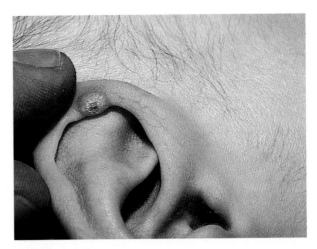

Fig. 12-25 Calcified nodule. Lesion on ear of infant.

smooth and glistening, but often it is ulcerated and crusted. The lesion bleeds easily when traumatized. Removal has resulted in the appearance of multiple satellite lesions in a few instances. Pyogenic granuloma may occur at any age, but in childhood it is most common in the first 5 years of life. The majority of patients have no history of a predisposing factor.[29]

Differential diagnoses

Pyogenic granuloma is often misdiagnosed as a hemangioma, glomus tumor, melanocytic nevus, wart, molluscum contagiosum, or malignant melanoma.[30] All of these lesions can ulcerate and crust if traumatized. Pathologic study will distinguish pyogenic granuloma from the other lesions.

Pathogenesis

Proliferation of capillaries within a circumscribed area with flattened or ulcerated epidermis on top and epidermal proliferation at the sides, producing a "collarette" of epidermis, is seen. Pyogenic granuloma may be caused by increased expression of vascular endothelial growth factor (VEGF).[31]

Treatment

Excision is the treatment of choice. Pulse dye laser treatment may be effective for smaller lesions.[32]

Patient education

The clinician should explain to the patient and parents that this growth is not malignant, will not disappear without treatment, and represents an abnormal healing response.

Follow-up visits

A visit 1 week after removal of the lesion is useful to inform the patient of the pathologic diagnosis and evaluate healing.

Smooth-Muscle Hamartoma

Smooth-muscle hamartomas are present a birth, but they may not be noted until later in infancy or childhood. The lesions may appear to have excess hair and may be hyperpigmented when compared with normal skin. On palpation, the lesional hairs may become erect as a result of the excess smooth muscle within the lesion. Biopsy of the lesion will show abundant smooth-muscle bundles within the dermis.[33]

Calcified Nodules

Cutaneous calcinosis results from precipitation of insoluble calcium salts within cutaneous tissues. This can occur in congenital or acquired lesions. Solitary or multiple lesions can be present that are firm or rock hard. They are usually asymptomatic but can be painful and discharge chalky material through the skin. Underlying metabolic disease, connective tissue disease, or malignancy may be associated, or the lesion can be idiopathic. In newborn infants, a solitary calcified nodule of the ear may form (Fig. 12-25), whereas in children with dermatomyositis or other collagen vascular diseases, multiple nodules may form on the extensor surfaces of hands and elbows. Biopsy confirmation is necessary before a comprehensive systemic evaluation is begun.[34]

Piezogenic Pedal Papules

Piezogenic pedal papules are common, sometimes painful papules that may occur on the feet (Fig. 12-26) and wrist.[35] The lesions represent herniations of fatty subcutaneous tissue into connective tissue. The herniations are seen when pressure is applied to the heel or wrist. Painful lesions can be excised or treated with orthopedic padding.[36]

Knuckle Pads

Knuckle pads are thickening of the skin overlying digital joints (Fig. 12-27). The lesions grow slowly and are asymptomatic.[37] The lesions are sporadic and idiopathic. They rarely are associated with trauma. The lesions can persist indefinitely. Treatment is usually unsuccessful and unnecessary because the lesions are asymptomatic.

Panniculitis

Inflammation in the subcutaneous fat may be first seen as painful lesions that feel as if they are deep beneath the skin. Biopsy will identify the inflammation within the fat. The cause of panniculitis may not be found, or it can be associated with infection, trauma, or metabolic or systemic disease.[38] Biopsy confirmation may be necessary before a comprehensive systemic evaluation is begun. One type of panniculitis, subcutaneous fat necrosis of the newborn infant, is described in Chapter 21.

Sarcoidosis

Sarcoidosis a systemic disease associated with granulomas. Skin lesions can occur with or without systemic symptoms. The skin lesions may appear as indurated papules or plaques. Skin biopsy showing the granulomas of sarcoid should prompt a systemic evaluation for sarcoidosis.[39]

Corns and Calluses
Clinical features

Corns and calluses are areas of thickened skin that appear on sites of prolonged pressure or friction. Patients who have these lesions often believe they are warts. Corns are more circumscribed (2 to 5 mm) and better demarcated than calluses (Fig. 12-28). Paring the surface off the lesions will reveal a central core in a corn. Corns are found primarily on the feet and are the result of poorly fitting shoes. Calluses are diffuse areas of thickened skin, 5 to 20 mm in diameter, on the palmar surfaces of hands or fingers or the weight-bearing areas of the feet. Paring the surfaces of these lesions will reveal normal skin grooves.

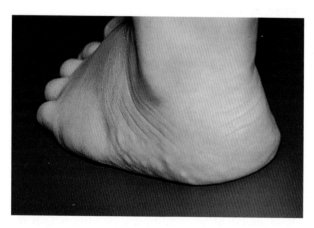

Fig. 12-26 Piezogenic pedal papules. Lesions on the foot are seen as multiple soft, compressible papules that appear when pressure is placed on the heel.

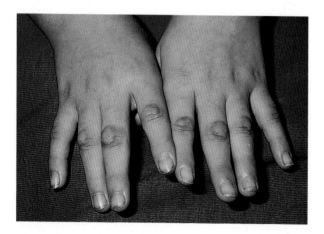

Fig. 12-27 Knuckle pads over the proximal interphalangeal joints of both hands.

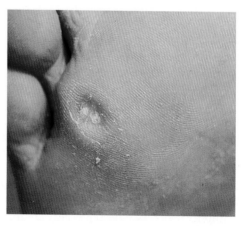

Fig. 12-28 Corn. Circumscribed epidermal thickening with central core.

Differential diagnosis

Plantar warts are most often confused with corns and calluses. Shaving off the skin surface with a razor blade will reveal interrupted skin ridges with a central area containing black dots in a wart, interrupted skin ridges with a central core of keratin in a corn, and normal skin ridges in a callus. Patients with unexplained focal or diffuse thickening of the palms or soles may have a variety of palmoplantar keratoderma. These conditions may be associated with metabolic or structural abnormalities and may require intensive investigation.

Pathogenesis

Prolonged pressure or friction from ill-fitting shoes produces corns and calluses on the feet. Playing a musical instrument, using playground equipment, or working with tools produces corns and calluses on the hands. The thickening is due to epidermal proliferation and an increase in the number of cells in the stratum corneum.

Treatment

Reducing the lesion with a razor blade by shaving off the excess stratum corneum and then covering the lesion with a salicylic acid 40% plaster for 1 to 7 days will relieve the discomfort of corns and calluses.

Patient education

The patient should be told that the lesion is not a wart and that prolonged pressure and friction are responsible for the genesis of the lesion.

Follow-up visits

Follow-up visits are unnecessary.

Histiocytosis

Clinical features

The histiocytoses include a group of benign and fatal disorders.[40-43] Lesions may be present at birth or appear during infancy or childhood (Figs. 12-29 to 12-31). The cutaneous lesions of Langerhans cell histiocytosis (LCH) may consist of discrete red, orange, and/or yellow-brown papules or nodules. The presenting symptom may be crusted, scaling dermatitis of the scalp, postauricular, perineal, and axillary areas. The presence of red-brown purpuric papules and nodules within or peripheral to areas of dermatitis should alert the clinician to a diagnosis of LCH.

Congenital self-healing reticulohistiocytosis consists of papules and nodular lesions present at birth that can look like the lesions of LCH or a pyogenic

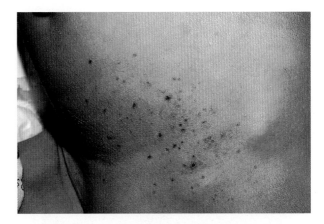

Fig. 12-29 Langerhans cell histiocytosis. Crusted purpuric papules on lower abdomen with underlying lymphadenopathy.

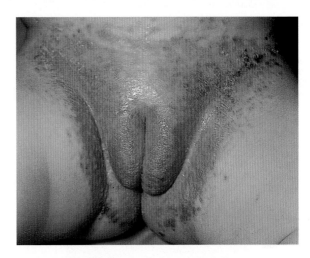

Fig. 12-30 Langerhans cell histiocytosis. Diaper dermatitis similar to Fig. 4-11.

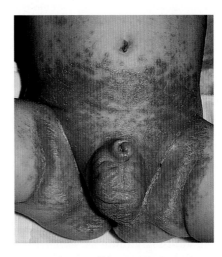

Fig. 12-31 Langerhans cell histiocytosis. More severe dermatitis in diaper area unresponsive to conventional therapy.

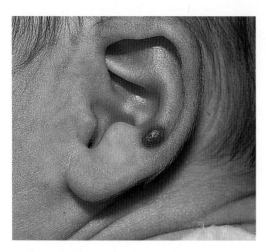

Fig. 12-32 Congenital self-healing reticulohistiocytosis. At birth, this lesion looks similar to a pyogenic granuloma.

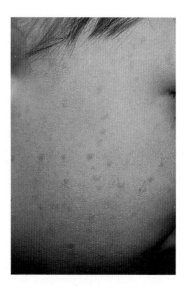

Fig. 12-34 Benign cephalic histiocytosis. Multiple tan papules on face.

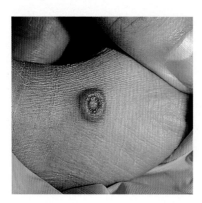

Fig. 12-33 Congenital self-healing reticulohistiocytosis. Nodule present at birth with crateriform central erosion.

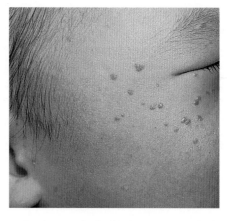

Fig. 12-35 Benign cephalic histiocytosis. Multiple red-tan papules on face.

granuloma (Fig. 12-32).[44-47] Larger lesions can demonstrate a crateriform central erosion (Fig. 12-33).

Benign cephalic histiocytosis consists of 2- to 5-mm, yellow-red to tan papules that develop on the face and upper part of the body (Figs. 12-34 and 12-35).[48,49] The lesions usually begin between 6 and 12 months of age. They consist of non-Langerhans cell histiocytes.

Differential diagnosis

Histiocytosis lesions include the differential diagnosis of juvenile xanthogranulomas, eczema, seborrheic dermatitis, diaper dermatitis, and scabies.[50] The pres-

ence of petechiae or purpura within or peripheral to areas of dermatitis suggests LCH.

Pathogenesis

The Langerhans cell is a specific monocyte-macrophage that expresses CD1, a glycoprotein, and contains Birbeck granules.[40] Langerhans cells are found within the epidermis of skin, regional lymph nodes, thymic epithelium, and bronchial mucosa. The histiocyte is a monocyte-macrophage. The associated histiocytic syndromes represent infiltrations with histiocytic cells that may or may not be Langerhans cells.

LCH is an umbrella term that includes the diseases previously called *histiocytosis X*. The diagnostic feature of LCH is the presence of lesional histiocytes, at least some of which are phenotypically like normal Langerhans cells.[51] The lesions may contain varying proportions of LCH cells, macrophages, lymphocytes, eosinophils, neutrophils, and plasma cells. Skin, bone, spleen, liver, lungs, and lymph nodes may be affected. Great clinical heterogeneity of LCH exists despite more uniform pathologic features. LCH may be localized to bone or skin, may be associated with diabetes insipidus and or exophthalmos, or may have lethal multi-organ involvement. Studies have considered a relationship of human herpesvirus 6 and LCH.[51-53]

Benign cephalic histiocytosis lesions consists of non-Langerhans cell histiocytes.

Treatment

Treatment of these disorders depends on the specific diagnosis and extent of disease. A biopsy is usually necessary to confirm the diagnosis. Additional biopsies may be needed for electron microscopic examination and immunohistochemistry to confirm the specific type of histiocytosis.

Benign cephalic histiocytosis usually requires no therapy and should resolve during childhood. Recently a patient was documented with diabetes insipidus and benign cephalic histiocytosis.[54] Congenital self-healing reticulohistiocytosis requires close clinical observation to confirm a benign course. LCH survival and therapy are dependent on the number of organs involved and the severity of the involvement.[43,55,56] Therapy for LCH may also involve surgical removal of lesions, chemotherapy, or observation. Chemotherapy may include corticosteroids, alkylating agents, cytokines, or immunoglobulin. Before therapy, a systemic evaluation is required to identify the extent and severity of disease.

Patient education

A thorough evaluation is necessary to identify the type and extent of histiocytic syndromes. Parents should be informed of the unusual nature of LCH and should be given information on the benign or malignant course that their child can expect.

Follow-up visits

Diagnosis and treatment of these conditions requires coordination with a pathologist, radiologist, pediatric oncologist, and primary care physician. Follow-up

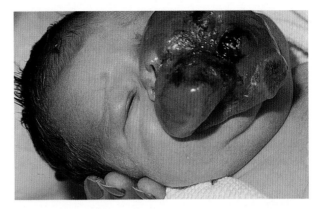

Fig. 12-36 Embryonal rhabdomyosarcoma on the face of an infant.

visits should be arranged to inform the patient and the patient's family of the severity and extent of disease and possible therapies directed by the pediatric oncologist.

Rhabdomyosarcomas
Clinical features

Rhabdomyosarcomas are the most common malignant soft-tissue tumors in childhood. They are far more common than melanomas in prepubertal children. The head (Fig. 12-36) and neck and urogenital tract are the usual sites of involvement. Two peaks of age in childhood have a higher incidence of rhabdomyosarcoma: ages 1 to 5 and during adolescence. The tumor usually appears as a mass lesion of the neck, face, or extremity, or is seen as a subcutaneous and/or intradermal nodule that has normal-appearing skin. Occasionally the surface of the skin covering the tumor becomes reddened. The lesion may produce local signs of destruction depending on the location. For example, in the orbit, it may produce exophthalmos or ptosis; in the ear canal, a bloody discharge with a polypoid ear mass; and in the nasal passages, obstruction of one of the airways and bleeding. In the genitourinary tract, it may appear as urinary obstruction. Grapelike masses of tumor protruding from the vagina are another presentation of rhabdomyosarcoma.

Rhabdomyosarcomas may spread either by local extension or by hematogenous or lymphatic metastases. Approximately 75% of the metastases will become apparent within 6 months of the appearance of the original lesion. The most frequent sites involved with metastases are the regional lymph nodes, lungs, liver, bone marrow, bone, and brain. Head and neck tumors have been reported to extend directly into the brain, and may occur as frequently as in one third of all cases.

Differential diagnosis

The feature of rapid, progressive growth will help distinguish rhabdomyosarcoma from the other skin nodules and cysts of infants and children listed in Table 12-1. Ulceration is not an early sign of rhabdomyosarcoma, but the tumor is fixed to deep fascia, is often greater than 3 cm, and is firm in consistency.

Pathogenesis

Rhabdomyosarcoma is a malignant tumor of striated muscles. There is no hereditary pattern and there are no known precipitating factors.[57]

Treatment

Therapy has included radiation and combination chemotherapy in the initial stages of disease after wide surgical excision. Debulking the tumor with wide surgical excision is the first treatment of choice. New therapeutic protocols are currently being evaluated.[58]

Patient education

Prognosis should be discussed with the family, keeping in mind that a number of factors are important in the survival rate. The prognosis is better for the embryonal type than the alveolar type of rhabdomyosarcoma.[59] The location of the original lesion is an important factor, with the best prognosis occurring in orbital lesions, the next best with bladder, and the worst with lesions beginning on the head and neck. Referral to a pediatric oncology facility as soon as the diagnosis is suspected is indicated.

Follow-up visits

Follow-up visits should be arranged for family support, but a pediatric oncologist should be involved in determining frequency of visits.

Neuroblastoma, Leukemia, and Lymphoma

Lymphoma, leukemia (Fig. 12-37), and neuroblastoma (Fig. 12-38) can present as inflamed cutaneous papules or nodules.[60-62] Neuroblastomas may blanch when stroked.[63] The lesions may appear as the primary manifestation of disease or as a metastases of known disease. Unknown nodules or lesions that demonstrate rapid progressive growth (see Box 12-1), should be biopsied for specific diagnosis. Therapy will need to be directed by a pediatric oncologist.

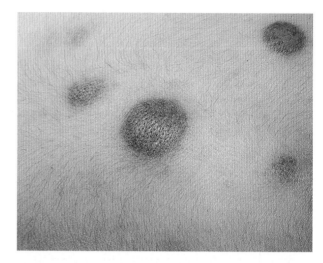

Fig. 12-37 Leukemia. Firm purple nodules on the back of an infant with congenital leukemia.

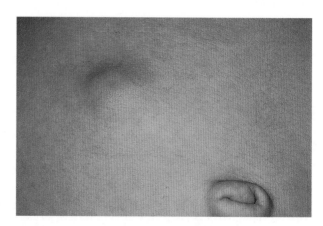

Fig. 12-38 Cutaneous neuroblastoma was the first sign of this infant's disease.

REFERENCES

1. Knight PJ, Reiner CB: Superficial lumps in children: what, when and why? *Pediatrics* 72:147, 1983.
2. Paller AS, Pensler JM, Tomimta T: Nasal midline masses in infants and children, *Arch Dermatol* 127:362, 1991.
3. Todd NW: Common congenital anomalies of the neck: embryology and surgical anatomy, *Surg Clin North Am* 73:599, 1993.
4. Covello SP et al: Keratin 17 mutations cause either steatocystoma multiplex or pachyonychia congenita type 2, *Br J Dermatol* 139(3):475, 1998.
5. Grimalt R, Gelmetti C: Eruptive vellus hair cysts: case report and review of the literature, *Pediatr Dermatol* 9:98, 1992.
6. Julian CG, Bowers PW: A clinical review of 209 pilomatricomas, *J Am Acad Dermatol* 39(2 Pt 1):191, 1998.
7. Chan EF et al: A common human skin tumour is caused by activating mutations in beta-carotenin, *Nat Genet* 21(4):410, 1999.

8. Pruzan DL, Esterly NB, Prose NS: Eruptive syringoma, *Arch Dermatol* 125:1119, 1989.

9. Price MA, Goldberg LH, Levy ML: Juvenile basal cell carcinoma, *Pediatr Dermatol* 11:176, 1994.

10. Howell JB: Nevoid basal cell carcinoma syndrome, *J Am Acad Derm* 11:98, 1984.

11. Shanley S et al: Nevoid basal cell carcinoma syndrome: review of 118 affected individuals, *Am J Med Genet* 50:282, 1994.

12. Kirchmann TT, Prieto VG, Smoller BR: CD34 Staining pattern distinguishes basal cell carcinoma from trichoepithelioma, *Arch Dermatol* 130:589, 1994.

13. Marrogi AJ, Wick MR, Dehner LP: Benign cutaneous adnexal tumors in childhood and young adults, excluding pilomatrixoma: review of 28 cases and literature, *J Cutan Pathol* 18:20, 1991.

14. Kraemer KH et al: Xeroderma pigmentosum and related disorders: examining the linkage between defective DNA repair and cancer, *J Invest Dermatol* 103:96, 1994.

15. Oro AE et al: Basal cell carcinomas in mice overexpressing sonic hedgehog, *Science* 2,276(5313):817, 1997.

16. Toftgard R: Hedgehog signaling in cancer, *Cell Mol Life Sci* 57(12):1720, 2000.

17. Lauri G et al: Recurrent digital fibromatosis of childhood, *J Hand Surg* 15A:106, 1990.

18. Ishii N et al: A case of infantile digital fibromatosis showing spontaneous regression, *Br J Dermatol* 121:129, 1989.

19. Hirshowitz B et al: Silicone occlusive sheeting (SOS) in the management of hypertrophic and keloid scarring, including the possible mode of action of silicone, by static electricity, *Eur J Plast Surg* 16:5, 1993.

20. Barron DF, Cootauco MH, Cohen BA: Granuloma annulare: a clinical review, *Lippincott's Prim Care Pract* 1(1):33, 1997.

21. Török E, Daróczy J: Juvenile xanthogranuloma: an analysis of 45 cases by clinical follow-up, light and electron microscopy, *Acta Derm Venereol* 65:167, 1985.

22. Fonseca E, Contreras F, Cuevas J: Papular xanthoma in children: report and immunohistochemical study, *Pediatr Dermatol* 10:139, 1993.

23. Hernandez-Martin A et al: Juvenile xanthogranuloma, *J Am Acad Dermatol* 36(3 Pt 1):355, 1997.

24. Karcioglu ZA, Mullaney PB: Diagnosis and management of iris juvenile xanthogranuloma, *J Pediatr Ophthalmol Strabismus* 34(1):44, 1997.

25. Freyer DR et al: Juvenile xanthogranuloma: forms of systemic disease and their clinical implications, *J Pediatr* 129(2):227, 1996.

26. Chang MW, Frieden IJ, Good W: The risk of intraocular juvenile xanthogranuloma: survey of current practices and assessment of risk, *J Am Acad Dermatol* 34(3):445, 1996.

27. Zvulunov A, Barak Y, Metzker A: Juvenile xanthogranuloma, neurofibromatosis, and juvenile chronic myelogenous leukemia: world statistical analysis, *Arch Dermatol* 131(8):904, 1995.

28. Azaña JM et al: Urticaria pigmentosa: a review of 67 pediatric cases, *Pediatr Dermatol* 11:102, 1994.

29. Patrice SJ, Wiss K, Mulliken JB: Pyogenic granuloma (lobular capillary hemangioma): a clinicopathologic study of 178 cases, *Pediatr Dermatol* 8:267, 1991.

30. Frieden IJ, Esterly NB: Pyogenic granulomas of infancy masquerading as strawberry hemangiomas, *Pediatrics* 90:989, 1992.

31. Bragado R et al: Increased expression of vascular endothelial growth factor in pyogenic granulomas, *Acta Derm Venereol* 79(6):422, 1999.

32. Tay YK, Weston WL, Morelli JG: Treatment of pyogenic granuloma in children with the flashlamp-pumped pulsed dye laser, *Pediatrics* 99(3):368, 1997.

33. Gagné EJ, Su WPD: Congenital smooth muscle hamartoma of the skin, *Pediatr Dermatol* 10:142, 1993.

34. Foster CM et al: Limited dermal ossification: clinical features and natural history, *J Pediatr* 109:71, 1986.

35. Laing VB, Fleischer AB: Piezogenic wrist papules: a common and asymptomatic finding, *J Am Acad Dermatol* 24:415, 1991.

36. Pontious J, Lasday S, Mele R: Piezogenic pedal papules extending into the arch: case reports and discussion, *J Am Podiatr Med Assoc* 80:444, 1990.

37. Paller AS, Hebert AA: Knuckle pads in children, *AJDC* 140:915, 1986.

38. Schuval SJ et al: Panniculitis and fever in children. *J Pediatr* 122:372, 1993.

39. Shetty AK, Gedalia A: Sarcoidosis in children, *Curr Probl Pediatr* 30(5):149, 2000.

40. Chu T, Jaffe R: The normal Langerhans cell and LCH cell, *Br J Cancer* 70:4S, 1994.

41. Willman CL et al: Langerhans' cell histiocytosis (histiocytosis x): a clonal proliferative disease, *N Engl J Med* 331:154, 1994.

42. Munn S, Chu AC: Langerhans cell histiocytosis of the skin, *Hematol Oncol Clin North Am* 12(2):269, 1998.

43. Bucsky P, Egeler RM: Malignant histiocytic disorders in children: clinical and therapeutic approaches with a nosologic discussion, *Hematol Oncol Clin North Am* 12(2):465, 1998.

44. Berger TG et al: A solitary variant of congenital self-healing reticulohistiocytosis: solitary Hashimoto-Pritzker disease, *Pediatr Dermatol* 3:230, 1986.

45. Herman LE et al: Congenital self-healing reticulohistiocytosis, *Arch Dermatol* 126:210, 1990.

46. Hashimoto K et al: Immunohistochemistry and electron microscopy in Langerhans cell histiocytosis confined to the skin, *J Am Acad Dermatol* 25:1044, 1991.

47. Jang KA et al: Histiocytic disorders with spontaneous regression in infancy, *Pediatr Dermatol* 17(5):364, 2000.

48. Barsky BL et al: Benign cephalic histiocytosis, *Arch Dermatol* 120:650, 1984.

49. Peña-Penabad C et al: Benign cephalic histiocytosis: case report and literature review, *Pediatr Dermatol* 11:164, 1994.

50. Talanin NY et al: Cutaneous histiocytosis with Langerhans cell features induced by scabies: a case report, *Pediatr Dermatol* 11:327, 1994.

51. Favara BE, Jaffe R: The histopathology of Langerhans cell histiocytosis, *Br J Cancer* 70:41S, 1994.

52. Leahy MA et al: Human herpesvirus 6 is present in lesions of Langerhans cell histiocytosis, *J Invest Dermatol* 101:643, 1993.

53. McClain K, Weiss RA: Viruses and Langerhans cell histiocytosis: is there a link? *Br J Cancer* 70:34S, 1994.

54. Willman CL, McClain KL: An update on clonality, cytokines, and viral etiology in Langerhans cell histiocytosis, *Hematol Oncol Clin North Am* 12(2):407, 1998.

55. Weston WL et al: Benign cephalic histiocytosis with diabetes insipidus, *Pediatr Dermatol* 17(4):296, 2000.

56. Ladisch S, Gardner H: Treatment of Langerhans cell histiocytosis: evolution and current approaches, *Br J Cancer* 70:41S, 1994.

57. Arceci RJ: Treatment options: commentary, *Br J Cancer* 70:58S, 1994.

58. Merlino G, Helman LJ: Rhabdomyosarcoma: working out the pathways, *Oncogene* 18(38):5340, 1999.

59. Ruymann FB, Grovas AC: Progress in the diagnosis and treatment of rhabdomyosarcoma and related soft tissue sarcomas, *Cancer Invest* 18(3):223, 2000.

60. Harms D: New entities, concepts, and questions in childhood tumor pathology, *Gen Diagn Pathol* 141(1):1, 1995.

61. Orozco-Covarrubias MDLL et al: Malignant cutaneous tumors in children, *J Am Acad Dermatol* 30:243, 1994.

62. Young G et al: Recognition of common childhood malignancies, *Am Fam Phys* 61(7):2144, 2000.

63. Maris JM, Matthay KK: Molecular biology of neuroblastoma, *J Clin Oncol* 17(7):2264, 1999.

CHAPTER THIRTEEN | Vascular Lesions

VASCULAR TUMORS AND MALFORMATIONS

Vascular birthmarks are one of the most common forms of birth defects. The classification of vascular birthmarks has in the past been confusing. We prefer the classification of Mulliken and Glowacki (Box 13-1), which divides vascular birthmarks into vascular tumors and vascular malformations.[1,2] Although they may occasionally appear similar at birth, the natural history of these lesions is quite distinct, and within a few months of age they can usually be differentiated (Table 13-1).

Vascular Tumors
Clinical features[3-5]

Hemangiomas. Although generally classified as vascular birthmarks, only 20% of hemangiomas are present at birth. The other 80% arise between 2 and 4 weeks of age. Approximately 1% to 3% of newborns will have a hemangioma noted at birth. By 1 year of age, 10% to 12% of children born at full term will have a hemangioma. Twenty percent of preterm babies weighing less than 1000 g will develop a hemangioma. Females are affected at least twice as often as males.

There are three major types of hemangioma presentations (Box 13-2). The most common is a pale white to gray-blue macule (Fig. 13-1). The other types are the telangiectatic (Fig. 13-2) and the papular (Fig. 13-3) forms. At the time of presentation it is impossible to predict what form the hemangioma will eventually take or its final size. Because all hemangiomas are derived from the same cell type, and all have the same natural history, the terms *strawberry* and *cavernous* should not be used to describe hemangiomas. These terms should be replaced by describing the location of the hemangioma within the skin (see Box 13-1). Bright-red, papular hemangiomas should be referred to as *superficial hemangiomas* (Fig. 13-4), whereas blue, nodular hemangiomas should be referred to as *deep hemangiomas* (Fig. 13-5). The majority of hemangiomas contain both a superficial and a deep component (Fig. 13-6) and should be labeled as *mixed hemangiomas* (see Box 13-1).

At 4 to 8 weeks of age, hemangiomas undergo a rapid growth phase that continues until the infant is 6 to 9 months of age. During this time the rate of growth of the hemangioma is much greater than the growth rate of the infant. This rapid growth phase is a characteristic feature of hemangiomas.[3] After the rapid growth phase, the hemangioma growth slows and approximates the growth rate of the infant. As they grow, most hemangiomas will feel soft and be easily compressible. The growth phase is eventually followed by regression of the hemangioma. This begins sometime in the second year of life. The regression phase begins with paling of the hemangioma (Fig. 13-7), followed by flattening of the tumor. This phase slowly continues, and by 5 years of age 50% of hemangiomas have reached maximal regression. By 9 years of age 90% of hemangiomas will have reached maximal regression. Maximal regression of the hemangioma does not define a return to normal skin. Residual post hemangioma regression includes hypopigmentation, telangiectasia (Fig. 13-8), fibrofatty deposits, and scarring if the hemangioma has previously ulcerated.

Although hemangiomas are usually benign lesions, they can be associated with certain local and systemic complications (Box 13-3). Ulceration and subsequent infection are the most common forms of complications of hemangiomas. Ulcerations (Fig. 13-9) occur during the rapid growth phase of hemangiomas primarily located in the diaper area.[6] Infection is usually with *Staphylococcus aureus,* but *Pseudomonas aeruginosa* may also be seen. Infants with periorbital hemangiomas should always be referred for ophthalmologic evaluation for amblyopia and/or astigmatism. Superficial cervicofacial hemangiomas in a "beard distribution" are associated with upper airway hemangiomas.[7] Large lumbosacral hemangiomas spanning the midline may be associated with underlying anomalies of the spine and spinal cord.[8] Large facial hemangiomas may be associated with central nervous system malformations (most commonly Dandy-Walker posterior fossa malformations), abnormal central nervous system arteries, cardiac and large vessel defects, and ophthalmologic abnormalities (PHACE syndrome [Posterior fossa malformation, Hemangiomas, Arterial anomalies,

Box 13-1 Classification of Hemangiomas and Vascular Malformations

HEMANGIOMAS
Superficial
Mixed
Deep

VASCULAR MALFORMATIONS
Capillary (port-wine stain)
Telangiectatic
Hypertrophic capillary (angiokeratoma)
Venous
Arteriovenous
Lymphatic
Cutis marmorata telangiectatica congenita
Mixed

Table 13-1 Differential Diagnosis of Hemangiomas and Vascular Malformations

Hemangiomas	Vascular Malformations
Tumor of endothelial cells	Developmental abnormality
Only 20% present at birth	Always present at birth
Undergo rapid growth	Stable growth
Always undergo regression	Never regress

Box 13-2 Clinical Presentation of Hemangiomas

Blue-gray macule
Telangiectatic
Papular

Box 13-3 Complications of Hemangiomas

LOCAL
Obstruction of vital function
Ulceration
Infection

SYSTEMIC
High-output cardiac failure

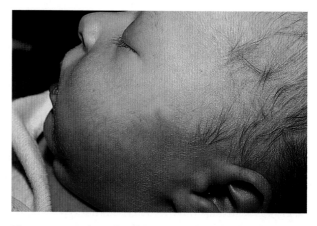

Fig. 13-1 Macular pale white presentation of a hemangioma.

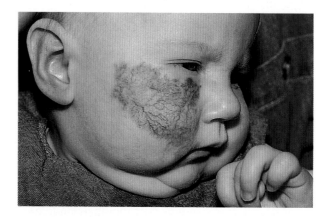

Fig. 13-2 Telangiectatic presentation of a hemangioma.

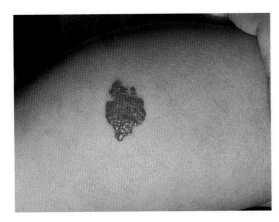

Fig. 13-3 Papular presentation of a hemangioma.

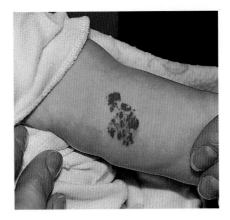

Fig. 13-4 Superficial hemangioma.

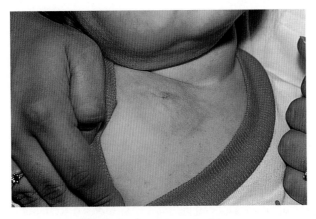

Fig. 13-5 Deep hemangioma.

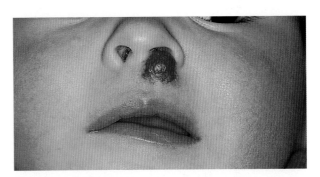

Fig. 13-6 Mixed superficial and deep hemangioma that obstructs breathing.

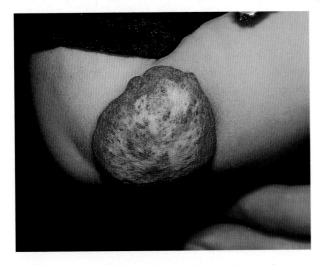

Fig. 13-7 Paling of a mixed superficial and deep hemangioma in an 18-month-old female. This is often the initial sign of regression of the hemangioma.

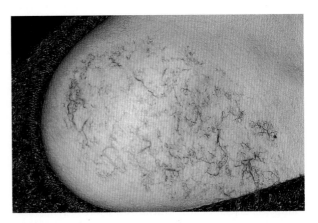

Fig. 13-8 Residual hypopigmentation and telangiectasia postregression of a hemangioma in a 17-year-old female.

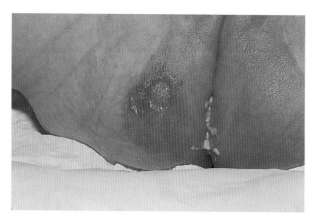

Fig. 13-9 Ulceration of a hemangioma on the buttock of a 3-month-old infant.

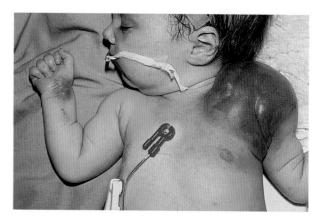

Fig. 13-11 Sudden change of a large superficial and deep hemangioma to deep purple as part of the Kasabach-Merritt syndrome.

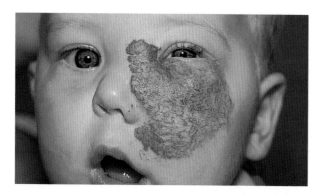

Fig. 13-10 Mixed superficial and deep hemangioma in a 4-month old male, leading to partial visual obstruction.

Coarctation of the aorta and other cardiac defects, and Eye abnormalities]).[9,10]

Magnetic resonance imaging (MRI) should be obtained on children with large lumbosacral hemangiomas. Brain and cardiac imaging should be performed if one is considering the possibility of the PHACE syndrome. Obstruction of a vital function (e.g., vision [Fig. 13-10], breathing [see Fig. 13-6], eating, urination, or defecation) and high-output cardiac failure may also be seen. A solitary cutaneous hemangioma causing high-output cardiac failure is an exceedingly rare event. Although historically described in hemangiomas, platelet trapping with consumption coagulopathy (Kasabach-Merritt syndrome) is rarely if ever seen with these tumors, but it is seen most commonly in association with kaposiform hemangioendothelioma or tufted angioma.[11,12]

Kaposiform hemangioendothelioma. Kaposiform hemangioendotheliomas are rare vascular tumors that often are present at birth and are usually seen before 2 years of age.[3,4,13] They occur equally in males and females. Mature lesions have a nodular and infiltrative growth pattern and a characteristic purple color. Lesions are usually solitary. They may be seen in the retroperitoneum and the skin, but hepatic kaposiform hemangioendothelioma has not been reported. These are very aggressive local tumors, and although not metastatic they can be fatal. As opposed to hemangiomas, kaposiform hemangioendotheliomas do not regress spontaneously.

Platelet trapping with consumption coagulopathy may occur. A large, rapidly growing, soft, compressible vascular tumor is noted to suddenly become firm and to become dark purple (Fig. 13-11).

Laboratory evaluation will show a decreased platelet count and abnormal blood clotting consistent with a consumption coagulopathy. Although quite rare, it is a medical emergency.

Histologically the tumor consists of a combination of plum- and spindle-shaped endothelial cells. The areas containing the spindle cells are slitlike vascular spaces resembling Kaposi's sarcoma. The cells are locally aggressive and form irregular lobules and sheets of cells that infiltrate the dermis and subcutaneous tissue.

Tufted angiomas. Tufted angiomas present as two distinct clinical patterns.[3,4,14] The most common of these are slowly expanding, dusky, reddish-blue vascular plaques. Greater than 50% occur on the head,

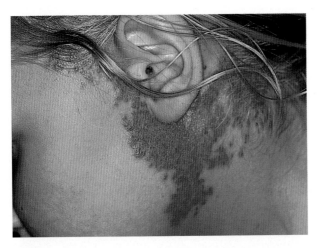

Fig. 13-12 Plaque-type tufted angioma on the neck of a 4-year-old girl.

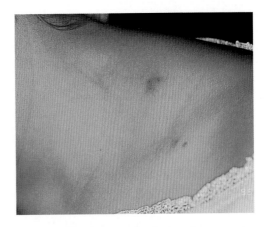

Fig. 13-13 Satellite lesions of tufted angioma on the neck of the same girl in Fig. 13-12.

neck, upper trunk, and upper arms (Fig. 13-12). Satellite lesions may be seen (Fig. 13-13). The majority arise within the first 2 decades of life. Regression in this type of tufted angioma is not expected. Kasabach-Merritt syndrome may also be seen with this tumor.

The less common form presents as a solitary vascular tumor on a lower extremity (Fig. 13-14). This type of tumor does not exhibit the slow expansion seen in the other clinical type of tufted angioma, and satellite lesions are not seen. Regression of this type of tufted angioma has been reported.

Histologically the blood vessels in tufted angiomas occur in discrete tufts (hence the name) described as "cannonball-like." The tufts consist of endothelial cells closely packed together.

Differential diagnosis

The differential diagnosis of a hemangioma depends on the time of presentation to the physician. A mature hemangioma that has undergone a rapid growth phase followed by the initiation of regression is difficult to confuse with anything else.[3-5] The greatest difficulty in the differential diagnosis of hemangiomas occurs with those present at birth. The telangiectatic presentation of hemangiomas can easily be confused with a telangiectatic vascular malformation.[15] Only observation over time will differentiate between these two types of birthmarks. Deep hemangiomas can be mistaken for lymphatic malformations, and again time will simplify the differential. Kaposiform hemangioendothelioma can be differentiated by the color and infiltrative growth pattern. Classic tufted angiomas are more plaquelike and are usually located

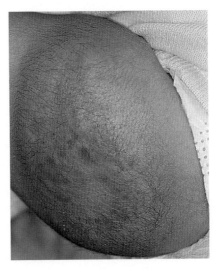

Fig. 13-14 Nodular-type tufted angioma on the thigh of a 2-week-old boy.

from the chest up. The nodular type of tufted angioma may be difficult to differentiate from certain types of venous malformations. Subcutaneous sarcomas are rare but should be considered when an infant presents with a firm, rather than rubbery-feeling, rapidly growing mass. MRI and biopsy may be required to obtain the correct diagnosis.

Pathogenesis

Hemangiomas are benign tumors of capillary endothelium.[3-5] Proliferating hemangiomas are associated with an overabundance of mast cells, and as the tumor regresses, the mast cell number also decreases.

It is not unusual for mast cells to be associated with blood-vessel growth, and it is unknown whether this is a primary or secondary event. Endothelial cell proliferation is enhanced by certain angiogenic factors, such as acidic and basic fibroblast growth factor, transforming growth factor a and b, and angiogenin. Regression in hemangiomas is asynchronous, with parts of the tumor regressing while other portions continue to grow. As with the beginning of growth of the tumor, the mechanism of initiation of regression remains unknown, although it is likely to be secondary to endothelial cell apoptosis. Kaposiform hemangioendotheliomas are aggressive tumors of endothelial cells. Tufted angiomas are also comprised of endothelial cells, but the mechanism of tuft formation is unknown.

Treatment

The first question that arises regarding treatment of hemangiomas is which ones should be treated (Box 13-4).[3-5] Certainly, all hemangiomas with the potential to interfere with a vital function should be treated. Periorbital hemangiomas may cause pressure on the eye, leading to astigmatism, or they may partially or totally obstruct vision, causing amblyopia. High-output cardiac failure, although rare, is a medical emergency and requires immediate attention. Hemangiomas in the diaper area frequently ulcerate,[6] and early treatment may minimize the risk of ulceration and decrease the likelihood of anal or urethral obstruction. Ulcerated hemangiomas are severely painful and at risk for superinfection. Recognition of the complications associated with hemangiomas in the diaper area and early treatment of these lesions can minimize complications and prevent the need for a diverting colostomy. Facial hemangiomas can be disfiguring, and early treatment minimizes the extent of hemangioma growth and the eventual residua. Other hemangiomas should be observed and treated only if complications arise.

For years the mainstay of treatment for hemangiomas has been oral glucocorticosteroids (Box 13-5).[3-5] From 30% to 60% of hemangiomas are reported to be responsive to glucocorticosteroid therapy. Treatment should be started at 2 mg/kg and adjusted depending on the response of the tumor. Some authors advocate using higher doses of glucocorticosteroids. Responsive hemangiomas will demonstrate an effect from treatment within 7 to 10 days, manifested as softening of the tumor, lightening in color, or a noticeable decrease in growth rate. Systemic glucocorticosteroids should be used as the first line of treatment for high-output car-

---

Box 13-4   Indications for Treatment of Hemangiomas

High-output cardiac failure
Obstruction of vital function
Ulceration
Infection
Facial location
Diaper area location

Box 13-5   Treatment Options for Hemangiomas

Oral glucocorticosteroids
Vascular-specific pulsed dye laser
Interferon alpha-2a

---

diac failure and those rapidly growing hemangiomas that threaten to interfere with a vital function. Systemic glucocorticosteroid therapy is not without side effects, and treatment should be maintained for as short a time as possible. The use of intralesional steroids has also been advocated for the treatment of hemangiomas, but we believe that this procedure should be done only by those with experience.

Interferon alpha-2a has been demonstrated to be effective for hemangiomas that are unresponsive to glucocorticosteroids.[3-5] Treatment is initiated daily by subcutaneous injection at a dose of 3 million U/m^2 and continued until the hemangioma is fully in a regressive state. On average, treatments have been continued for 9 to 12 months. Treatment with interferon alpha-2a is expensive and potentially toxic. Fever and myalgias occur in almost every case, as do reversible elevation of liver function tests, neutropenia, and anemia. The most worrisome side effect of interferon alpha-2a is spastic diplegia, which may persist after cessation of therapy. Therefore use of interferon alpha-2a should be reserved for truly endangering or life-threatening hemangiomas unresponsive to glucocorticosteroids.[3-5]

The vascular-specific pulsed dye laser has added another option for the treatment of hemangiomas.[16] This form of therapy is excellent for the treatment of ulcerated hemangiomas, leading to a rapid decrease in the pain associated with the ulceration and complete healing of 75% of the ulcerations within 2 weeks

(Figs. 13-15 and 13-16).[6] Superficial papular hemangiomas treated before or early in the rapid growth phase also respond well to treatment.[9] The treatment is simple and fast, and side effects are nearly nonexistent. Vascular-specific pulsed dye laser therapy should be considered for facial and diaper-area hemangiomas because it minimizes the eventual residua and decreases the risk for ulceration in at-risk tumors. It also has a role as an adjunct to steroid therapy in rapidly growing hemangiomas. The limitation of vascular pulsed dye lasers in the treatment of hemangiomas is their minimal depth of penetration into the skin. Vascular pulsed dye laser treatment minimally alters the long-term outcome of mixed or deep hemangiomas.[16] Nonspecific laser therapy, such as the carbon dioxide or the neodymium:yttrium, aluminum, garnet (Nd:YAG) laser, although effective in destroying hemangiomas, often leads to scarring and a worse outcome than natural regression.

The response of kaposiform hemangioendotheliomas to treatment is unpredictable.[3,4,13] Multiple therapies have been used, including surgery, glucocorticosteroids, interferon, antiplatelet aggregating agents, embolization, and radiotherapy. Heparin is contraindicated for the treatment of disseminated intravascular coagulopathy associated with kaposiform hemangioendotheliomas because it has been shown to increase the growth rate of the tumor and worsen the clinical situation. Patients should be referred for comprehensive multispecialty care.

The response of tufted angiomas to treatment is also variable, but treatment with either vascular pulsed dye laser or interferon alpha-2a has been reported to be succesful.[3,4] Fortunately, this tumor is not as aggressive as kaposiform hemangioendothelioma and does not always require treatment.

Systemic glucocorticosteroids should be used as the first line of treatment for Kasabach-Merritt syndrome. Heparin and fresh frozen plasma may also be needed to control bleeding. Heparin is contraindicated in Kasabach-Merritt secondary to kaposiform hemangioendothelioma. Combination chemotherapy may be beneficial.[17]

Patient education

The natural history and potential complications of hemangiomas should be discussed with the patient's family. They should be aware of the difficulty of predicting the eventual size and type of the hemangioma, the final outcome, and the need for treatment. The need for frequent follow-up visits, until the hemangioma growth and complication pattern is evident,

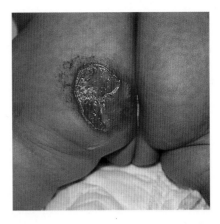

Fig. 13-15 Ulceration of a hemangioma on the buttock of a 5-month-old infant.

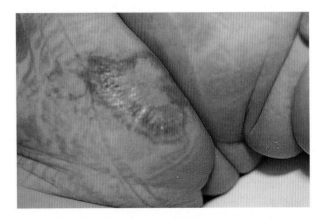

Fig. 13-16 Same hemangioma 4 weeks later after one pulsed dye laser treatment.

should be emphasized. Parents should be told of the aggressive nature of kaposiform hemangioendotheliomas and the need for prompt treatment. The chronic nature of tufted hemangiomas and poor response to most treatments should be discussed.

Follow-up visits

Hemangiomas need to be followed closely during the rapid growth phase. Initially visits should be every 2 weeks, and if no complications occur and the hemangioma growth has stabilized the time between visits can be lengthened.

Children with periorbital hemangiomas should be referred for ophthalmologic evaluation and management. Measurement of the size of the lesions allows a more accurate measure of actual growth than observation alone. Once regression has begun and no complications have been noted, follow-up should be on a yearly basis.

Patients with hemangioendotheliomas will need to be treated aggressively until the tumor is under control.

The follow-up of tufted hemangiomas will depend on their location, rate of growth, and response to chosen treatment.

Vascular Malformations
Clinical features

Vascular malformations are developmental errors of blood and/or lymphatic vessel formation. By definition, vascular malformations are always present at birth.[1] They do not undergo a rapid growth phase, but rather grow proportionally with the child. Vascular malformations should be classified according to the predominant vessel type within the birthmark (see Box 13-1).[1]

Capillary malformations (port-wine stains) are the most common type of vascular malformation. Eyelid, occipital, and nuchal vascular birthmarks are very common in light-skinned newborns. Small lesions over the eyelids often fade, but the occipital and nuchal lesions will remain. Excluding these, port-wine stains occur in 3 per 1000 births. The name *port-wine stain* derives from the dark red color that is common in mature capillary malformations (Fig. 13-17). However, most port-wine stains present as light pink macules (Fig. 13-18). The dark red color (port-wine) slowly develops as the patient ages. Along with the darkening in color, maturing port-wine stains develop progressive nodularity and blebbing, and may lead to overgrowth of the underlying soft tissue and bone.[18,19] The rate of progression of any individual port-wine stain cannot be predicted, but approximately 67% of patients with facial port-wine stains will develop these changes by the fifth decade.[18,19]

In patients with facial port-wine stains, the possibility of the Sturge-Weber syndrome should be considered. The Sturge-Weber syndrome is the association of a facial port-wine stain with central nervous system (seizures, mental retardation, hemiplegia) and ophthalmologic (glaucoma) abnormalities. The overall risk of a facial port-wine stain having the associated abnormalities of the Sturge-Weber syndrome is 8%, but the chances increase with increasing size of the facial port-wine stain (Fig. 13-19). Infants with bilateral facial port-wine stains are at the highest risk (33%).[20] Patients with a port-wine stain or any other type of vascular malformation covering an extremity are at risk for the development of overgrowth of that extremity (Klippel-Trenaunay syndrome) (Fig. 13-20). As the child gets older the overgrowth can become enormous

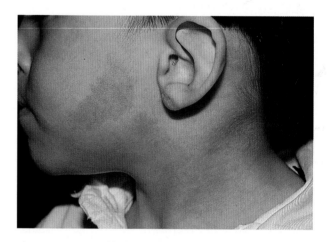

Fig. 13-18 Typical light pink port-wine stain in a 3-year-old male.

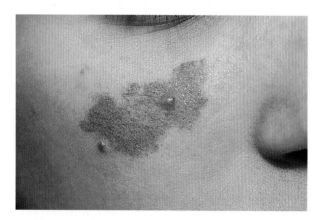

Fig. 13-17 Dark red port-wine stain with central blebbing in a 14-year-old female.

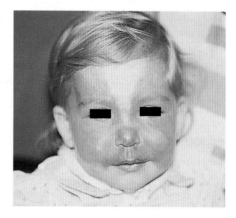

Fig. 13-19 Bilateral port-wine stain in a 2-year-old female with the Sturge-Weber syndrome.

and can be associated with severe varicosities, venous stasis, ulceration, and recurrent infection, leading to a state of chronic lymphedema. Occasionally, port-wine stains are extensive and cover large areas of skin.

Telangiectatic vascular malformations are capillary malformations in which individual rather than confluent telangiectasias are the presenting feature.[15] They should be considered a variant of port-wine stains. The risk of development of Sturge-Weber and Klippel-Trenaunay syndromes in association with telangiectatic malformations is unknown.

Hyperkeratotic capillary malformations (angiokeratomas) are distinguished by their acanthotic, hyperkeratotic epidermis overlying a capillary malformation. Five separate conditions are classified as angiokeratomas, but only angiokeratoma circumscriptum is congenital.[21] Angiokeratomas should be considered a mixed developmental abnormality of vessels and epidermis. They are most commonly seen on an extremity as unilateral bands or as palm-sized plaques composed of blue-black papules or nodules with a warty, hyperkeratotic surface (Fig. 13-21).

Venous malformations are developmental errors in vein formation.[22,23] These malformations may contain any size vessel from venules to large draining veins. Their distinct venous pattern is often obvious at presentation (Fig. 13-22). Occasionally, large nodules will develop within these lesions (Fig. 13-23).

Arteriovenous malformations (fistulae) are direct connections between an artery and the venous system, bypassing the capillary bed.[23] They are often initially

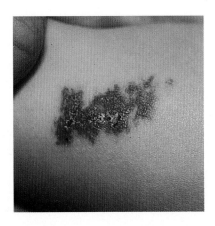

Fig. 13-21 Angiokeratoma circumscriptum in a 6-month-old female demonstrating thickened epidermis overlying a capillary malformation.

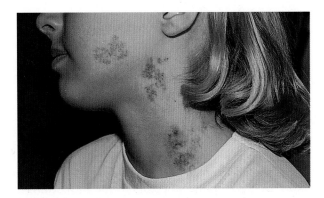

Fig. 13-22 Distinct blue venous pattern of a venous malformation in an 11-year-old female.

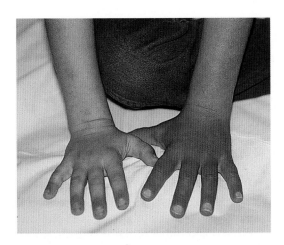

Fig. 13-20 Hypertrophy of the left arm and hand in a 6-year-old male with the Klippel-Trenaunay-Weber syndrome.

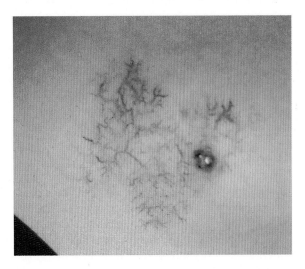

Fig. 13-23 Venous malformation with a large nodule in a 9-year-old male.

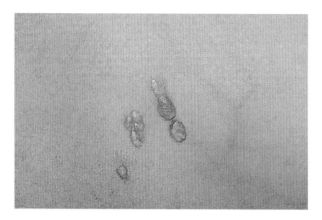

Fig. 13-24 Lymphangioma circumscriptum. Grouping of gelatinous skin-colored papules on the abdomen.

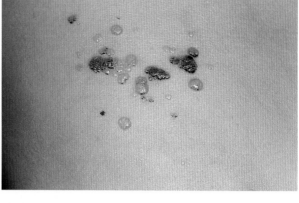

Fig. 13-25 Lymphangioma circumscriptum. After minor trauma, lesions may darken, the result of bleeding into the lesion.

trivial-appearing lesions but with time may expand rapidly. They are high-flow lesions and may have a notable pulsation and/or thrills and bruits. Localized pain, hyperhidrosis, hypertrichosis, and hyperthermia of a relatively banal-looking vascular lesion should raise the suspicion of an arteriovenous malformation. Arteriovenous malformations are the rarest type of vascular malformation.

Lymphatic malformations are in general referred to as *lymphangiomas*—a misnomer because the lesions are developmental errors in the formation of lymphatic vessels and not tumors as the suffix *-oma* designates. There are three clinical types of lymphatic malformations: solitary simple, circumscriptum, and cavernous. Solitary simple lymphatic malformations present as dermal or subcutaneous squishy nodules. Lymphangioma circumscriptum consists of multiple clusters of small vesicles covering limited skin areas, usually less than 10 cm in diameter (Figs. 13-24 and 13-25). Cavernous lymphatic malformations (cystic hygromas) present as large, ill-defined, grotesque, rubbery, skin-colored, subcutaneous nodules that may underlie areas of more superficial lymphatic malformations.[24] They are usually solitary and involve the face, trunk, and extremities.

In cutis marmorata telangiectatica congenita, two clinical presentations may be seen. The first is a mottled pattern of blue or dusky-red erythema present at birth (Fig. 13-26). In the second form there is atrophy of the skin and larger, depressed, blue venous malformations (congenital phlebectasia) (Fig. 13-27). Both types may be seen in the same patient. Often a single extremity is involved, but the lesions may occur bilaterally on the extremities or on the

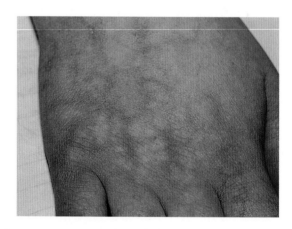

Fig. 13-26 Permanent mottled appearance of cutis marmorata telangiectatica congenita.

trunk. A gradual increase in the size of the lesions is expected as the child grows, but the lesions become less noticeable within the first few years of life.[25-27] Associations with musculoskeletal or other vascular malformations may occur.

Occasionally, vascular malformations will contain a mixture of many different types of vascular components. They present as a composite of the presentation of each individual component.

Differential diagnosis

In older children, port-wine stains and telangiectatic malformations are rather characteristic and are seldom confused with other lesions. At birth, port-wine stains and telangiectatic vascular malformations must be differentiated from the macular and telangiectatic presentations of hemangiomas.[3-5,15] These lesions will

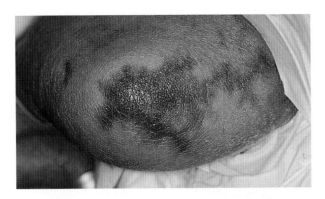

Fig. 13-27 Venous pattern of cutis marmorata telangiectatica congenita (congenital phlebectasia).

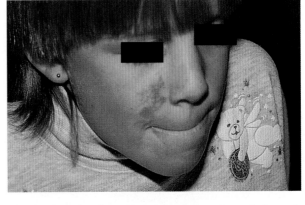

Fig. 13-28 Before laser treatment of port-wine stain in an 8-year-old female.

eventually be distinguished by the presence or absence of a rapid growth phase.

Congenital solitary angiokeratomas and angiokeratoma circumscriptum must be differentiated historically from the acquired forms of angiokeratoma. Although quite rare, the development of numerous angiokeratomas at a young age should alert the clinician to the possibility of either Fabry's disease or α-fucosidosis.

As with the capillary malformations, venous and arteriovenous malformations are usually quite characteristic. Rarely, these lesions are disfiguring and can be mistaken for vascular malignancies such as Kaposi's sarcoma and angiosarcomas.

Lymphangioma circumscriptum may be mistaken for a disorder with grouped vesicles, such as herpes simplex, herpes zoster, or dermatitis herpetiformis. There is no erythematous base in circumscribed lymphangioma, however, and the lesions appear gelatinous, not fluid-filled. As noted, hemorrhage into such lesions results in darkening, which may be confused with melanoma.

Cavernous lymphatic malformations may be confused with lipomas, plexiform neurofibromas, and other soft subcutaneous masses.

In contrast to cutis marmorata telangiectatica congenita, mottling of newborn skin is a transient vasodilatation and is relieved by rewarming the skin. The livedo reticularis pattern of collagen vascular disease is flat, is not depressed over the discolored areas, is always bilateral, and is associated with systemic signs and symptoms.

Pathogenesis

All vascular malformations should be considered developmental errors in vessel formation. Most are sporadic and are likely caused by genetic mosaicism.

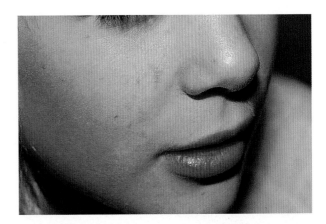

Fig. 13-29 Same patient shown in Fig. 13-28, 2 years later, after 10 laser treatments.

Treatment

The vascular-specific (585 nm) pulsed (450 msec) dye laser is recognized as the treatment of choice for capillary and telangiectatic vascular malformations.[28] Vascular-specific pulsed dye lasers capable of emitting longer wavelengths and longer pulse duration are now available. Theoretically, they have the advantage of deeper depth of penetration into the dermis and the ability to destroy larger-caliber vessels. Comparative studies of different wavelengths and pulse duration have not been performed. Response of these lesions to treatment depends on the age of the patients at the beginning of treatment and the size of the lesion.[29] The younger the child at the beginning of treatment and the smaller the lesion, the increased likelihood of complete removal (Figs. 13-28 and 13-29). Treatments can safely be started as early as 2 weeks of

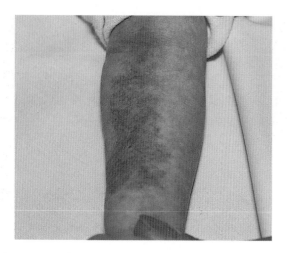

Fig. 13-30 Telangiectatic malformation in a 4-month-old female.

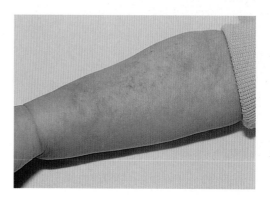

Fig. 13-32 Same patient shown in Fig. 13-30, after second laser treatment.

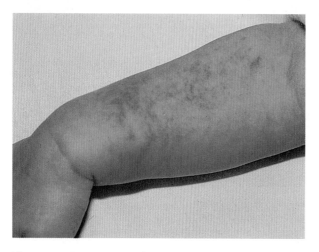

Fig. 13-31 Same patient shown in Fig. 13-30, 2 months after initial laser treatment.

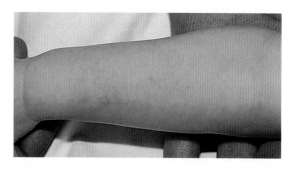

Fig. 13-33 Same patient shown in Fig. 13-30, 10 months after initial laser treatment. Only three laser treatments were required to achieve almost total clearing of the telangiectatic malformation.

age.[29,30] Large lesions are improved by treatment, but total removal is less likely. Response to treatment is slow, and even small lesions in very young infants will frequently take 1 to 3 years for complete removal. The vascular-specific (585 nm) pulsed (450 msec) dye laser is very safe, and side effects are minimal. Treatment has been greatly improved by the introduction of topical EMLA and other topical anesthetic creams, which significantly decrease the pain associated with the procedure.

Unlike port-wine stains, telangiectatic vascular malformations have a much smaller vessel load to destroy to return the skin to normal. Most of these le-sions will be completely removed in three to six treatments (Figs. 13-30 through 13-33).[15]

Treatment of all other types of vascular malformations, including the Klippel-Trenaunay syndrome, is difficult and must be handled on an individual basis.[31-33] Referral to a multidiscipline specialty clinic with specific expertise in dealing with these types of birth defects is optimal.

Patient education

Parents of babies with capillary and telangiectatic malformations should be told about the possibility of treatment with vascular-specific pulsed dye lasers.

They should be referred to the nearest treatment center as soon as possible.

If a large facial port-wine stain is present, the possibility of the Sturge-Weber syndrome should be discussed, and the patient should be referred for neurologic and ophthalmologic consultation.

For other types of vascular malformations, the difficulty of treatment should be discussed, and, if possible, the child should be referred to a specialty clinic with expertise in managing these type of lesions.

Follow-up visits

The frequency of follow-up visits is determined by the degree of complications associated with a given malformation.

ACQUIRED VASCULAR LESIONS
Pyogenic Granuloma
Clinical features

Pyogenic granulomas are most common in acral areas, such as the hands and fingers, and on the face (Fig. 13-34).[34] They appear as solitary, dull-red, firm nodules that are 5 to 6 mm in diameter. The surface may be smooth and glistening, but often it is ulcerated and crusted. The lesion bleeds easily when traumatized. Removal by surgical excision followed by suturing has resulted in the appearance of multiple satellite lesions in a few instances. Pyogenic granuloma may occur at any age, but in childhood it is most common in the first 5 years of life. The majority of patients have no history of a predisposing factor.

Differential diagnosis

Pyogenic granuloma is often misdiagnosed as a hemangioma, glomus tumor, melanocytic nevus, wart, molluscum contagiosum, or malignant melanoma. All of these lesions can ulcerate and crust if traumatized. Pathologic study distinguishes pyogenic granuloma from the other lesions.

Pathogenesis

Proliferation of capillaries within a circumscribed area, with flattened or ulcerated epidermis on top and epidermal proliferation at the sides, producing a "collarette" of epidermis, is seen. Pyogenic granuloma is believed to be caused by an abnormal healing response.

Treatment

Excision by curettage with electrocautery to the base is the treatment of choice. Pulse dye laser treatment is effective for smaller lesions.[35]

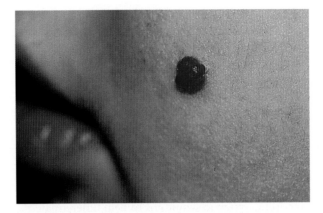

Fig. 13-34 Pyogenic granuloma. Smooth, glistening surface of the erythematous papule.

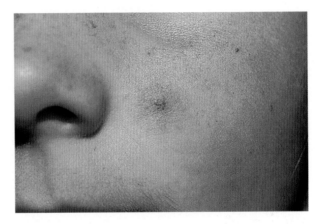

Fig. 13-35 Vascular spider with prominent central feeding vessel on the cheek of a child.

Patient education

It should be explained to the patient and family that this growth is not malignant but will not disappear without treatment and represents an abnormal healing response.

Follow-up visits

A visit 1 week after removal of the lesion is useful to inform the patient and family of the pathologic diagnosis and evaluate healing.

Spider Telangiectasia
Clinical features

A spider telangiectasia is a small lesion consisting of a central arteriole from which superficial blood vessels radiate peripherally (Fig. 13-35). They usually appear between ages 2 and 6 years and are located in sun-exposed areas, usually on the cheeks, nose, dorsa of the hands, and forearms. Sometimes the central arteriole is raised and prominent and it may be pulsatile on diascopy. Approximately 40% of light-skinned children will have these lesions.

Differential diagnosis

Spider telangiectasia must be differentiated from the telangiectatic mats of the autosomal dominant Osler-Weber-Rendu syndrome, in which confluent telangiectasia compose each lesion and multiple lesions are seen over the dorsum of the hands, lips, and face. Associated epistaxis, peptic ulcer–like symptoms, or both may be important systemic symptoms to help differentiate the two conditions. Spider telangiectasia may be confused with the telangiectatic mats seen in collagen vascular diseases such as scleroderma and lupus erythematosus.

Pathogenesis

The cause of these lesions is unknown.

Treatment

If the cosmetic appearance is a concern to the child, lesions may be removed without scarring using the pulsed dye laser at 585 nm. A single treatment is over 90% effective.[36]

Patient education

The common and nonserious nature of these lesions should be emphasized.

Follow-up visits

Follow-up visits are unnecessary.

Cherry Angiomas and Diffuse Angiokeratomas
Clinical features

True cherry angiomas are rare in childhood and usually appear as 1- to 3-mm solid-red, dome-shaped, blanching papules (Fig. 13-36).[37] The appearance of multiple cherry angiomas around the umbilicus and scrotum, which increases progressively with age, should bring to mind two diagnoses: Fabry's disease and α-fucosidosis. In Fabry's disease, attacks of pain, numbness, and tingling of the hands and feet often accompany the eruption.[38] The usual onset of the eruption is between 4 and 12 years of age. In α-fucosidosis, severe mental retardation and neuromuscular spasticity accompany the disorder.

Differential diagnosis

Cherry angiomas and angiokeratomas must be differentiated from small pyogenic granulomas and small

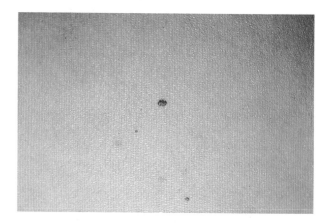

Fig. 13-36 Cherry angioma on the trunk of a child.

superficial hemangiomas. Usually the differentiation is quite simple. Cherry angiomas are small (2 to 5 mm) and dome-shaped with a normal epithelium over them. Pyogenic granulomas have a friable, often crusted surface and bleed easily. When they first appear, angiokeratomas have a smooth surface but later will develop a rough, scaly surface.

Pathogenesis

Fabry's disease is an X-linked recessive disorder in which activity of a specific lysosomal hydrolase, α-galactosidase A, is deficient. The glycosphingolipid, ceramide trihexoside, accumulates within endothelial cells and produces the cutaneous vascular lesions. Rearrangements or point mutations in the gene encoding α-galactosidase have been found. On electron microscopy the endothelial cells of the affected vessels are shown to contain multiple laminated inclusions diagnostic of the disease. In α-fucosidosis the lysosomes of the endothelial cells are widely dilated, but the material is washed out during fixation so the cells appear empty. Fibroblast culture and analysis of α-galactosidase A activity may be performed to confirm the diagnosis of Fabry's disease. In α-fucosidosis, an autosomal recessive trait, fibroblast cultures may also be useful in confirming the diagnosis.

Treatment

There is no effective treatment for either Fabry's disease or α-fucosidosis. Renal transplantation has resulted in improvement in some patients with Fabry's disease. Cherry angiomas may be easily treated with the pulsed dye laser at 585 nm, if desired.

Patient education

The patient and family should be informed about the seriousness of each of these conditions and referred for genetic counseling. They should be advised that prenatal diagnosis is possible for future pregnancies, and that molecular probes are available to screen carrier females. Pediatric neurologic care is usually advisable. Because the condition of patients with Fabry's disease progresses to severe renal disease, and they may succumb to renal failure, evaluation of renal function with appropriate consultation should be recommended to the parents.

Follow-up visits

Follow-up visits should be arranged with the appropriate pediatric care specialists.

REFERENCES

1. Mulliken JB, Fishman SJ, Burows PE: Vascular anomalies, *Curr Probl Surg* 37:517, 2000.
2. Enjolras O, Mulliken JB: Vascular tumors and vascular malformations (new issues), *Adv Dermatol* 13:375, 1997.
3. Metry DW, Hebert AA: Benign cutaneous vascular tumors of infancy: when to worry, what to do, *Arch Dermatol* 136:905, 2000.
4. Mueller BU, Mulliken JB: The infant with a vascular tumor, *Semin Perinatol* 23:332, 1999.
5. Drolet BA, Esterly NB, Frieden IJ: Hemangiomas in children, *N Engl J Med* 341:173, 1999.
6. Morelli JG et al: Treatment of ulcerated hemangiomas in infancy, *Arch Pediatr Adol Med* 148:1104, 1994.
7. Orlow SJ, Isakoff MS, Blei F: Increased risk of symptomatic hemangiomas of the airway in association with cutaneus hemangioma in a "beard" distribution, *J Pediatr* 131:643, 1997.
8. Albright AL, Gartner JC, Weiner GS: Lumar cutaneous hemangiomas as indicators of tethered spinal cords, *Pediatrics* 83:977, 1989.
9. Coats DK, Paysse EA, Levy ML: PHACE: a neurocutaneous syndrome with important ophthalmologic implications: case report and literature review, *Ophthalmol* 106:1739, 1999.
10. Frieden IJ, Reese V, Cohen D: PHACE syndrome: the association of posterior fossa brain malformations, hemangiomas, arterial anomalies, coarctation of the aorta and cardiac defects and eye abnormalities, *Arch Dermatol* 132:307, 1996.
11. Enjolras O et al: Residual lesions after Kasabach-Merritt phenomenon in 41 patients, *J Am Acad Dermatol* 42:225, 2000.
12. Enjolras O et al: Infants with Kasabach-Merritt syndrome do not have "true" hemangiomas, *J Pediatr* 130:631, 1997.
13. Quante M et al: Epithelioid hemangioendothelioma presenting in the skin: a clinicopathologic study of eight cases, *Am J Dermatopathol* 20:541, 1998.
14. Jones EW, Orkin M: Tufted angioma (angioblastoma): a benign progressive angioma, not to be confused with Kaposi's sarcoma or low-grade angiosarcoma, *J Am Acad Dermatol* 20:214, 1989.
15. Morelli JG, Huff JC, Weston WL: The treatment of congenital telangiectatic vascular malformations with the vascular specific pulsed dye laser, *Pediatrics* 92:603, 1993.
16. Richards KA, Garden JM: The pulsed dye laser for cutaneous vascular and nonvascular lesions, *Semin Cutan Med Surg* 19:276, 2000.
17. Hu B et al: Kasabach-Merritt syndrome-associated kaposiform hemangioendothelioma successfully treated with cyclophosphamide, vincristine, and actinomycin D, *J Pediatr Hematol/Oncol* 20:567, 1998.
18. Geronemus RG, Ashinoff R: The medical necessity of evaluation and treatment of port wine stains, *J Dermatol Surg Oncol* 117:76, 1991.
19. Klapman MH, Yao JF: Thickening and nodules in port-wine stains, *J Am Acad Dermatol* 44:300, 2001.
20. Tallman B et al: Location of port wine stains and the likelihood of ophthalmic and/or CNS complications, *Pediatrics* 87:323, 1991.
21. Schiller PI, Itin PH: Angiokeratomas: an update, *Dermatology* 193:275, 1996.
22. Enjolras O et al: Extensive pure venous malformation in the upper or lower limb: a review of 27 cases, *J Am Acad Dermatol* 36:219, 1997.
23. Upton J et al: Vascular malformations of the upper limb: a review of 270 patients, *J Hand Surg* 24:1019, 1999.
24. Gallagher PG, Mahoney MJ, Gosche JR: Cystic hygroma in the fetus and newborn, *Semin Perinatol* 23:341, 1999.
25. Amitai DB et al: Cutis marmorata telangiectasia congenita: clinical findings in 85 patients, *Pediatr Dermatol* 17:100, 2000.
26. Gerritsen MJ et al: Cutis marmorata telangiectasia congenita: report of 18 cases, *Br J Dermatol* 142:366, 2000.
27. Devillers AC, de Waard-van der Spek FB, Oranje AP: Cutis marmorata telangiectasia congenita: clinical features in 35 cases, *Arch Dermatol* 135:34, 1999.
28. Richards JA, Garden JM: The pulsed dye laser for cutaneous vascular and nonvascular lesions, *Semin Cutan Med Surg* 19:276, 2000.
29. Nguyen CM et al: Facial port wine stains in childhood: prediction of the rate of improvement as a function of the age of the patient, size and location of the port wine stain and the number of treatments with the pulsed dye (585) laser, *Br J Dermatol* 136:821, 1998.
30. Ashinoff RA, Geronemus RG: Flashlamp-pumped pulsed tunable dye laser for port-wine stains in infancy: earlier versus later treatment, *J Am Acad Dermatol* 24:467, 1991.
31. Noel AA et al: Surgical treatment of venous malformations in Klippel-Trenaunay syndrome, *J Vasc Surg* 32:840, 2000.
32. Fliegelman LJ et al: Lymphatic malformation: predictive factors for recurrence, *Otolaryngol Head Neck Surg* 123:706, 2000.
33. Berry SA et al: Klippel-Trenaunay syndrome, *Am J Med Genet* 79:319, 1998.
34. Harris MN et al: Lobular capillary hemangiomas: an epidemiologic report, with emphasis on cutaneous lesions, *J Am Acad Dermatol* 42:1012, 2000.
35. Tay Y-K, Weston WL, Morelli JG: Treatment of pyogenic granulomas in children with the flashlamp-pumped pulsed dye laser, *Pediatrics* 99:368, 1997.
36. Tan E, Vinciullo C: Pulsed dye laser treatment of spider telangiectasia, *Austral J Dermatol* 38:22, 1997.
37. Plunkett A et al: The frequency of common nonmalignant skin conditions in adults in central Victoria, Australia, *Int J Dermatol* 38:901, 1999.
38. Peters FP et al: Fabry's disease: a multidisciplinary disorder, *Postgraduate Med J* 73:710, 1997.

Vascular Reactions: Urticaria, Erythemas, and Purpuras

Urticaria, erythemas, and purpuras are considered together in a single chapter because they represent a spectrum of disease characterized by progressive signs of injury to cutaneous blood vessels. All are accompanied by vasodilation (erythema) and leakage of fluid from blood vessels (edema). Leakage of red blood cells also occurs in the purpuras as a further sign of vascular insult. A complex interplay of chemical mediators may be involved. Histamine is involved in urticaria, as are complement fragments with vasoactive properties, such as C3a and C5a. Eicosanoids, kinins, neuropeptides, serotonin, and certain cytokines may also participate.[1] In addition, other immunoreactants may be involved, such as immunoglobulin E (IgE), antibodies directed against the epsilon receptor I, and circulating antigen-antibody complexes, particularly in the initial stages of vascular injury.[1,2] Immune complex disease seems to be particularly important in the reactive erythemas and vasculitis. Included is pyoderma gangrenosum, a rare but life-threatening dermatosis.

URTICARIA

Urticarial states are common in infancy and childhood, although the exact incidence is not known. Several large studies indicate that 3% of preschool children and about 2% of older children suffer from urticaria.[2-6] Children that have atopic dermatitis in infancy have an increased incidence of urticaria.[4] The high incidence of urticaria in healthy children undoubtedly includes children with a single episode of short-lived urticaria rather than persistent urticaria.[2,6] Interestingly, of all children with urticaria, only 3% to 5% have what can be documented as immunoglobulin E (IgE)-mediated allergic urticaria. In contrast, approximately 15% of children with urticaria have a physical urticaria, with the bulk of these diagnoses classified as "idiopathic."[2,5] Rarely, children with persistent idiopathic urticaria may have urticarial vasculitis. For purposes of presenting a clinical approach to urticaria, transient urticaria and persistent urticaria are discussed separately.

Transient Urticaria and Angioedema
Clinical features

Transient urticaria in children often follows infection,[2,3,5,6] encounters with stinging or biting insects,[2,5,7] ingestion of medications[8,9] (see Chapter 22) or certain foods,[6,10] or occurs with inflammatory systemic diseases such as collagen vascular disease or thyroiditis[2,11] (Box 14-1). The eruption is sudden in onset and pruritic, with erythematous raised wheals scattered over the body.[2,6] The wheals are usually 2 to 15 mm in diameter, flat-topped, and have tense edema (Fig. 14-1). The edema can be appreciated by stretching the skin slightly to demonstrate whitish centers. The erythematous borders with pale centers can be quite large and mistaken for target lesions of erythema multiforme.[12] Occasionally, giant urticarial lesions up to 30 cm in diameter with polycyclic borders will appear (Figs. 14-2 and 14-3). Such wheals commonly last from 20 minutes to 3 hours, disappear, then reappear in other areas. The entire episode of transient urticaria often lasts 24 to 48 hours; rarely, it lasts as long as 3 weeks. Transient urticaria, as it resolves, may leave flat dusky areas lasting several days that mimic bruises (Fig. 14-4).[2,5,6,8]

Subcutaneous extension of lesions, called *angioedema*, may occur.[2,6] These lesions appear as large, deep swellings with indistinct borders around the eyelids and lips. They may also appear on the face, trunk, genitalia (Fig. 14-5), and extremities. The face, hands, and feet are involved in 85% of patients, and other areas are involved in 15%. Up to half of children with transient urticaria may have angioedema, with swelling of the hands and feet commonly seen. When examined within the first 4 weeks of illness, all of the persistent urticarias may be indistinguishable from transient urticaria.

Box 14-1   Transient Urticaria

INFECTIOUS ASSOCIATIONS
Streptococcus
Infectious mononucleosis (Epstein-Barr virus)
Hepatitis
Adenovirus
Enterovirus
Parasites

BITES AND STINGS
Bees
Wasps
Scorpions
Spiders
Jellyfish

DRUGS
Penicillin
Cephalosporins
Salicylates
Morphine, codeine, and other opiates
Nonsteroidal antiinflammatory drugs
Barbiturates
Amphetamines
Atropine
Hydralazine
Insulin

BLOOD AND BLOOD PRODUCTS

FOODS
Nuts
Eggs
Shellfish
Strawberries
Tomatoes

SYSTEMIC DISEASES
Collagen vascular diseases
Lupus erythematosus
Juvenile rheumatoid arthritis
Polyarteritis nodosa
Dermatomyositis
Neonatal lupus syndrome
Sjögren's syndrome
Rheumatic fever
Inflammatory bowel diseases
Crohn's disease
Ulcerative colitis

MISCELLANEOUS
Aphthous stomatitis
Behçet's disease
Thyroiditis

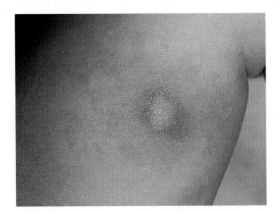

Fig. 14-1 Central wheal with red border in acute urticaria.

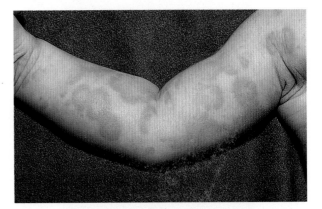

Fig. 14-2 Multiple polycyclic red wheals of different sizes in a child with urticaria. Commonly mistaken for erythema multiforme.

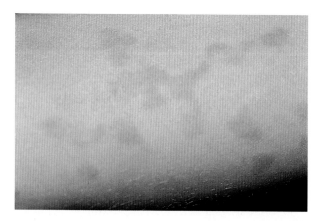

Fig. 14-3 Multiple shapes of urticarial lesions in a child.

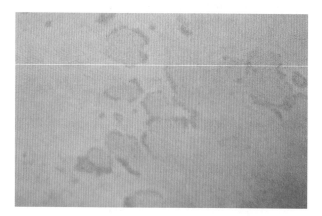

Fig. 14-4 Dusky centers with red borders in resolving childhood urticaria.

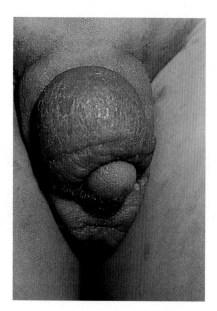

Fig. 14-5 Angioedema of the scrotum and foreskin in an infant.

Hereditary angioedema accounts for only 0.4% of cases of urticaria, but its specific diagnostic tests and high mortality deserve special mention. It is an autosomal dominant condition with repeated attacks of swelling of the extremities, face, and throat, accompanied by abdominal pain.[13] The onset usually follows trauma, such as surgery, dental manipulation, or accidents. It presents as a diffuse, brawny swelling of the extremities in 75% of patients, abdominal pain in 52%, and swelling of the face and throat in 30%. Its onset is usually in adolescence, with the more severe symptoms associated with the menses. Abdominal pain eventually becomes a major complaint in 93% of patients. They do not have typical urticarial wheals, but 26% have lesions resembling erythema multiforme. Severe airway edema accounts for the mortality of almost 30% in untreated patients. Only 25% of patients give a positive family history. The diagnosis should be suspected if the serum C4 level is persistently low. It is confirmed by functional assay of the C1 esterase inhibitor. In some children hereditary angioedema is associated with lupus erythematosus or other collagen vascular diseases.[14]

Differential diagnosis

The conditions to be considered in the differential diagnosis of urticaria are listed in Box 14-2. A skin biopsy is recommended in atypical forms of urticaria.[5] Urticaria, especially giant urticaria, is frequently confused with erythema multiforme.[12] Urticarial lesions may blanch in the center, showing a red border and thus concentric zones of color change, as is seen in erythema multiforme. However, it should be remembered that individual urticarial lesions are transient, usually lasting less than 3 hours, whereas erythema multiforme lesions are fixed and stay in place at least 7 to 14 days. Also, the target lesions of erythema mul-

---

Box 14-2   Differential Diagnosis of Urticaria

Erythema multiforme
Mastocytosis
Flushing
Reactive erythemas
Juvenile rheumatoid arthritis
Vasculitis
Guttate psoriasis
Pityriasis rosea (early lesions)

tiforme reveal disruption of the epidermis in the center, with blisters, crusts, or scabs. Frequently when polycyclic urticarial wheals of different sizes and shapes accompany edema of the hands and feet, erythema multiforme is incorrectly diagnosed.[12] Urticarial lesions often clear with the administration of subcutaneous epinephrine; erythema multiforme does not. A skin biopsy will also distinguish the two. Urticaria can be differentiated from mastocytosis by a skin biopsy because increased numbers of mast cells are seen in mastocytosis. Flushing states are flat rather than elevated. In juvenile rheumatoid arthritis, faint erythematous macules with a clear center are present and are associated with a spiking fever. Vasculitis lesions have nonblanching purpuric centers, whereas psoriasis and pityriasis rosea demonstrate scaling overlying the erythematous papules.

Angioedema (deep hives) (Box 14-3) should be differentiated from cellulitis and erysipelas, which are tender, warm, red lesions. Chronic thickening of tissues occurs in lymphedema, in contrast to the acute stretching of tissue seen in angioedema. Angioedema of the hands and feet, which accompanies urticaria, may be confused with erythema multiforme.[12] A skin biopsy will distinguish. Persistent angioedema of the face or lip should bring to mind lupus erythematosus or other collagen vascular diseases.[14] Considerable deep edema can develop in acute contact dermatitis, but vesiculation of the overlying epidermis and epidermal papules will help distinguish it from angioedema. Idiopathic scrotal edema of children and the Melkersson-Rosenthal syndrome are rare and can be distinguished from angioedema by the furrowed tongue and cranial nerve palsies of Melkersson-Rosenthal syndrome and the limitation of angioedema to the scrotum in idiopathic scrotal edema.

Box 14-3 Differential Diagnosis of Angioedema

Cellulitis and erysipelas
Lymphedema
Acute contact dermatitis
Idiopathic scrotal edema of children
Melkersson-Rosenthal syndrome

Pathogenesis

Histamine is undoubtedly the major chemical mediator of transient urticaria, and the mast cell is central in all forms of transient urticaria and angioedema. Histamine may be directly released from cutaneous mast cells in the case of certain foods or opiate drugs. Specific IgE antibodies bound to mast cell surfaces that "recognize" certain antigens, such as penicillin and other drugs, foods, and venom of certain stinging insects, result in the release of histamine after combination with antigen. In some, autoantibodies to the epsilon receptor on skin mast cells may be responsible.[1,5,6] Rechallenge studies are few, and in suspected urticarial reactions to drugs, only 4% could be reproduced.[14]

Complement fragments, activated by immune complexes, may activate mast cells to release histamine or exert vasoactive effects of their own on cutaneous blood vessels. The latter mechanism is most often associated with infection, but careful documentation of the mechanism of histamine release involved with each inciting substance is not available. Eicosanoids may induce mast cell mediator release and have been implicated in exacerbations of urticaria,[6,15] and other cytokines have been implicated in urticaria.

In hereditary angioedema, a deficiency of the C1 esterase inhibitor permits unregulated cleavage of complement proteins once the complement system is activated, with particular consumption of C4. A C2 kinin activates the clotting system via the Hageman factor in hereditary angioedema.[13] Complement cleavage products may be responsible for the edema and erythema.

Treatment

Oral antihistamines are valuable in symptomatic control of urticaria. Hydroxyzine hydrochloride, 1 to 2 mg/kg/day in a single dose, or diphenhydramine hydrochloride, 5 mg/kg/day in four divided doses, is the most prescribed.[2,6] If urticaria at night is the problem, administration of hydroxyzine 1 hour before bedtime may allow a single treatment per day. Combinations of H1 blocking agents such as cetirizine in the morning and hydroxyzine at bedtime may be effective. Nonsedating antihistamines are less effective in controlling urticaria. In angioedema not controlled by antihistamines, the addition of pseudoephedrine, 4 mg/kg/day in four divided doses, is useful but nightmares and sleep disturbances and sympathomimetic side effects limit its use to older children.[6] The same drugs may be used to treat chronic angioedema. In acute angioedema of the airway, epinephrine 1:1000,

0.01 ml/kg/dose to a maximum dose of 0.5 ml, or albuterol inhalers may be used.[2,6] There is no evidence to support the use of systemic glucocorticosteroids in urticaria or angioedema. The addition of H2 blocking drugs to H1 antihistamines is of little additional benefit, and H2 blockers are ineffective when used alone.[6] Cromolyn sodium preparations, which may be efficacious in treatment of airway or bowel reactions, have not been particularly useful in skin. Leukotriene antagonists, such as zafirlukast or montelukast, may be useful in treating exacerbations that result from nonsteroidal antiinflammatory usage.[15] Allergen avoidance is an important strategy if the allergen can be identified. Virtually any drug may produce urticaria, but certain drugs are more frequently implicated. Drugs such as penicillin and aspirin account for most drug-induced urticaria, and they should be specifically questioned in review of the patient's history. Cephalosporins produce an urticarial serum-sickness–like reaction. Foods suspected of causing the urticaria could be avoided if nutrition is not compromised. Restriction diets are of little value if a suspected food factor has not been identified.

In hereditary angioedema, acute attacks are managed by intravenous fluid replacement and airway maintenance.[13] Administration of danazol or stanozolol, synthetic attenuated testosterones, increases C1q esterase inhibitor levels and prevents the attacks of angioedema. Fresh-frozen plasma or ε-aminocaproic acid may be useful before surgical procedures.[13]

Patient education

It should be explained that cause-and-effect relationships often cannot be found in transient urticaria and angioedema, but that lesions can be expected to resolve by 1 month in most instances. One should emphasize that control of symptoms is possible with the use of antihistamines. An extensive and expensive allergy workup is not indicated in children who have had urticaria less than 6 weeks, and workup of chronic urticaria should be guided by history.

Patients with angioedema should have an adrenergic agent available for airway attacks, and patients with hereditary angioedema should be advised of the high mortality rate and the need to continue taking prophylactic drugs.

Follow-up visits

In transient urticaria and angioedema a visit 1 week after the initial evaluation is useful for monitoring the course of the disease. In chronic urticaria it is useful to reevaluate precipitating factors periodically if a factor has not been identified. Patients with hereditary angioedema should be seen after 1 month of therapy to remeasure the C1 esterase inhibitor and adjust the drug dosage.

Persistent Urticaria
The physical urticarias

Urticaria that persists for over 4 weeks may be simply prolonged common urticaria or may be caused by one of the physical urticarias, urticarial vasculitis, or mastocytosis. The physical urticarias, which account for 15% of this group, consist of dermatographism, heat- and exercise-induced urticaria, delayed-pressure urticaria, cold urticaria, and familial cold urticaria.[2,16-18]

Clinical features

DERMATOGRAPHISM. Dermatographism occurs in 1% of adolescents and is characterized by wheal and erythema after minor stroking of or pressure on the skin (Fig. 14-6).[1,18] It often results in mild itching. The wheal reaches maximal size in 6 to 7 minutes and persists for 10 to 15 minutes. Wheals are commonly found around the belt area and may follow widespread insect bites and transient episodes of urticaria. The wheal is seen in comatose children (e.g., in encephalitis, meningitis, drug overdose) and has been termed *tache cérébrale.* Dermatographism is also seen in about half of children with mastocytosis. Dermatographism may persist for years, but most patients can expect spontaneous regression within 2 years.

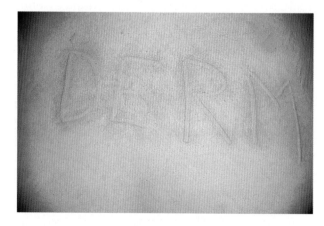

Fig. 14-6 Dermatographism. Light stroking of the skin evokes intense wheal and flare reaction.

HEAT- AND EXERCISE-INDUCED URTICARIA. Heat- and exercise-induced urticaria (cholinergic urticaria) is characterized by a large (10 to 20 mm), blotchy erythema surrounding tiny (1 to 3 mm) central wheals (Fig. 14-7).[2,17,18] It occurs in up to 3% of adolescents. Heating of the skin or exercise sufficient to raise the body temperature 0.5° C will induce attacks of multiple wheals with itching. Hot or spicy foods, febrile illnesses, and hot baths may also initiate attacks. The onset is characteristically in adolescence, but the condition tends to persist into young adult years.

DELAYED PRESSURE URTICARIA. Delayed pressure urticaria, which occurs primarily in adolescents, appears after prolonged pressure with a heavy weight.[2,18] A 7-kg weight suspended from an extremity by a strap for 15 minutes will reproduce the disease. Painful, deep swellings begin 4 to 6 hours after pressure and last up to 24 hours. Spontaneous remissions have been reported, but the natural history is unknown.

COLD URTICARIA. Cold urticaria appears in three forms: it may be associated with cryoglobulins and immune complex disease, it may appear as an acquired form not associated with cryoproteins, or it may occur as autosomal dominant familial cold urticaria.[2,17,18] In the form associated with cryoglobulins the signs and symptoms of collagen vascular disease are often present. This disease is uncommon in children. The acquired form occurs after rewarming an area of skin exposed to cold. Wheals appear, and itching is severe. Cooling the entire body may result in

widespread wheals and fainting. To test for acquired cold urticaria, an ice cube is applied to the patient's skin for 2 to 10 minutes, and the skin is allowed to rewarm. The wheal appears during the rewarming. There may be a spontaneous remission, but the natural history is not known.

FAMILIAL COLD URTICARIA. Familial cold urticaria is an autosomal dominant condition beginning shortly after birth.[19] The gene has been localized to chromosome 1q.[19] Erythematous macules appear in exposed areas 30 minutes after exposure to a cold wind, but not after ingestion of iced drinks or ice. Older children complain of burning in the skin. Fever and chills, arthralgias, and headaches appear and last up to 48 hours. A leukocytosis occurs during the attacks. The patient tends to suffer these attacks throughout life.

Differential diagnosis. The physical urticarias are often confused with other forms of urticaria (see Box 14-2). The role of light pressure in dermatographism and deep pressure in delayed-pressure urticaria should help distinguish these disorders from the other forms of urticaria. Heat- and exercise-induced urticarias may be distinguished from other types of urticaria by the characteristic tiny central wheal with a large rim of erythema. The cold urticarias may be distinguished by the history of cold exposure, and in the familial form, by the systemic symptoms accompanying the skin lesions. Box 14-4 lists the conditions to be considered in the differential diagnosis of cold urticaria.

Pathogenesis. The physical urticarias differ from other urticarial states in that histamine does not appear to be the chemical mediator of the disease. Histamine skin levels are normal in dermatographism,

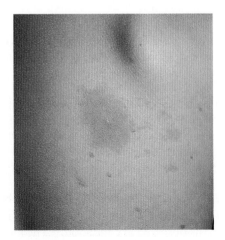

Fig. 14-7 Heat- and exercise-induced urticaria. Pinpoint central wheal surrounded by large, blotchy erythema.

Box 14-4 Differential Diagnosis of Cold Urticaria
Cryoglobulinemia and immune complex diseases Systemic lupus erythematosus and other collagen vascular diseases Macroglobulinemia Mycoplasma infections (cold hemagglutinins) Syphilis Familial cold urticaria Acquired cold urticaria

heat- and exercise-induced urticaria, cold urticaria with cryoglobulins, urticarial states, and familial cold urticaria. Histamine has been implicated in acquired cold urticaria and delayed-pressure urticaria.[2,6,18] In dermatographism and heat- and exercise-induced urticaria, mediation through cholinergic fibers of the autonomic nervous system has been implicated. The vasoactive split products of the complement system may be involved in the cryoglobulinemic and familial cold urticarial forms.

Treatment. Many patients with physical urticaria require no therapy. If symptoms are severe enough to require therapy, H1 blocking antihistamines such as hydroxyzine hydrochloride, 1 to 2 mg/kg/day in a single evening dose, or cetirizine, 2.5 to 5.0 μg daily, may reduce the symptoms in dermatographism and heat- and exercise-induced urticaria.[2,18] This is surprising because histamine is not involved in the pathogenesis. There is little additional benefit from adding an H2 blocking agent. Delayed-pressure urticaria does not respond to antihistamines but may respond to prednisone, 1 mg/kg/day for 4 to 5 days, but prednisone is generally not required.[2] There is no satisfactory treatment for cold urticaria other than cold avoidance, although cyproheptadine, 2 to 4 mg three times a day, has been reported to provide relief in some patients.[6,18]

Patient education. Patients with the physical urticarias must be instructed to reduce their exposure to the precipitating factors. Patients with dermatographism and delayed-pressure urticaria should not wear backpacks or carry other heavy weights and should avoid tight-fitting clothing and excessive friction or pressure on the skin. Patients with heat- and exercise-induced urticaria need to avoid excessive heating of the skin, vigorous exercise, hot baths, and other factors resulting in increased body heat. Patients with cold urticaria should avoid ice-cold food or drinks, dress warmly in cold weather, and avoid swimming in cold water.

Follow-up visits. A visit 2 weeks after the initial evaluation will be useful to monitor the progress of the disease and the therapeutic response.

Urticarial vasculitis

Clinical features. Urticarial vasculitis is characterized by fixed wheals distributed symmetrically over the extremities.[2] It is rare in childhood and may be associated with systemic symptoms. Lesions remain fixed in the same area for 24 to 72 hours and may be accompanied by mild arthralgias or malaise.[2,5] Most patients have an elevated erythrocyte sedimentation rate and depressed serum complement levels. The natural history is not known. Although the findings are similar to those in necrotizing vasculitis with palpable purpura, most patients do not progress to palpable purpura.

Differential diagnosis. Urticarial vasculitis may be distinguished from other conditions (see Box 14-2) by the elevated erythrocyte sedimentation rate, depressed serum complement levels, the finding of small-vessel vasculitis on skin biopsy, and the associated systemic symptoms.

Pathogenesis. Urticarial vasculitis has been associated with circulating immune complexes, resulting in injury to postcapillary venules in the upper dermis. Immunofluorescence has demonstrated immunoglobulins and complement split products around inflamed venules.[2] Neutrophils and degenerating neutrophil nuclei are seen around the venules on skin biopsy, with swelling of the venule wall and fibrin deposition. The inflammatory events are most probably mediated through the interaction of immune complexes with the complement and clotting systems.

Treatment. If a cause for immune complex disease, such as streptococcal infection, can be determined, it can be eliminated, but such associations are difficult to document. There is no known effective treatment. Antihistamines, indomethacin, dapsone, colchicine, and low-dose prednisone therapy have been utilized, with variable success.[2]

Patient education. Patients should be advised of the difference between urticarial vasculitis and other urticarias.

Follow-up visits. Monthly visits are advisable to determine whether the disorder has progressed to involve vessels of other organs. Urinalysis, erythrocyte sedimentation rate, and complement levels may be used to follow the course of the disease.

Mastocytosis (including urticaria pigmentosa)

Clinical features. There are four distinct forms of mastocytosis observed in childhood.[20] The most common are the solitary mastocytoma (discussed in Chapter 12) and urticaria pigmentosa. The uncommon forms are diffuse cutaneous mastocytosis (bullous mastocytosis) and the rare telangiectasia macularis eruptiva perstans.[21] The blotchy macular and nodular pigmented lesions of urticaria pigmentosa appear in the first 8 months of life (Fig. 14-8). One or two lesions are noted initially, but numerous lesions accumulate during the next few months (Fig. 14-9). The majority of lesions appear on the trunk, although some may appear on the face and extremities. Individual lesions are often red at first and may easily become blistered (Fig. 14-10).[20] The characteristic blotchy, brown pigmentation may not appear until 6 months after the onset of the lesions. Stroking the pigmented lesion will result in tense edema within the lesion and an erythematous flare surrounding the area (Darier's sign). Half of the patients with mastocytosis will demonstrate dermatographism in uninvolved skin. Skin biopsy will confirm the diagnosis.[20,21]

Spontaneous bulla formation within lesions may occur or be induced by a variety of drugs (Box 14-5). These drugs, or rubbing of the skin, may induce enough histamine release to produce systemic symptoms, such as flushing, tachycardia, hypotension with fainting, diarrhea, and vomiting. As the child ages, it becomes more difficult to urticate the lesions, or to induce blisters, or both. Often by age 5 these lesions are asymptomatic, and by adolescence only residual flat pigmentation remains.[20]

Enlargement of the liver and spleen, systemic flushing episodes, and peptic ulcer symptoms should suggest systemic mastocytosis. Systemic mastocytosis occurs in up to 2% of infants with urticaria pigmentosa.[20] Bony involvement can be documented by radiologic examination, and bone-marrow examination will reveal increased numbers of mast cells. Extreme infiltration of the liver sufficient to produce cirrhosis may occur. In the infant who has urticaria pigmentosa without systemic symptoms, skeletal surveys and bone marrow examinations are not warranted.

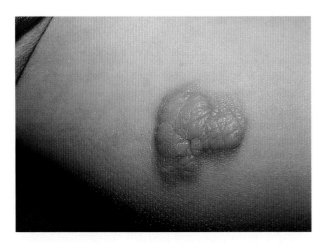

Fig. 14-8 Mastocytoma. Pink plaque on the skin of an infant.

Box 14-5 Drugs Producing Histamine Release in Mastocytosis
Opiates (codeine, meperidine [Demerol], morphine) Polymyxin B Acetylsalicylic acid

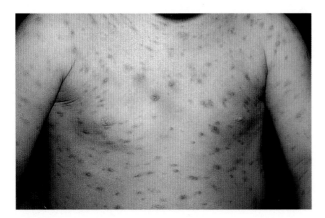

Fig. 14-9 Urticaria pigmentosa. Multiple, blotchy, brown macules on the chest of an infant.

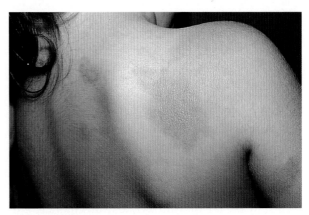

Fig. 14-10 Tense edema within tan macule of urticaria pigmentosa after stroking.

Diffuse cutaneous mastocytosis (bullous mastocytosis) presents as blisters in the neonatal period, often accompanied by flushing episodes.[20] The blisters are often large and they peel, leaving large, eroded bases. After a severe blistering episode, 5 to 10 days may be required to regranulate mast cells, and the baby experiences recurrent episodes. When the baby is evaluated, marked dermatographism is present. A leathery thickening with yellow-tan skin usually does not appear until 3 to 8 months of age. Severe syncopal episodes and death from prolonged hypotension have been reported.[20] Gastrointestinal symptoms are seen as the child becomes older, including chronic diarrhea states and recurrent episodes of vomiting associated with abdominal pain. In addition to gastrointestinal involvement, bone marrow involvement is more likely. It is an autosomal dominant disorder.

Differential diagnosis. Mastocytosis can be differentiated from other conditions by skin biopsy (see Box 14-1). The bullous lesions must be differentiated from other bullous diseases of infancy. Diffuse cutaneous mastocytosis has been confused with staphylococcal scalded skin syndrome, especially recurrent scalded skin syndrome, and with epidermolysis bullosa.

Pathogenesis. Excessive numbers of mast cells accumulate with the dermis in mastocytosis.[20] It is believed that mastocytosis represents reactive mast-cell hyperplasia caused by activating mutations in the c-kit receptor in response to stem cell factor.[22,23] Excessive histamine release from these mast cells results in whealing or blister formation. The blister is subepidermal and may bleed. Histamine is undoubtedly responsible for the local and systemic effects. Flushing and syncopal episodes are due to prostaglandin D2 release, and bleeding is caused by heparin release by cutaneous mast cells.[20] Increased bone marrow apoptosis and cluster formation is observed in c-kit mutations as it is in other myelodysplastic disorders.[23] Recently, it has been appreciated that children with systemic mastocytosis demonstrate chromosomal abnormalities in the bone marrow cells demonstrating genetic instability of hematopoietic cells.[24]

Treatment. Most infants with solitary mastocytomas or urticaria pigmentosa require no treatment.[2,20,25] Flushing episodes or other systemic symptoms may be controlled by the use of hydroxyzine hydrochloride, 2 to 4 mg/kg/day divided into four doses. Solitary mastocytomas may be treated with 2 weeks of superpotent topical steroids. Oral cromolyn sodium has been reported to be valuable in infants with gastrointestinal involvement. Diffuse cutaneous mastocytosis may respond to psoralen ultraviolet A-range (PUVA) therapy.[26]

Patient education. It is essential that the child with mastocytosis not be given cough syrups with codeine or other medications with opiates. Parents should be provided the list in Box 14-5 of medications to be avoided. If surgery is contemplated, preoperative medications should be carefully selected. Substitution of other antipyretics for aspirin is also advised. The natural course should be emphasized. Genetic counseling is valuable for diffuse cutaneous mastocytosis.

Follow-up visits. A follow-up visit in 2 weeks is useful in determining the presence or absence of systemic symptoms. If treatment is given, monthly visits are advisable.

ERYTHEMAS

Erythemas of the skin without wheal production are uncommon in infants and children. Often called the *reactive erythemas,* they include the annular erythemas (including erythema chronicum migrans, erythema marginatum, and erythema annulare), erythema multiforme, and erythema nodosum. Erythema multiforme is covered in detail in Chapter 11 and erythema chronicum migrans in Chapter 5.

Annular Erythemas
Clinical features

Annular, polycyclic, and partially marginated lesions are called annular erythemas. One should remember that giant urticaria can assume annular shapes.

Erythema annulare. In erythema annulare the lesions have erythematous borders, a trailing scale, and a dusky center (Fig. 14-11). These lesions may occur anywhere on the skin.[27] Multiple lesions are usually present, and they slowly enlarge. They last for several months and tend to recur. In infants the lesions may be associated with a maternal collagen vascular disorder, particularly with Sjögren's syndrome. A distinct annular erythema is *erythema annulare centrifugum,* which has a fine, white scale just inside the red zone ("trailing scale") and may be associated with hidden infection such as urinary tract infections.[28]

Erythema marginatum. Erythema marginatum is a transient eruption consisting of curvilinear, migrating

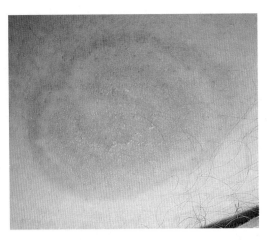

Fig. 14-11 Erythema annulare. Concentric zones of red and dusky skin.

<table>
<tr><td colspan="2">**Box 14-6   Differential Diagnosis of Annular Erythemas**</td></tr>
</table>

Box 14-6	Differential Diagnosis of Annular Erythemas

Erythema annulare
Erythema annulare centrifugum
Erythema chronicum migrans
Erythema marginatum
Tinea corporis
Pityriasis rosea
Subacute cutaneous lupus erythematosus
Neonatal lupus syndrome
Sarcoidosis
Syphilis
Juvenile rheumatoid arthritis

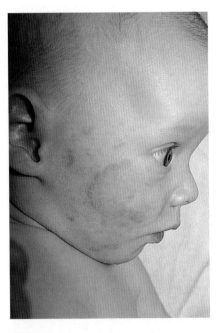

Fig. 14-12 Erythema marginatum. Fleeting, semiannular erythema on the face of an infant with acute rheumatic fever.

areas of erythema that form incomplete circles (Fig. 14-12). The marginated lesions may move rapidly over the skin within several hours and disappear.[29] Inducing cutaneous vasodilation may make the lesions more visible. It is found in only 10% of children with acute rheumatic fever, despite being one of the Jones criteria for diagnosis, and is associated with the fever and well-established carditis. A thorough evaluation for acute rheumatic fever is indicated. It may also be seen after streptococcal infections without evidence of acute rheumatic fever.[29]

Differential diagnosis

Conditions to be considered in the differential diagnosis of annular erythemas are listed in Box 14-6. Dermatophyte lesions have a scaly border and may be diagnosed by potassium hydroxide (KOH) examination and fungal cultures. Granuloma annulare lesions have a distinct nodular and papular border without epidermal change. The lesions of pityriasis rosea may be annular on occasion and have central clearing. Lupus erythematosus, sarcoidosis, and syphilis may also present with annular lesions. The transient urticarial lesions of juvenile rheumatoid arthritis tend to be limited to the abdomen, and clear slightly in the center.

Pathogenesis

Two of the erythemas demonstrate infectious agents within the skin lesions, with an attendant host response. In erythema chronicum migrans, *Borrelia burgdorferi* is found (see Chapter 5); in erythema multiforme, herpes simplex virus is noted (see Chapter 11). In erythema annulare and in erythema marginatum, the mechanism of disease is unknown. Dense accumulation of lymphocytes that surround superficial dermal blood vessels is seen on skin biopsy, which helps distinguish annular erythemas from urticaria.

Treatment

No treatment is useful for erythema annulare. Children with erythema marginatum are treated with penicillin.

Patient education

Clinicians should emphasize to the patient and family that these eruptions are skin reactions that do not require treatment but serve as a clue to a systemic disorder.

Follow-up visits

A visit 1 week after the initial evaluation is useful to discuss the results of laboratory evaluation for systemic disorders. The need for follow-up care is determined by the nature of the associated systemic disorder.

Erythema Nodosum
Clinical features

Erythema nodosum is characterized by the abrupt onset of symmetric, very tender, erythematous nodules on the extensor surface of the extremities (Fig. 14-13).[30-32] Occasionally, lesions will involve other areas of skin, such as the soles of the feet, eyelids, hands, or trunk. Widespread involvement is more characteristic of infants (Fig. 14-14). The nodules have indistinct borders. Occasionally, it will be unilateral at presentation. The lesions may be so painful that the patient will limp. A prodrome of cough, sore throat, and fever will occur in about 25% of children. It occurs most commonly in adolescents and is uncommon before age 2 years. Females predominate at a ratio of 1.7:1. Lesions last from 2 to 6 weeks. Re-

currences are reported in 4% of children. Lesions resolve as a bruise, with a color change to purple, then yellow-brown. Infectious causes, such as β-hemolytic streptococcal infections, tuberculosis, sarcoidosis, histoplasmosis, tularemia, Epstein-Barr virus (EBV), hepatitis B, Yersinia, and coccidioidomycosis, are the most common associations.[30-32] Streptococcal infections account for 30% of cases.[30-32] A careful history should be obtained for preceding infections.

Inflammatory bowel disease and Hodgkin's disease are uncommon associations.[30-32] Drugs may uncommonly produce erythema nodosum, particularly oral contraceptives in adolescent females.

Differential diagnosis

Erythema nodosum may be confused with many other processes involving the subcutaneous fat. In contrast to erythema nodosum, thrombophlebitis usually occurs on the lateral or flexor surface of the lower legs and heals with fibrosis. The nodose lesions of polyarteritis nodosa are associated with an exaggerated dusky, mottling pattern called *livedo reticularis*. Giant insect-bite reactions may be confused with erythema nodosum, but a central punctum will help differentiate. Panniculitis can be distinguished on biopsy of skin to include subcutaneous fat. Vasculitis and eosinophilic cellulitis may also mimic erythema nodosum.[30] The lesions of erythema nodosum are usually so characteristic that they are seldom confused with those of other disorders.

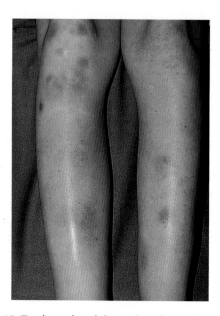

Fig. 14-13 Tender red nodules with indistinct borders in a teenage girl with erythema nodosum.

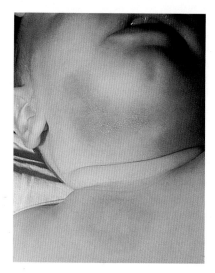

Fig. 14-14 Atypical location of erythema nodosum in an infant.

Pathogenesis

Erythema nodosum is a chronic injury of the blood vessels of the lower dermis and subcutaneous fat. Initially the perivascular inflammation is neutrophilic, then lymphocytic, then granulomatous as the lesions age. There is increasing evidence to implicate circulating immune complexes in the pathogenesis of erythema nodosum as a part of the host immune response to an infectious agent. Fat cell destruction usually does not occur in erythema nodosum, so it is not a true panniculitis.

Treatment

Symptomatic treatment with acetylsalicylic acid or antihistamines may suffice because in many cases the erythema nodosum resolves within 3 weeks. In patients with acutely tender lesions that interfere with walking, nonsteroidal antiinflammatory agents, such as indomethacin, may be tried.[30-34] Although some relief can be obtained with prednisone, oral steroids are not generally recommended and should not be used chronically. Thalidomide, effective in erythema nodosum associated with leprosy, has been used successfully in erythema nodosum of other causes.[34,35] The restricted availability of thalidomide in the United States limits its use.

Patient education

It should be emphasized that erythema nodosum is a response to infection or to certain inflammatory diseases. A search for such associations should be guided by the history and should not involve expensive laboratory tests. Parents should be reassured that most children recover within 3 weeks.

Follow-up visits

A return visit in 1 week is useful to ascertain the need for, or response to, therapy.

Gustatory Flushing
Clinical features

Gustatory flushing usually develops in early infancy and may first present when solid foods are introduced. An erythematous flush of one cheek occurs during or just after eating, lasting from 5 to 60 minutes.[36-38] Sweating may develop within the flushed area, and tearing of the adjacent eye may occur.[37] Frequently the infant is misdiagnosed as having a food allergy. Spontaneous remission has been reported after several years.

Differential diagnosis

Urticaria and food allergy are often considered in the diagnosis. However, gustatory flushing always occurs in the same site and does not move from skin area to skin area as urticaria would. Food allergy reactions should occur with specific foods and be widespread and not localized. Gustatory flushing occurs with any foods that stimulate the taste buds. Herpes facialis may be considered, but it presents with persistent erythema that lasts for at least 3 days and usually evolves to vesicle formation. Contact dermatitis also produces a persistent erythema on the cheek.

Pathogenesis

Gustatory flushing is caused by cross-linking of the parasympathetic nerve fibers innervating the parotid gland to the sympathetic fibers supplying the sweat glands and cutaneous vessels along the distribution of the auriculotemporal nerve. Foods that would ordinarily stimulate salivation instead produce flushing and sweating.[36,37] In infancy, cases are believed to be due to a congenital malformation resulting in cross-linking of nerve fibers. It may result from nerve regeneration after parotid surgery or injury in older children.

Treatment

There is no known effective treatment. Topical antiperspirants will control the sweating. If antiperspirants fail, injections of botulinum toxin have been effective.[38]

Patient education

Clinicians should emphasize that the condition does not represent allergy, and that spontaneous remission can be expected in most infants. Allergy evaluation should be discouraged.

Follow-up visits

Routine follow-up visits are unnecessary.

PURPURAS

Purpuric lesions always prompt investigation into bleeding states. They may involve small areas (e.g., petechiae) or large areas (e.g., ecchymoses). Palpable purpura (purpuric papules), dissecting purpura, and chronic pigmented purpura are presented in this section. Neonatal purpura (Box 14-7), acral petechiae and purpura (Box 14-8), and flat generalized petechiae and purpura (Box 14-9) are not discussed, but

Box 14-7   Differential Diagnosis
            of Neonatal Purpura

Congenital infection
    Toxoplasma
    Enterovirus
    Rubella
    Cytomegalovirus
    Herpes simplex
    Syphilis
Coagulation defects
Autoimmune disorders (systemic lupus
    erythematosus and erythroblastosis fetalis)
Hemangioma with platelet trapping syndrome

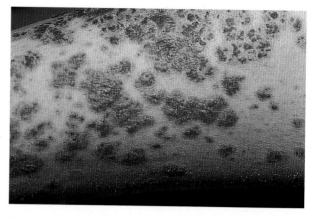

Fig. 14-15 Papules with petechial centers on the leg of a child with necrotizing vasculitis (Henoch-Schönlein purpura).

Box 14-8   Differential Diagnosis
            of Flat Acral Purpura

Rocky Mountain spotted fever
Meningococcemia
Atypical measles
Coagulation disorders
Progressive pigmentary purpura

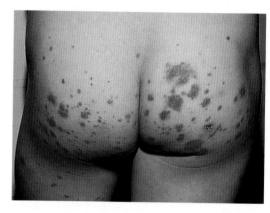

Fig. 14-16 Numerous purpuric macules and papules on the buttocks of a child with necrotizing vasculitis.

Box 14-9   Differential Diagnosis
            of Flat Generalized Purpura

Thrombocytopenic states (idiopathic
    thrombocytopenic purpura, leukemia)
Coagulation disorders
Trauma (including child abuse)

are presented to aid the reader in making a differential diagnosis of these lesions.

Palpable Purpura (Purpuric Papules)
Clinical features

Discrete 1- to 5-mm papules with petechial centers or those that are completely purpuric characterize palpable purpura (Fig. 14-15).[39-42] They are usually found on the extremities and are symmetric and numerous (Fig. 14-16). Palpable purpura should imme-

diately bring to mind vasculitis or septicemia. The vasculitis that occurs is called *cutaneous necrotizing venulitis* (anaphylactoid purpura, Henoch-Schönlein purpura [HSP]) and may be associated with vasculitis of renal, gastrointestinal, joint, or cerebral vessels.[39-44] The lesions may begin as discrete urticarial wheals,[45] then progress to papular purpura and pustular purpura. Occasionally, cutaneous infarcts, purpuric bullae, and gangrene with subsequent ulceration and scarring will occur. Arthralgia or arthritis of the knees and ankles is found in 80% of patients.[40-42] Cramping abdominal pain, vomiting, hematemesis, and melena signal gastrointestinal involvement. Abdominal pain is common but in most children lasts less than 24 hours. The kidney is involved in 70% of children.[3] Most have asymptomatic microscopic hematuria, but only 25% on the first visit. Some children may present with a nephrotic syndrome. Up to 10% of children may progress to chronic renal failure. Rarely, seizures, paresis, or coma occur, with involvement of the central nervous system vessels.

Most episodes of necrotizing venulitis have skin changes that last from 4 to 6 weeks and then resolve. In addition to necrotizing vasculitis, septicemic states also present with palpable purpura, which may evolve to pustules. Lesions are acral, symmetric, and few in number. Palpable purpura is seen in chronic meningococcemia, gonococcemia, and subacute bacterial endocarditis and is frequently associated with arthritis or arthralgias of the large joints.[29] Blood cultures or genital cultures will confirm the diagnosis. It is difficult to culture organisms from lesions, but they may be identified by specific immunofluorescence from smears of lesions. Rarely, Pseudomonas, staphylococcal, deep fungal, or gram-negative septicemia is responsible. Palpable purpura is also seen in collagen vascular diseases of childhood, especially juvenile rheumatoid arthritis and lupus erythematosus.[40-42] It occurs in long-standing disease, often years after the diagnosis was confirmed. It is also seen in the periodic fevers.[43]

Differential diagnosis

Biopsy plus bacterial and fungal culture will distinguish infectious causes of palpable purpura from one another (Box 14-10). Immunofluorescent examination of a skin biopsy will reveal immunoglobulin A (IgA) deposits surrounding superficial cutaneous blood vessels in HSP.[40-42] Antineutrophil cytoplasmic antibodies (ANCAs) may help in the diagnosis.[40-42] Associated collagen vascular disease is usually already established, and diagnostic serologies are not required.

Pathogenesis

In necrotizing venulitis and in septicemic states, circulating immune complexes have been implicated in the production of lesions through their interaction with the complement and clotting systems. The prodrome of upper respiratory tract infection, and sometimes positive streptococcal throat cultures, has implicated infectious agents as likely triggers of immune complex formation in HSP. An association with parvovirus B19, hepatitis B and C and vaccination against hepatitis B, pneumococci, and influenza in childhood HSP may also be found.[40-44] Drugs such as propylthiouracil, hydralazine, and zafirlukast have been associated with necrotizing venulitis.[40]

Box 14-10	Differential Diagnosis of Palpable Purpura

Necrotizing venulitis (anaphylactoid [Henoch-Schönlein] purpura)
Meningococcemia
Gonococcemia
Staphylococcal sepsis
Pseudomonas sepsis
Subacute bacterial endocarditis

Fibrinoid necrosis of venule walls in the upper dermis, with perivascular accumulation of neutrophils, nuclear fragments, and extravasation of red blood cells, is seen on skin biopsy.[41] Organisms may also be detected with Gram's stains of skin biopsies in the septicemic states.

Treatment

In necrotizing venulitis with skin involvement only, no treatment is required. The skin lesions are unlikely to respond to corticosteroids. Prednisone, 2 mg/kg/day, may be indicated with internal organ involvement, particularly bowel disease. The administration of systemic antibiotics, with the choice of agent based on appropriate cultures, is indicated for septicemic states. In severe prolonged necrotizing venulitis, pulse therapy with intravenous methylprednisolone and plasmapheresis or cyclophosphamide orally or pulsed intravenously may be useful.[46] Azathioprine has been successfully used for maintenance therapy.[46]

Patient education

The serious nature of vasculitis of internal organs and septicemic states should be emphasized. Future upper respiratory tract illnesses should be brought to the physician's attention promptly, and appropriate cultures should be obtained. Early treatment of an associated streptococcal infection may be required.

Follow-up visits

In necrotizing venulitis, weekly follow-up visits are recommended for the first 4 weeks to monitor internal involvement, particularly of the kidney. Microscopic examination of the urinary sediment and protein determination are required. Thereafter, evaluations of renal function every 3 months are valuable to identify the children at risk of renal failure.

Nodular Purpura With Livedo: Polyarteritis Nodosa (Periarteritis Nodosa)

Clinical features

There are three polyarteritis syndromes in childhood: infantile polyarteritis nodosa, Kawasaki disease, and chronic cutaneous polyarteritis nodosa. The infantile form may represent Kawasaki disease without cutaneous findings and is considered with Kawasaki disease in Chapter 11.

The cutaneous findings of livedo reticularis plus palpable, tender, linear, purple nodules are found in children with chronic cutaneous polyarteritis nodosa (Fig. 14-17).[40-42] Typically, older children rather than toddlers are affected. Fever, myalgias, arthralgias, and gastrointestinal symptoms are observed in 70%.[40-42] Hypertension, renal disease, pulmonary involvement, and localized neuropathy (mononeuritis multiplex) may be observed. The skin lesions are usually located symmetrically on the proximal extremities and persist for weeks, with recurrent crops of new nodules appearing (Fig. 14-18). Exacerbations may occur on cold exposure. Focal areas of skin infarction and ulceration may accompany the nodules. The course is quite chronic and may last for years.[40-42,44] Newborns of mothers with long-standing polyarteritis nodosa may develop a transient polyarteritis nodosa with lesions lasting 3 months. ANCAs may be present, and the affected child may have a positive antinuclear antibody test. The erythrocyte sedimentation rate is virtually always elevated.

Differential diagnosis

Livedo patterns must be distinguished from mottling, which may be seen transiently with cold exposure. Mottling disappears on rewarming and livedo patterns do not. Cutis marmorata telangiectasia congenita has a livedo pattern but is present from birth, not acquired. Careful palpation of the skin within the livedo area may be required to detect the linear nodules of periarteritis nodosa. Selection of a site for skin biopsy is critical. A biopsy specimen must include a linear nodule, with subcutaneous fat, to detect the characteristic pathology because artery involvement is segmental. Biopsy of the livedo area or a shallow biopsy may miss the pathology.

Pathogenesis

Polyarteritis nodosa is an inflammatory segmental disease of the walls of cutaneous arteries. Neutrophilic infiltration of the arterial wall and adjacent periarterial tissue is seen. Thrombosis of vessels may be found. In children there is an association with parvovirus B19, hepatitis B and C, and with streptococcal infection.[40-42,44] Mixed cryoglobulinemia may be found.[40]

Treatment

Most children respond well to low-dose oral steroids (0.5 mg/kg prednisone).[46] In children who require high-dose oral steroids, low-dose once-weekly methotrexate, pulsed intravenous cyclophosphamide, and oral azathioprine have been used successfully.[46]

Patient education

Avoiding cold exposure is advisable. The child and the family should be informed about the chronic and persistent nature of this condition and advised of potential systemic complications and the need for monitoring of renal, gastrointestinal, and pulmonary involvement.

Follow-up visits

Initially follow-up visits should be every 2 weeks until disease control is established. After the disease is

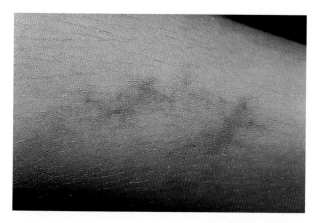

Fig. 14-17 Livedo pattern of purple lacy macules in childhood polyarteritis nodosa.

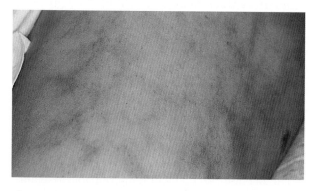

Fig. 14-18 Linear tender red nodules and livedo reticularis in childhood polyarteritis nodosa.

stabilized, evaluation of renal status and other systemic complications should be performed every 4 to 6 weeks.

Nodular Purpura: Pernio
Clinical features

Pernio is characterized by asymptomatic purple to purple-red nodules, several days to weeks after exposure to wetness and cold.[47] The nodules are usually on the digits and may be accompanied by a livedo pattern of the adjacent skin (Fig. 14-19). Other acral areas, such as the ears, may also be involved (Fig. 14-20). The livedo pattern slowly fades and the nodules remain for weeks. Occasionally the nodules will ulcerate and are then quite painful. The cold exposure may seem trivial rather than severe, and associated wetness is required. Pernio has been associated with anorexia nervosa in adolescent girls.

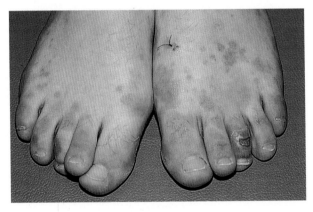

Fig. 14-19 Purple oval nodules on the toes in a child with pernio.

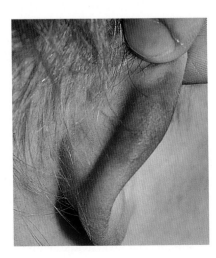

Fig. 14-20 Purple nodule on the ear of toddler with pernio.

Differential diagnosis

The nodules of pernio must be differentiated from lymphoma or leukemia states, which also produce red-purple nodules. Pernio lesions have an insidious onset rather than the abrupt onset of lymphomas and, once established, do not grow but remain stable. Polyarteritis nodosa nodules are linear rather than oval and tender rather than nontender. A skin biopsy will distinguish the two conditions.

Pathogenesis

The exact mechanism of the response to cold injury is not known. Some children may have cryoproteins.[47] Pathology shows middermal inflammation, including a lymphohistiocytic infiltrate around blood vessels, but is not specific.

Treatment

In most circumstances no treatment is required.

Patient education

Protection against cold and wetness is critical.

Follow-up visits

A follow-up visit in 2 weeks may be useful to ascertain the course of the condition and to reinforce the cold and wetness avoidance.

Dissecting Purpura (Disseminated Intravascular Coagulation)
Clinical features

Dissecting purpura, or disseminated intravascular coagulation, has an acute onset, with high fever and extensive, large, dissecting purpuric areas on the extremities.[48-50] The purpuric "lakes" are large and are not associated with petechiae (Fig. 14-21). The

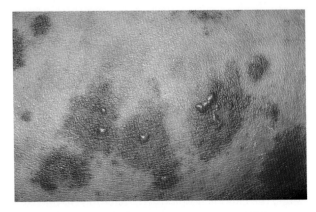

Fig. 14-21 Purpuric lakes with hemorrhagic blisters in a child with disseminated intravascular coagulation.

condition has been associated with overwhelming infections, such as meningococcemia, Escherichia coli septicemia, and Rocky Mountain spotted fever, or it may follow common childhood infections, such as streptococcal pharyngitis or varicella, by 5 to 10 days.[29,49,50] Vascular collapse is common, and mortality is high in untreated patients. Even in those who survive, large areas of infarcted skin require long-term management.

Differential diagnosis

The large purpuric lakes are so characteristic that they are not confused with other purpuric diseases.

Pathogenesis

The syndrome is triggered by the massive release of tissue thromboplastin with widespread fibrin deposition in the blood vessels of skin, lungs, and kidneys; fibrinolysis; and consumption of coagulation factors, leading to secondary bleeding.[49,50] Proteins C and S are particularly consumed by the infections as well. Protein C is a vitamin K–dependent plasma serine protease that acts as an anticoagulant by inactivating clotting factors Va and VIIIa after clotting is initiated. Protein S acts as a cofactor for protein C in the inactivation of clotting factor Va. When protein C or protein S is deficient, intravascular hypercoagulability results, with widespread thrombosis.[49,50]

Treatment

Replacement of consumable clotting factors with fresh plasma, protein C concentrate, or platelet concentrates is the treatment of choice.[48-50] Most children require hospitalization. With persistent disseminated intravascular coagulation, heparin, 100 U/kg intravenously every 4 to 6 hours, may be given. Antibiotic treatment of the triggering bacterial infection is necessary. With extensive areas of skin necrosis, admission to a burn unit with appropriate debridement, prevention of secondary infection, and biologic dressings may be useful.[49,50]

Patient education

Advice to the patient and family depends on the nature of the triggering disease. Counseling regarding the grave prognosis and need for long-term care should be provided.

Follow-up visits

While the child is hospitalized, daily follow-up visits are useful to evaluate response to therapy.

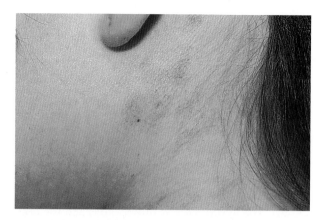

Fig. 14-22 Golden-brown and cayenne-pepper macules on the neck of a child with progressive pigmentary purpura.

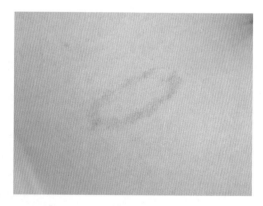

Fig. 14-23 Annular pigmented macules in progressive pigmentary purpura.

Chronic Pigmented Purpura
Clinical features

Chronic pigmented purpura is characterized by an insidious onset and slow progression of grouped nonpalpable petechiae over the extremities, trunk, or neck (Fig. 14-22) in adolescents.[51,52] Individual lesions show fresh and old petechiae intermixed and an interplay of red, brown, and yellow spots. Lesions are usually flat (Fig. 14-23), but a lichenified epidermis may overlie the lesions. The grouped petechiae are oval and may begin unilaterally[51] but progress to become symmetric (Fig. 14-24). The lower extremities are most commonly involved, with more lesions in dependent areas.[51,52] Lesions may progress to involve the entire trunk and upper extremities. Itching is usually mild or absent, and no systemic symptoms are associated with chronic pigmented purpura. Sponta-

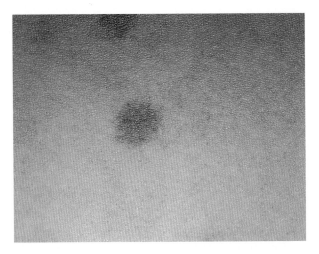

Fig. 14-24 Pigmented macule in progressive pigmentary purpura.

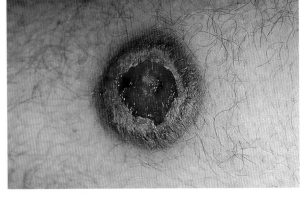

Fig. 14-25 Pyoderma gangrenosum. Ulceration with characteristic loosely-attached epidermis and purple border.

neous remission occurs within 1 to 2 years, but the natural course of the disease is not well documented.

Differential diagnosis

The lesions of grouped petechiae of multiple ages are so characteristic that this type of purpura is seldom confused with other disorders. Occasionally trauma (e.g., child abuse) or a mild bleeding disorder is suspected.

Pathogenesis

A mild capillaritis is seen in these disorders, with extravasation of red blood cells, hemosiderin deposits, and a mild perivascular lymphocytic infiltration of superficial dermal blood vessels.[52] The vascular injury is mild, and its cause is unknown.

Treatment

There is no specific therapy. Reduction of venous stasis may be helpful.

Patient education

The expected remission and the mild nature of this disorder should be emphasized.

Follow-up visits

Follow-up visits are unnecessary.

Pyoderma Gangrenosum
Clinical features

Pyoderma gangrenosum begins as a 3- to 8-mm red papule that progresses within hours to a pustule, then to an ulceration surrounded by edematous, loosely at-

tached epidermis (Fig. 14-25).[53,54] The ulceration rapidly and relentlessly enlarges to greater than 2 cm or more. Often, a history of preceding trauma is obtained.[53,54] Ulcers can appear anywhere, but the legs are most common and are seen in 80% of cases.[53,54] Skin ulceration at sites of trauma (pathergy) such as venipuncture sites or attempts at surgical debridement may be seen. A history of an associated disease, such as inflammatory bowel disease, rheumatoid arthritis, or myelodysplastic disease may be obtained.[53,54] The mortality rate is 10%.

Differential diagnosis

Spider or other insect bites are often misdiagnosed.[54] Infections such as herpes simplex virus (HSV) or ecthyma gangrenosum are often mistaken for pyoderma gangrenosum.[53] The presence of the characteristic purple, loosely-attached, epidermal edges to the ulcer distinguishes pyoderma gangrenosum.[53,54] A skin biopsy to include the loosely-attached epidermal edge will distinguish.

Pathogenesis

Pyoderma gangrenosum is considered one of the neutrophilic dermatoses because sheets of neutrophils replacing the reticular dermis and undermining the adjacent epidermis are found. Activated neutrophils are believed responsible for the tissue damage.[54] The association with other disorders with activated neutrophils, such as inflammatory bowel disease, rheumatoid arthritis, and myelodysplasia, reinforces the concept. Recently, one associated form of pyoderma gangrenosum has been mapped to chromosome 15q.[55]

Treatment

Immunosuppressive drugs, such as cyclosporine and tacrolimus, are the most effective in controlling the disease.[54,56] The condition is often responsive to high-dose glucocorticosteroids, but steroid side-effects from long-term usage limit their usefulness. Antineutrophil drugs, such as dapsone and colchicine, may be useful in combination. Topical tacrolimus may be a useful adjunct.[55] Many cytotoxic agents have been used, but no rigorous evaluation is avaliable.[54]

Patient education

The clinician should explain to the patient and family the life-threatening nature of the disease and the requirement of days to weeks to accomplish a remission. He or she should also emphasize that an endoscopic examination for inflammatory bowel disease, a bone marrow examination for myelodysplasia, and an arthritis consultation are required, and that long-term immunosuppressive therapy will be required.

Follow-up visits

Weekly visits are required until remission is accomplished, after which monthly visits are necessary. Frequent monitoring of side-effects of the immunosuppressive agents is required.

REFERENCES

1. Doutre M: Physiopathology of urticaria, *Eur J Dermatol* 9:601, 1999.
2. Greaves MW: Chronic urticaria in childhood, *Allergy* 55:3090, 2000.
3. Legrain V, Taieb A, Sagi T: Urticaria in infants: a study of forty patients, *Pediatr Dermatol* 7:101, 1990.
4. Gustafsson D, Sjoberg O, Foucard T: Development of allergies and asthma in infants and young children with atopic dermatitis: a prospective follow-up to seven years of age, *Allergy* 55:240, 2000.
5. Greaves MW: Chronic urticaria, *J Allergy Clin Immunol* 105:664, 2000.
6. Kwong KY, Maalouf N, Jones CA: Urticaria and angioedema: pathophysiology, diagnosis and treatment, *Pediatr Ann* 27:719, 1998.
7. Janniger CK, Schutzer SE, Schwartz RA: Childhood insect bite reactions to ants, wasps, and bees, *Cutis* 54:14, 1994.
8. Knowles S, Shapiro L, Shear NH: Drug eruptions in children, *Adv Dermatol* 14:399, 1999.
9. Bircher AJ: Drug-induced urticaria and angioedema caused by non-IgE mediated pathomechanisms, *Eur J Dermatol* 9:657, 1999.
10. Jarisch R, Beringer K, Hemmer W: Role of food allergy and food intolerance in recurrent urticaria, *Curr Problems Dermatol* 28:64, 1999.
11. Heymann WR: Chronic urticaria and angioedema associated with thyroid autoimmunity: review and therapeutic implications, *J Am Acad Dermatol* 40:229, 1999.
12. Weston WL: What is erythema multiforme? *Pediatr Ann* 25:106, 1996.
13. Laurent J, Guinnepain MT: Angioedema associated with C1 inhibitor deficiency, *Clin Rev Allergy Immunol* 17:513, 1999.
14. Pacheco T et al: Three generations of lupus erythematosus and hereditary angioedema, *Am J Med* 109:256, 2000.
15. Asero R: Leukotriene receptor antagonists may prevent NSAID-induced exacerbations in patients with chronic urticaria, *Ann Allergy Asthma Immunol* 85:156, 2000.
16. Martin-Munoz F et al: Evaluation of drug-related hypersensitivity reactions in children, *J Invest Allerg Clin Immunol* 9:172, 1999.
17. Friedmann PS: Assessment of urticaria and angioedema, *Clin Exp Allergy* 29(suppl)3:109, 1999.
18. Greaves MW, O'Donnell BF: Not all chronic urticaria is "idiopathic," *Exp Dermatol* 7:11, 1998.
19. Hoffman HM et al: Identification of a locus on 1q44 for familial cold urticaria, *Am J Hum Genet* 66:1693, 2000.
20. Katsamba AD et al: Mastocytosis with skin manifestations: current status, *J Eur Acad Dermatol Venereol* 13:155, 1999.
21. Gibbs NF, Friedlander SF, Harpster EF: Telangiectasia macularis eruptiva perstans, *Pediatr Dermatol* 17:194, 2000.
22. Longley BJ Jr et al: Activating and dominant inactivating c-KIT catalytic domain mutations in distinct clinical forms of human mastocytosis, *Proc Natl Acad Sci* 96:1609, 1999.
23. Dror Y et al: Mastocytosis cells bearing a c-kit point mutation are characterized by hypersensitivity to stem cell factor and increased apoptosis, *Br J Haematol* 108:729, 2000.
24. Swolin B, Rodjer S, Roupe G: Cytogenetic studies in patients with mastocytosis, *Cancer Genet Cytogenet* 120:131, 2000.
25. Kissling S et al: Strategies in childhood and adult mastocytosis, *Dermatology* 198:426, 1999.
26. Smith MB et al: Photochemotherapy of dominant diffuse cutaneous mastocytosis, *Pediatr Dermatol* 7:251, 1990.
27. Helm TN, Bass J, Chang LW: Persistent annular erythema of infancy, *Pediatr Dermatol* 10:46, 1993.
28. Borbujo J et al: Erythema annulare centrifugum and *Escherichia coli* urinary infection, *Lancet* 347:897, 1996.
29. Report of the Committee on Infectious Disease: *Red book 2000,* Elk Grove Village, Ill, 2000, American Academy of Pediatrics.
30. Kakourou T et al: Erythema nodosum in children: a prospective study, *J Am Acad Dermatol* 44:17, 2001.
31. Picco P et al: Clinical and biological characteristics of immunopathological-disease related erythema nodosum in children, *Scand J Rheumatol* 28:27, 1999.
32. Cribier B et al: Erythema nodosum and associated diseases, *Int J Dermatol* 37:667, 1998.
33. Garty BZ, Poznanski O: Erythema nodosum in Israeli children, *Israel Med Assoc J* 2:145, 2000.
34. Winter HS: Treatment of pyoderma gangrenosum, erythema nodosum and aphthous ulcerations, *Inflamm Bowel Dis* 4:71, 1998.
35. Calabrese L, Fleischer AB: Thalidomide: current and potential clinical applications, *Am J Med* 108:487, 2000.
36. Cliff S et al: Frey's syndrome without hyperhidrosis, *J Roy Soc Med* 91:388, 1998.
37. Dulguerov P et al: New objective and quantitative tests for gustatory sweating, *Acta Otolaryngol* 119:599, 1999.

38. Dulguerov P et al: Frey syndrome treatment with botulinum toxin, *Otolaryngol Head Neck Surg* 122:821, 2000.

39. Ansell BM, Falcini F: Cutaneous vasculitis in children, *Clin Dermatol* 17:577, 1999.

40. Savage COS et al: Vasculitis, *Br Med J* 320:1325, 2000.

41. Scott DG, Watts RA: Systemic vasculitis: epidemiology, classification and environmental factors, *Ann Rheum Dis* 59:161, 2000.

42. Sorensen SF et al: A prospective study of vasculitis patients collected in a five year period: evaluation of the Chapel Hill nomenclature, *Ann Rheum Dis* 59:4787, 2000.

43. Tekin M et al: Clinical, laboratory and molecular characteristics of children with Familial Mediterranean Fever-associated vasculitis, *Acta Paediatr* 89:177, 2000.

44. Campanile G, Hautmann G, Lotti TM: The etiology of cutaneous necrotizing vasculitis, *Clin Dermatol* 17:505, 1999.

45. Cadnapaphornchai MA, Saulsbury FT, Norwood VF: Hypocomplementemic urticarial vasculitis: report of a pediatric case, *Pediatr Nephrol* 14:328, 2000.

46. Brogan PA, Dillon MJ: The use of immunosuppressive and cytotoxic drugs in non-malignant disease, *Arch Dis Child* 83:259, 2000.

47. Weston WL, Morelli JG: Childhood pernio and cryoproteins: *Pediatr Dermatol* 17:97, 2000.

48. Finn A et al: Infectious purpura fulminans: caution needed in the use of protein C, *Br J Haematol* 106:253, 1999.

49. Faust SN, Heyderman RS, Levin M: Disseminated intravascular coagulation and purpura fulminans secondary to infection, *Bailliere's Best Practice Clin Haematol* 13:179-197, 2000.

50. Smith OP, White B: Infectious purpura fulminans: diagnosis and treatment, *Br J Haematol* 106:253, 1999.

51. Mar A, Fergin P, Hogan P: Unilateral pigmented purpuric eruption, *Austr J Dermatol* 40:211, 1999.

52. Crowson AN, Magro CM, Zahochak R: Atypical pigmentary purpura: a clinical, histopathologic and genotypic study, *Hum Pathol* 30:1004, 1999.

53. Graham JA et al: Pyoderma gangrenosum in infants and children, *Pediatr Dermatol* 11:10, 1994.

54. Powell FC, Collins S: Pyoderma gangrenosum, *Clin Dermatol* 18:283, 2000.

55. Yeon HB et al: Pyogenic arthritis, pyoderma gangrenosum and acne syndrome maps to chromosome 15q, *Am J Hum Genet* 66:1443, 2000.

56. Jolles S, Niclasse S, Benson E: Combination oral and topical tacrolimus in therapy-resistant pyoderma gangrenosum, *Br J Dermatol* 14:564, 1999.

CHAPTER FIFTEEN

Hair Disorders

Hair loss is far more common in children than is excessive hair. This chapter is divided into two sections: hair loss and excessive hair.

COMMON FORMS OF HAIR LOSS

When evaluating hair loss in children, one should determine whether it is congenital or acquired, circumscribed or diffuse. This results in four diagnostic categories of hair loss (Box 15-1). Hair loss, or *alopecia*, accounts for approximately 3% of children's visits to a dermatologist. It causes the parents and the child considerable anxiety and the health team considerable frustration. Among the numerous causes of hair loss in children, three types account for the great majority of visits to the clinician: alopecia areata, tinea capitis (see Chapter 6), and traumatic alopecia. All three are forms of acquired, circumscribed hair loss (Box 15-2). These three conditions should always be considered in the differential diagnosis of hair loss.

Alopecia Areata
Clinical features

Alopecia areata is characterized by complete or almost complete hair loss in circumscribed areas (Fig. 15-1). Usually from one to three areas are involved.[1] It is most commonly seen (in 80% of patients) in the frontal or parietal scalp, but body hair, sexual hair, eyelashes, and eyebrows may be involved.[1] The appearance of a circumscribed area that is completely devoid of hair without any scalp change is a constant feature. Scalp erythema or scaling may occur in alopecia areata after sunburn. A positive family history for alopecia areata is found in 10% to 42% of the patients.[1,2]

Nail disease occurs in 10% to 46% of children with alopecia areata.[1-3] Nail pitting is the most common change and appears as shallow, wide (1 to 2 mm) depressions in the nail plate. The pits are wider than those seen in psoriasis (Fig. 15-2).

The prognosis for most children is excellent. Complete regrowth of the hair occurs within a year in the majority of children with alopecia areata.[1,2] Spontaneous remission is the rule. Approximately 30% will have a future episode of alopecia areata with 7% to 10% having chronic disease.[2]

Ophiasis, an unusual subtype involving less than 5% of all patients with alopecia areata, begins in the occiput or along the frontal scalp and spreads, with many patches of alopecia along the hair margins (Fig. 15-3). Ophiasis is likely to eventuate in loss of all of the scalp hair (alopecia totalis) (Fig. 15-4), or all of the scalp and body hair (alopecia universalis). When this occurs, the prognosis for regrowth is extremely poor.[2]

Differential diagnosis

Hair pulling or other forms of traction alopecia may mimic alopecia areata. Broken-off hairs, scalp petechiae, and a history of trauma are features that help distinguish these conditions. Tinea capitis, particularly the black-dot form, may be confused with alopecia areata. Careful examination of the scalp will reveal broken-off hairs within the follicle, and microscopic examination of these hairs in potassium hydroxide (KOH) 10% will reveal hyphae within the hair shaft. A fungal culture will help confirm the diagnosis. Much has been made of the importance of exclamation point hairs in the differential diagnosis of circumscribed hair loss, but this change is not specific.[4] Although a scalp biopsy may be helpful in difficult cases, it is rarely necessary.

The scarring alopecias may present circumscribed areas of hair loss, but a history of inflammation or injury and the scalp thickening and color change seen in these conditions will help distinguish them from alopecia areata.

Circumscribed alopecia may be congenital and present from birth. It is characteristic of certain birthmarks in the scalp, particularly sebaceous nevus and aplasia cutis congenita. These alopecias are usually not difficult to differentiate from alopecia areata. The history of onset at birth, and the yellow plaques or scarred areas in the scalp, will differentiate congenital circumscribed alopecias from alopecia areata.

Pathogenesis

It has been presumed that alopecia areata represents an immune mechanism because a dense perifollicular accumulation of lymphocytes precedes the hair loss.[5,6] The exact mechanism of hair loss is not un-

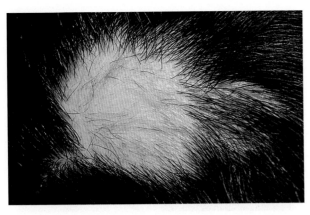

Fig. 15-1 Alopecia areata. Circumscribed patch of completely bald scalp.

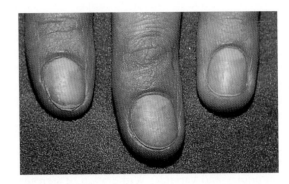

Fig. 15-2 Nail pitting in a child with alopecia areata.

Box 15-1 Diagnostic Categories of Hair Loss in Children

Congenital circumscribed alopecia
Acquired circumscribed alopecia
Congenital diffuse alopecia
Acquired diffuse alopecia

Box 15-2 Major Types of Acquired, Circumscribed Alopecia in Childhood

Alopecia areata
Tinea capitis
Traction alopecia (including trichotillomania)

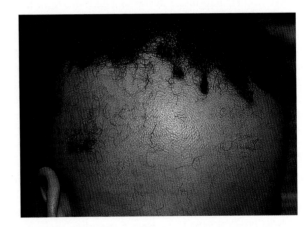

Fig. 15-3 Ophiasis pattern of alopecia areata, with hair loss starting in occiput.

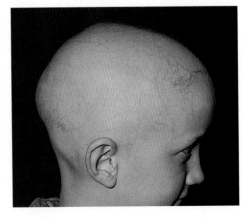

Fig. 15-4 Alopecia totalis. Ophiasis progressing to a completely bald scalp.

derstood, but direct lymphocyte injury to the hair matrix has been postulated, and 100% of alopecia areata patients compared with 44% of controls have autoantibodies to as yet unidentified hair follicle antigens.[7]

The injury to the growing hair results in premature conversion of growing hairs to resting hairs that are shed. Evaluation of clinically normal scalp hairs to determine the anagen (growing) to telogen (resting) ratio can be used to predict the likelihood of short-term hair regrowth.[8]

Treatment

There is no specific treatment for alopecia areata. Because spontaneous regrowth occurs in 95% of cases, the prognosis is good in most patients. Many forms of local therapy, including intralesional or superpotent topical steroids, anthralin, minoxidil, contact sensitizers, and combinations of the above, have demonstrated short-term hair regrowth, but they do not alter the long-term course of alopecia areata.[9-12] The administration of systemic glucocorticosteroids or cyclosporine has been advocated for their antiinflammatory effect. However, the suppression of inflammation and hair regrowth is temporary and variable. Withdrawal of steroids or cyclosporine results in prompt loss of the hair that has grown back. Thus the risks of side effects outweigh the benefits of temporary hair growth.

In complete hair loss, referral to a dermatologist may be useful, and prompt attention should be given to obtaining a wig for the child. Excellent children's wigs are manufactured, and a physician's prescription may allow the family to obtain a wig at reduced prices. A support group, the National Alopecia Areata Foundation, has a number of North American chapters that provide excellent psychological support and the latest treatment information for persons with alopecia areata.

Patient education

Parents should be informed that there is no specific treatment regimen for alopecia areata. However, in children with the usual type of alopecia areata, with one to three circumscribed patches of complete scalp hair loss, it is important to emphasize the excellent prognosis even without treatment. Explaining the proposed mechanism of the disease and the excellent chances for spontaneous recovery will greatly aid understanding of the problem. Ophiasis patients should be told of the poor prognosis. Considerable effort should be devoted at the first visit to answering questions for the child and the family. The risks and benefits of all current therapy should be explained in detail, and the psychological benefits of wearing a wig should be discussed.

The clinician should provide the patient and family with information about the National Alopecia Areata Foundation, which can be contacted by mail at P.O. Box 150760, San Rafael, CA 94915-0760, 710 C Street, Suite 11, San Rafael, CA 94901; by email at www.alopeciaareata.com; or by phone at 415-456-4644.

Follow-up visits

In the usual type of alopecia areata, a visit every 3 months is useful to check on progress and the

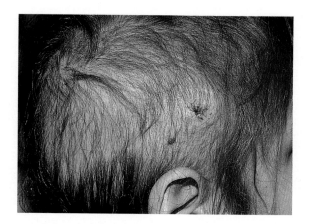

Fig. 15-5 Trichotillomania. Hair broken at many different lengths associated with scalp excoriations.

chances for spontaneous regression. In the ophiasis type, a visit in 2 weeks to re-explain the illness and encourage the use of a wig is most helpful. Frequent visits may be necessary to establish the proper physician-patient relationship.

Tinea Capitis

Tinea capitis is a major cause of acquired, circumscribed hair loss in children. It is covered in detail in Chapter 6.

Traumatic Alopecia

Traumatic alopecia results from hair injury produced by traction, friction, chemical, or other injury to hair. The common types seen in childhood include trichotillomania (hair pulling) and the traction alopecia seen with various popular hairstyles.

Hair Pulling
Clinical features

Circumscribed areas of hair loss with irregular borders and hairs broken off at different lengths are seen in hair pulling. Frequently scalp excoriations and perifollicular petechiae are present (Fig. 15-5). Commonly, only one area of the scalp is involved, with the frontoparietal and frontotemporal scalp being the most usual sites. Rarely, the eyebrows or eyelashes may be plucked (Fig. 15-6). Hair pulling in children should be divided into three categories: acute hair pulling associated with stress, trichotillomania, and hair pulling associated with other psychiatric conditions. Children who outgrow the habit of hair pulling without any major intervention do not have true trichotillomania. The estimated lifetime prevalence of trichotillomania is 0.5% to 1% or higher, with the majority of patients

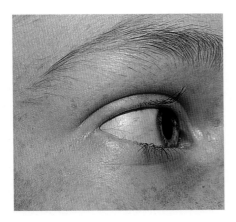

Fig. 15-6 Trichotillomania of the eyelashes.

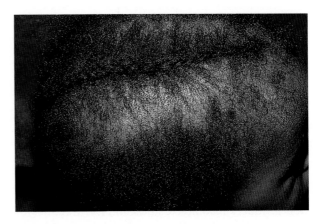

Fig. 15-7 Traction alopecia. Hair loss caused by tight braiding.

exhibiting onset of trichotillomania before the age of 18 years.[13] The mean age of onset is 8 years for males and 12 years for females.[13] The condition is more common in females but is not rare in males.[13]

Differential diagnosis

The diseases considered in the differential diagnosis of hair pulling are the same as those for alopecia areata and tinea capitis (see Box 15-2). One should also consider the possibility that someone other than the affected child, such as a sibling, playmate, parent, or baby-sitter, is doing the hair pulling. Hair cutting (which is associated with other artefactual skin diseases) must be differentiated from hair pulling.

Pathogenesis

Traumatic events, such as the death of a family member or close friend, separation or divorce of parents, or difficulties in school, may precipitate acute hair pulling. Trichotillomania is an impulse control disorder leading to chronic hair pulling.[13] Hair pulling may be associated with a large variety of psychiatric diagnoses and symptoms.[13] Parents often vehemently deny such hair pulling because they have not personally observed it.

Treatment

The search for antecedent traumatic events is helpful. In children in whom a precipitating event can be identified, relief of stress will result in ending the nervous habit. Application of oils to the hair makes it more difficult to pull. Psychodynamic therapy, chemical treatments with antidepressants, and behavior modification have all been used to treat trichotillomania. However, it is difficult to evaluate which therapy is most effective and which patients will benefit most from whatever

form of therapy is chosen. Some children persist with trichotillomania into adult life. In severe forms that are associated with other signs of emotional stress, psychiatric referral may be indicated.

Patient education

A careful search for a precipitating event, and an explanation of the complex nature of the process, are crucial to patient and parent education. The clinicians and others should avoid blaming the child or one or more family members. If a precipitating event can be identified, the clinician should suggest that remedying the circumstances surrounding that event will likely lead to cessation of the hair pulling. If no precipitating event can be demonstrated, the clinician should explain that this may be a difficult problem to treat. He or she should also emphasize that hair pulling may just be a reaction to acute stress or a nervous habit; however, it may be a sign of significant chronic stress or other emotional problems, and if the child is having other psychosocial difficulties, counseling may be useful.

Follow-up visits

A follow-up visit in 1 to 2 months is useful in evaluating progress. Continued reassurance should be given. If the problem persists, referral to a child psychologist or psychiatrist is indicated.

Traction Alopecia
Clinical features

Thinning of hair in particular areas of the scalp may result from constant traction or friction. Very few fractured hairs are found in the involved areas, although the hairs may be smaller in diameter than those found in adjacent areas (Fig. 15-7). The thinning is often patchy, depending on the nature of the trauma. The history of methods of hair care and types of hairstyle is crucial for the diagnosis.[14]

Differential diagnosis

The differential diagnosis is the same as for alopecia areata and tinea capitis (see Box 15-2).

Pathogenesis

Several different sources of traction or friction have been identified as responsible for traction alopecia.[14] The hairstyle, chemical or thermal treatment, or friction produces incomplete and complete fractures of hair. One should always consider child abuse (e.g., pulling the child by the hair). Neonatal occipital alopecia is physiologic hair loss exacerbated by the rubbing of the baby's head on the sheet or mattress. Massage alopecia may occur from vigorous scalp massage and frequent shampooing. Marginal alopecia is seen with hair straightening or tight hair curlers. Cornrow alopecia, ponytail alopecia, and braid alopecia are all related to tight hairstyles. Hot-comb alopecia occurs on the vertex of the scalp and may involve scarring. It is the result of use of a hot comb to straighten or style hair. Marginal alopecia is sometimes seen in hot-comb alopecia.

Treatment

Discontinuation of the trauma to the hair is the obvious treatment of choice. The use of mild shampoos and wide-toothed combs with rounded ends, infrequent shampooing, and gentle brushing are all important components of therapy. Recovery may take 3 to 6 months.

Patient education

The susceptibility of certain hair types to such trauma should be explained and the benefits of being gentle with the hair emphasized.

Follow-up visits

A follow-up visit in 3 to 6 months is useful to assess hair regrowth.

UNCOMMON FORMS OF HAIR LOSS

The remaining types of hair loss are uncommon or rare. No attempt is made to consider these numerous conditions in detail, but an orderly approach to them is presented. The clinician should first determine whether the hair loss is circumscribed or diffuse, then determine whether it has been present from birth or

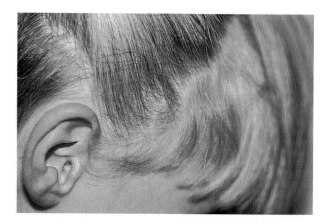

Fig. 15-8 Nevus sebaceous. Absence of hair in the area of yellow-orange plaque of a birthmark.

acquired later in life. This results in four diagnostic categories: congenital circumscribed alopecia, acquired circumscribed alopecia, congenital diffuse alopecia, and acquired diffuse alopecia (see Box 15-1). In congenital diffuse alopecia, a further diagnostic step, the hair mount examination, is necessary. Only the general clinical features of each group and the differential diagnoses are given. Telogen effluvium is discussed in more detail later in this chapter.

The mechanisms of hair loss in most of these unusual forms of alopecia have not been uncovered. However, certain associations are of therapeutic importance. An extraordinary number of clinical conditions are associated with hair loss, and hair loss should be characterized into one of the preceding four types to permit proper diagnosis and therapy.

Congenital Circumscribed Alopecia
Clinical features

Localized areas of scalp hair loss present from birth usually overlie a birthmark, such as a sebaceous or epidermal nevus.[15] The scalp surface is smooth, particularly in newborns or infants with circumscribed hair loss, and yellow to tan (Fig. 15-8). As the child gets older, a plaque is noted. A congenital circumscribed alopecia may also occur in aplasia cutis congenita (Fig. 15-9). Aplasia cutis congenita occurs most commonly as an isolated defect, but it may be associated with other malformations or genetic syndromes.[15-17]

Differential diagnosis

A scalp biopsy will help to identify and characterize these birthmarks, which represent hyperplasia of epidermal cells or sebaceous structures. Aplasia cutis

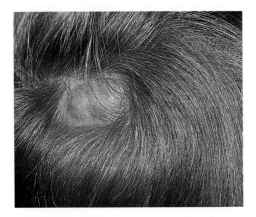

Fig. 15-9 Localized scarring of the scalp in aplasia cutis congenita.

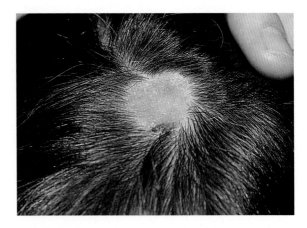

Fig. 15-10 Acquired circumscribed inflammatory scarring alopecia.

Box 15-3	Differential Diagnosis of Congenital Circumscribed Hair Loss

Sebaceous nevus
Aplasia cutis congenita (scarlike)
Epidermal nevus
Hair follicle hamartomas
Triangular alopecia of the frontal scalp

Box 15-4	Differential Diagnosis of Acquired, Scarring, Circumscribed Hair Loss

Postinfectious
  Kerion caused by tinea capitis
  Pyoderma
  Varicella
Postinflammatory
  Lichen planus
  Lupus erythematosus
Postinjury
  Physical trauma (e.g., abrasion, cuts)
  Chemical or thermal burns
  Radiation injury

congenita demonstrates scarring of the scalp in a circumscribed area and represents failure of formation of one or more layers of the scalp. In the other rare forms, circumscribed patches of hair loss without scalp changes are present. The differential diagnosis of this type of alopecia is given in Box 15-3.

Acquired Circumscribed Alopecia: Scarring Forms
Clinical features

Circumscribed hair loss acquired during childhood, other than alopecia areata, tinea capitis, and traction alopecia, is usually scarring in nature (Fig. 15-10)—that is, the hair follicles are replaced by fibrous tissue following injury to the hair follicles after infection, trauma, or inflammatory skin disease.

Differential diagnosis

Box 15-4 presents the conditions to be considered in the differential diagnosis.

Congenital Diffuse Alopecia
Clinical features

Diffuse scalp hair loss present from birth usually results in the complaint that the child's hair simply will not grow. Such children never require haircuts. Included in this group are hair shaft defects in which the failure of hair growth is the result of structural defects that cause the breaking off of hairs (Figs. 15-11 through 15-16).[15] The child has short, broken hairs of equal length. In many forms of ectodermal dysplasia, reduced numbers or absence of hair follicles produce the clinical picture of congenital diffuse alopecia. Children with genetic diseases associated with photosensitivity, premature aging, and early cancer development will often have diffusely thin hair.

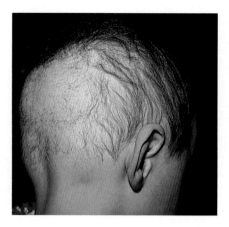

Fig. 15-11 Three-year-old male with congenital trichorrhexis nodosa.

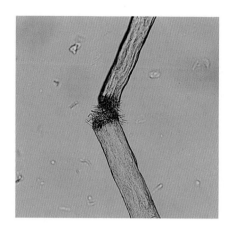

Fig. 15-12 Photomicrograph of hair mount demonstrates broomstick fracture of trichorrhexis nodosa.

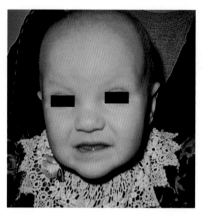

Fig. 15-13 Two-year-old female with monilethrix.

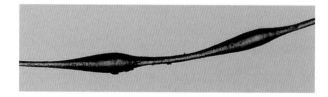

Fig. 15-14 Photomicrograph of hair mount demonstrates beading of the hair in monilethrix.

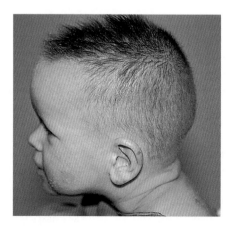

Fig. 15-15 Child suffering from trichorrhexis invaginata in Netherton's syndrome.

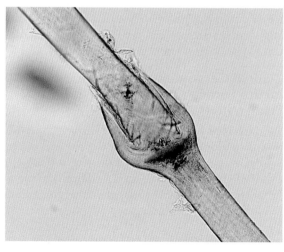

Fig. 15-16 Photomicrograph of hair mount demonstrates bamboo hair in trichorrhexis nodosa.

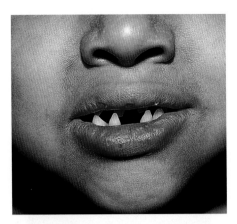

Fig. 15-17 Cone-shaped teeth in a child with hypohidrotic ectodermal dysplasia.

Differential diagnosis

Removing hairs and placing them on a microscope slide with mounting fluid will allow demonstration of the particular type of structural hair defect. Many rare forms of diffuse congenital hair loss are associated with syndromes, and complete examination of the child is necessary for accurate diagnosis (Figure 15-17). The differential diagnosis of this type of hair loss is given in Box 15-5.

Acquired Diffuse Alopecia

Diffuse hair loss with onset in childhood after a period of normal hair growth is rare. It usually results from telogen effluvium or cancer chemotherapy. In other children with diffuse hair loss a careful search for endocrine, chemical, and nutritional abnormalities is warranted (Box 15-6). In these children a rigorous and detailed history should be taken and appropriate laboratory studies ordered if the clinical data so indicate. Because most of the endocrine, chemical, and nutritional causes are correctable, the clinician should consider undertaking a thorough laboratory evaluation in such children.

Telogen Effluvium

Telogen effluvium is the name given to the acquired diffuse alopecia that results from rapid conversion of scalp hairs from the growing state to the resting state (Fig. 15-18).[18] In physiologic circumstances an infant or child has 88% of scalp hair in a growing, or anagen, state and only 12% of hair in a resting, or telogen, state. Each individual scalp hair grows for 3 years, then regresses over 2 or 3 weeks, and rests for

---

Box 15-5   Differential Diagnosis of Congenital Diffuse Hair Loss

HAIR SHAFT DEFECTS
Trichorrhexis nodosa (broomstick fractures)
Familial form
Argininosuccinic aciduria
Pili torti (twisted hair)
Classic form
Menkes' syndrome
Monilethrix (beaded hair)
Trichorrhexis invaginata (bamboo hair)
Netherton's syndrome

ABSENT OR SPARSE HAIR
Atrichia congenita
Ectodermal dysplasias
Photosensitivity disorders
Premature aging disorders
Premature cancer disorders

Box 15-6   Differential Diagnosis of Acquired Diffuse Hair Loss

TELOGEN EFFLUVIUM

ENDOCRINE
Hypothyroidism
Hypopituitarism
Hypoparathyroidism
Diabetes mellitus

ANDROGENETIC ALOPECIA
Male pattern in adolescents

CHEMICAL
Thallium poisoning (rat poison)
Antithyroid drugs
Heparin
Coumarin
Antimetabolites (e.g., cyclophosphamide)

NUTRITIONAL
Hypervitaminosis A
Acrodermatitis enteropathica (zinc deficiency)
Maramus

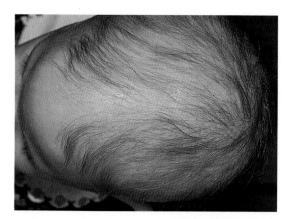

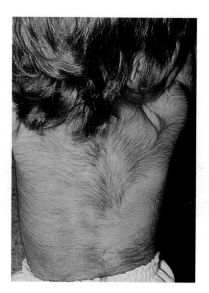

Fig. 15-18 Acquired diffuse nonscarring alopecia in telogen effluvium.

Fig. 15-19 Hypertrichosis lanuginosa.

3 months. This growth throughout the scalp is asynchronous in that the majority of hairs are growing at any time of observation. Acutely stressful events, such as birth, auto accidents, illnesses with high fever, and acute psychiatric problems, may result in a rapid conversion of growing hairs to resting hairs. Following the event by 2 to 4 months, the hairs are shed and usually continue to shed over 3 to 4 months. Each hair shed is a resting hair and will be replaced by a normal growing hair. In the newborn, the hairs are shed in two phases from the frontal scalp to the occipital scalp and are not asynchronous in growth phase until about 12 months of age.

Diagnosis of telogen effluvium can be made by plucking at least 50 hairs from a child's scalp and examining the roots to determine whether they are growing or resting. This is best done by cutting away the remainder of the hairs and mounting the roots in a commercial slide-mounting medium. A growing, or anagen, hair will have a pigmented core and a bulbous root that is larger in diameter than the hair shaft. Often the external root sheath is present. In a telogen, or resting, hair, the external root sheath is absent or fragmented, pigment is often absent, and the root of the hair is narrower than the caliber of the other hair and frequently curved. One can reassure the patient with telogen effluvium that complete regrowth is possible. Telogen effluvium has been reported after surgery, crash diets, and the use of anticoagulants and antithyroid drugs.

Anagen effluvium, in which growing hairs are lost, is an expected result of cancer treatment in children in which the antimetabolites interfere with hair growth, or radiation to the head injures the growing hair.

EXCESSIVE HAIR

Excessive hair may be congenital or acquired.

Congenital Hypertrichosis
Clinical features

Excessive hair may be generalized (hypertrichosis lanuginosa) or circumscribed (nevoid hypertrichosis). Excessive body hair in the newborn may be a transient problem, especially in premature infants, and resolves by 6 months of age, or may represent the rare hypertrichosis lanuginosa in which long, fine lanugo hairs cover the entire glabrous skin (Fig. 15-19). Hypertrichosis lanuginosa is thought to be autosomal dominant, but most cases are sporadic.[19] Congenital hypothyroidism may also demonstrate excessive body hair. Circumscribed hypertrichosis may be seen as one to six patches of excessive, long hair over various body regions. It is usually persistent, but spontaneous remission has been reported.[20] When in the midline, circumscribed hypertrichosis may be associated with nervous system abnormalities. Hypertrichosis over the lumbosacral spine (the "human tail") may be a clue to spina bifida; over the occiput it may indicate a meningocele or encephalo-

---

Box 15-7   Syndromes With Hypertrichosis

Cornelia de Lange's syndrome
Rubinstein-Taybi syndrome
Gingival hyperplasia with hypertrichosis
Winchester syndrome
Recessive dystrophic epidermolysis bullosa
Fetal hydantoin syndrome
Erythrohepatic porphyria

Box 15-9   Conditions Resulting in Hirsutism

Racial hirsutism
Polycystic ovaries
Ovarian tumors
Congenital adrenal hyperplasia
Cushing's syndrome
Exogenous androgens

Box 15-8   Differential Diagnosis of Circumscribed Congenital Hypertrichosis

Congenital pigmented nevus
Pilar and smooth muscle hamartoma
Nevoid hypertrichosis
Midline nevoid hypertrichosis with spinal or central
    nervous system malformations

---

cele. Facial hypertrichosis may be seen in a number of syndromes listed in Box 15-7.

Differential diagnosis

Circumscribed areas of hypertrichosis must be differentiated from congenital smooth muscle and pilar nevus and congenital pigmented nevi (Box 15-8). Differentiating hypertrichosis lanuginosa from the transient lanugo overgrowth may be difficult in the first few months of life, although the body and facial hairs in hypertrichosis lanuginosa are longer, often reaching 2 inches in length.

Pathogenesis

In nevoid hypertrichosis, excessive numbers of hair follicles are found. In hypertrichosis lanuginosa, body hairs appear as terminal hairs. Endocrine evaluations are normal.

Treatment

The treatment options for either diffuse or circumscribed hypertrichosis include cutting or shaving, depilatories, electrolysis,[21] or laser.[22,23] The best option for any individual will depend on the degree of excess hair. Shaving, cutting, and depilatories are the simplest

and cheapest, but have to be done recurrently. Electrolysis is slow and somewhat painful, but permanent. Laser is faster and less painful than electrolysis, but is more expensive and may not be permanent.

Patient education

In circumscribed hypertrichosis, the clinician should explain that a malformation has taken place, with excessive follicular structures in that segment of skin. In hypertrichosis lanuginosa, genetic counseling may be useful.

Follow-up visits

Support and counseling are very useful for parents and children, and regularly scheduled visits are useful.

Acquired Excessive Hair (Hirsutism)
Clinical features

Hirsutism is the growth of terminal hair in part or all of the male sexual pattern. It is observed predominantly in adolescent females. In Mediterranean races, females may have some male pattern hair, and it may be impossible to distinguish clinically from true hirsutism. Asian females, in contrast, have no racial pattern of hirsutism. Excessive facial hair in the beard or moustache area may be accompanied by excessively long body hairs. Other features of virilization may be seen, such as increased muscle mass, clitoral hypertrophy, and deepening of the voice. A history of abnormal menses is often obtained.

Differential diagnosis

Racial forms that mimic hirsutism lack other signs of virilization, have female family members with similar findings, and lack endocrine abnormalities (Box 15-9). Patients with porphyrias may have facial hirsutism, but they usually have a history of photosensitivity and scars from previous skin lesions.

Pathogenesis

Hirsutism is androgen dependent, and a careful gynecologic and endocrine evaluation will detect underlying disease. Hyperandrogenism should be considered in any female with hirsutism (see Box 15-9).[24-27] Normal testosterone production by the female is 50% adrenal and 50% ovarian. Although the skin does not produce androgens from cholesterol, it is capable of metabolizing weaker androgens to more potent androgens such as dihydrotestosterone. Most patients with moderate to severe hirsutism, and 50% of those with mild hirsutism, will demonstrate elevated levels of plasma free testosterone.[27]

Treatment

Screening evaluation for hyperandrogenism should include measurements of free testosterone, androstenedione, and dehydroepiandrosterone.[24-27] Treatment depends on the underlying endocrine abnormality and whether it is of ovarian or adrenal origin. Treatment options include hormonal suppression to decrease androgen production, administration of antiandrogens, and physical methods of hair removal.

Patient education

The clinician should explain to the patient and family that hirsutism is just one feature of an endocrine disorder, and that correcting the underlying endocrine disease is required.

Follow-up visits

Follow-up 2 weeks after gynecologic or endocrine consultation is obtained is useful.

UNMANAGEABLE HAIR

The uncombable hair syndrome, woolly hair, and woolly hair nevus result in hair that is difficult to comb. In the uncombable hair syndrome, an autosomal dominant condition, the entire scalp hair is blond or silvery and does not lay flat when combed (Fig. 15-20).[28] Generalized woolly hair is tightly curled hair differing considerably from that of other family members.[29] In woolly hair nevus there are one to three patches of scalp hair that are curly and coarse, different from the remaining hair.[30] Also, the cowlick of long, straight hairs over the scalp vertex is seen in 7% of children.

SCALP WHORLS

A single whorl in the parietal scalp is found in 98% of children. In 45% it is in the midline, in 40% to

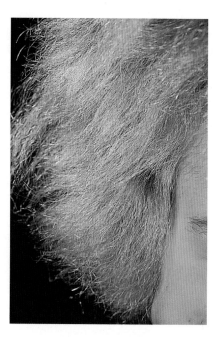

Fig. 15-20 Unmanageable hair.

the right of midline, and to the left in the remainder. Abnormal locations of scalp whorls may be clues to central nervous system disease.[31] For example, Down syndrome, trisomy 13, Prader-Willi syndrome, and Rubinstein-Taybi syndrome show anterior scalp whorls, whereas malformations of cranial bones often display widely spaced biparietal whorls.

REFERENCES

1. Sharma VK, Kumar B, Dawn G: A clinical study of childhood alopecia areata in Chandigarh, India, *Pediatr Dermatol* 13:372, 1996.
2. Mandini S, Shapiro J: Alopecia areata update, *J Am Acad Dermatol* 42:549, 2000.
3. Tosti A et al: Prevalence of nail abnormalities in children with alopecia areata, *Pediatr Dermatol* 11:112, 1994.
4. Ihm CW, Han JH: Diagnostic value of exclamation mark hairs, *Dermatology* 186:99, 1993.
5. Ghersetich I, Canpanile G, Lotti T: Alopecia areata: immunochemistry and ultrastructure of infiltrate and identification of adhesion molecule receptors, *Int J Dermatol* 35:28, 1996.
6. Whiting DA: Histopathology of alopecia areata in horizontal sections of scalp biopsies, *J Invest Dermatol* 104(S5):26S-27S, 1995.
7. Tobin DJ et al: Antibodies to hair follicles in alopecia areata, *J Invest Dermatol* 102:721, 1994.
8. Peereboom-Wynia JD et al: The trichogram as a prognostic tool in alopecia areata, *Acta Derm Venereol* 73:280, 1993.
9. Meidan VM, Touitou E: Treatments for androgenetic alopecia and alopecia areata: current options and future prospects, *Drugs* 61:53, 2001.

10. Cotelessa C et al: The use of topical diphenylcyclopropenone for the treatment of extensive alopecia areata, *J Am Acad Dermatol* 44:73, 2001.

11. Charuwichitratana S, Wattanakrai P, Tanrattanakorn S: Randomized double-blind placebo-controlled trial in the treatment of alopecia areata with 0.25% desoximetasone cream, *Arch Dermatol* 136:1276, 2000.

12. Camacho FM, Garcia-Hernandez MJ: Zinc aspartate, biotin, and clobetasol propionate in the treatment of alopecia areata, *Pediatr Dermatol* 16:336, 1999.

13. Messinger ML, Cheng TL: Trichotillomania, *Pediatr Rev* 20:249, 1999.

14. Whiting DA: Traumatic alopecia, *Int J Dermatol* 38(suppl)1:34, 1999.

15. de Berker David: Congenital hypotrichosis, *Int J Dermatol* 38(suppl)1:25, 1999.

16. Blunt K et al: Aplasia cutis congenita: a clinical review and associated defects, *Neonatal Netw* 11:17, 1992.

17. Kruk-Jeromin J, Janik J, Rykala J: Aplasia cutis congenita, *Dermatol Surg* 24:549, 1998.

18. Rebora A: Telogen effluvium, *Dermatology* 195:209, 1997.

19. Lee JJ, Im SB, Kim DK: Hypertrichosis universalis congenita: a separate entity, or the same as gingival fibromatosis, *Pediatr Dermatol* 10:263, 1993.

20. Dudding TE et al: Nevoid hypertrichosis with multiple patches of hair that underwent almost complete spontaneous resolution, *Am J Med Genet* 79:195, 1998.

21. Richards RN: Electrolysis for the treatment of hypertrichosis and hirsutism, *Skin Ther Lett* 4:3, 1999.

22. Littler CM: Laser hair removal in a patient with hypertrichosis lanuginosa congenita, *Dermatol Surg* 23:705, 1997.

23. Hobbs L, Ort R, Dover J: Synopsis of laser assisted hair removal systems, *Skin Ther Lett* 54:1, 2000

24. Shaw JC: Hormonal therapy in dermatology, *Dermatol Clin* 19:169, 2001.

25. Hock DL, Seifer DB: New treatments of hyperandrogenism and hirsutism, *Obstet Gynecol Clin North Am* 27:567, 2000.

26. Bergfeld WF: Hirsutism in women: effective therapy that is safe for long term, *Postgrad Med* 107:93, 99, 2000.

27. Rosenfield RL, Lucky AW: Acne, hirsutism, and alopecia in adolescent girls, *Endocrinol Metab Clin North Am* 22:507, 1990.

28. Ang P, Tay YK: What syndrome is this? Uncombable hair syndrome (Pili triangulati canaliculi), *Pediatr Dermatol* 15:475, 1998.

29. Sarkar R et al: Hereditary wooly hair in an Indian family, *J Dermatol* 27:220, 2000.

30. Amichai B, Grunwald MH, Halevy S: A child with a localized hair abnormality: woolly hair nevus, *Arch Dermatol* 132:573, 1996.

31. Samlaska CP, James WD, Sperling LC: Scalp whorls, *J Am Acad Dermatol* 21:553, 1989.

CHAPTER SIXTEEN | Nail Disease

Nail disorders are uncommon in children. However, nail changes may be useful in the clinical identification of systemic disorders. Normal variations are important to recognize and distinguish from nail disease. Concave nail shapes are normal from birth to 3 years of age.[1,2] Normal nails may have a few small pits in the nail plate. Scattered white spots are common in the nail plate and are caused by minor trauma.[1,2] Longitudinal ridging is also common in normal nails and worsens with age.

DISRUPTION OF THE NAIL SURFACE
Clinical Features

Changes in the surface of the nail that occur in childhood include pitting, scaling, longitudinal ridging, transverse ridges, or splitting (Fig. 16-1).[1,2] Pitting is predominantly seen in psoriasis and alopecia areata.[1-5] Pitting is the most common nail change seen in psoriasis.[1-4] At least 50% of children with alopecia areata will have pitting.[1,2,5] Pits are more numerous in alopecia areata, but it is often difficult to distinguish between the nail pitting of alopecia areata and psoriasis. Roughening and splitting of the nail surface (trachyonychia) is seen in idiopathic trachyonychia (20-nail dystrophy),[1,2,6] psoriasis,[1,4] alopecia areata,[1,2,5,7] lichen planus,[1,2,8-10] lichen striatus,[11] trauma[1,2] (Fig. 16-2), dermatitis of the digits,[1,2] and in some of the ectodermal dysplasias.[1,2] Transverse ridges (Beau's lines) are seen after a severe illness,[1,2] hand-foot-and-mouth disease,[12] a toxic event such as cancer chemotherapy,[13] or from a nervous habit of nail picking.[1,2,14,15] Multiple transverse ridges from repeated nail self-trauma (Fig. 16-3) may weaken the nail plate and lead to central splitting (Fig. 16-4).[1,2,14,15] This is particularly seen on the thumbnails of children and is associated with disruption of the cuticle.

Differential Diagnosis

When a disturbance of the nail surface is seen, onychomycosis is often considered in the differential diagnosis. Onychomycosis is uncommon in children and usually affects nails by producing thickening and surface roughening.[1,2,16-18] A potassium hydroxide (KOH) examination and fungal culture will help differentiate.

Pathogenesis

Injury to the germinative cells of the nail is the cause of disturbances of the nail surface, whether from inflammation, trauma, toxins, or chemotherapeutic agents.

Treatment

Treatment is difficult. If trauma is identified, behavior modification may help. Recovery is likely from all causes.

Patient Education

If self-trauma is the cause, open discussion with the patient regarding alternative habits is recommended. Reassurance that eventual recovery will occur should be given.

Follow-up Visits

A follow-up visit in 4 to 6 weeks may be useful in determining the course of disease.

THICK NAILS
Clinical Features

Nails thicken in proliferative epidermal disease. In psoriasis, alopecia areata, and lichen planus of children, all 20 nails may be involved.[1-11] In psoriasis, thickening begins distally and is associated with distal nail separation (onycholysis), giving a yellow color to the nails (Fig. 16-5).[1-4] The entire nail plate may then be involved. Pitting of the nail surface also occurs (Fig. 16-6). In lichen planus there is thickening of the nails, with a pinched-up central ridge and synechia formation over the nail surface (Fig. 16-7).[1,2,8-10]

In idiopathic trachyonychia[6] the child has thickened nails with exaggerated longitudinal ridges (Fig. 16-8). At least in some children, this disease may be a hereditary disorder. Trachyonychia of all 20 nails may be the presenting sign of alopecia areata, lichen planus, or psoriasis. Long-term follow-up is required to determine the development of associated features.[1,10]

Psoriasis, lichen planus, and idiopathic trachyonychia account for most cases of thick nails.[1-10] Nails may be thickened, shiny, and contain horizontal

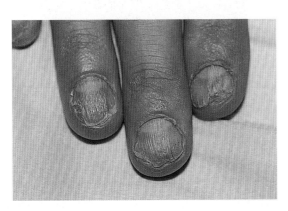

Fig. 16-1 Trachyonychia. Disruption of the nail surface.

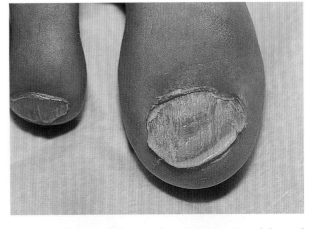

Fig. 16-2 Trachyonychia. Scaling and grooving of the nail in childhood idiopathic trachyonychia.

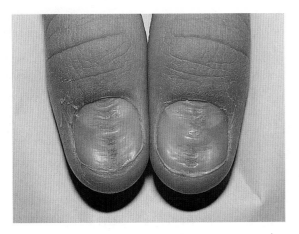

Fig. 16-3 Median nail dystrophy. Multiple medial transverse grooves from repeated self-trauma.

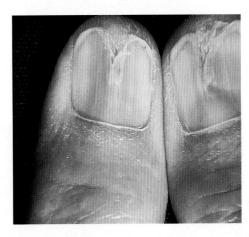

Fig. 16-4 Central splitting of the nail from repeated self-trauma.

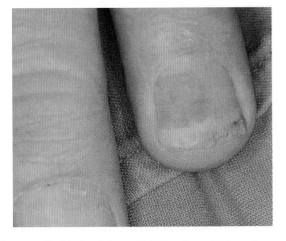

Fig. 16-5 Psoriasis of the nail. Yellowing within nail represents separation of the nail plate from the nail bed.

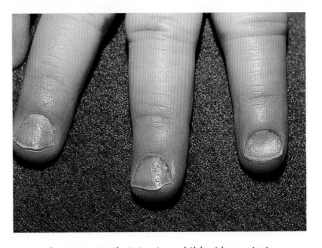

Fig. 16-6. Nail pitting in a child with psoriasis.

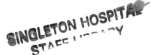

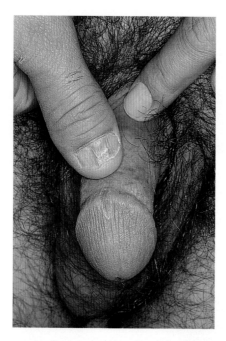

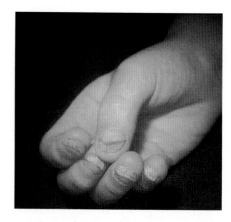

Fig. 16-9 Pachyonychia congenita type I. Distal thickening and elevation of the nails.

Fig. 16-7 Lichen planus of the nail. Trichoonychotic deformity with lichen planus lesion of the penis.

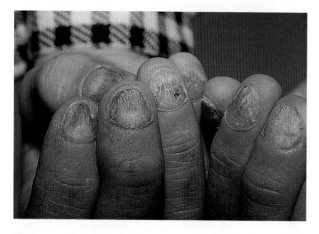

Fig. 16-8 Idiopathic trachyonychia. Exaggerated longitudinal ridging and rough surface of all 20 nails.

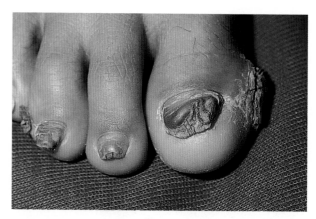

Fig. 16-10 Pachyonychia congenita type II. Distal thickening of the nails associated with painful circumscribed keratoses of the feet.

Differential Diagnosis

Conditions to be considered in the differential diagnosis of thick nails are listed in Box 16-1. Longitudinal nail biopsy may be useful in differentiating nail disorders. Involvement of all 20 nails should suggest psoriasis, alopecia areata, lichen planus, or idiopathic trachyonychia but not fungal infection. Finding characteristic papulosquamous skin lesions will help in the diagnosis of psoriasis and lichen planus. Thickened nails may be seen in children with scabies who cannot scratch.

Pathogenesis

The increased turnover time in the nail matrix results in a thickened, often dystrophic nail.[11] This occurs primarily in psoriasis and lichen planus. Pachyonychia

ridges in dermatitis that involves the hands and cuticular skin.[1,2] In pachyonychia congenita, an autosomal dominant disorder, thickened nails that are present at birth will become even thicker by age 2 or 3 years (Fig. 16-9). Dermatophyte infections of the nail (onychomycosis) will also thicken the nails. However, these infections are unusual in children, having a prevalence of 0.5%, and will usually involve only one or two nails (Fig. 16-10).[1,2,16-18]

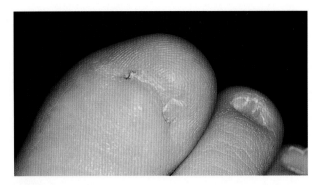

Fig. 16-11 Thin, hypoplastic nail in ectodermal dysplasia.

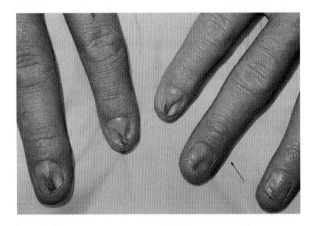

Fig. 16-12 Thin nails with trichoonychotic nail deformity in a child with hidrotic ectodermal dysplasia.

congenita is caused by mutations in keratins 6a, 6b, 16 and 17.[19]

Treatment

There is no satisfactory treatment for hypertrophic disorders of the nail. In dermatophyte infection, itraconazole pulsed therapy is effective in the majority of cases.[18] Itraconazole is given at a dose of 3 to 5 mg/kg/day for 1 week followed by 3 weeks without treatment. This regimen is repeated, and then a third and final week of treatment is given. Terbinafine, 3 to 5 mg/kg daily for 6 weeks for fingernails and 12 weeks for toenails may also be used.[17]

Patient Education

The clinician must be careful to explain to the patient and family that nail thickening merely reflects overgrowth of nail cells and that it does not represent a specific disease.

Follow-up Visits

Visits every 6 months may be useful in following the course of these conditions.

THIN OR ATROPHIC NAILS
Clinical Features

Poorly developed or absent nails are characteristic of a wide variety of congenital syndromes.[1,2,20-24] All babies' nails are normally thin until 3 to 4 years of life, at times making the diagnosis of thin or atrophic nail difficult early in life. These nail-plate abnormalities generally reflect nail matrix disorders. Most often this is the result of ectodermal dysplasia (Figs. 16-11 and 16-12), but intrauterine injury to the nail, such as that caused by epidermolysis bullosa, may be responsible. Usually most or all of the nails are affected. The nails are often narrow, and the nail plate is thin and fragile.

Congenital anonychia, or complete absence of some or all nails, has been described as an isolated dominant or sometimes recessive condition, or associated with other congenital ectodermal defects.[22] With anonychia, neither the nail plate nor the nail bed is present.

The nail-patella syndrome deserves special comment. It is thought to be an autosomal dominant syndrome with both ectodermal and mesodermal manifestations.[24] The nail matrix of usually the thumb, index fingers, and great toes is hypoplastic (Fig. 16-13). Occasionally it is absent. Other nails may be involved. The lunula is often characteristically triangular. In addition, there are multiple bone abnormalities: rudimentary or absent patellae, bony spurs on the posterior iliac crest, subluxation of the elbows, and thickening of the scapulae are seen. Other anomalies

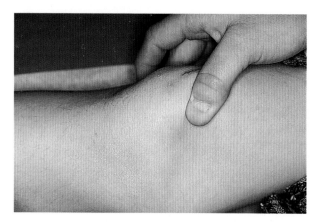

Fig. 16-13 Thin, hypoplastic thumbnail and dislocated patella in nail-patella syndrome.

described include skin laxity, heterochromia irides, and proteinuria. Periodic shedding of one or more nails is inherited as an autosomal dominant trait. This is a rare problem, and during the period of regrowth the nails may be dystrophic.

The more important causes of acquired thin or atrophic nails include trauma, infection, lichen planus, erythema multiforme, and bullous drug eruptions. Poor acral circulation, such as in Raynaud's disease or vascular malformations, may also contribute.

Differential Diagnosis

The clinician must first determine whether the nail disorder is congenital or acquired. Most often the associated clinical features are very useful in distinguishing one cause of nail disease or atrophy from another. Box 16-2 lists the conditions to be considered in the differential diagnosis of thin or atrophic nails.

Treatment

There is no treatment.

Patient Education

The clinician should emphasize to the patient and family that the cells responsible for nail growth are poorly formed or injured.

Follow-up Visits

Follow-up visits are unnecessary.

PARONYCHIA
Clinical Features

Acute paronychia is most often caused by *Staphylococcus aureus* or *Candida albicans*.[1,2,25] Occasionally, gram-negative organisms such as Pseudomonas and

---

> **Box 16-2 Differential Diagnosis of Thin, Absent, or Atrophic Nails**
>
> **CONGENITAL**
> Ectodermal dysplasia (anhidrotic, hidrotic)*
> Epidermolysis bullosa
> Incontinentia pigmenti
> Nail-patella syndrome*
> Acrodermatitis enteropathica
> Anonychia with or without ectrodactyly*
> Coffin-Siris syndrome*
> Hallermann-Streiff syndrome*
> Progeria
>
> **ACQUIRED**
> Trauma
> Infection
> Lichen planus
> Erythema multiforme
> Focal dermal hypoplasia
> Ellis–van Creveld syndrome (chondroectodermal dysplasia)
> Turner's syndrome
> Dyskeratosis congenita
> Trisomy 13
> Periodic shedding
> Severe Raynaud's phenomenon
> Vascular disease
> Bullous drug eruptions

*May be absent from birth.

Proteus are implicated. This is a common, painful infection of the nail fold in which the red, inflamed, swollen periungual tissue has a purulent exudate. Herpes simplex infection may also occur in the paronychial area (herpetic whitlow) and is distinguished by grouped vesicles on an erythematous base.[1,2,25]

Chronic paronychia is a difficult but common problem, primarily in children who are thumb suckers, nail biters, and nail pickers.[1,2,15,25] It appears as dull-red swelling of the cuticle area that is usually not tender. Hobbies and habits that recurrently traumatize the nail fold are important causes. Chronic or recurrent dermatitis often occurs around the nail folds and may be the underlying cause. The nail fold is red, indurated, and raised, and the cuticle margin is lost (Fig. 16-14). Often there is proximal separation of the nail plate from the nail bed. *C. albicans* is the most important causative organism.[2,25]

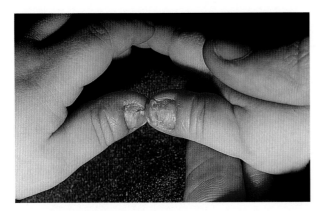

Fig. 16-14 Candida-related paronychia. Swelling and redness of the proximal nail fold in child who is a thumb sucker.

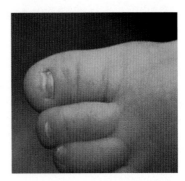

Fig. 16-15 Ingrown toenails with lateral nail-fold hypertrophy

Differential Diagnosis

Paronychia is so characteristic that it is not easily confused with other conditions.

Pathogenesis

Alterations in the integrity of the cuticle area, such as maceration and trauma, alter the epidermal barrier and allow microbial invasion.

Treatment

Treatment is complicated by the fact that avoiding the underlying cause may be extremely difficult. Systemic antibiotics are required in acute bacterial paronychia. Treatment with nystatin is useful in Candida infection, and good success may be achieved with the nightly application of nystatin cream followed by airtight occlusion. Aspiration of occluding material by children who are thumb suckers must be avoided by covering the thumb with a cotton sock and taping it around the wrist. Imidazole antiyeast agents will also be effective.[2] Other topical agents, such as gentamicin cream, sulfonamide solutions, and gentian violet, have limited efficacy.

Patient Education

Elimination or reduction of the causes of maceration and trauma should be emphasized.

Follow-up Visits

A visit in 1 month will be useful to determine the response to therapy.

INGROWN TOENAILS
Clinical Features

The large toes have a particular predilection for penetration of their nails into the lateral nail fold, producing a tender and sometimes erythematous swelling (Fig. 16-15). In infants this may appear at 1 to 2 months of age, with hypertrophy of the lateral nail folds.[1,2,26,27] Limping and discomfort on walking are frequent complaints. Purulence is occasionally seen secondary to bacterial invasion, usually due to *S. aureus.*

Differential Diagnosis

An ingrown toenail is usually so characteristic that it is not confused with other processes.

Pathogenesis

Ingrown toenails are caused by the penetration of ragged edges of the nail plate into the lateral nail fold, giving rise to a foreign body inflammatory response with eventual formation of granulation tissue.[1,2,26,27] Tight-fitting shoes and improper nail cutting promote crowding of the nail plate. In infants, asynchronous growth of the nail plate and the lateral nail folds may produce the penetration of the edge of the nail plate within the nail fold.[1,2,26,27]

Treatment

The majority of cases resolve with simple local measures.[28] In infants these include minimization of pressure by wearing loose-fitting shoes, proper trimming of the nails, soaking of the foot, and using cotton to prevent the nail edge from penetrating the skin.[27] The foreign body, namely the ragged lateral spicules of the nail plate, must be removed. This can be done by excising the lateral portion of the nail plate and inserting a small cotton wad to keep the nail plate separated from the inflamed area. Frequent soaking softens the indurated area. Systemic antibiotics are required only rarely.[29] When granulation tissue is present, it can be surgically curetted, then cauterized. Occasionally, surgical removal of the lateral one fourth of the nail plate

Box 16-3 Causes of Specific Color Changes in Nails

BLACK
Peutz-Jeghers syndrome
Vitamin B deficiency
Pinta
Ammoniated mercuric sulfide
Hair dyes
Film developer
Irradiation
Junctional nevus
Malignant melanoma
Fungus

BLUE LUNULAE
Antimalarials
Wilson's disease
Purpura
Cyanosis
Antimalarials
Argyria

GREEN
Pseudomonas
Aspergillus

RED
Resorcinol (nail lacquer)
Hemorrhage
Half-and-half nail of renal disease

YELLOW
Yellow nail syndrome
Onycholysis

RED LUNULAE
Collagen vascular diseases
Systemic lupus erythematosus
Rheumatoid arthritis
Carbon monoxide poisoning
Cardiac failure
Cirrhosis
Psoriasis
Idiopathic trachyonychia

GRAY
Silver salts
Phenolphthalein
Malignant melanoma

WHITE
Arsenic (Mees' lines)
Partial onycholysis
Leukonychia (hereditary, traumatic, idiopathic)
Hypoalbuminemia

BROWN
Resorcinol (nail lacquer)
Film developer
Fungus infection
Tobacco staining

is necessary to reduce the size of the nail plate.[26,28] Avulsion of the complete nail is unnecessary.

Patient Education

Instructions in cutting the toenails are invaluable. The lateral margins must remain smooth. One should not cut the toenail until it grows beyond the distal end of the lateral nail fold. Trimming the nail straight across rather than in an arc is required. Patients and family should be instructed to avoid tight-fitting shoes. For infants, the clinician should explain to the family that a slow-growing nail plate penetrates a rapidly growing lateral nail fold.

Follow-up Visits

A visit in 1 month is useful in evaluating therapy and reemphasizing toenail care.

COLOR CHANGES IN THE NAIL

It is beyond the scope of this chapter to discuss nail color changes in detail, but Box 16-3 lists the disorders to be considered when specific color changes in the nail are encountered.

REFERENCES

1. Noronha PA, Zubkiv B: Nails and nail disorders in children and adults, *Am Fam Physician* 55:2129, 1997.

2. Pappert AS, Scher RK, Cohen JL: Nail disorders in children, *Pediatr Clin North Am* 38:921, 1991.

3. Farber EM, Nall L: Nail psoriasis, *Cutis* 64:309, 1999.

4. Akinduro OM, Venning VA, Burge SM: Psoriatic nail pitting in infancy, *Br J Dermatol* 130:800, 1994.

5. Tosti A et al: Prevalence of nail abnormalities in children with alopecia areata, *Pediatr Dermatol* 11:112, 1994.

6. Tosti A et al: Idiopathic trachyonychia (twenty-nail dystrophy): a pathological study of 23 patients, *Br J Dermatol* 131:866, 1994.

7. Tosti A et al: Trachyonychia associated with alopecia areata: a clinical and pathologic study, *J Am Acad Dermatol* 25:266, 1991.

8. Tosti A et al: Nail lichen planus: clinical and pathologic study of twenty-four patients, *J Am Acad Dermatol* 28:714, 1993.

9. Peluso AM et al: Lichen planus limited to the nails in childhood: case report and literature review, *Pediatr Dermatol* 10:36, 1993.

10. de Berker D, Dawber R: Childhood lichen planus, *Clin Exp Dermatol* 16:233, 1991.

11. Tosti A et al: Nail lichen striatus: clinical features and long-term follow up of five patients, *J Am Acad Dermatol* 36:908, 1997.

12. Clementz GC, Mancini AJ: Nail matrix arrest following hand-foot-mouth disease: a report of five children, *Pediatr Dermatol* 17:7, 2000.

13. Ben-Dayan D et al: Transverse nail ridgings (Beau's lines) induced by chemotherapy, *Acta Haematol* 91:89, 1994.

14. Griego RD, Orengo IF, Scher RK: Median nail dystrophy and habit tic deformity: are they different forms of the same disorder? *Int J Dermatol* 34:799, 1995.

15. Lubitz L: Nail biting, thumb sucking and other irritating behaviours in childhood, *Aust Fam Physician* 21:1090, 1992.

16. Huang PH, Paller AS: Itraconazole pulse therapy for dermatophyte onychomycosis in children, *Arch Pediatr Adolesc Med* 154:614, 2000.

17. Gupta AK et al: Onychomycosis in children: prevalence and management, *Pediatr Dermatol* 15:464, 1998.

18. Gupta AK et al: Onychomycosis in children: prevalence and treatment strategies, *J Am Acad Dermatol* 36:395, 1997.

19. Munro CS: Pachyonychia congenita: mutations and clinical presentation, *Br J Dermatol* 144:929, 2001.

20. McCarthy DJ: Congenital anomalies of the nail unit, *Clin Pod Med Surg* 12:319, 1995.

21. Telfer NR: Congenital and hereditary nail disorders, *Semin Dermatol* 10:2, 1991.

22. Krebsova A et al: Assignment of the gene for a new hereditary nail disorder, congenital nail dysplasia, to chromosome 17p13, *J Invest Dermatol* 115:664, 2000.

23. Akoz T et al: Congenital anonychia, *Plast Reconstr Surg* 101:551, 1998.

24. Knoers NV et al: Nail-patella syndrome: identification of mutations in the LMXB1 gene in Dutch families, *J Am Soc Nephrol* 11:1762, 2000.

25. Rockwell PG: Acute and chronic paronychia, *Am Fam Physician* 63:1113, 2001.

26. Piraccini BM et al: Congenital hypertrophy of the lateral nail folds of the hallux: clinical features and follow-up of seven cases, *Pediatr Dermatol* 17:348, 2000.

27. Katz AM: Congenital ingrown toenails, *J Am Acad Dermatol* 34:519, 1999.

28. Lazar L, Erez I, Katz S: A conservative treatment for ingrown toenails in children, *Pediatr Surg Int* 15:121, 1999.

29. Reyzelman AM et al: Are antibiotics necessary in the treatment of locally infected ingrown toenails? *Arch Fam Med* 9:930, 2000.

CHAPTER SEVENTEEN

Disorders of Pigmentation: The White Lesions and the Brown Lesions

An infant's skin color is always light at birth and becomes darker with age. Hyperpigmentation of the scrotum and of the linea alba is common in dark-skinned infants. Pigmentary changes are very common in infants and children. Loss of skin color or increase in skin color in an infant or child may cause concern in parents. Mongolian spots are expected in dark-skinned newborns and café-au-lait spots are very common. Hypopigmented lesions, in contrast, are uncommon in infants, with piebaldism or ash-leaf macules occurring in less than 1% of babies. Alterations in skin color in an infant or child are often the earliest clues to genetic diseases, such as the hypopigmented macules in tuberous sclerosis and café-au-lait spots in neurofibromatosis. Acquired pigmentary changes are also common. This chapter is divided into discussions of white lesions and brown lesions.

WHITE LESIONS
Congenital Circumscribed Flat Hypopigmentation or Depigmentation

Localized areas of hypopigmented or depigmented skin are uncommon in infants and newborns. A hypopigmented area of the skin is found in approximately 8 per 1000 live births, and a hypopigmented tuft of hair is found in 3 per 1000 live births (Fig. 17-1).[1]

Piebaldism and Waardenburg's syndrome

Clinical features. *Piebaldism* is the name designated to circumscribed areas of absence of pigment in the newborn.[2] This disorder is transmitted in an autosomal dominant pattern. Although completely devoid of melanocytes, the white patches of skin may be difficult to detect at birth because of the light color of most newborn skin. The use of a Wood's lamp to examine the infant's skin may accentuate differences in

color. A depigmented tuft of hair, usually in the frontal region, may also be seen.

Waardenburg's syndrome is an autosomal dominant syndrome that exhibits a white forelock, white patches on the skin, heterochromia of the irises, sensorineural deafness in one or both ears, and other defects.[3] There are four types of Waardenburg's syndrome. Type II does not exhibit dystopia canthorum but is more likely to have sensorineural hearing loss and heterochromia iridis than type I. In addition to the typical features of Waardenburg's type I, type III exhibits musculoskeletal abnormalities, and type IV is associated with Hirschsprung's disease.[3]

Differential diagnosis. The differential diagnosis of congenital circumscribed depigmentation includes piebaldism, Waardenburg's syndrome, ash-leaf or hypopigmented macules, nevus depigmentosus, and nevus anemicus. It is at times difficult in the newborn to distinguish hypopigmented macules from totally depigmented macules. Examination of the skin with a Wood's lamp will help accentuate the color differences. Biopsy of a depigmented lesion will reveal a total lack of melanocytes, whereas melanocytes will be present in a hypopigmented macule. A family history of piebaldism, Waardenburg's syndrome, or tuberous sclerosis is very helpful. Nevus depigmentosus is a congenital localized area of hypopigmentation secondary to hypofunctional melanocytes, whereas nevus anemicus is a hypopigmented macule caused by alterations in vascular tone. Nevus anemicus can be differentiated by loss of the borders by pressing with a glass microscope slide.

Pathogenesis. Piebaldism is caused by mutations in the *c-kit* protooncogene, which encodes for a transmem-

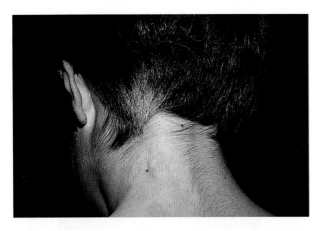

Fig. 17-1 Piebaldism. Segmental white patch on the neck with a tuft of white hair present from birth.

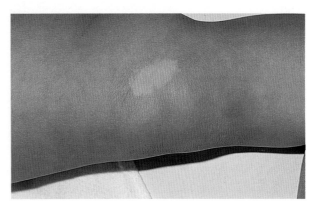

Fig. 17-2 Ash-leaf white macule of tuberous sclerosis.

brane tyrosine kinase cell surface receptor for stem cell factor.[2] Waardenburg's syndrome types I and III are caused by mutations in the *pax*-3 gene.[3] Type II is caused by a mutation in the MITF gene, and type IV is created by a mutation in either the EDN3, EDNRB, or SOX10 genes.[3] These genes are all involved in embryonic migration and survival of the organs affected in these syndromes.

Treatment. There is no treatment for the depigmentation of skin or hair in piebaldism or Waardenburg's syndrome. Patients with Waardenburg's syndrome should be referred to the appropriate specialists, depending on their associated problems.

Patient education. The genetic nature of these diseases should be explained to the patient and family. Those with Waardenburg's syndrome should be told of the associated difficulties.

Follow-up visits. No follow-up visits are necessary for the skin changes. Follow-up of a patient with Waardenburg's syndrome depends on the associated features.

White patches of tuberous sclerosis (ash-leaf macules)

Clinical features. The white spots of tuberous sclerosis appear as hypopigmented macules, which may be lance-ovate (ash-leaf macules), polygonal (thumbprint), or confetti-shaped (Fig. 17-2).[4,5] The macules range in size from 0.1 to 12 cm at their greatest diameter.[4,5] In the newborn period they may be the only sign of tuberous sclerosis, and in families in which this condition

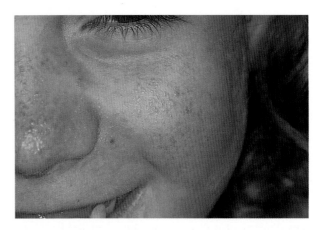

Fig. 17-3 Facial angiofibromas of tuberous sclerosis that mimic acne.

occurs, involvement of the newborn infant may be first suspected by the presence of these lesions. A Wood's lamp examination is often necessary to detect the lesions in the newborn. They may be found anywhere on the skin but are most predominant on the posterior trunk and the extremities. Hypopigmented macules by themselves are not diagnostic of tuberous sclerosis because 2 to 3 per 1000 otherwise normal newborns and 5% of Caucasians under age 45 years will also demonstrate these patches.[1,6] However, less than 1% of people will have two hypopigmented macules, and greater than three is exceedingly rare.[6]

The other signs and symptoms of tuberous sclerosis do not appear until later in life.[4,5] The angiofibromas found on the nose and face, which may mimic acne, usually begin to appear between the ages of 2 and 10 years (Fig. 17-3). Seizure disorders usually

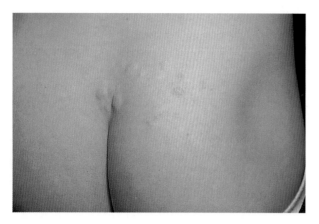

Fig. 17-4 Shagreen patch on sacral skin (tuberous sclerosis).

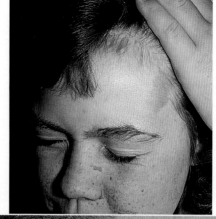

A

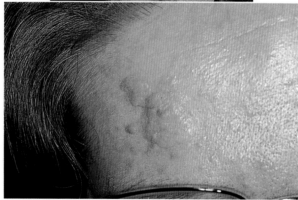

B

appear within the first year of life, but renal tumors and periungual fibromas usually appear after adolescence. A large connective tissue nevus, designated as a shagreen patch, is seen in almost half of the patients.[4,5] It may be present at birth, or it may become more apparent as the child becomes older. It is skin-colored to ivory-colored and feels thickened (Fig. 17-4). The fibrous forehead plaque present in 20% of patients (Fig. 17-5, A and B) is also one of the major features of tuberous sclerosis (Box 17-1).[4]

Differential diagnosis. The differential diagnosis of hypopigmented macules in the newborn includes nevus depigmentosus, nevus anemicus, piebaldism, and hypomelanosis of Ito. Nevus depigmentosus is generally a larger segmental area of hypopigmentation. The involved skin in piebaldism is totally depigmented. The areas of hypopigmentation in hypomelanosis of Ito are swirled and may cover a large portion of the body. In an infant without a family history of tuberous sclerosis, other criteria must be present to establish the diagnosis (see Box 17-1).[4-6]

Pathogenesis. Tuberous sclerosis is an autosomal dominant condition with nearly 100% penetrance.[4] Often a family history is difficult to obtain. The spontaneous mutation rate is as high as 60%.[4] Tuberous sclerosis is caused by mutations in the genes coding for the proteins hamartin (TS1) and tuberin (TS2). Similar phenotypes are seen with mutations in either gene.[4]

Treatment. There is no effective treatment for the hypopigmented macules. Although these lesions do contain melanocytes, they are hypofunctional; therefore they are more susceptible to ultraviolet radiation

Fig. 17-5 A, Red forehead plaque of tuberous sclerosis. **B,** Flesh-colored forehead plaque of tuberous sclerosis.

(UVR) and should be protected from excess sunlight. Children in whom the diagnosis of tuberous sclerosis has been documented are best managed in an appropriate multispecialty clinic.

Patient education. For those children with a family history of tuberous sclerosis and hypopigmented macules, the family should be told that it is highly likely that the child has tuberous sclerosis. In families without a history of tuberous sclerosis, discussion should be based on the number of hypopigmented macules present. A child with three or more hypopigmented macules is likely to have tuberous sclerosis and should be referred to the appropriate multispecialty clinic for evaluation for other stigmata of the disease. A child with one hypopigmented macule is less likely to have tuberous sclerosis. The parents should be told about the other findings associated with tuberous sclerosis.

Follow-up visits. Infants likely to have tuberous sclerosis should be followed in a multispecialty clinic. In-

Box 17-1 Diagnostic Criteria for Tuberous Sclerosis

MAJOR FEATURES
Facial angiofibromas or forehead plaque
Nontraumatic ungual or periungual fibroma
Hypomelanotic macules (three or more)
Shagreen patch
Multiple retinal nodular hamartomas
Cortical tuber
Subependymal giant-cell astrocytoma
Cardiac rhabdomyoma (single or multiple)
Lymphangiomatosis
Renal angiolipoma

MINOR FEATURES
Multiple, randomly distributed enamel pits in dental enamel
Hamartomatous rectal polyps
Bone cysts
Cerebral white matter radial migration lines
Gingival fibromas
Nonrenal hamartoma
Retinal achromic patch
Confetti skin lesions
Multiple renal cysts§

DEFINITE TUBEROUS SCLEROSIS COMPLEX
Either two major features or one major feature plus two minor features

PROBABLE TUBEROUS SCLEROSIS COMPLEX
One major plus one minor feature

POSSIBLE TUBEROUS SCLEROSIS COMPLEX
Either one major or two or more minor features.

Box 17-2 Differential Diagnosis of Patchy Pigment Loss in Children

Postinflammatory hypopigmentation
Pityriasis alba
Tinea versicolor
Vitiligo
White spots (ash-leaf macules), with or without tuberous sclerosis
Halo nevus
Piebaldism
Scleroderma morphea
Lichen sclerosus et atrophicus
Hypomelanosis of Ito
Waardenburg's syndrome
Chediak-Higashi syndrome

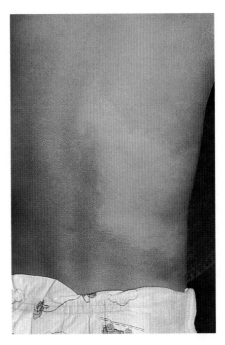

Fig. 17-6 Nevus depigmentosus. Quasidermatomal hypopigmentation.

fants with one or two hypopigmented macules should be evaluated on a yearly basis.

Nevus depigmentosus

Clinical features. Nevus depigmentosus generally presents at birth as a unilateral, localized, quasidermatomal patch of hypopigmentation (Fig. 17-6).[7,8] The borders may be regular or irregular and at times the lesions may be whorled. A negative family history for hypopigmented birthmarks is usually obtained.

Differential diagnosis. The differential diagnosis of nevus depigmentosus is the same as that for hypopigmented macules (Box 17-2).

Pathogenesis. Nevus depigmentosus should be considered a birthmark consisting of hypofunctional melanocytes.[7] In general, hypofunctioning melanocytes produce and transfer less melanin to the surrounding keratinocytes. Therefore the skin supplied by these melanocytes appears lighter than normal skin.

Treatment. As with the other forms of congenital hypopigmentation, there is no effective treatment. Because of the hypopigmentation in these areas, they should be chronically protected from excess UVR.

Patient education. Parents should be informed of the chronicity and benign nature of this birthmark. They should be told that the involved area of skin will be more sensitive to UVR than the child's normal skin, and that the area should be protected from excess sunlight.

Follow-up visits. Follow-up visits are not necessary.

Hypomelanosis of Ito

Clinical features. Newborns with hypomelanosis of Ito have bizarre hypopigmented swirls on their skin that follow Blaschko's lines (Figs. 17-7 and 17-8). The hypopigmentation may be quite extensive, involving an entire half of the body, or in some circumstances it may even be found bilaterally. Patients with hypomelanosis of Ito may have associated neurologic, skeletal, and/or ocular abnormalities. Because it is not a single entity, but a cutaneous sign of mosaicism, the exact incidence is unknown.[9,10]

Differential diagnosis. The differential diagnosis of hypomelanosis of Ito is the same as that for hypopigmented macules, but it is distinguished by the whorled pattern following Blaschko's lines and by involvement of an extensive portion of the body. Hypomelanosis of Ito is often confused with incontinentia pigmenti, linear and whorled hypermelanosis, or the linear hypermelanosis associated with the *Proteus* syndrome, all of which follow Blaschko's lines and have sharp midline demarcation of pigmentation. Hypomelanosis is lighter than normal skin color, rather than darker. Rarely, patients with incontinentia pigmenti will also have whorled hypopigmentation, making differentiation from hypomelanosis of Ito difficult.

Pathogenesis. The hypopigmentation is secondary to hypofunctioning of melanocytes. It is thought that a mishap early in embryogenesis is responsible for mosaicism, with two distinct genetically different melanocyte populations produced. *Hypomelanosis of Ito* is a nonspecific, descriptive term applied to individuals with extensive areas of whorled pigmentation but without a consistent genetic defect.[9,10]

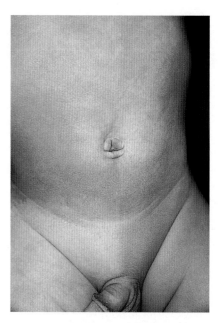

Fig. 17-7 Hypomelanosis of Ito. Whorls of hypopigmentation of the trunk with demarcation at midline.

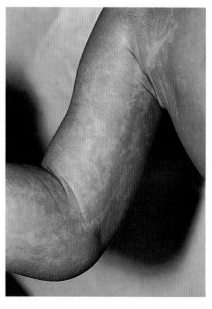

Fig. 17-8 Hypomelanosis of Ito. Whorls of hypopigmentation extending down an extremity.

Treatment. As with the other hypopigmented and depigmented problems, no treatment is available for the pigmentary changes. Associated neurologic, skeletal, or ophthalmologic problems should be referred to the appropriate specialist.

Patient education. The clinician should inform the parents that the number of infants who will have associated problems is unknown. They should also be told that no specific genetic defect has been identified.

Follow-up visits. Follow-up will depend on the associated abnormalities.

Nevus anemicus

Clinical features. Nevus anemicus presents as a solitary, localized, hypopigmented macule (Fig. 17-9).[11]

Differential diagnosis. Nevus anemicus is separated from the other forms of congenital hypopigmentation by diascopy. This will cause blanching of the surrounding normal skin and obscure the original borders of the lesion.

Pathogenesis. Unlike the other congenital hypopigmented macules, nevus anemicus is a problem of vascular control and not of melanocytes. The defect is thought to be a localized vascular hypersensitivity to catecholamines via α-adrenergic receptors.[11] Injection of α-blocking agents will temporarily return the skin to normal color.

Treatment. No treatment is necessary.

Patient education. The benign nature of the disorder should be discussed.

Follow-up visits. No follow-up visits are necessary.

Acquired Circumscribed Flat Hypopigmentation or Depigmentation
Vitiligo

Clinical features. Vitiligo is a patchy loss of skin pigment. The patches are flat, completely depigmented, and have distinct borders (Fig. 17-10). A small percentage of patients will have inflammatory vitiligo with raised erythematous borders. In dark-skinned patients, hypopigmented skin can be seen between the depigmented and normal skin (trichrome vitiligo). Hair within the patch of vitiligo is often depigmented as well. Fifty percent of cases of vitiligo start before the age of 18 years.[12] Vitiligo may be divided into generalized or segmental types. Generalized vitiligo usually begins acrally and symmetrically (Fig. 17-11). The extensor surface of the extremities and the face and neck are the areas most commonly involved. Generalized vitiligo continues to spread and develop new lesions for years,

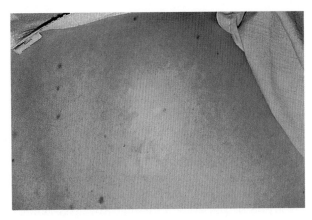

Fig. 17-9 Nevus anemicus. Hypopigmented macule that disappears with pressure on the surrounding skin.

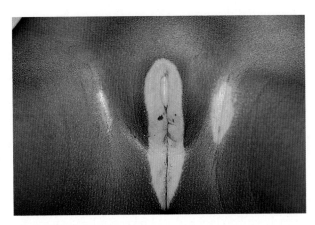

Fig. 17-10 Generalized vitiligo. Involvement of perineal and inguinal skin. Note the distinct borders.

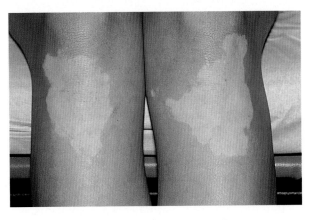

Fig. 17-11 Symmetric acral vitiligo.

although most patients will have less than 20% of the body surface involved.[13] Generalized vitiligo is associated with other autoimmune diseases, but they are rarely seen in childhood, and random screening should not be performed. Generalized vitiligo is the most common form seen in children, although segmental vitiligo is more common in children than in adults.[12] Segmental vitiligo affects only one part of the body. It spreads rapidly in that area and then stabilizes, usually within 1 year (Fig. 17-12). It is not associated with autoimmune diseases. Vitiligo of the face, eyelashes, and scalp hair in association with uveitis, dysacousis, and alopecia areata occurs in the rare Vogt-Koyanagi-Harada syndrome. Complete spontaneous repigmentation is unusual in vitiligo. Pigmentation returns first around hair follicles. In black and other dark-skinned children, vitiligo produces great distress.

Differential diagnosis. The conditions to be considered in the differential diagnosis of vitiligo are listed in Box 17-2. In contrast to vitiligo, the abnormally pigmented areas of pityriasis alba and tinea versicolor are hypopigmented rather than depigmented and often have scaling and indistinct borders. In postinflammatory hypopigmentation, irregular mottling of both hyperpigmented and hypopigmented areas is often seen. In piebaldism, lesions are present from birth. Patients with morphea and lichen sclerosus et atrophicus have immobilized skin and hypopigmentation.

Pathogenesis. An infiltrate of T lymphocytes is seen in early vitiligo lesions.[14,15] Long-standing inactive lesions of vitiligo always lack melanocytes.[15] Several theories have been postulated to explain the cause of vitiligo.[16] These include the autoimmune, autocytotoxic, neural, and genetic theories. It is likely that vitiligo is a heterogenous disorder with portions of all theories being correct in a given subset of patients.

Treatment. There is no entirely satisfactory treatment, and not all children will want treatment. Desire for treatment will depend on the age of the patient, location and extent of the disease, and cultural beliefs. Patients not wishing therapy should be advised about the lack of natural protection from the sun and the need for photoprotection. Cover-up cosmetics that match the child's skin color may be very beneficial for cosmetically sensitive areas. Potent topical steroids are effective in many patients.[17]

Psoralen, a furocoumarin derived from plants, is a potent stimulator of melanocytes. In combination

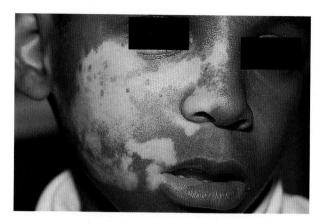

Fig. 17-12 Rapidly progressing segmental vitiligo.

with ultraviolet A radiation (PUVA [psoralen ultraviolet A-range]), psoralen has resulted in successful repigmentation in over half of the patients treated.[18] Even in those patients with a good result, repigmentation is seldom complete (Fig. 17-13, *A* and *B*). Psoralen is best used by an experienced dermatologist because it is easy to produce severe sunburns with this photosensitizing drug. Psoralens may be given either topically, if less than 20% of the body surface is involved, or orally. Topical psoralens must be used cautiously because of the high risk of phototoxic burns even when treatment is supervised by an experienced dermatologist. If systemic therapy is to be used, an ophthalmologic examination, complete blood cell count, liver function tests, and an antinuclear antibody test should be obtained before therapy. PUVA therapy requires 6 months of biweekly treatment to evaluate efficacy. If repigmentation occurs, treatments are often continued up to 1 year. Because the use of a photosensitizer combined with UVR enhances photoaging and increases the risk for the development of skin cancer, PUVA therapy is not recommended for children under 12 years of age.[18] Older, motivated children achieve the best results. Narrow band UVB (UVB 311 nm) has been successfully used to treat children with vitiligo.[19] It may be as effective as PUVA without many of the associated side effects.

Patient education. The clinician should discuss the natural history of vitiligo with the child and family and should also emphasize the need to follow a strict regimen in those motivated to undergo therapy.

Follow-up visits. During therapy, monthly visits are advisable.

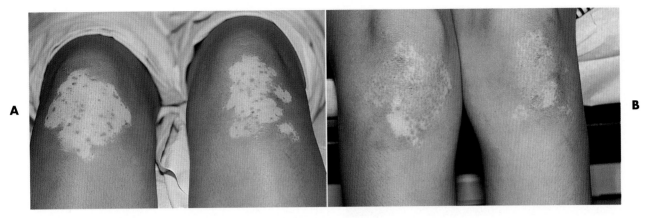

Fig. 17-13 A, Symmetric acral vitiligo before PUVA treatment. **B,** Same patient shows perifollicular pattern of repigmentation during PUVA therapy.

Pityriasis alba

Clinical features. Pityriasis alba is characterized by multiple oval, scaly, flat, hypopigmented patches on the face, extensor surface of arms, and upper trunk (Fig. 17-14).[20] The lesions range from 5 to 50 mm in diameter, and multiple patches may be seen. The borders are indistinct. Pityriasis alba occurs predominantly between the ages of 3 and 16 years, and up to 40% of all children may be affected. The lesions do not itch, and medical help is sought because of the child's appearance. It is particularly distressing in dark-skinned children. It is a chronic dermatitis and may be recurrent over several years.

Differential diagnosis. Pityriasis alba most closely mimics tinea versicolor, which can be excluded by findings in a negative potassium hydroxide (KOH) examination. (See Box 17-2 for the list of conditions to be considered in the differential diagnosis.)

Pathogenesis. On pathologic examination the lesion resembles that seen in chronic dermatitis. Hyperkeratosis, parakeratosis, spongiotic edema, and a lymphocytic infiltrate are seen. The cause of the hypopigmentation is not known, but it is likely related to inflammatory mediators that inhibit melanocyte function. Some regard this as a form of atopic dermatitis, but in many children it occurs without the features of atopic dermatitis.

Treatment. There is no satisfactory treatment for pityriasis alba. Bland lubricants and topical glucocorticosteroids have some influence on the disorder.

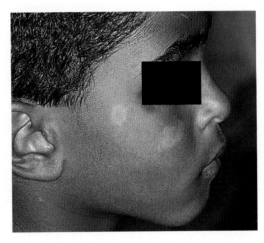

Fig. 17-14 Pityriasis alba. White, slightly scaly patches with indistinct borders on child's cheek.

Patient education. The natural history of this disorder should be emphasized.

Follow-up visits. Follow-up visits should be scheduled at monthly intervals if a treatment program is considered.

Postinflammatory hypopigmentation

Clinical features. After any inflammatory skin disease or injury to the skin, irregular hypopigmented areas may appear. The hypopigmentation is most obvious in dark-skinned people. The hypopigmented blotches are usually in a mottled pattern and may be associated with hyperpigmented areas (Figs. 17-15

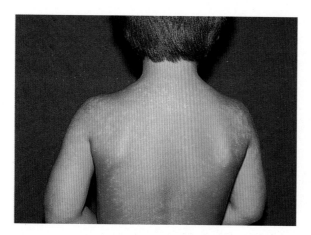

Fig. 17-15 Postinflammatory hypopigmentation with numerous hypopigmented patches on child's back.

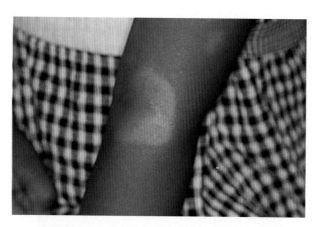

Fig. 17-16 Blotchy hypopigmentation after treatment for atopic dermatitis.

and 17-16). They resolve several months after the inflammatory disorder.

Differential diagnosis. Blotchy hypopigmentation associated with hyperpigmentation, and a history of a preceding inflammatory dermatosis differentiate this form of hypopigmentation (see Box 17-2).

Pathogenesis. Inflammatory injury to melanocytes and epidermal cells results in decreased pigment production and transfer.

Treatment. Treatment is not necessary.

Patient education. The patient should be informed of the nature of the pigment loss and told that recovery is expected.

> **Box 17-3 Classification of Oculocutaneous Albinism**
>
> **OCA1**
> Tyrosinase related
> No tyrosinase activity OCA1A
> Residual tyrosinase activity
> Yellow OCA1B
> Minimal pigment OCA1MP
> Temperature-sensitive OCA1TP
>
> **OCA2**
> Pink-eyed dilution
>
> **OCA3**
> TRP-1
>
> **DEFECTS IN MELANOSOMES AND OTHER LYSOSOMAL-LIKE STRUCTURES**
> Hermansky-Pudlak syndrome
> HPS1 gene
> β-3A subunit of Ap3
> Chediak-Higashi syndrome
> CHS-1 gene

Follow-up visits. Follow-up visits are unnecessary.

Diffuse hypopigmentation or depigmentation: albinism

Clinical features. Albinism can be separated into those individuals with eye, skin, and hair abnormalities (oculocutaneous albinism [OCA]) and those with only eye involvement (ocular albinism [OA]). There are at least four classes of OCA, with multiple subsets within each class (Box 17-3).[21-23] All variants of OCA have defects in melanin synthesis, resulting in reduction or total absence of pigmentation (Fig. 17-17). Regardless of the pigment defect, all patients with OCA will have visual abnormalities.[21] All newborns with OCA1 have fine white hair, pink skin, blue irides, severe nystagmus, and photophobia. The skin and hair in patients with OCA1A will remain white their entire life. Patients with variants of OCA1 may develop darker hair, skin, and eyes; freckles; lentigines; and nevi. In the other classes of OCA, hair and skin pigment may be present at birth and increase with age. Pigmented nevi and freckles commonly develop in these patients. The phenotypic expression of these forms of OCA is quite variable. Hermansky-Pudlak is albinism associated with bleed-

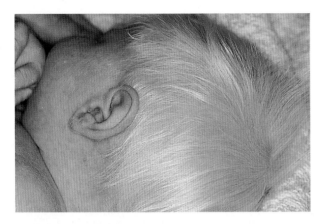

Fig. 17-17 OCA1. Newborn with hair and skin totally devoid of pigmentation.

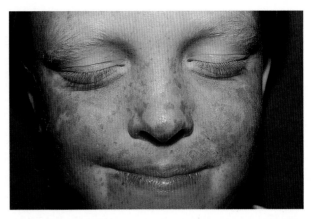

Fig. 17-18 Freckles. Note the sunburn between freckled areas.

ing caused by abnormal platelet aggregation, whereas Chediak-Higashi is albinism associated with susceptibility to infection as a result of dysfunctional leukocyte degranulation.

Differential diagnosis. The diagnosis of OCA1 in a child with white skin and hair and blue eyes is usually obvious. The other classes may be difficult to diagnose in light-skinned whites. The major differential is between the classes of OCA.

Pathogenesis. OCA1 is caused by mutations in the genes encoding for the protein tyrosinase.[21-23] OCA1A is due to complete lack of functional tyrosinase. In the variants of OCA1, partial tyrosinase function remains. Tyrosinase is a major enzyme necessary for the formation of the pigment melanin. OCA2 is caused by defects in the human homologue to the mouse pink-eyed dilution *(p)* gene.[24] The function of this gene product has not yet been determined, but may be involved in the regulation of melanosomal pH.[24] OCA3 is caused by mutations in the gene coding for the protein TRP-1. TRP-1 is another enzyme involved in the formation of melanin. Hermansky-Pudlak syndrome is caused by mutations in either the HPS1 gene or the gene encoding the β-3A sub unit of AP3. Chediak-Higashi syndrome is caused by mutations in the CHS1 gene. Patients with Hermansky-Pudlak syndrome or the Chediak-Higashi syndrome have defects in melanosomes and other lysosomal-like structures.

Treatment. No treatment is available for the pigmentary changes. Because of the lack of pigmentation, sun protection is required for all children with albinism.

Patient education. The family should be referred to an ophthalmologist and to the appropriate specialists for genetic counseling and identification of the class of OCA expressed. The need for photoprotection should be stressed.

Follow-up visits. Follow-up visits are determined by the type of OCA and the degree of ocular involvement.

BROWN LESIONS

In considering a hyperpigmented state, one should first determine whether the hyperpigmentation is circumscribed or diffuse.

Circumscribed Flat Hyperpigmentation
Clinical features

Freckles. Freckles are small, 1- to 5-mm, light brown, pigmented macules that are UVR responsive and occur in sun-exposed skin (Fig. 17-18).[25,26] They are autosomal dominant and first appear at age 3 to 5 years, predominantly on the face and extensor surface of the extremities. They are most frequent in fair-skinned, light-haired, blue-eyed children. They become less common with age.

Lentigines. Lentigines are brown or brown-black, 1- to 2-mm macules found sparsely scattered over the body, including the mucous membranes (Fig. 17-19).[27] They do not change with sun exposure. They usually first appear during school age. Lentigines on the lips (Fig. 17-20) are also seen in the autosomal dominant Peutz-Jeghers syndrome associated with multiple bowel polyps and an increased risk of gastrointestinal and genitourinary carcinomas.[28]

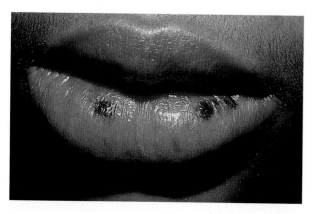

Fig. 17-19 Lip lentigines not associated with the Peutz-Jeghers syndrome.

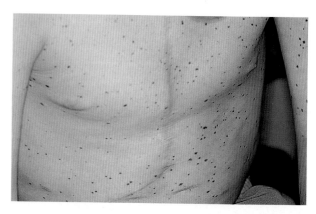

Fig. 17-21 Infant with multiple lentigines and the LEOPARD syndrome. Note scars from repair of pulmonary stenosis.

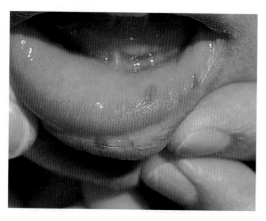

Fig. 17-20 Lip lentigines in an adolescent with the Peutz-Jeghers syndrome.

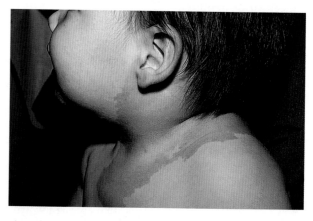

Fig. 17-22 Café-au-lait spot. Large lesion on a child's neck.

Multiple lentigines are associated with cardiac abnormalities in the so-called *LEOPARD syndrome* (*l*entigines, *e*lectrocardiograph abnormalities, *o*cular hypertelorism, *p*ulmonary stenosis, *a*bnormalities of the genitalia, growth *r*etardation, *d*eafness) (Fig. 17-21).[29] Central facial lentigines have been described in association with cardiac defects and malignancies in the NAME (Carney complex) syndrome (*n*evi, *a*trial myxomas, *m*yxoid neurofibroma, *e*phelides).[30]

Café-au-lait spots. Café-au-lait spots are tan, flat, oval macules with distinct borders (Fig. 17-22). They frequently have a diameter greater than 0.5 cm. Multiple café-au-lait spots occur in type 1 neurofibromatosis (NF-1) (Box 17-4). In children age 6

or older, café-au-lait macules over 0.5 cm are a major criterion for NF-1 (see Box 17-4) (Figs. 17-23 and 17-24).[4] Rarely, families have autosomal-dominant, multiple, café-au-lait macules without other stigmata of neurofibromatosis.[31] Café-au-lait spots are rarely present at birth, but increase in number with age through the teen years. They are seen in 25% to 35% of children between the ages of 4 and 18 years.[31,32] They are also seen in Albright's syndrome, tuberous sclerosis, and the *Proteus* syndrome.[33] The *Proteus* syndrome can be mistaken for NF-1 because of the skeletal overgrowth and large hamartomas that are confused with plexiform neurofibromas.[34] In NF-1, more café-au-lait spots appear with age and may be accompanied by soft cutaneous neurofibromas (Fig. 17-25).

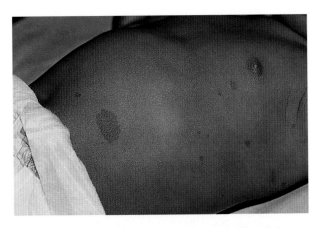

Fig. 17-23 Numerous café-au-lait spots on the abdomen and chest of a child with neurofibromatosis type 1.

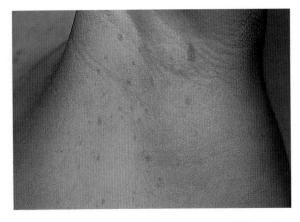

Fig. 17-24 Numerous café-au-lait spots in a child's axilla in neurofibromatosis type 1.

Box 17-4 Diagnostic Criteria for Neurofibromatosis Type 1

Two or more of the following must be found:
- Six or more café-au-lait spots greater than 5 mm in diameter in prepubertal children; greater than 1.5 mm in postpubertal children
- Two or more neurofibromas of any type
- One plexiform neurofibroma
- Axillary freckling
- Inguinal freckling
- Two or more Lisch nodules (iris hamartomas)
- Distinctive osseous lesion, such as sphenoid dysplasia or thinning of a long bone, with or without pseudoarthrosis
- A first-degree relative with NF-1

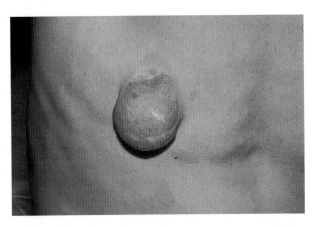

Fig. 17-25 Soft cutaneous neurofibroma surrounded by café-au-lait spots in an adolescent with neurofibromatosis type 1.

Mongolian spots. The mongolian spot is a blue-black macule found over the lumbosacral area in up to 90% of Asian, black, and American Indian babies. They are occasionally noted over the shoulders and back and may extend over the buttocks and extremities (Fig. 17-26).[35] The difference in the pigmentation from normal skin pigment becomes less obvious as a newborn's skin darkens in color. Some traces of mongolian spots may persist into adult life.

Nevus of Ota, Nevus of Ito. Flat, blue-black, speckled pigmentary discoloration may be noted in the skin surrounding the eye (nevus of Ota) (Fig. 17-27) or around the chest and shoulder (nevus of Ito). Most

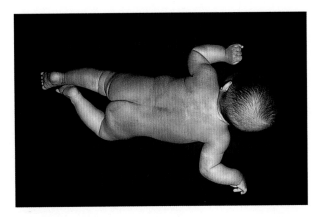

Fig. 17-26 Mongolian spots. Extensive lesions over the back and buttocks.

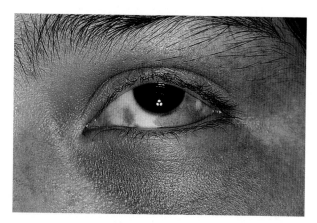

Fig. 17-27 Nevus of Ota. Speckled blue macules in the periorbital skin and sclera.

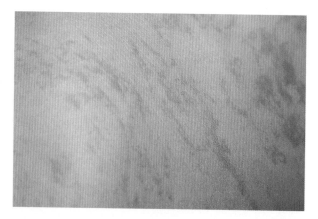

Fig. 17-28 Linear and whorled hypermelanosis. Brown whorls over the trunk of a child.

cases are present at birth, but some are acquired.[36] The sclera may be involved in nevus of Ota.

Linear and whorled nevoid hypermelanosis. Hypermelanotic macules arranged in streaks corresponding to Blaschko's lines, with sharp demarcation at the midline, characterize linear and whorled nevoid hypermelanosis (Fig. 17-28).[37]

Postinflammatory hyperpigmentation. In children with dark skin, any inflammatory skin disorder may heal with hyperpigmentation. Often the pigmentation persists for months.

Differential diagnosis

Freckles are small, acquired, sun-responsive macules, whereas lentigines and café-au-lait macules are not related to sun exposure. Café-au-lait macules are larger

---

> **Box 17-5** Differential Diagnosis of Circumscribed, Flat Pigmented Lesions
>
> **ACQUIRED**
> Freckles
> Lentigo
> Café-au-lait spot
> Junctional melanocytic nevi
> Postinflammatory hyperpigmentation
>
> **CONGENITAL**
> Mongolian spot
> Nevus of Ota, Ito
> Linear and whorled nevoid hypermelanosis

and lighter brown than lentigines. Skin biopsy may differentiate the acquired flat pigmented lesions from one another, but should only be done if it will help delineate one of the associated genetic syndromes. Mongolian spots, nevus of Ota, and nevus of Ito are blue-black, with location being used to differentiate.[38] Linear and whorled nevoid hypermelanosis is obvious by the extent of the condition and the pigmentation occurring along the lines of Blaschko. Unlike incontinentia pigmenti, linear and whorled nevoid hypermelanosis is not preceded by a vesicular or verrucous stage. The conditions to be included in the differential diagnosis are listed in Box 17-5.

Pathogenesis

Freckles. Freckles are areas with increased pigment secondary to sun exposure.[22]

Lentigines. In lentigines, increased numbers of melanocytes are dispersed along the basal layer of the epidermis, and the epidermal rete ridges are elongated. The majority of cases of Peutz-Jeghers syndrome are caused by mutations in the LKB1 gene, which encodes a multifunctional serine-threonine kinase.[39] The Carney complex is caused by mutations in the PRKAR1A gene, which encodes for the type 1A regulatory subunit of protein kinase A.[40] The gene for the LEOPARD syndrome has not yet been identified.

Café-au-lait spots. In café-au-lait spots, melanocyte activity is increased, as is the melanin in melanocytes and in epidermal cells. The number of melanocytes is not increased. Despite this in vivo increase in function, no differences have been demonstrated in vitro in melanocytes grown from café-au-lait macules compared with melanocytes from normal skin. Neurofibromatosis is an autosomal dominant disease caused by mutations in the gene that encodes a protein, neurofibromin, which acts as a tumor suppressor.

Mongolian spots. The pathology of mongolian spots consists of spindle-shaped cells that contain pigment and are located between collagen fibers deep within the dermis.

Nevus of Ota, nevus of Ito. Similar to mongolian spots, nevus of Ota and nevus of Ito have spindle-shaped melanocytes found within the dermis.

Linear and whorled nevoid hypermelanosis. With linear and whorled nevoid hypermelanosis, epidermal melanocytes are increased in number and keratinocytes have increased melanin in the affected area. It is thought that two genetically distinct populations of melanocytes are produced.

Postinflammatory hyperpigmentation: With postinflammatory hyperpigmentation, the excess pigment is related to loss of pigment from damaged epidermal keratinocytes and melanocytes into the dermis, where the large polymer melanin sits free in the dermis or is engulfed by macrophages to form melanophages. Breakdown of the dermal pigment is slow.

Treatment

No treatment is necessary, but cosmetically bothersome lesions may be treated with any of the q-switched lasers.[41]

Patient education

The common and benign nature of these pigmented areas should be emphasized. Parents of children with multiple café-au-lait macules should be told of the possibility of NF-1.

Follow-up visits

Children with multiple café-au-lait macules should be referred for evaluation for NF-1, otherwise follow-up visits are unnecessary.

Melanocytic Nevi

There are two distinct forms of melanocytic nevi with entirely different natural histories. These are congenital melanocytic nevi (CMN) and acquired nevi. They will be considered separately.

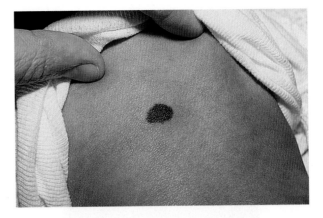

Fig. 17-29 Small congenital nevus.

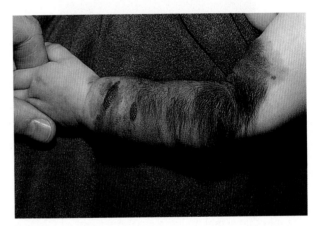

Fig. 17-30 Large congenital nevus with long, pigmented hair and a mixture of tan, brown, and blue within the lesion.

Congenital melanocytic nevi

Clinical features. Skin-colored to tan, or brown, solitary papules with smooth surfaces represent CMN. Most such nevi present at birth are small, measuring less than 1.5 cm at their greatest diameter (Fig. 17-29).[42,43] Large melanocytic nevi, which are defined as being greater than 5% of the body surface area, are very uncommon, occurring in 1 in 20,000 live births. Large melanocytic nevi are often not uniform in color and may contain flat tan areas, brown areas, blue-black plaques, and pigmented, long, thick hair (Fig. 17-30 and 17-31). Numerous smaller nevi located at skin sites distant from the large nevi are found. These "satellite lesions" are more often uniform in color and may arise throughout childhood. Neurocutaneous melanosis is the association of a giant CMN overlying the scalp or spine, with central

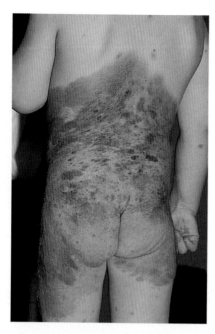

Fig. 17-31 Large congenital nevus in the so called "bathing suit" distribution.

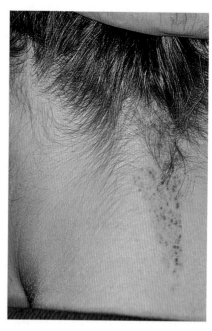

Fig. 17-32 Nevus spilus. Flat, tan lesion containing numerous small, dark brown areas.

nervous system involvement. The results of magnetic resonance imaging of the brain are abnormal in approximately 25% of these children, but only 1% to 2% will be symptomatic.[44] Erosions and ulcerations may be seen in neonates with large CMN, but these are not changes that signal malignancy.[45] A variant of CMN is the nevus spilus.[46] Nevus spilus is a café-au-lait macule studded with small, dark, raised nevi (Fig. 17-32).

Differential diagnosis. Occasionally, a congenital melanocytic nevus will be flat at birth and will appear as a café-au-lait macule, but with time it becomes raised. Congenital smooth muscle and pilar hamartomas may also present as light brown plaques with fine hair and may be difficult to distinguish from CMN. Histological examination will differentiate.

Pathogenesis. Nests of pigment cells are found within the epidermis and dermis. Sometimes the pigment cells are large and unusually shaped, making it difficult to distinguish benign from malignant changes.[47] In giant CMN, pigment cells may populate the entire dermis and extend around hair and eccrine sweat structures. Most authorities consider congenital nevocellular nevi to be developmental errors in pigment-cell proliferation and migration. The pathogenesis of CMN is unknown. There is a slightly increased fre-

quency of large, congenital pigmented lesions in blacks and in those infants born to mothers with acute illnesses. There is no correlation of large pigmented nevi with gender, twins, parental consanguinity, parental age, birth order, radiation exposure, or drug intake.

Treatment. The management of large CMN is controversial. Patients with large CMN are at risk for the development of melanoma; however, many of these melanomas do not occur in the skin.[43,47,48] In these instances removal of the CMN from the skin would not be beneficial. Currently it is advisable to take into consideration the potential for cosmetic improvement and surgical risk before recommending removal of such lesions. There is no compelling reason to remove these in the child's first year. Small lesions can be removed during adolescence. There is no urgency to remove small congenital nevi before puberty. There is a very small risk of melanoma arising in a small congenital nevus in late adolescence or in young adults.[43,49]

Patient education. There is no uniform agreement among authorities as to the best management for congenital nevi, and the clinician should explain to the parents both the positive and negative reasons for treatment. CMN will grow proportionately with the child, and this should not be a concern. Satellite lesions may continue to develop throughout childhood. Any change in one portion of the CMN should be evaluated to determine the need for biopsy. In patients with large CMN overlying the scalp and spine, the small risk of neurocutaneous melanosis should be discussed.

Follow-up visits. Yearly visits are recommended for treatment of large CMN, and additional visits are recommended any time there is a nonproportional change in the birthmark. Children with large CMN overlying the scalp or spine should be evaluated by a neurologist if there are any signs of CNS or developmental abnormalities.

Acquired melanocytic nevi (common moles)

Clinical features. The development of acquired melanocytic nevi in white children is related to genetic susceptibility and sun exposure. This is not true for nonwhite children, who develop fewer nevi.[50] There are families in which members develop numerous, atypical nevi beginning in childhood. Members of these families are at markedly increased risk for the development of melanoma.[43,51] In white families not affected by the atypical mole syndrome, the development of moles is related to skin type, hair and eye color, freckles, and sun exposure.[52-54] Those children with light skin, light hair and eye color, many freckles, and a history of numerous sunburns develop the highest number of nevi.[54] Children with similar genetic backgrounds who are exposed to more UVR will develop more nevi.[54]

To differentiate benign moles from melanoma, it is important to understand the changes that occur during the development of common acquired nevi.[55] Acquired melanocytic nevi begin as flat, well-demarcated, brown to brown-black lesions (Fig. 17-33). These are called *junctional melanocytic nevi.* They characteristically have regular borders and may have a light brown rim (rim mole) and/or a dark brown center. Rim moles are commonly seen in the scalp. They usually measure 2 to 5 mm but may occasionally be larger. Most nevi found in infants and children are junctional nevi. If many nevi appear before age 5 years, the child is likely to have a large number of moles after puberty. After puberty the number of moles continues to increase. Enlargement and darkening of nevi with growth spurts and puberty is also a common event.

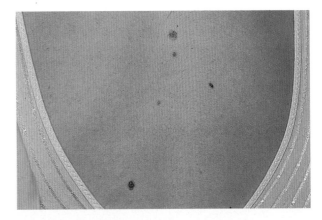

Fig. 17-33 Back of an adolescent with multiple benign junctional and compound nevi.

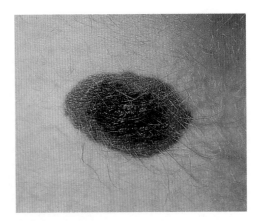

Fig. 17-34 Intradermal nevus, darker in the center.

Approximately 20% of junctional melanocytic nevi will progress to compound melanocytic nevi, which appear as small, raised, dome-shaped, brown to brown-black papules (see Fig. 17-33). There are several frequent clinical variants of compound nevi. In some of these the center will be raised and darker than the periphery (fried egg mole) (Fig. 17-34). Compound nevi may also appear skin-colored, with little melanin production (Fig. 17-35). Neither of these changes is worrisome.

Dermal nevi are usually few in number before the preadolescent growth period, averaging one or two. A less-common type of dermal nevi is the so called *Becker's nevus.* This is a large, pigmented, hairy nevus that occurs most commonly over the shoulder and is often first noticed in adolescence (Fig. 17-36). It may be seen in other locations.

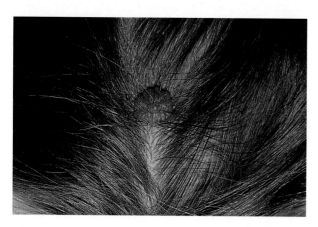

Fig. 17-35 Nonpigmented intradermal nevus of the scalp.

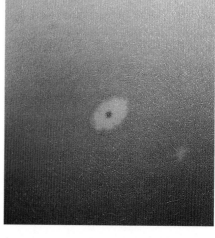

Fig. 17-37 Halo nevus. Loss of pigment around regressing central intradermal nevus.

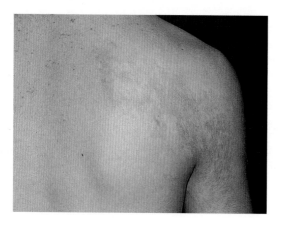

Fig. 17-36 Becker's nevus on the back and arm of an adolescent male.

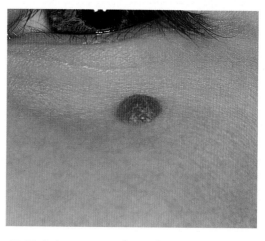

Fig. 17-38 Spitz nevus. Red papule on the face of a child.

A halo may appear around a nevus that is regressing in childhood (Fig. 17-37), producing the "halo nevus." This change may occur during any stage of nevus development. Multiple halo nevi may be seen in an individual, and this is at times associated with vitiligo.

There are two other uncommon types of benign nevi that are sometimes confused with melanoma.

The Spitz nevus begins as a solitary red or red-brown nodule, usually on the extremities or face (Fig. 17-38). Blue nevi are blue to blue-black, 4- to 10-mm solitary papules (Fig. 17-39).

ATYPICAL NEVI. No single change takes place when a common nevus becomes malignant, but rather a spectrum of changes are encompassed by the so called *atypical* or *dysplastic nevus*.[56] Clinically, these lesions are usually over 5 mm in diameter, with a variegated tan to brown color on a pink background and an impalpable, irregular ill-defined border (Fig. 17-40). They occur in the familial melanoma syndrome and in patients with melanoma who do not have a family history of melanoma or the clinical phenotype of the familial melanoma syndrome. They may also be seen as isolated moles occurring in the general population.

MALIGNANT MELANOMA. Malignant melanomas are rare in childhood, and although still uncommon they are being seen with increased frequency in adolescents.[57]

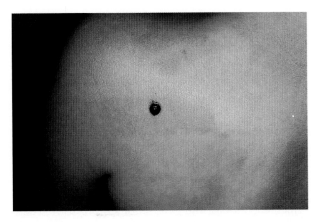

Fig. 17-39 Blue nevus. Blue-black papule on a child's shoulder.

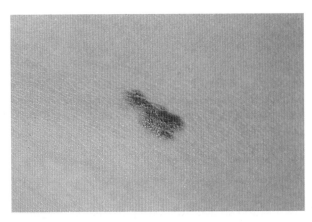

Fig. 17-41 Severely atypical nevus with marked abnormalities in symmetry and borders.

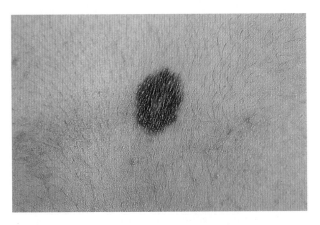

Fig. 17-40 Atypical nevus with irregular borders and pink background.

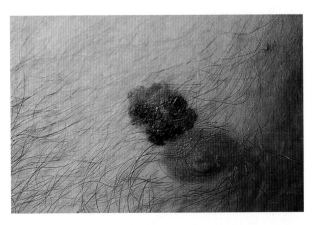

Fig. 17-42 Malignant melanoma on the chest of an adolescent male.

One must be familiar with the ABCDs of melanoma (Box 17-6), but at times these characteristics can be difficult to apply to prepubertal children (Fig. 17-41). Some pigmented nevi in children will be asymmetrical with irregular borders. Changes in color must also be evaluated carefully. The pigmented lesion that changes from light brown to dark brown is not cause for worry. Within a single brown lesion the appearance of red, white, and blue colors (Fig. 17-42) is a worrisome change. The most important clinical feature is rapid, progressive growth of a pigmented lesion disproportionate to the other nevi. Ulceration and bleeding are far-advanced signs. In familial malignant melanoma, multiple primary melanomas may be found, usually first appearing in late adolescence or early adult life.[51] There is a correlation with skin type,

---

Box 17-6   ABCDs of Melanoma Detection

Asymmetry: the lesion is not round, but has an irregular shape
Border: the border is not even, but notched and irregular
Color: areas of red, white, and/or blue within a brown area
Diameter: greater than 10 mm
A rapid change in any of these parameters over a few weeks is a matter for concern.

large numbers of nevi, and a history of excess sun exposure in childhood and melanoma later in life.[43,53,56]

Differential diagnosis. The conditions to be considered in the differential diagnosis of circumscribed, acquired pigmented lesions are listed in Box 17-7. Histology will differentiate these pigmented lesions from one another.

Pathogenesis

JUNCTIONAL, COMPOUND, AND DERMAL MELANOCYTIC NEVI. Clumps of increased numbers of melanocytes are located at the dermal-epidermal junction in junctional nevi. Dermal melanocytic nevi represent accumulations of groups of immature melanocytes within the mid to upper dermis. When associated with clumps of melanocytes at the dermal-epidermal junction, such a nevus is called a *compound nevus.* Development of these types of nevi is related to genetic background and amount of sun exposure. Spitz nevi are composed of collections of melanocytes with irregular cytoplasmic and nuclear shapes and are located throughout the dermis. These nevi are associated with a proliferation of blood vessels. The bizarre nuclear shapes often result in confusion with melanoma. These histologic changes are categorized as *spindle* and *epithelioid.* Not all spindle and epithelioid nevi are Spitz nevi. Therefore when a pathology report indicates a spindle and epithelioid nevus, clinical correlation is extremely important.

Box 17-7	**Differential Diagnosis of Circumscribed, Acquired Pigmented Lesions**

Junctional melanocytic nevus
Dermal melanocytic nevus
Compound melanocytic nevus
Atypical melanocytic nevus
Spitz nevus
Blue nevus
Malignant melanoma
Pyogenic granuloma
Mastocytoma
Dermatofibroma
Juvenile xanthogranuloma

Atypical nevi display architectural atypia and cytologic dysplasia. These changes encompass a wide spectrum between common nevi and melanoma.

In malignant melanomas the tumor originates at the dermal-epidermal junction and has a radial growth phase before it demonstrates a vertical growth phase. The tumor cells within a melanoma show great variation in size and shape and invade epidermal structures. The depth of invasion is an important prognostic factor and is the basis for histologic classifications of melanomas. Familial melanoma has been linked to the cell cycle regulator CDKN2A gene, which encodes for the p16 tumor suppressor.[50] There are compelling data to support a role of sunlight in melanomas. An experienced dermatopathologist should review all pigmented lesions in which the diagnosis of melanoma is considered.

A blue nevus represents clumps of mature melanocytes located in the deep dermis.

Becker's nevus is considered a hamartoma of hair follicles and associated arrector pilae muscles. In Becker's nevus the number of melanocytes is slightly increased, and melanin is seen throughout the epidermis.

Treatment. In any raised pigmented lesion in which melanoma is suspected, surgical excision is the treatment of choice. Although malignant melanoma is rare in childhood it is becoming more common in adolescents. Therefore a high index of suspicion of malignant melanoma should be maintained for any rapidly growing pigmented skin lesion in postpubertal children. Any excised skin lesion, particularly pigmented skin lesions, should be sent to a pathologist. In childhood or adolescence it is unnecessary to remove common melanocytic nevi that are uniform in shape and color.

Patient education. Families with familial melanoma traits and with sporadic melanomas must be counseled regarding the high risk for the development of melanoma, the importance of routine follow-up, and the need for excision of any changing lesion. Parents of children with light skin, light hair, blue eyes, and freckles need to be told of the correlation between sun exposure in childhood and the increased risk of developing melanoma later in life. Proper sun protection programs should be discussed. The risk of melanoma in a child who has a solitary atypical nevus without a family history of melanoma is unknown. If a lesion is removed, the nature of the lesion can be explained to the patient after confirmation by the pathologist.

Follow-up visits. Adolescents with the familial melanoma syndrome or with a family history of sporadic melanoma should be followed yearly. If a lesion has been excised, a visit 1 to 2 weeks after surgical removal is necessary to inform the patient of the diagnosis and suggested further treatment, if any.

Acanthosis Nigricans
Clinical features

Acanthosis nigricans is characterized by hyperpigmentation and a velvety thickening of irregular folds of skin of the posterior neck and the axilla (Figs. 17-43 and 17-44). It is common in Native American,

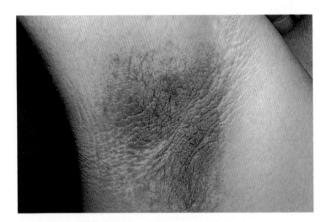

Fig. 17-43 Acanthosis nigricans of a child's axilla. Velvety, brown rows of hyperpigmentation.

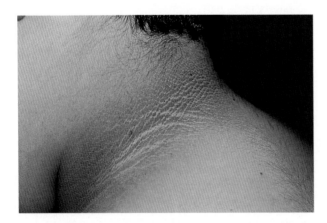

Fig. 17-44 Acanthosis nigricans of a child's neck.

African American, and Hispanic adolescents.[58] Often parents complain that their child's skin is dirty and cannot be cleaned. Small papillomatous growths (skin tags) may be found within the irregular folds. Acanthosis nigricans also can be found in other skin areas, such as elbows, inguinal creases, areolae, and knuckles. It is associated with obesity and correlates well with hyperinsulinemia and insulin resistance.[59] With obesity, the age of onset correlates with the onset of obesity. Less commonly it is associated with other endocrinologic abnormalities and with various syndromes.[60]

Differential diagnosis

Acanthosis nigricans is so distinctive that it is seldom misdiagnosed. A lichenified chronic dermatitis may mimic.

Pathogenesis

The epidermis is papillomatous with no abnormality of pigmentation. The majority of children with acanthosis nigricans will have obesity and insulin resistance.[59,60]

Treatment

In obese adolescents, weight loss has resulted in reversal of the acanthosis nigricans and may decrease the risk for future problems associated with type II diabetes mellitus.[61,62]

Patient education

Parents should be told that acanthosis nigricans is not dirt and is unrelated to hygiene. If the child is obese, the relationship of the skin condition to obesity should be emphasized, and the institution of a weight-control program should be considered. Nonobese children with signs of associated hyperandrogenism should be referred for endocrine evaluation.

Follow-up visits

Follow-up visits should be determined by therapy.

Diffuse Hyperpigmentation

Diffuse hyperpigmentation is rare in infancy and childhood. Pigmentation of the scrotum, linea alba, and palmar creases may occur. Diffuse hyperpigmentation may occur as a result of endocrine disturbances, such as adrenal insufficiency, with overproduction of adrenocorticotropic hormone (ACTH) and its melanocyte-stimulating fragments,

> ### Box 17-8   Differential Diagnosis of Diffuse Hyperpigmentation
>
> Addison's disease
> Acromegaly
> Cushing's syndrome of pituitary origin
> Thyrotoxicosis
> ACTH administration
> Subacute bacterial endocarditis
> Lymphomas and leukemia
> Scleroderma, dermatomyositis
> Renal failure
> Hemochromatosis
> Familial progressive hyperpigmentation
> Chronic arsenism
> Argyria

or hyperfunction of the pituitary. Box 17-8 lists the conditions to be included in the differential diagnosis of diffuse hyperpigmentation.

REFERENCES

1. Alper JC, Holmes LB: The incidence and significance of birthmarks in a cohort of 4641 newborns, *Pediatr Dermatol* 1:58, 1983.
2. Richards KA et al: A novel KIT mutation results in piebaldism with progressive depigmentation, *J Am Acad Dermatol* 44:288, 2001.
3. Dourmishev AL et al: Waardenburg syndrome, *Int J Dermatol* 38:656, 1999.
4. Arbuckle HA, Morelli JG: Pigmentary disorders: update on neurofibromatosis-1 and tuberous sclerosis, *Curr Opin Pediatr* 12:354, 2000.
5. Jozwiak S et al: Skin lesions in children with tuberous sclerosis complex: the prevalence, natural course and diagnostic significance, *Int J Dermatol* 37:911, 1998.
6. Vanderhooft SL et al: Prevalence of hypopigmented macules in a healthy population, *J Pediatr* 129:355, 1996.
7. Lee HS, Chun YS, Hann SK: Nevus depigmentosus: clinical features and histopathologic characteristics in 67 patients, *J Am Acad Dermatol* 40:21, 1999.
8. DiLernia V: Segmental nevus depigmentosus: analysis of 20 patients, *Pediatr Dermatol* 16:349, 1999.
9. Ruggieri M, Pavone L: Hypomelanosis of Ito: clinical syndrome or just phenotype? *J Child Neuro* 15:635, 2000.
10. Kuster W, Konug A: Hypomelanosis of Ito: no entity, but a cutaneous sign of mosaicism, *Am J Med Genet* 85:348, 1999.
11. Ahkami RN, Schwartz RA: Nevus anemicus, *Dermatology* 198:327, 1999.
12. Morelli JG: Vitiligo in children: treatment options, *Dermatol Ther* 2:93, 1997.
13. Handa S, Kaur I: Vitiligo: clinical findings in 1436 patients, *Int J Dermatol* 26:653, 1999.
14. van den Wijngaard R et al: Local immune response in skin of generalized vitiligo patients: destruction of melanocytes is associated with the prominent presence of CLA+ T cells at the perilesional site, *Lab Invest* 80:1299, 2000.
15. Le Poole IC et al: Presence of T cells and macrophages in inflammatory vitiligo parallels melanocyte disappearance, *Am J Pathol* 148:1219, 1996.
16. Kovacs SO: Vitiligo, *J Am Acad Dermatol* 38:647, 1998.
17. Njoo MD et al: Nonsurgical repigmentation therapies in vitiligo: meta-analysis of the literature, *Arch Dermatol* 134:1532, 1998.
18. Halder RM, Young CM: New and emerging therapies for vitiligo, *Dermatol Clin* 18:79, 2000.
19. Njoo MD, Bos JD, Westerhof W: Treatment of generalized vitiligo in children with narrow-band (TL-01) UVB radiation, *J Am Acad Dermatol* 44:634, 2000.
20. Galan EB, Janniger CK: Pityriasis alba, *Cutis* 61:11, 1998.
21. Oetting WS: Albinism, *Curr Op Pediatr* 11:565, 1999.
22. Oetting WS, King RA: Molecular basis of albinism: mutations and polymorphisms of pigmentation genes associated with albinism, *Hum Mutat* 13:99, 1999.
23. Biswas S, Lloyd IC: Oculocutaneous albinism, *Arch Dis Child* 80:565, 1999.
24. Brilliant MH: The mouse p (pink-eyed dilution) and human P genes oculocutaneous albinism type 2 (OCA2), and melanosomal pH, *Pigment Cell Res* 14:86, 2001.
25. Bastiaens MT et al: Ephelides are more related to pigmentary constitutional host factors than solar lentigines, *Pig Cell Res* 12:316, 1999.
26. McClean DI, Gallagher RP: "Sunburn" freckles, café-au-lait macules, and other pigmented lesions of schoolchildren: the Vancouver Mole Study, *J Am Acad Dermatol* 32:565, 1995.
27. Okulicz JF, Schwartz RA, Jozwiak S: Lentigo, *Cutis* 67:367, 2001.
28. Wirtzfeld DA, Petrelli NJ, Rodriguez-Bigas MA: Hamartous polyposis syndromes: molecular genetics, neoplastic risk, and surveillance recommendations, *Ann Surg Oncol* 8:319, 2001.
29. Coppin BD, Temple IK: Multiple lentigines syndrome (LEOPARD syndrome or progressive cardiomyopathic lentiginosis), *J Med Genet* 34:582, 1997.
30. Stratakis CA: Clinical genetics of multiple endocrine neoplasias, Carney complex and related syndromes, *J Endocrinol Invest* 24:370, 2001.
31. Abeliovich D et al: Familial café-au-lait spots: a variant of neurofibromatosis type I, *J Med Genet* 32:985, 1995.
32. Cohen JB, Janniger CK, Schwartz RA: Café-au-lait spots, *Cutis* 66:22, 2000.
33. Landau M, Krafchik BR: The diagnostic value of café-au-lait macules, *J Am Acad Dermatol* 40:877, 1999.
34. Biesecker LG: The multifaceted challenges of Proteus syndrome, *JAMA* 285:2240, 2001.
35. Leung AK, Kao CP: Extensive mongolian spots with involvement of the scalp, *Pediatr Dermatol* 16:371, 1999.
36. Leung AK et al: Scleral melanocytosis and oculodermal melanocytosis (nevus of Ota) in Chinese children. *J Pediatr* 137:581-584, 2000.
37. Mendiratta V et al: Linear and whorled nevoid hypermelanosis, *J Dermatol* 28:58, 2001.
38. Stanford DG, Georgouras KE: Dermal melanocytosis: a clinical spectrum, *Austr J Dermatol* 37:19, 1996.

39. Olschwang S, Boisson C, Thomas G: Peutz-Jeghers families unlinked to STK11/LKB1 gene mutation are highly predisposed to primitive biliary adenocarcinoma, *J Med Genet* 38:356, 2001.

40. Kirschner LS et al: Genetic heterogeneity and spectrum of mutations of the PRKAR1A gene in patients with the Carney complex, *Hum Mol Genet* 12:3037, 2000.

41. Carpo BG, Grevelink JM, Grevelink SV: Laser treatment of pigmented lesions in children, *Semin Cutan Med Surg* 18:233, 1999.

42. Schaffer JV, Bolognia JL: The clinical spectrum of pigmented lesions, *Clin Plast Surg* 27:391, 2000.

43. Kanzler MH, Mraz-Gernhard S: Primary cutaneous malignant melanoma and its precursor lesions: diagnostic and therapeutic overviews, *J Am Acad Dermatol* 45:260, 2001.

44. Foster RD et al: Giant congenital melanocytic nevi: the significance of neurocutaneous melanosis in neurologically asymptomatic children, *Plast Reconstr Surg* 107:933, 2001.

45. Giam YC et al: Neonatal erosions and ulcerations in giant congenital melanocytic nevi, *Pediatr Dermatol* 16:354, 1999.

46. Schaffer JV, Orlow SJ, Lazova R, Bolognia JL: Speckled lentiginous nevus: within the spectrum of congenital melanocytic nevi, *Arch Dermatol* 137:172, 2001.

47. Egan CL et al: Cutaneous melanoma risk and phenotypic changes in large congenital nevi: a follow-up study of 46 patients, *J Am Acad Dermatol* 39:923, 1998.

48. Bittencourt FV et al: Large congenital melanocytic nevi and the risk for development of malignant melanoma and neurocutaneous melanocytosis, *Pediatrics* 106:736, 2000.

49. Sahin S et al: Risk of melanoma in medium-sized congenital melanocytic nevi: a follow-up study, *J Am Acad Dermatol* 39:428, 1998.

50. Gallagher RP et al: Melanocytic nevus density in Asian, Indo-Pakistani and white children: the Vancouver mole study, *J Am Acad Dermatol* 25:507, 1991.

51. Greene MH: The genetics of hereditary melanoma and nevi, *Cancer* 86(suppl 11):2464, 1999.

52. Bataille V et al: Genetics of risk factors for melanoma: an adult twin study of nevi and freckles, *J Nat Can Inst* 92:457, 2000.

53. Bataille V et al: The association between nevi and melanoma in populations with different levels of sun exposure: a joint case-control study of melanoma in the UK and Australia, *Br J Can* 77:505, 1998.

54. Gallagher RP et al: Suntan, sunburn, and pigmentation factors and the frequency of acquired melanocytic nevi in children, *Arch Dermatol* 126:770, 1990.

55. Morelli JG, Weston WL: Sun, kids, moles, and melanoma, *Contemp Pediatr* 16:61,65,73, 1999.

56. Kim JC, Murphy GF: Dysplastic melanocytic nevi and prognostically indeterminate nevomelanomatoid proliferations, *Clin Lab Med* 20:691, 2000.

57. Silverberg NB: Update on malignant melanoma in children, *Cutis* 67:393, 2001.

58. Stuart CA et al: Acanthosis nigricans, *J Basic Clin Phys Pharm* 9:407, 1998.

59. Taylor SJ, Arioglu E: Syndromes associated with insulin resistance and acanthosis nigricans, *J Basic Clin Phys Pharm* 9:419, 1998.

60. Schwartz RA, Janniger CK: Childhood acanthosis nigricans, *Cutis* 55:337, 1995.

61. Kuroki R et al: Acanthosis nigricans with severe obesity, insulin resistance and hypothyroidism: improvement by diet control, *Dermatology* 198:164, 1999.

62. Katz AS, Goff DC, Feldman SR: Acanthosis nigricans in obese patients: presentation and implications for prevention of atherosclerotic disease, *Dermatol Online J* 6:1, 2000.

Immobile and Hypermobile Skin

Certain skin changes are distinguished by palpation rather than by visual assessment of morphology. Skin mobility and elasticity are two qualities that are distinguished by this method.

Skin that is immobile is fixed to the underlying fascia and sometimes to muscle or bone. A growth or nodule that is fixed to the underlying fascia might indicate a malignant tumor in childhood. Far more common, however, are fibrous thickenings that attach the dermis to the fascia, as in the various types of morphea. Testing for this feature is performed by grasping the skin with the thumb and forefinger and determining its movement. Hypermobile skin is often associated with hypermobile joints and brings to mind the various forms of the Ehlers-Danlos syndrome.

SKIN THICKENINGS

Skin may become thickened and immobile in certain areas. Nodules are not formed, but the thickened, slightly raised, or slightly depressed area can be appreciated on palpation.

LOCALIZED SCLERODERMA (MORPHEA)
Clinical Features

Localized thickening of the skin should be called *morphea*. The classifications of morphea are listed in Box 18-1. Circumscribed areas of morphea may occur as solitary or multiple oval lesions, or as a linear lesion (Fig. 18-1).[1] The majority of children will have either plaque type or linear morphea.[1,2] Atrophy of an extremity, digital contracture, or facial hemiatrophy (Parry-Romberg syndrome) may occur (Fig. 18-2).[1] Linear lesions of the forehead often extend into the frontal scalp, producing a scarring hair loss (en coup de sabre) (Fig. 18-3).[1] The immobile area will be exaggerated by having the child wrinkle the forehead. The surface of the immobile, bound-down skin of morphea is often shiny and hypopigmented (Fig. 18-4), and it may be surrounded by a violaceous hue (lilac) or a brown border (Fig. 18-5).[1] Guttate morphea may present with a depressed, dusky-appearing, slightly thickened area that is not completely bound down (Fig. 18-6).[1-3] Some children have lesions of guttate morphea and linear morphea simultaneously. Concurrent lesions of morphea and lichen sclerosus et atrophicus (LSA) have also been noted in childhood. About one third of children with morphea have arthralgias.[1]

Deep morphea consists of subcutaneous morphea, eosinophilic fasciitis, and pan sclerotic morphea. Subcutaneous morphea and eosinophilic fasciitis may represent the same entity. There is often diffuse thickening of the skin in an irregular surface pattern, leading to a "lumpy-bumpy" skin appearance.[1,3] Children with eosinophilic fasciitis often progress to scleroderma-like fibrosis of the skin with sparing of distal areas.[3]

Differential Diagnosis

LSA has many features that overlap those of morphea, but its characteristic epidermal thinning and lichenoid papules help differentiate it from morphea. Atrophoderma may mimic morphea and is differentiated by the characteristic well-demarcated areas with cliff-drop borders, which are usually seen on the trunk. Progressive systemic sclerosis is rare in childhood and usually presents with severe acral and orofacial sclerosis.[3]

The dusky lesions of early morphea often appear slightly depressed, and only with the evolution of

---

Box 18-1 Classification of Morphea

Plaque	Generalized
Guttate	Bullous
Linear	Deep
Nodular	

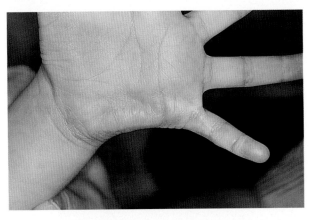

Fig. 18-1 Linear morphea (scleroderma). White, bound-down plaque extending down the left hand and fifth finger.

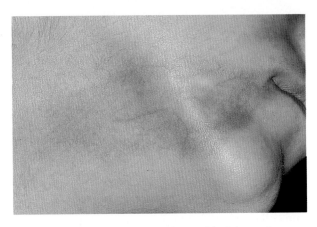

Fig. 18-2 Hyperpigmentation and facial atrophy.

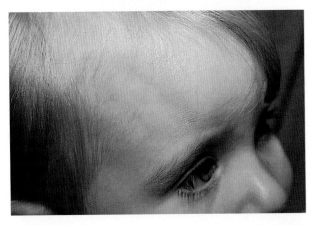

Fig. 18-3 Linear scleroderma of the forehead in a child.

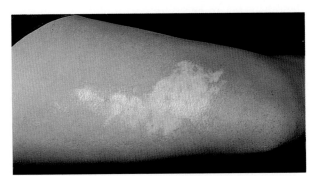

Fig. 18-4 Residual hypopigmentation following linear morphea on the leg.

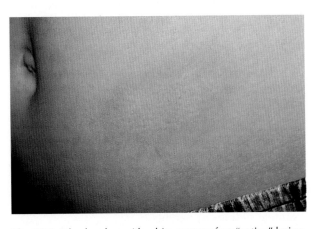

Fig. 18-5 Lilac borders with white center of an "active" lesion.

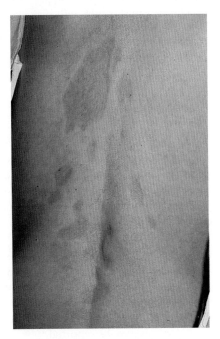

Fig. 18-6 Slightly depressed, tan, slightly bound-down lesions of early morphea.

lesions such that some become "bound down" will the diagnosis be certain. An excisional skin biopsy down to and including fascia may be diagnostic.

Pathogenesis

The mechanism of the disease is unknown, but the debate over the role of *Borrelia burgdorferi* infection continues.[4-6] An inflammatory stage precedes the sclerotic stage and is characterized by a predominantly lymphocytic infiltrate around dermal blood vessels and collagen bundles. In the sclerotic stage, thickened dermal collagen replaces the subcutaneous fat. Injury to the underlying muscle fibers, with separation and inflammation of muscle, occurs in linear forms. In eosinophilic fasciitis, thickening and inflammation of the fascia is diagnostic.[4] The inflammation often demonstrates an excess of eosinophils. Fibrous replacement of the subcutaneous fat may be minimal.

Treatment

There is no specific treatment. Topical calcipotriene ointment, with and without occlusion; UVA1, alone or in combination with calcipotriene ointment; low-dose broad band UVA; and topical PUVA have all been demonstrated to be effective treatments.[2,7-11]

Patient Education

The duration of lesion activity is 3 to 5 years, followed by softening of the skin. Residual pigmentary changes may last several years longer.[1-3] Atrophy of the limbs or facial hemiatrophy will persist.

Follow-up Visits

Examination at 3-month intervals is useful to determine whether systemic symptoms or signs have appeared.

LICHEN SCLEROSUS ET ATROPHICUS
Clinical Features

The white papules and immobile plaques of LSA occur primarily in the anogenital area in grade-school age or adolescent girls.[12,13] LSA is 5 to 10 times more common in girls (Fig. 18-7).[12,13] Purpura, vesicles, and telangiectasia may be seen within the plaques in the genital area. As the lesions age, the skin surface becomes thinned and finely wrinkled. Bleeding may occur.[12-14] Ulcerations and excoriations may be superimposed on these primary lesions. The anogenital lesions in girls tend to surround both the vulva and the anus in a figure-eight pattern.[12,13] Itching and burning of the skin are frequent complaints. Painful defecation, constipation, bloody stools, and encopresis may be reported.[12,13]

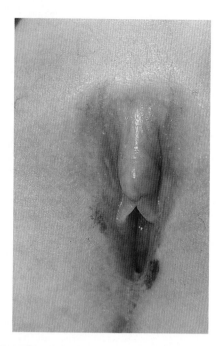

Fig. 18-7 Lichen sclerosus et atrophicus of a child's vulva.

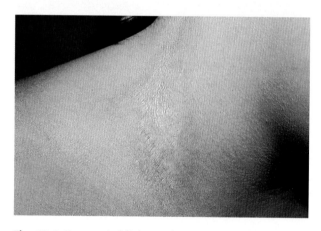

Fig. 18-8 Extragenital lichen sclerosus et atrophicus of the neck. Telangiectasia and fine wrinkling within the white area.

Extragenital lesions appear as asymptomatic white papules on the upper back or upper chest (Fig. 18-8) and occasionally on the face or extremities.[12] About one fourth of the patients with anogenital lesions will also have distal lesions. The isomorphic phenomenon occurs in LSA, and lesions may develop in surgical scars or other sites of skin trauma. Coexistence of LSA with morphea is observed in children.[1] Familial cases have been documented, and it may be useful to examine siblings or parents.[12]

Table 18-1	Subtypes of Ehlers-Danlos Syndrome and Their Clinical Features			
Subtype	**Inheritance**	**Skin/Joints**	**Other**	**Gene Defect**
I Classical	AD	Hyperextensible, lax skin and joints	Hernias, scars, varicosities	Col 5A1 or 5A2
II Hypermobility	AD	Hyperextensible, lax hands and feet		Col 5A1 or 5A2
III Vascular	AD	Pale, thin, prominent veins, ecchymoses	Bowel and/or aortic rupture	Col 3A1
IV Kyphoscoliosis	AR	Hyperextensible skin, lax joints	Ocular globe rupture	Lysyl hydroxylase
V Arthrochalasis	AD	Lax joints, congenital hip dislocation	Bruising	Col 1A1 or 1A2
VI Dermatosparaxis	AR	Skin fragility, sagging skin	Premature fetal membrane rupture	Procol I n-terminal peptidase

AD, Autosomal dominant; *AR*, autosomal recessive.

Differential Diagnosis

Skin immobility suggests localized scleroderma, but atrophic skin, the white color, and papular lesions help distinguish it from scleroderma. Anogenital lesions may be confused with sexual abuse, and abuse investigations may be incorrectly initiated.[12] In LSA, the hymen is never involved, whereas it may reveal injury in sexual abuse. Also, candidiasis, intertrigo, or irritant dermatitis may be confused with LSA. Atrophic areas of lichen planus may mimic LSA, but the purple papular border of lichen planus is a useful differentiating feature.

Pathogenesis

In LSA the dermis is sclerotic and thickened and the epidermis is thinned and atrophic.[12] A bandlike accumulation of lymphocytes is present in the middermis, and features of epidermal injury are also seen. Atrophy of the epidermis and hydropic degeneration of the basal epidermal cells are present.[12] Hyperkeratosis occurs, so that the stratum corneum layer is much thicker than the remainder of the epidermis.[12] Edema and homogenization of collagen in the upper dermis are also seen. As the lesions progress, the collagen of the lower dermis thickens, mimicking circumscribed scleroderma. The mechanism of this inflammatory disease is unknown.

Treatment

Without treatment the majority of patients will improve by puberty.[12,13] There is no specific treatment. Itching often responds to potent topical glucocorticosteroid ointments applied two times daily.[12,13] Topical lubricants may relieve the symptoms. Cleanliness of the anogenital area is useful in preventing superimposed infection. For bleeding telangiectatic vessels, the vascular-specific pulsed dye laser at 585 nm has been useful.[14]

Patient Education

It is helpful to explain to patients that the course of LSA is irregularly progressive, although lesions may remain stable for long periods. The clinician should emphasize that by puberty most children will have spontaneous clearing.[12,13] Patients should be informed that areas of whitish thickening (leukoplakia) may appear on the mucosa or adjacent mucosal surfaces, and that these may progress to carcinoma. Carcinomas have been reported in childhood, but they are exceedingly rare.[15]

Follow-up visits

Yearly examinations are useful to monitor the progress of the disease and examine lesions for possible malignant changes, which require biopsy.

EHLERS-DANLOS SYNDROME
Clinical Features

Ehlers-Danlos syndrome is a phenotype in which there is excessive stretching of skin and joints.[15-18] Six different subtypes of Ehlers-Danlos syndrome have been described, with most forms having autosomal dominant inheritance (Table 18-1).[16,17] The increase in skin stretchability is often spectacular; however, the skin returns to its normal position (Fig. 18-9). Skin fragility is a major problem, and slow healing is very common.[16,17] Skin injury often results in large hematomas that heal with a fibrotic nodule covered by thin, wrinkled epidermis. These are usually prominent over the lower part of the legs (Fig. 18-10). These nodules may calcify. Wound dehiscence is observed in at least one third of these lesions. Easily visible veins and epistaxis are also noted. Hyperextensible joints may result in subluxation of the joints, particularly of the shoulders, elbows, hips, and knees. Flat feet, kyphosis, and scoliosis may occur (Fig.

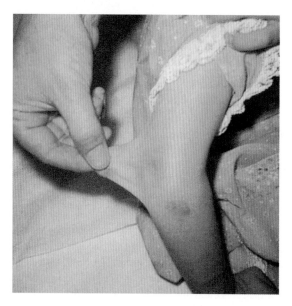

Fig. 18-9 Hyperextensible skin in a child with Ehlers-Danlos syndrome.

18-11). Back pain may become a problem with age, and weakness, muscle cramps, and arthritis may eventuate.[18] Jaw pain or jaw clicking is common.[18]

Hematemesis and bleeding in the lower intestine may occur. Menorrhagia may be seen. Aortic aneurysms, arteriovenous fistula, retinal detachment, lens abnormalities, and myopia have been described.[16,17] Premature births and miscarriages are common.

Differential Diagnosis

The hyperextensible skin is characteristic and usually is not confused with other disorders.

Pathogenesis

The common problem in all six subtypes is faulty formation of collagen.[13] Because collagen limits the stretchability of skin, joints, and blood vessels, defective collagen results in hyperextensible skin and joints and fragile blood vessels. The genetic defects have now been identified for all six types of Ehlers-Danlos (see Table 18-1).

Treatment

Protective measures to prevent skin trauma, particularly during the toddler stage, are most useful. Pediatric orthopedic and ophthalmologic care is recommended. Otherwise, no satisfactory treatment is available.

Patient Education

Informed genetic counseling should be given if a parent is affected. The expectation of premature birth should be emphasized. The skeletal and eye difficulties that may occur as the child grows should also be stressed.

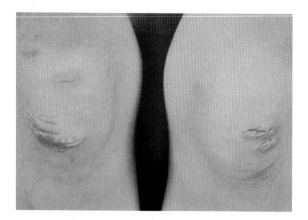

Fig. 18-10 Large "fish mouth" scars on the knees of a child with Ehlers-Danlos type 1.

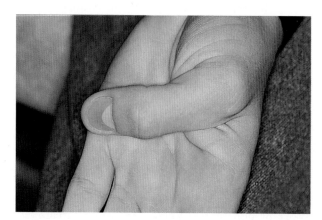

Fig 18-11 Hyperextensible, lax joints of a child with Ehlers-Danlos syndrome.

Follow-up Visits

Yearly ophthalmologic and orthopedic examinations are recommended.

REFERENCES

1. Krafchik BR: Localized morphea in children, *Adv Exp Med Biol* 455:49, 1999.
2. Kreuter A et al: Combined treatment with calcipotriol ointment and low-dose ultraviolet A1 phototherapy in childhood morphea, *Pediatr Dermatol* 18:241, 2001.
3. Nelson AM: Localized scleroderma including morphea, linear scleroderma and eosinophilic fasciitis, *Curr Probl Pediatr* 26:318, 1996.
4. Weide B et al: Morphea is neither associated with features of *Borrelia burgdorferi* infection, nor is this agent detectable in skin lesions by polymerase chain reaction, *Br J Dermatol* 143:780, 2000.
5. Ozkan S et al: Evidence for Borrelia burgdorferi in morphea and lichen sclerosus, *Int J Dermatol* 39:278, 2000.
6. Weide B, Walz T, Garbe C: Is morphea caused by *Borrelia burgdorferi?* A review, *Br J Dermatol* 142:636, 2000.
7. Cunninghan BB et al: Topical calcipotriene for morphea/linear scleroderma, *J Am Acad Dermatol* 39:211, 1998.
8. Kerscher M et al: Low dose UVA1 phototherapy for treatment of localized scleroderma, *J Am Acad Dermatol* 38:21, 1998.
9. Stege H et al: High-dose UVA1 radiation therapy for localized scleroderma, *J Am Acad Dermatol* 36:938, 1997.
10. El-Mofty M et al: Low-dose broad-band UVA in morphea using a new method for evaluation, *Photodermatol Photoimmunol Photomed* 16:43, 2000.
11. Kershcer M et al: PUVA bath photochemotherapy for localized scleroderma, *Arch Dermatol* 132:1280, 1996.
12. Powell JJ, Wojnarowska F: Childhood vulvar lichen sclerosus: an increasingly common problem, *J Am Acad Dermatol* 44:803, 2001.
13. Powell JJ, Wojnarowska F: Lichen sclerosus, *Lancet* 353:1777, 1999.
14. Rabinowitz LG: Lichen sclerosus et atrophicus treatment with the 585-nm flashlamp-pumped pulsed dye laser, *Arch Dermatol* 129:381, 1993.
15. Carlson JA et al: Vulvar lichen sclerosus and squamous cell carcinoma: a cohort, case control, and investigational study with historical perspective; implications for chronic inflammation and sclerosis in the development of neoplasia, *Human Pathol* 29:932, 1998.
16. Reichel JL et al: What syndrome is this? *Pediatr Dermatol* 18:156, 2001.
17. Mao J-R, Bristow J: The Ehlers-Danlos syndrome: on beyond collagens, *J Clin Invest* 107:1063, 2001.
18. Stanitski DF et al: Orthopaedic manifestations of Ehlers-Danlos syndrome, *Clin Ortho Related Res* 376:213, 2000.

There are hundreds of hereditary skin diseases, and the discussion of all of them is beyond the scope of this textbook. The most common genodermatoses are considered in other chapters: the neurocutaneous disorders in Chapter 17, genetic nail disorders in Chapter 16, genetic hair disorders in Chapter 15, photodermatoses in Chapter 10, and vascular lesions in Chapter 14. There are uncommon types of hereditary skin diseases that may be encountered in practice. Comprehensive textbooks and atlases may assist diagnosis of less common skin disorders.[1,2] In addition, access is available to large databases of genetic mutations and laboratories, which can confirm the specific mutation.[3]

More common conditions are considered here because they are important in the differential diagnosis and they are life-long problems for the affected individuals. Included in this chapter are the disorders of keratinization, including the ichthyoses and Darier's disease, the mechanobullous diseases, and ectodermal dysplasias. Acrodermatitis enteropathica is also included in this chapter, although it is separate from the three major categories.

ICHTHYOSIS

Ichthyosis is a term used to describe excessive scaling of the skin, which may be "fish scale like." Although normal infants born after 40 to 42 weeks of gestation will display some thin scales and mild peeling of skin, as will the postmature infant, the scaling in the forms of ichthyosis is usually generalized and the scales are thick. Four major hereditary types of ichthyosis have been described and characterized (Fig. 19-1).[4] Lamellar and bullous types of ichthyosis usually present at birth with severe scaling.[4] Ichthyosis vulgaris and X-linked ichthyosis may be present in the neonate or may present later in childhood.[4,5]

Clinical Features
Ichthyosis vulgaris

Ichthyosis vulgaris is inherited as an autosomal dominant disease that may be as frequent as 1 in 250 individuals.[4] Fine scales usually become prominent by 6 months to 1 year of age.[4] The scales are most prominent over the lower legs (Figs. 19-1 and 19-2) and buttocks. Dry, follicular, horny plugs (keratosis pilaris) are present on the extensor extremities and may be widespread. Palms and soles show an increased number of skin creases. The entire skin surface is dry. Water retention by the stratum corneum is minimal.[6] Some children may have associated atopic dermatitis.[5] The skin in ichthyosis vulgaris usually remains normal throughout the newborn period.

X-Linked ichthyosis

X-linked ichthyosis may appear at birth but usually presents in infancy with scales over the posterior neck, upper trunk, and extensor surfaces of the extremities.[4] As the child ages, the scales often become thicker and a dirty-yellow or brown color (Fig. 19-3). The antecubital and popliteal fossae may be spared (Fig. 19-4). Scaling is usually mild during the first 30 days of life, and the skin is a normal color. Palms and soles are spared, in contrast to the other forms of ichthyosis. The incidence is thought to be in the range of 1 in 2000 to 6000 males.[4] The cause for this disorder is a mutation in the enzyme steroid sulfatase, which is localized to the distal short arm of the X chromosome.[7]

Lamellar ichthyosis and congenital nonbullous ichthyosiform erythroderma

Although both lamellar ichthyosis and congenital nonbullous ichthyosiform erythroderma appear to be caused by an autosomal recessive trait, two separate disease entities exist.[4] Individuals with nonbullous congenital ichthyosiform erythroderma have generalized fine scales on erythematous skin.[1,2] Those with lamellar ichthyosis have larger, darker, platelike scales, with or without erythematous skin. Patients with lamellar ichthyosis have been associated with a gene defect in transglutaminase (Tgase 1) located on chromosome 14.[4] With either condition the affected baby can be born with a collodion membrane, and the two conditions may not be able to be distinguished in neonates.[4] Severe water and electrolyte imbalance may develop.[8] The erythroderma may fade during childhood in some of the infants (Fig. 19-5). Ectropion and eclabium may be present at birth or appear

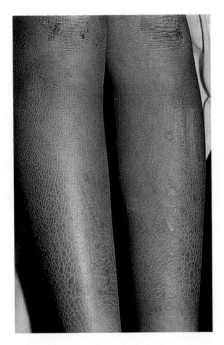

Fig. 19-1 Ichthyosis vulgaris. Scales over the lower legs in a toddler.

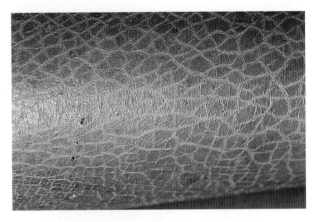

Fig. 19-2 Ichthyosis vulgaris. Prominent scales over the lower legs in a 12-year-old.

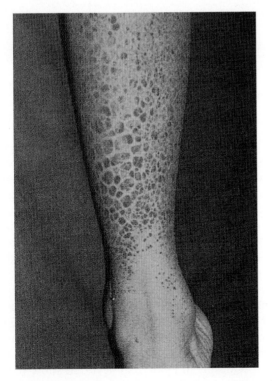

Fig. 19-3 X-linked ichthyosis. Large, dark, platelike scales on lower leg.

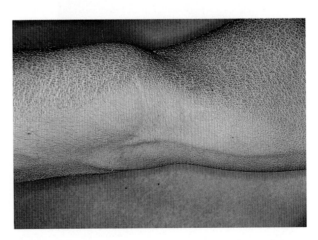

Fig. 19-4 X-Linked ichthyosis. Darkened scales with sparing of antecubital fossa.

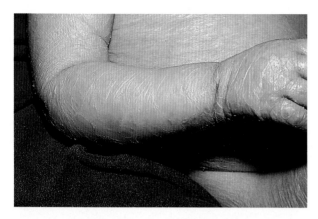

Fig. 19-5 Lamellar ichthyosis. Thickened, shiny skin without erythema in child.

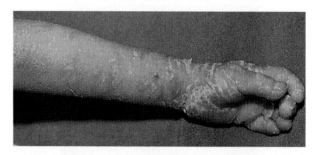

Fig. 19-7 Epidermolytic hyperkeratosis. Thickened scales plus numerous erosions on arm of child.

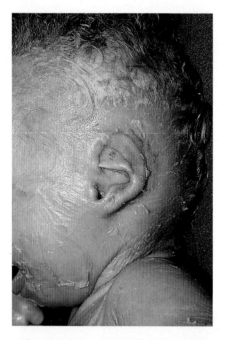

Fig. 19-6 Lamellar ichthyosis. Thickened scales in scalp and shiny, thickened skin of ear and face in toddler.

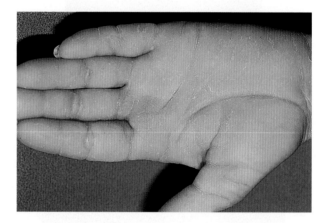

Fig. 19-8 Epidermolytic hyperkeratosis. Hyperkeratosis of palms and deep fissures of creases.

shortly after in patients with lamellar ichthyosis.[4,9] The palms and soles in these patients may be greatly thickened. Skin biopsy after the collodion membrane is shed will demonstrate hyperkeratosis but is otherwise not diagnostic.[4,9]

Bullous ichthyosis (congenital bullous ichthyosiform erythroderma, epidermolytic hyperkeratosis)

Epidermolytic hyperkeratosis, an autosomal dominant disorder, is characterized by extensive scaling at birth, erythroderma, and recurrent episodes of bullae for-

mation (Figs. 19-6 to 19-8).[4,8,9] The blisters represent lysis of the epidermal granular layer, and secondary infection with *Staphylococcus aureus* becomes a major difficulty in the neonatal period and during infancy. As the child ages, the involvement becomes more limited in extent. By school age, thick, warty, dirty-yellow scales with malodorous excessive bacterial colonization of the skin will have developed on the palms, soles, elbows, and knees (Fig. 19-9). Skin biopsy will reveal enlargement of the granular cell layer with bizarre vacuolization of the epidermal granular cells.[4,9,10] A related autosomal dominant condition called *bullous ichthyosis of Siemens* demonstrates similar but milder findings, with more superficial bullae.[11] Widespread epidermal nevi that show pathologic changes of epidermolytic hyperkeratosis (EHK), such as ichthyosis hystrix and systematized epidermal nevi, may show histologic changes similar to EHK.[9,10]

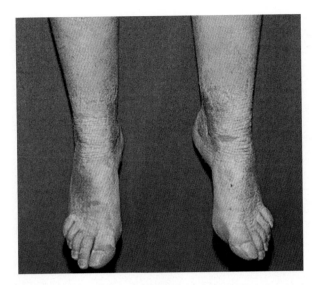

Fig. 19-9 Epidermolytic hyperkeratosis. Thickened, malodorous skin on legs and ankles.

Differential Diagnosis

At birth, lamellar and bullous types of ichthyosis may be difficult to distinguish from one another. The hereditary pattern and skin biopsy may help.[9] If an individual with ichthyosis has corneal opacities and sparing of the palms and soles, the diagnosis is likely to be X-linked ichthyosis. If an ectropion and eclabium are present, it is likely to be lamellar ichthyosis; and recurrent bullous episodes will distinguish epidermolytic hyperkeratosis. Measurement of steroid sulfatase activity in red blood cells may be useful in the diagnosis of X-linked ichthyosis.[7]

Ichthyosis vulgaris in its mild form may be difficult to distinguish from dry skin, but the extensive distribution of scales, particularly scaling over the buttocks and lower legs, increased palmar creases, and skin biopsy will differentiate ichthyosis vulgaris from dry skin.[10] Scaling disorders similar to lamellar ichthyosis are present in many ichthyosis syndromes associated with neurologic disease.[12]

Pathogenesis

Skin biopsy in the ichthyosis syndromes will often be of diagnostic value. In ichthyosis vulgaris there is a thin or absent granular cell layer in addition to the hyperkeratosis.[4,8] X-linked ichthyosis demonstrates hyperkeratosis with an otherwise normal-appearing epidermis.[4,8] Vacuolization and separation of the granular cell layer with blister cavity formation are associated with the hyperkeratosis in bullous ichthyosis.[4,8,9] Similar findings in the more superficial epidermis are found in bullous ichthyosis of Siemens.[9-11] Lamellar ichthyosis may demonstrate hyperkeratosis, acanthosis, and a mild chronic inflammatory infiltrate.[4,8]

Increased epidermal turnover has been demonstrated in nonbullous congenital ichthyosiform erythroderma and bullous ichthyosis, such that excessive numbers of stratum corneum cells are produced.[4] In contrast, X-linked ichthyosis and ichthyosis vulgaris demonstrate normal epidermal turnover, and the accumulated scale is felt to be caused by faulty shedding of the stratum corneum.

Molecular diagnosis is most useful, if available (Fig. 19-10).[3] In ichthyosis vulgaris, gene abnormalities of profilaggrin and filaggrin have been identified.[13] In X-linked ichthyosis, mutations in the gene coding for steroid sulfatase are described.[7] In bullous ichthyosis, mutations in the genes encoding the paired keratins 1 and 10 have been uncovered.[14,15] These keratin proteins are expressed in differentiated keratinocytes, and with mutations develop an unstable keratin scaffolding within the suprabasilar keratinocytes. The cytoskeleton collapses, resulting in separation of affected cells from one another and blister formation.[10] In bullous ichthyosis of Siemens, mutations in the gene encoding keratin 2e, a cytoskeletal protein expressed superficial to the granular layer, have been identified.[11] In lamellar ichthyosis, mutations in the gene encoding transglutaminase 1 have been found.[16] Transglutaminase 1 is important in the cross-linking of the proteins forming the cornified envelope of the differentiated keratinocyte, and the failure to form the envelope may result in loss of regulation of keratinocyte proliferation. Epidermal nevi with pathology of EHK may represent mosaicism for epidermolytic hyperkeratosis, with the affected skin showing the gene mutation for keratins 1 or 10 and the unaffected intervening skin displaying normal keratins.[17]

Treatment

There is no satisfactory treatment for the ichthyosis. In ichthyosis vulgaris and X-linked ichthyosis, hydration of the skin twice daily and the generous use of lubricants will control the dryness and scaling. The use of alpha-hydroxy acids such as lactic acid 5% ointment or 12% ammonium lactate lotion applied once or more daily may be helpful in the more severe ichthyoses, although many such patients do as well with bland lubricants alone. In bullous ichthyoses, systemic antistaphylococcal antibiotics are required to treat the infectious episodes.

In ichthyosis great caution must be used in applying therapy to the skin of an affected infant or child.

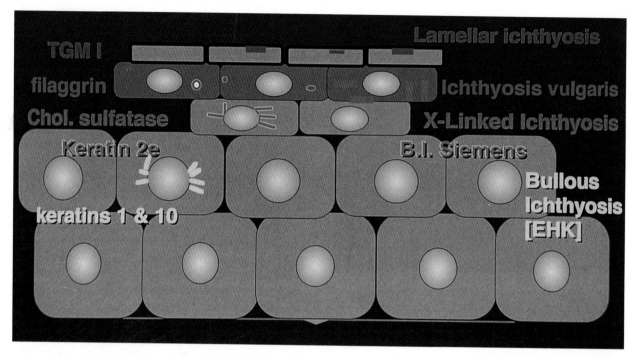

Fig. 19-10 Gene mutations in the ichthyoses.

Because of the larger surface area per body weight, systemic toxicity and side effects can be seen and acidosis can occur secondary to topical therapy. The clinician should recognize that both the active medication and the vehicle for the medication could cause significant toxicity in the infant with ichthyosis.

The synthetic retinoids given orally have shown promise in management of ichthyosis, but their use is restricted by long-term effects on growing bones.[18-20]

Patient Education

The genetic nature of the ichthyoses and the methods of controlling these disorders should be emphasized to the family by the clinician. Good supportive relationships should be established with these patients.

Follow-up Visits

A visit 1 week after discharge from the newborn nursery is useful in evaluating therapy. Thereafter, the routine visits for pediatric care and additional visits may be necessary depending on the severity of the ichthyosis.

NETHERTON SYNDROME

Netherton syndrome is a severe, autosomal recessive disorder characterized by congenital ichthyosis with defective cornification. These children have a specific hair shaft defect (trichorrhexis invaginata, or "bamboo hair") (see Chapter 15, Figs. 15-15 and 15-16) and severe atopic manifestations including atopic dermatitis and hay fever, with high serum IgE levels and hypereosinophilia. In addition, infants with Netherton's syndrome may have severe failure to thrive, infections, and hypernatremic dehydration, which result in high postnatal mortality. The genetic cause of this disease is a mutation in SPINK5, which encodes the serine protease inhibitor LEKTI. SPINK5 appears to play a critical role in epidermal barrier function and immunity.[21]

EPIDERMOLYSIS BULLOSA

Epidermolysis bullosa is a term used to describe a group of inherited skin conditions associated with blister formation after mild trauma. This condition can be associated with defects of any of many different proteins present at the junction of the dermis and epidermis or within the epidermis or dermis. The severity of the disease may not only be associated with the specific proteins involved, but also the specific mutation associated with the gene encoding that protein. Epidermolysis bullosa can be divided into nonscarring and scarring types. The nonscarring types include those with intraepidermal separation and junctional separation, whereas the scarring (dystrophic) form includes the subepidermal types. The disease is uncommon but potentially life-threatening to newborns and infants. Correct diagnosis in the newborn period can be difficult and depends on a combination of clinical, histologic, and molecular biology techniques.[22,23] In all forms of epidermolysis bullosa, evolution of clinical lesions during the first 30 days of life may make the diagnosis difficult. A family history of childhood blistering diseases is often absent, and the clinician must depend on the findings in the affected baby.[22] Extreme care must be taken to obtain a biopsy of an induced blister and not an old or established blister. Induction of a blister with a pencil eraser or a suction device is the most reliable method.[22,23] A shave biopsy taken from the normal skin into the induced blister is preferred. Optimally the biopsy specimen should be examined by light and electron microscopy plus immunofluorescent mapping.[17]

Clinical Features
Nonscarring types of epidermolysis bullosa

Epidermolysis bullosa simplex. Epidermolysis bullosa simplex is dominantly inherited and may be generalized or localized.[22] The most common form is localized to the hands and feet (Fig. 19-11) and often is not present at birth. This form, which causes recurrent blisters on the hands and feet, is called Weber-Cockayne disease. Blisters of the hands and feet first occur in late childhood or adolescence, when the child experiences minor frictional trauma (Fig. 19-12). It often has its onset in warm weather.

Epidermolysis bullosa simplex may also be generalized, with lesions present at birth or, more likely, the appearance of blisters at 6 to 12 months of age.[22] These lesions are more numerous on the distal extremities but may also be seen on elbows and knees. The condition is autosomal dominant and worsens in warm weather. In the Koebner type of generalized epidermolysis bullosa simplex, the lesions are discrete (Fig. 19-13), and in the Dowling-Meara type they are grouped (Fig. 19-14).[22]

Junctional epidermolysis bullosa. A generalized, often-fatal form (Herlitz) and a milder form of junctional epidermolysis bullosa are recognized.[22,23] Both will present at birth with very few lesions (Fig. 19-15). Mucous membrane lesions appear within the first month of life in the lethal form and are absent or minimal in the milder form. Oral mucosa becomes severely affected in the lethal form (Fig. 19-16), interfering with eating and often resulting in failure to thrive.[22] Nonhealing granulation tissue may develop over bony

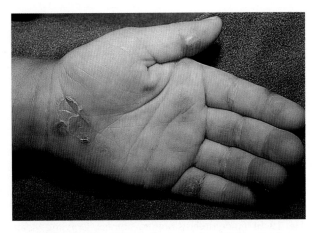

Fig. 19-11 Epidermolysis bullosa simplex, Weber-Cockayne type. Minor trauma on playground equipment induced blisters of the palms.

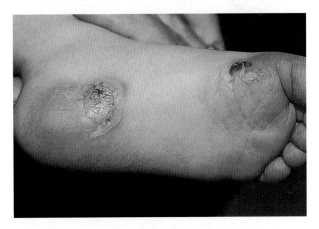

Fig. 19-12 Epidermolysis bullosa simplex, Weber-Cockayne type. Painful blisters on the foot of a child after a run.

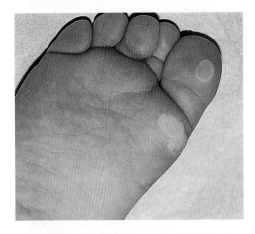

Fig. 19-13 Epidermolysis bullosa simplex, Koebner type. Discrete blisters on a toddler's foot.

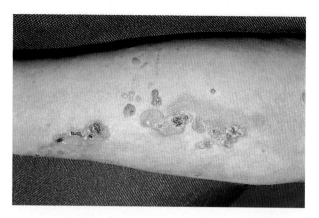

Fig. 19-14 Epidermolysis bullosa simplex, Dowling-Meara type. Grouped blisters on the leg of a child.

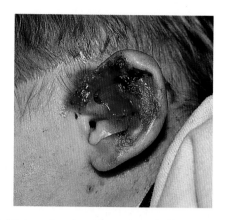

Fig. 19-17 Junctional epidermolysis bullosa. Nonhealing granulation tissue at blister site on child's ear.

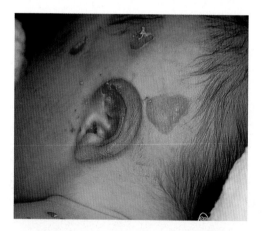

Fig. 19-15 Junctional epidermolysis bullosa. Newborn with a few scattered blisters.

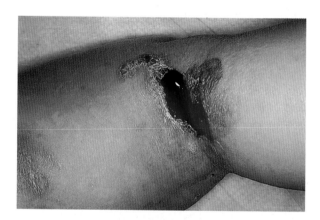

Fig. 19-18 Dystrophic epidermolysis bullosa, recessive. Hemorrhagic blister on newborn.

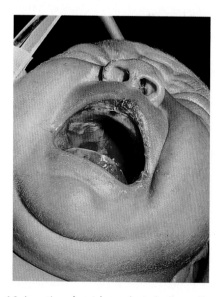

Fig. 19-16 Junctional epidermolysis bullosa. Severe oral erosions in an infant.

prominences such as the spine, ear, or mid-face (Fig. 19-17).[22] Secondary bacterial infection can be severe. The majority of lesions heal without scarring, but lateral extension of large bullae can result in hemorrhage and healing with scarring.

Scarring (dystrophic) forms of epidermolysis bullosa

In epidermolysis bullosa of the recessive dystrophic type, hemorrhagic bullae appear on the skin at birth or shortly after (Fig. 19-18).[22,23] Removal of the blister roof leaves a raw, bleeding base that heals with scar formation. Healing scars often entrap islands of epithelium, producing milia that appear as tiny white cysts within scars (Fig. 19-19).[22] Scarring is sufficiently severe to result in replacement of nails and pseudowebbing of all digits, leading eventually to a clublike appearance of hands and feet (Fig. 19-20).[22] Scarring alopecia of the scalp will develop. Severe scarring of the eyelid may occur.[22] Blisters and erosions of the oral

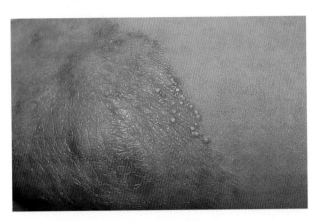

Fig. 19-19 Recessive dystrophic epidermolysis bullosa. Multiple white milia at border of scar.

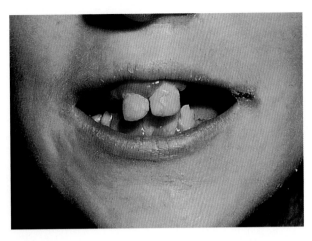

Fig. 19-21 Recessive dystrophic epidermolysis bullosa. Loss of teeth and restriction of mouth opening in child.

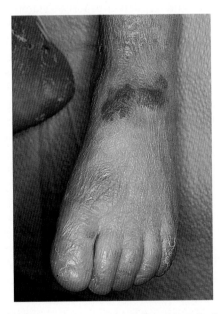

Fig. 19-20 Recessive dystrophic epidermolysis bullosa. Loss of toenails, pseudowebbing of digits, and new blisters.

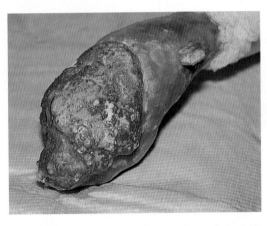

Fig. 19-22 Recessive dystrophic epidermolysis bullosa. Huge verrucous growth on hand of adolescent represents squamous cell carcinoma.

mucosa result in limitation of eating, immobilization of the tongue, and esophageal stricture with resultant dysphagia in 76% of cases.[22-24] Laryngeal bullae will produce respiratory stridor.[22] The teeth may be malformed and carious (Fig. 19-21). Anemia caused by chronic blood loss and malnutrition occurs, and failure to thrive will commonly develop.[22] Secondary bacterial or Candidal infection of the skin is frequent. In adolescent years, squamous cell carcinoma may arise in atrophic scars of the skin (Fig. 19-22) or in leukoplakic areas of the mucous membranes.[22]

In epidermolysis bullosa of the dominant dystrophic type, hemorrhagic bullae are seen at birth, and erosions caused by intrauterine blister formation may be observed at delivery.[22,23] Intrauterine erosions are frequently found over the dorsa of the feet and the anterior lower legs. As the child ages, atrophic scars and milia appear (Fig. 19-23). Mucous membrane involvement is less common than in the recessive dystrophic type and when present is quite mild.[22,24] Ichthyosis, keratosis pilaris, thickened nails, and hyperhidrosis may develop. Nails may be shed and

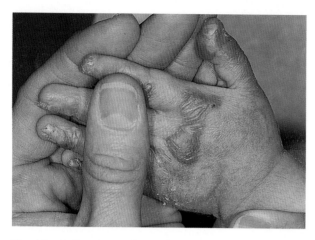

Fig. 19-23 Dominant dystrophic epidermolysis bullosa. Blister, scar formation, milia, and loss of a fingernail in infant.

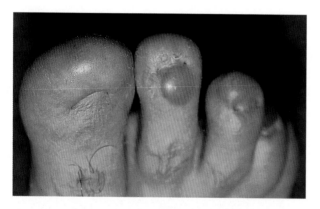

Fig. 19-24 Dominant dystrophic epidermolysis bullosa. Loss of toenails, active blisters, but no pseudowebbing in adolescent.

replaced by scars (Fig. 19-24), but pseudowebbing does not occur.[22] Scarring alopecia is absent, and anemia and failure to thrive are rarely seen.[22,24]

A variant, also dominantly inherited, characterized by white atrophic lesions without clinical blister formation, is called *albopapuloid form*.[22] Numerous milia and hypopigmented scars are seen predominantly on the trunk rather than the extremities.

Differential Diagnosis

The ease of blistering skin by suction or friction will differentiate epidermolysis bullosa from friction blisters or spontaneous blistering disease.[22] At birth, obstetric injuries are frequently confused because of the hemorrhagic blisters and eroded, raw areas.[22] Urinary uroporphyrins will distinguish porphyria cutanea tarda from epidermolysis bullosa. The forms of epidermolysis bullosa may be differentiated from one another by the inheritance pattern, with a skin biopsy specimen examined by electron microscopy or by molecular genetic analysis.[22,23]

Pathogenesis

The mechanism of epidermolysis bullosa is known to be due to gene mutations encoding structural proteins: keratin 5, keratin 14, or plectin in epidermolysis bullosa simplex; laminin 5, BP180, or $\alpha 6 \beta 4$ integrin in junctional epidermolysis bullosa and collagen VII in dystrophic forms of epidermolysis bullosa (Fig. 19-25).[23] They are distinguished by ultrastructural examination of the skin biopsy specimen. Recurrent bullous eruption of the hands and feet demonstrates a separation of epidermal cells just above the basal layer. Epidermolysis bullosa simplex separates the basal cells within the basal layer. In junctional epidermolysis bullosa, the separation occurs just below the plasma membrane of the basal cells and above the basal lamina of the dermis.[22,23] The scarring forms show a separation below the basal lamina in the dermis. In epidermolysis bullosa dystrophica, recessive type, the anchoring fibrils, which support the basal lamina, are missing.[22]

The severity and clinical presentation of the different types of epidermolysis bullosa not only depend on the specific gene involved but also specific mutations on that gene. Mutations in the evolutionarily conserved regions of the gene may produce more severe clinical disease than mutations that do not involve the conserved region. This is specifically seen in epidermolysis bullosa-Dowling-Meara, in which the mutations are in the highly conserved region of the keratin genes.[22] Patients who have premature termination type of mutations usually have more severe disease than those patients that have structural mutations of the same gene.[23]

Treatment

Treatment is symptomatic and supportive.[22,25] One of the United States centers for epidermolysis bullosa may be consulted for a comprehensive care program. For the scarring and junctional forms, skilled nursing and general health care are required. For the newborn infant, small, frequent feedings with a soft nipple are indicated. Gentle handling; soft, loose-fitting clothing; gentle sponge baths; cotton diapers; and a sheepskin pad for the crib should be instituted. Large blisters

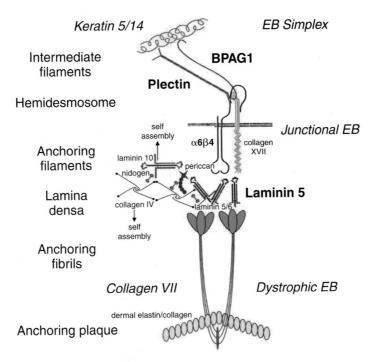

Keratin 5/14

Intermediate
filaments

BPAG1

Plectin

EB Simplex

Hemidesmosome

self
assembly

Junctional EB

Anchoring
filaments

$\alpha6\beta4$ collagen
XVII

laminin 10

periccan

nidogen

Lamina
densa

collagen IV

laminin 5/6

Laminin 5

self
assembly

Anchoring
fibrils

Collagen VII   *Dystrophic EB*

dermal elastin/collagen

Anchoring plaque

Fig. 19-25 Gene mutations in epidermolysis bullosa. (*From Marinkovich MP: Protein-protein interactions at the dermal-epidermal BMZ. In Barker J, McGrath J (editors): Cell adhesion and migration in skin disease, Amsterdam, 2001, Harwood Academic Publishers.*)

can be opened with sterile scissors and the roof allowed to collapse by gently compressing out the fluid. Blisters and erosions should have a topical antibiotic (mupirocin) applied gently to the surface (a wooden tongue depressor is useful). Rotating topical antibiotics over months will be useful to reduce the likelihood of bacterial resistance.[22,25]

For infants and children, a passive physical therapy program should be instituted. Water beds, eggcrate padding, or sheepskin is useful for sleep.[25] Keeping the room cool will reduce blistering and the accompanying pruritus. Wound dressings, such as Vigilon, Second Skin, and DuoDerm, may be useful for large nonhealing erosions. Keratinocyte-cultured autografts have been successful in severe nonhealing areas.[26] If anemia is present, vitamin supplements and iron may be required. Protein and caloric requirements may be twice that recommended for size because of ongoing skin or mucosal losses. Fluids should be lukewarm, and acidic juices should be avoided. Ensure or other nutritional supplements may be considered. Whole-grain breads and cereals may reduce constipation, which can be a major problem. A

multidisciplinary approach is required in the scarring forms to deal with problems such as esophageal strictures, dental disease, pseudodactyly, laryngeal disorders, urethral meatal stenosis, conjunctival scarring, and psychosocial problems.

In recurrent bullous eruption of the hands and feet, resistance to friction may improve by painting the hands and feet one to two times a week with tincture of benzoin or spray preparations such as Tuff-Skin.

Patient Education

Much support is required for parents and patients with these disorders, which are chronic, frustrating, and in the dystrophic form, severely debilitating. Patients and family members should be provided with a checklist of steps to reduce friction, and they should be instructed by persons skilled in nursing techniques. Lay support groups, DEBRA (Dystrophic Epidermolysis Bullosa Research Association) of America, Inc. (http://www.debra.org/), and the Epidermolysis Bullosa Medical Research Foundation (http://www.ebkids.org) have excellent information available for parents and a North American network of local support groups to help families with children who have epidermolysis bullosa. Future therapy using gene transfer technology may be helpful and give hope for the patients who are most severely involved.[27]

Follow-up Visits

A regular schedule of visits is required to monitor anemia and secondary infections. After birth, visits should be weekly or biweekly. Routine immunizations and well baby care are needed.

ECTODERMAL DYSPLASIAS

There are dozens of ectodermal dysplasias but the ones most frequently seen include incontinentia pigmenti, hypohidrotic and hidrotic forms of ectodermal dysplasia, Goltz syndrome, the palmoplantar keratodermas, and Darier's disease. Ectodermal dysplasias have defects of skin, hair, teeth, nails, and sweating. Skin defects include ichthyosis changes, pigmentary abnormalities, and hypoplasias or aplasias. Sparse or absent scalp or other hair may be found. Ichthyosis with sparse hair is a frequent combination and is seen in Conradi's disease, Netherton's syndrome, and the keratitis-ichthyosis deafness syndrome, for example. Teeth may be cone-shaped, sparse, or absent. Nails may be thickened, thinned, or hypoplastic. Sweating is usually diminished, but hypohidrosis may be patchy and difficult to detect.

INCONTINENTIA PIGMENTI
Clinical features

Four distinct stages of skin changes occur in incontinentia pigmenti. First, linear rows of blisters on the extremities are seen (Fig. 19-26).[28] These blistering episodes recur over the first 3 months of life and are replaced by warty linear areas that may last until 1 year of age (Fig. 19-27).[28] Rows of brown pigmentation are then left (Fig. 19-28). In addition, swirls of brown pigmentation are found on the trunk and in areas where the blisters and warty lesions did not occur (Fig. 19-29).[28,29] The lesions may follow along the lines of Blaschko. The pigmentation fades as the child ages and is usually not seen after adolescence. Hypopigmented scarred areas may develop afterward.

Incontinentia pigmenti is believed to be an X-linked trait that is lethal to the male, which explains the female predominance in this disorder.[28-30] Mental retardation, seizures, microcephaly, and other central nervous system disorders occur in up to 30% of the reported patients,[28] although it is our experience that the association is much less. Ocular and skeletal anomalies may also be noted.

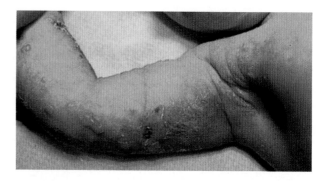

Fig. 19-26 Incontinentia pigmenti. Linear vesicles and crust in affected newborn girl.

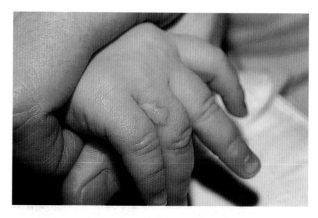

Fig. 19-27 Incontinentia pigmenti. Warty, linear growths at site of previous blisters.

Differential diagnosis

In the blistering stage, herpes simplex or bullous impetigo may be confused with incontinentia pigmenti, but the linear arrangement of its blisters and appropriate cultures will distinguish it from these two disorders. The warty phase may mimic linear epidermal birthmarks or warts. The hyperpigmentation is uniquely arranged in whorls and is unlikely to be confused with other causes of hyperpigmentation.

Pathogenesis

Skin biopsy demonstrates an inflammatory dermatitis with subcorneal vesicles filled with numerous eosinophils.[29] The warty stage merely demonstrates hyperkeratosis and chronic inflammation in the dermis. In the pigmentary stage, melanin is found free in the dermis or engulfed by dermal macrophages, which accounts for the term *incontinentia pigmenti*.[28,29] Two distinct genes have been implicated, one mapped to

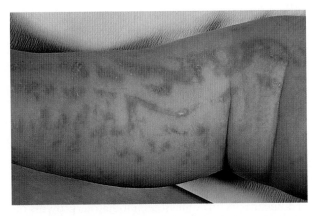

Fig. 19-28 Incontinentia pigmenti. Whorled pigmentation of extremity in sites of previous blisters.

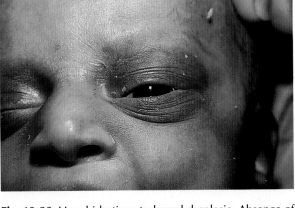

Fig. 19-30 Hypohidrotic ectodermal dysplasia. Absence of eyebrows and lashes and darkened eyelids in newborn.

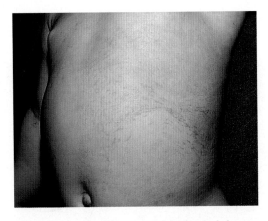

Fig. 19-29 Incontinentia pigmenti. Whorled, brown-pigmented streaks on abdominal skin where no prior blisters were noted.

Xp11 and the other to Xq28.[30] The etiology of this acute dermatitis and its peculiar linear arrangement is not known.

Treatment

There is no satisfactory treatment.

Patient education

The clinician should emphasize that the disorder is inherited and describe the expected future cutaneous stages.

Follow-up visits

Routine infant care visits should be scheduled. Additional visits may be necessary based on complications that arise.

Hypohidrotic and Hidrotic Ectodermal Dysplasias
Clinical features

Two common forms of ectodermal dysplasia have been recognized, the hypohidrotic form and the hidrotic form.[31] The anhidrotic form is also commonly called *hypohidrotic* because sweating may be markedly decreased but not absent. In each there is sparse scalp hair. In addition, a number of other uncommon and rare forms of ectodermal dysplasias have thin or absent hair.[31] Absence of the eyebrows and eyelashes in the newborn may be an important clue to the diagnosis (Fig. 19-30).[31,32] Other clinical findings may be less obvious.

In hypohidrotic ectodermal dysplasia, sweating is reduced or completely absent.[31,32] Such infants may present with fever of unknown origin or recurrent high fevers. The facies of such children are very distinctive, with everted lips, prominent frontal ridges, a saddle nose, and absence of eyebrows and eyelashes.[31,32] Temporary and permanent teeth are reduced in number or may be entirely absent. If teeth erupt, they are often cone-shaped, and this may be observed by dental radiographs even in the preeruptive stage. Atrophic rhinitis and frequent upper respiratory symptoms may lead to the mistaken diagnosis of respiratory allergy.[31] Scalp hair is seldom totally absent, but it is very sparse and is often the first concern of the parents. Fingernails and toenails are normal in at least half of the cases but may be thin or brittle. A careful genetic history should be obtained.

The hidrotic form is characterized by nail dystrophy as the most prominent clinical finding. The nails are thickened, slow growing, and brittle. Thick nails may be apparent early in infancy. In one third of the families, the only feature present is nail disease. As in the hypohidrotic form, the scalp hair is thin and sparse and eyebrows are thin, but sweating is normal. Teeth are often normal. The palms and soles may be diffusely thickened, and thickening over the knuckles, knees, and elbows may be prominently observed.

Differential diagnosis

The major conditions to be considered in the differential diagnosis are listed in Box 15-5, p. 229. The findings of disorders of nails, skin, and teeth in the same patient in addition to the hair loss will suggest ectodermal dysplasia. Within a single family with ectodermal dysplasia, the features may be quite variable. To diagnose abnormalities of sweating, a combination of tests may be required.[33] Sweat pore counting using silicone rubber plastic imprints and silver nitrate staining is reliable but does not take into account functional sweating, which can be quantified by 0-phthaldialdehyde stains of induced sweating.[33]

Pathogenesis

Hypohidrotic ectodermal dysplasia is inherited in an X-linked recessive pattern by a defect in the protein ectodysplasin, a transmembrane protein.[34] The hidrotic form is inherited as an autosomal dominant condition and has been observed in a large French-Canadian family surnamed Clouston. The gene for the hidrotic form is associated with the connexin gene GJB6.[35] In the hypohidrotic form, sweat glands are absent or rudimentary, as are scalp hair follicles, sebaceous glands, and the mucous glands of the respiratory passages. Lack of sweating results in poor thermal control and high fevers. Lack of hair follicles is expressed as sparse hair, and lack of respiratory mucus produces frequent infections and watery rhinorrhea. A disorder of keratinization is thought to be important in the hidrotic form to explain the nail disease and hyperkeratosis of the palms and soles.

Treatment

Fever control through the use of cool compresses is vital in the newborn or infant with recurrent fevers. There is no specific therapy otherwise available.[31] The use of wigs and dental corrective devices may be necessary.

Patient education

Genetic counseling is very useful to the patient and family, as is the explanation of the cause of the febrile responses and respiratory symptoms in the infant.

Follow-up visits

At least one follow-up visit within 4 weeks of the initial visit is most useful to re-explain the genetic factors and the symptoms of disease.

Focal Dermal Hypoplasia (Goltz Syndrome)
Clinical features

The hallmark of Goltz syndrome are linear, red, swirly streaks in the skin that represent the areas of focal dermal hypoplasia (Fig. 19-31).[33,36] Atrophy, scarring areas, hypopigmentation (Fig. 19-32), and telangiectasias are seen. There may be yellow nodules in a linear pattern.[36] Small papillomatous growths on periorificial or intertriginous areas are found.[33] In the oral mucosa or perineal area they may be mistaken for warts. Nails may be hypoplastic, short, or brittle. Hair is sparse. Teeth are sparse, and enamel defects are frequently found.[36]

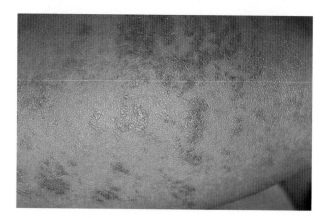

Fig. 19-31 Focal dermal hypoplasia. Linear and whorled red streaks on female infant.

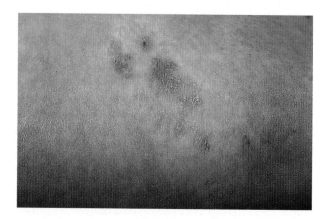

Fig. 19-32 Focal dermal hypoplasia. Atrophic and scarred skin with hypopigmented patch in child.

Syndactyly, polydactyly, and a variety of other bony malformations are seen (Fig. 19-33). Lip pits, hemihypoplasia of the tongue, cleft lip, strabismus, colobomas, cataracts, neurosensory hearing loss, and mental retardation are common.[33,36]

Differential diagnosis

Many other ectodermal dysplasias will demonstrate some features in common with Goltz syndrome, but will not show the characteristics of focal dermal hypoplasia.[36] Sometimes aplasia cutis congenita or intrauterine erosions of epidermolysis bullosa are mistaken for dermal hypoplasia, but a skin biopsy will distinguish. In focal dermal hypoplasia, a normal epidermis overlies subcutaneous fat with a rudimentary dermis present. In aplasia cutis, the epidermis is absent or effaced, and subcutaneous fat is diminished; in dystrophic epidermolysis bullosa, the sweat glands and hair follicles are present in a normal dermis with a loss of epidermis.

Pathogenesis

An X-linked dominant inheritance pattern is described with many sporadic cases. In a variant with microphthalmia, a deletion of Xp22 is described.[36]

Treatment

There is no available treatment. Consultation with, or referral to, a multidisciplinary genetics clinic may be of great assistance in assessment.

Patient education

The genetics of the disease should be discussed with the patient and family, including the likelihood of a great variety of bony, eye, and central nervous system disturbances.

Follow-up visits

The frequency of review should be determined by the associated defects.

The Hereditary Palmoplantar Keratodermas

Some children are born with thickening of the palms and soles or develop thickening later in childhood. There are many genetic types and phenotypic patterns of hereditary palmoplantar keratodermas. Thickening can be diffuse, involving the entire surface (Fig. 19-34); round and linear (Fig. 19-35); or multiple discrete 1- to 2-mm papules (Fig. 19-36).[37] Mutations in palmoplantar-specific keratin K9 can cause an epidermolytic type of palmoplantar keratoderma, whereas K16 mutations can present as focal nonepidermolytic palmoplantar keratoderma.[38]

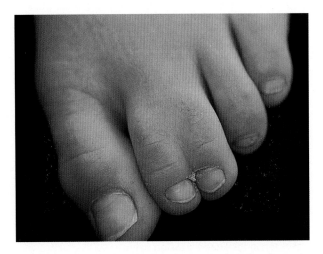

Fig. 19-33 Focal dermal hypoplasia. Syndactyly of toes in child.

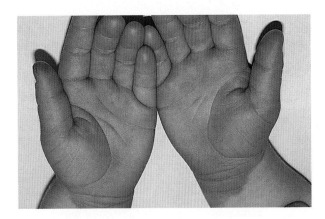

Fig. 19-34 Diffuse palmoplantar keratoderma. All of child's palmar skin is thickened.

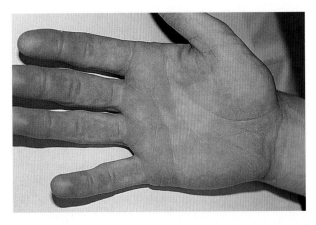

Fig. 19-35 Oval and linear palmoplantar keratoderma. Child's palms have linear and oval plaques of thickening.

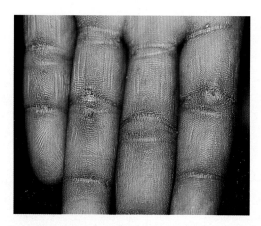

Fig. 19-36 Punctate palmoplantar keratoderma. Adolescent has discrete thickened areas on palms.

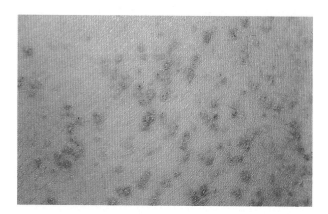

Fig. 19-38 Keratosis follicularis. Discrete brown, "greasy-feeling" keratotic papules.

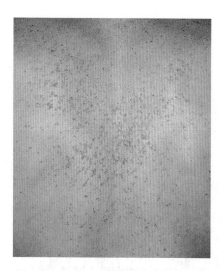

Fig. 19-37 Keratosis follicularis. Numerous keratotic papules on adolescent's upper back.

Keratosis Follicularis (Darier-White Disease)
Clinical features

Keratosis follicularis is characterized by skin-colored to red-brown, keratotic 2- to 5-mm papules on the face, neck, scalp, chest, back (Figs. 19-37 and 19-38), and proximal extremities.[39] The skin changes usually begin between the ages of 5 to 10 years, but the age of onset is variable. Over the tops of the hands, the skin changes involve skin-colored, flat-topped papules; 0.1-mm punctate papules may be seen on the palms. There are longitudinal streaks of the nails, which terminate in a wedge-shaped split in the free end of the nail. Heat sensitivity is severe, with exacerbations in hot weather or after sun exposure. Severe bacterial or herpes simplex skin infections may occur. Hypopig-

mented macules on the trunk and extremities are seen. The course often worsens during adolescence.[39]

Differential diagnosis

Inflamed lesions of keratosis pilaris can mimic keratosis follicularis, except that they are usually localized to the extensor proximal arms and legs. The lesions of keratosis pilaris are often much smaller, white, and likely to be dome-shaped. A biopsy may be required to distinguish. Keratosis follicularis has focal areas of acantholytic dyskeratosis, whereas keratosis pilaris reveals a follicular keratotic plug in the body hair channel.

Pathogenesis

Keratosis follicularis is associated with mutations in ATP2A2, a gene that encodes the sarco/endoplasmic reticulum Ca^{2+}-ATPase isoform 2. Abnormalities in the function of this calcium pump are hypothesized to interfere with cell growth and differentiation calcium-dependent signaling processes.[40]

Treatment

Keeping the skin surface cool, sometimes with wet dressings is helpful. Oral retinoids, such as isotretinoin at 0.5 to 1.0 mg/kg/day, during hot months may be useful. Oral antibiotics for bacterial superinfections should be used.

ACRODERMATITIS ENTEROPATHICA
Clinical Features

Acrodermatitis enteropathica is an autosomal recessive disorder of zinc transport.[41,42] It is not apparent at birth, but begins at 1 to 2 months of age, with acral skin erosions, intermittent diarrhea, and failure to

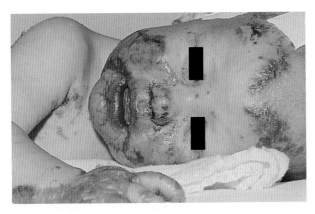

Fig. 19-39 Acrodermatitis enteropathica. Perioral erosions, scalp crusting, and hand erosions in infant.

thrive.[42] The erosions appear as red, moist areas over the distal extremities, including the hands and feet, and in the perioral and perineal areas (Fig. 19-39). Often, the cutaneous features precede the diarrhea by several weeks to several months. As the disorder continues, weight loss occurs, along with photophobia, apathy, irritability, anorexia, anemia, alopecia, thrush, and paronychia caused by *Candida albicans*. If the child survives the complications of malnutrition, the skin lesions become erythematous plaques with silvery scales that mimic psoriasis.[42]

Measuring serum or plasma zinc levels affirms the diagnosis.[42,43] There are many sources of zinc contamination in rubber stoppers and glass tubes and other blood-collecting devices that produce falsely high zinc levels. Thus the diagnosis may be obscured. Therefore blood samples should be collected in acid-washed sterile plastic tubes, using acid-washed plastic syringes.

Zinc deficiency can also be seen in premature and term infants who are fed a diet deficient in zinc. Occasionally human breast milk can be low in zinc, allowing zinc deficiency in the totally breast-fed infant.[42] Acquired zinc deficiency can be seen in organic acidurias, during hyperalimentation, and a variety of severe gastrointestinal disturbances.[41]

Differential Diagnosis

The lesions of acrodermatitis enteropathica are often mistaken for mucocutaneous candidiasis associated with an immune deficiency such as human immunodeficiency virus (HIV) infection. Measuring plasma or serum zinc levels will distinguish between the two. Often, protein-calorie malnutrition states are considered, but lesions usually develop in such patients after 6 months of age, and the nutritional history may

distinguish between the two. Cystic fibrosis can present with loose stools and acral erythematous eruption.[44] Histiocytosis X will present with intertriginous erosions in infancy. Acquired zinc deficiency states, such as seen with prolonged parenteral hyperalimentation, will mimic acrodermatitis enteropathica. Necrolytic migratory erythema, seen with a glucagonoma, will also mimic the lesions of acrodermatitis enteropathica.[41]

Pathogenesis

Depletion of body zinc stores caused by faulty transport of zinc is responsible for the symptoms and signs of acrodermatitis enteropathica.[42,43] It is not known whether this is due to the lack of a zinc carrier protein or to some defect of zinc absorption in the intestine. Zinc is stored in the same tissues as iron and serves as an important cofactor for a variety of enzymes, such as alkaline phosphatase and carbonic anhydrase. The zinc deficiency is the result of depletion of total body stores. It is believed that zinc deficiency results in impairment of metalloenzyme activity, which produces the clinical features.[39,40] The genetic defect has been localized to 8q24.3 region.[45]

Treatment

Oral zinc sulfate, 5 mg/kg/day given twice daily, produces rapid clinical improvement.[42] Apathy disappears within 24 hours, and the skin lesions and diarrhea resolve within 7 to 14 days. Photophobia, alopecia, and growth failure are reversed over the ensuing months.

Patient Education

The hereditary inability to absorb zinc should be explained to the patient and family. It is not known whether lifetime maintenance with supplemental zinc is required.

Follow-up Visits

A visit 2 weeks after diagnosis is useful to repeat measurement of zinc levels and to evaluate the response to treatment. The measurement of plasma or serum zinc levels at monthly intervals is useful to monitor supplemental zinc requirements.

REFERENCES

1. Spitz JL: *Genodermatoses: a full-color clinical guide to genetic skin disorders,* Baltimore, 1996, Williams & Wilkins.
2. Sybert VP: *Genetic skin disorders,* New York, 1997, Oxford University Press.

3. http://www.genetests.org

4. Ammirati CT, Mallory SB: The major inherited disorders of cornification: new advances in pathogenesis, *Dermatol Clin* 16(3):497, 1998.

5. Rabinowitz LG, Esterly NB: Atopic dermatitis and ichthyosis vulgaris, *Pediatr Rev* 15:220, 1994.

6. Mukerjee S, Gupta AB: A statistical study on the in vivo sorption and desorption of water in ichthyosis vulgaris, *J Dermatol* 21:78, 1994.

7. Hernandez-Martin A, Gonzalez-Sarmiento R, De Unamuno P: X-linked ichthyosis: an update, *Br J Dermatol* 141(4):617, 1999.

8. Buyse L et al: Collodion baby dehydration: the danger of high transepidermal water loss, *Br J Dermatol* 129:86, 1993.

9. Niemi KM et al: Clinical light and electron microscopic features of recessive congenital ichthyosis type I, *Br J Dermatol* 130:626, 1994.

10. Anton-Lamprecht I: Ultrastructural identification of basic abnormalities as clues to genetic disorders of the epidermis, *J Invest Dermatol* 103:6s, 1994.

11. Basarab T et al: Ichthyosis bullosa of Siemens: report of a family with evidence of a keratin 2e mutation, and a review of the literature, *Br J Dermatol* 140(4):689, 1999.

12. Bale SJ, Doyle SZ: The genetics of ichthyosis: a primer for epidemiologists, *J Invest Dermatol* 102:49s, 1994.

13. Burton JL: Keratin genes and epidermolytic hyperkeratosis, *Lancet* 344:1103, 1994.

14. Fuchs E et al: Genetic basis of epidermolysis bullosa simplex and epidermolytic hyperkeratosis, *J Invest Dermatol* 103:25s, 1994.

15. DiGiovanna JJ, Bale SJ: Epidermolytic hyperkeratosis: applied molecular genetics, *J Invest Dermatol* 102:390, 1994.

16. Huber M et al: Mutations of keratinocyte transglutaminase in lamellar ichthyosis, *Science* 267:525, 1995.

17. Paller AS et al: Genetic and clinical mosaicism in a type of epidermal nevus, *N Engl J Med* 331:1408, 1994.

18. Steijlen PM, Van Dooren-Greebe RJ, Van de Kerkhof PC: Acitretin in the treatment of lamellar ichthyosis, *Br J Dermatol* 130:211, 1994.

19. Paige DG et al: Bone changes and their significance with ichthyosis on long-term etretinate therapy, *Br J Dermatol* 127:387, 1992.

20. Ruiz-Maldonado R, Tamayo-Sanchez L, Orozco-Covarrubias ML: The use of retinoids in the pediatric patient, *Dermatol Clin* 16(3):553, 1998.

21. Chavanas S et al: Mutations in SPINK5, encoding a serine protease inhibitor, cause Netherton syndrome, *Nat Genet* 25(2):141, 2000.

22. Fine J-D et al: Epidermolysis bullosa: clinical, epidemiologic, and laboratory advances and the findings of the National Epidermolysis Bullosa Registry, Baltimore, 1999, The Johns Hopkins University Press.

23. Marinkovich MP: Update on inherited bullous dermatoses, *Dermatol Clin* 17(3):473, 1999.

24. Travis SPL et al: Oral and gastrointestinal manifestations of epidermolysis bullosa, *Lancet* 340:1505, 1992.

25. Pessar A, Verdicchio JF, Caldwell D: Epidermolysis bullosa: the Pediatric Dermatological Management and Therapeutic Update, *Adv Dermatol* 3:99, 1988.

26. Falabella AF et al: The use of tissue-engineered skin (Apligraf) to treat a newborn with epidermolysis bullosa, *Arch Dermatol* 135(10):1219, 1999.

27. Robbins PB et al: In vivo restoration of laminin 5β3 expression and function in junctional epidermolysis bullosa, *PNAS* 98:5193, 2001.

28. Landy SJ, Donnai D: Incontinentia pigmenti (Bloch-Sulzberger syndrome), *J Med Genet* 30:53, 1993.

29. Ashley JR, Burgdorf WHC: Incontinentia pigmenti: pigmentary changes independent of incontinence, *J Cutan Pathol* 14:248, 1987.

30. Shastry BS: Recent progress in the genetics of incontinentia pigmenti (Bloch-Sulzberger syndrome), *J Hum Genet* 45(6):323, 2000.

31. Masse JF, Perusse R: Ectodermal dysplasia, *Arch Dis Child* 71:1, 1994.

32. Zonana J et al: Detection of de novo mutations and analysis of their origin in families with X linked hypohidrotic ectodermal dysplasia, *J Med Genet* 31:287, 1994.

33. Berg D et al: Sweating in ectodermal dysplasia syndromes, *Arch Dermatol* 126:1075, 1990.

34. Elomaa O et al: Ectodysplasin is released by proteolytic shedding and binds to the EDAR protein, *Hum Mol Genet* 10(9):953, 2001.

35. Lamartine J et al: Mutations in the human connexin gene GJB6 cause hidrotic ectodermal dysplasia (Clouston syndrome), *Nat Genet* 26:142, 2000.

36. Kilmer SL, Grix AW Jr, Isseroff RR: Focal dermal hypoplasia: four cases with widely varying presentations, *J Am Acad Dermatol* 28:839, 1993.

37. Lucker GPH, Van De Kerkhof PCM, Steijlen PM: The hereditary palmoplantar keratoses: an updated review and classification, *Br J Dermatol* 131:1, 1994.

38. Corden LD, McLean WH: Human keratin diseases: hereditary fragility of specific epithelial tissues, *Exp Dermatol* 5(6):297, 1996.

39. Burge S: Darier's disease: the clinical features and pathogenesis, *Clin Exp Dermatol* 19:193, 1994.

40. Sakuntabhai A et al: Mutations in ATP2A2, encoding a Ca²⁺ pump, cause Darier disease, *Nat Genet* 21(3):271, 1999.

41. Black CK, Piette WW: The multisystem spectrum of necrolytic migratory erythema, *Curr Opin Dermatol* 1:87, 1995.

42. Van Wouve J: Clinical and laboratory diagnosis of acrodermatitis enteropathica, *Eur J Pediatr* 149:2, 1989.

43. Sandstrom B et al: Acrodermatitis enteropathica, zinc metabolism, copper status and immune function, *Arch Pediatr Adolesc Med* 148:980, 1994.

44. Darmstadt GL et al: Dermatitis as a presenting sign of cystic fibrosis, *Arch Dermatol* 128(10):1358, 1992.

45. Wang K et al: Homozygosity mapping places the acrodermatitis enteropathica gene on chromosomal region 8q24.3, *Am J Hum Genet* 68(4):1055, 2001.

CHAPTER TWENTY | Drug Eruptions

There is an enormous variety of cutaneous reactions to drugs, with many different clinical patterns.[1-13] The uncommon, but life-threatening drug eruptions include Stevens-Johnson syndrome, toxic epidermal necrolysis (see Chapter 11),[3,7,13] widespread bullous reactions, and angioedema/anaphylaxis (see Chapter 14).[2,3,5,7] Common patterns include morbilliform eruptions, urticarial eruptions, and fixed drug eruptions. Vasculitic, lichenoid, purpuric, scarlatiniform, the exfoliative dermatitis/fever/hepatitis/lymphadenopathy syndrome, phototoxic, photoallergic, Sweet's syndrome, and acute generalized erythematous pustular (AGEP) eruptions have all been described in children.[1-13] Acneiform reactions and pigmentary disturbances are discussed in Chapters 3 and 16.

The diagnosis of a drug eruption is usually based on clinical suspicion and not confirmed by rechallenge studies. Evaluation of the possibility of a drug eruption depends on the patient's previous experience with specific drugs and the experience of the general population with drugs to which the patient has been exposed. The morphology of the patient's lesions, and the relative frequency of similar-type reactions in the general population, are of assistance. Specific medications have a higher frequency of drug eruptions and specific types of a drug eruption than other medications. The timing of the eruption in relationship to the commencement of drug therapy may assist in establishing the association of the drug with the eruption. The onset of disease after ingestion of the drug varies from a few hours in urticarial reactions to as long as 3 months in exfoliative dermatitis and lichenoid reactions (Table 20-1). The clinician should look for alternate explanations for the eruption, including infection or the primary illness. This is especially true in erythema nodosum[11,12] and exfoliative dermatitis in infants and children,[14] in which drugs rarely are the cause. Withdrawal of the suspected drug may help in the diagnosis. However, removal of the suspected drug from the patient may not always result in rapid resolution of the drug eruption. Clearing is slow in the exfoliative dermatitis/hepatitis/fever/lymphadenopathy reactions to anticonvulsants. Fortunately the incidence of adverse drug reactions in infants and children appears to be less than in adults.[3,7] For a few drugs, the relative risk of a particular reaction is known (Table 20-2), but for many drug reactions, it is undetermined.

CLINICAL FEATURES
Commonly Seen Types of Drug Eruptions
Morbilliform drug eruptions

Cutaneous drug reactions often have specific patterns. The morbilliform (so-called *maculopapular eruption*) or exanthematous eruption is probably the most common of all drug-induced eruptions in children.[2-5] The term *morbilliform* means measles-like because of the development of a maculopapular erythematous rash that becomes confluent (Figs. 20-1 and 20-2). This rash often starts on the trunk and extends onto the extremities. It is frequently symmetric and often has areas of totally normal skin that are surrounded by the eruption (Fig. 20-3). The initial macules may become papular, and then large plaques may form from the confluence of the individual lesions. The eruption typically lasts 7 to 14 days and may be associated with pruritus during that time. The patient may have associated fever, malaise, and arthralgias. Box 20-1 lists drugs associated with morbilliform drug eruptions; Table 20-3 lists the frequency of morbilliform rash to specific drugs.

Urticarial drug eruptions

Drug eruptions associated with hives are called *urticarial drug eruptions*. These present as edematous, flat, erythematous papules that usually last less than 24 hours (Fig. 20-4). New lesions appear almost continuously. The lesions may begin as small discrete papules that become confluent, large, figurate plaques (Fig. 20-5). Occasionally, the edema can be so intense in the center of the erythematous papules and plaques that the center appears less erythematous than the periphery, giving a target appearance. Lesions may resolve, leaving a macular blue-brown appearance that looks like a bruise. The absence of epidermal injury and more typical urticarial papules and plaques on the rest of the body confirm that this is an urticarial drug eruption and not erythema multiforme. Box 20-2 lists the drugs associated with urticarial drug eruptions.

Table 20-1	Onset of Drug Eruption After Ingestion of Medication

Reaction	Time
Acute generalized erythematous pustulosis	Hours to 2 days
Urticaria	Hours to 7 days
Phototoxic eruptions	Hours to 7 days
Fixed drug eruption	1 to 7 days
Generalized pustular eruptions	1 to 21 days
Morbilliform eruptions	7 to 21 days
Scarlatiniform eruptions	7 to 21 days
Bullous drug reactions	7 to 21 days
Erythema nodosum eruptions	14 to 56 days
Stevens-Johnson syndrome	14 to 56 days
Toxic epidermal necrolysis	14 to 56 days
Exfoliative dermatitis/fever/ hepatitis/lymphadenopathy syndrome	30 to 100 days
Lichenoid eruptions	30 to 100 days

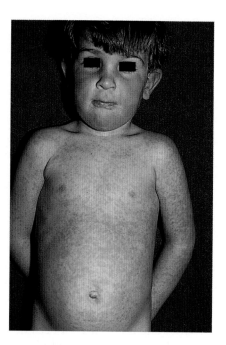

Fig. 20-1 Morbilliform drug eruption. Trimethoprim-sulfamethoxazole–induced eruption with discrete macules and papules on the trunk and confluent erythema on the face.

Table 20-2	Relative Risk of Life-threatening Drug Reactions* Among Anticonvulsants

Drug	Relative Risk
Carbamazepine	120
Phenytoin	91
Phenobarbital	57
Lamotrigine	25
Valproic acid	24

*Stevens-Johnson syndrome and toxic epidermal necrolysis.

Table 20-3	Frequencies of Drug Morbilliform Rash With Antibiotic Treatment

Drug	Frequency (%)
Cefaclor	12.3
Sulfonamides	8.5
Penicillins	7.4
Other cephalosporins	2.6

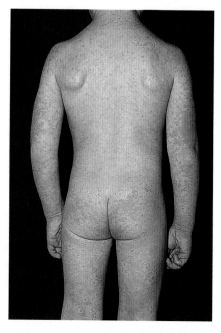

Fig. 20-2 Morbilliform drug eruption. Trimethoprim-sulfamethoxazole–induced eruption with confluence of lesions on the upper arms and buttocks.

Box 20-1 Drugs Associated With Morbilliform Drug Eruptions

ANTIBIOTICS
Amoxicillin
Ampicillin
Cephalosporins
Chloramphenicol
Erythromycin
Gentamicin sulfate
Isoniazid
Penicillins
Sulfonamides
Trimethoprim
Trimethoprim-sulfamethoxazole combinations

NONSTEROIDAL ANTIINFLAMMATORY DRUGS (NSAIDs)
Ibuprofen
Meclofenamate sodium
Piroxicam

Sulindac
Zomepirac sodium

ANTICONVULSANTS
Barbiturates
Carbamazepine
Phenytoin
Tacrolimus
Allopurinol
Alprazolam

ANTIFUNGALS
Fluconazole
Ketoconazole
Itraconazole
Infliximab

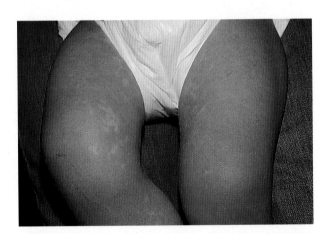

Fig. 20-3 Morbilliform drug eruption. Confluent intense erythema with islands of normal skin in a patient treated with both phenobarbital and trimethoprim-sulfamethoxazole.

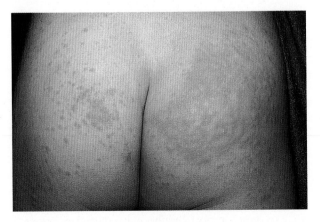

Fig. 20-4 Mixed urticarial and morbilliform drug eruption. Trimethoprim-sulfamethoxazole–induced urticarial plaques on the left buttock with maculopapular lesions on the right buttock.

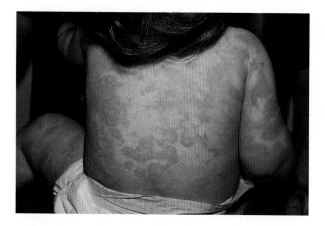

Fig. 20-5 Urticarial drug eruption. Large urticarial plaques in a child treated with cefaclor.

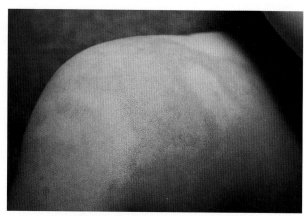

Fig. 20-6 Serum-sickness–like reaction to cefaclor. The urticarial lesions resolve with a dusky, bruised appearance. Note the swelling and edema involving the knee.

Box 20-2 Drugs Commonly Associated With Urticarial Drug Eruptions
NSAIDs, especially ibuprofen Cephalosporins, especially Ceclor Acetylsalicylic acid Antibiotics Amoxicillin Ampicillin Penicillins Sulfonamides Trimethoprim-sulfamethoxazole Asparaginase

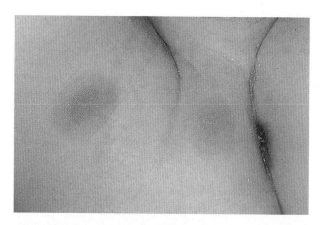

Fig. 20-7 Fixed drug eruption. Trimethoprim-sulfamethoxazole–induced oval, erythematous macules with diffuse hyperpigmentation within several lesions.

If the lesions show a deep extension with induration and swelling of the subcutaneous tissue, the reaction is called *angioedema*. If angioedema involves the mucous membranes, it can become life threatening secondary to airway obstruction.

One variant of urticaria is the serum-sickness–like reaction that clinically initially appears to resemble urticaria, often accompanied by angioedema (Fig. 20-6). The child may develop fever, pruritus, arthritis, and/or arthralgias. As in urticaria, the large plaques may resolve with dusky to purple centers, giving the skin a bruised appearance. The affected child may appear severely ill and be very uncomfortable. Cephalosporins are most commonly reported to cause this type of drug eruption.[2-5]

Fixed drug eruptions

Fixed drug eruptions may present as solitary or multiple, sharply demarcated, erythematous lesions that go on to give an intense macular hyperpigmentation (Fig. 20-7).[8,9] The lesions may initially appear edematous, like urticaria, or become bullous (Fig. 20-8). Over several days the edema and erythema will frequently decrease within the lesion, leaving a macular hyperpigmentation with sharply demarcated outlines in a figurate pattern. Rechallenges with the same medication may cause lesions in precisely the same spot and lesions on new locations as well. Box 20-3 lists the drugs that commonly cause fixed drug eruptions. Trimethoprim-sulfa, sulfonamides, and acetaminophen are the drugs that account for most childhood fixed drug eruptions.[8,9]

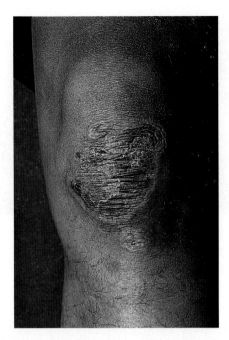

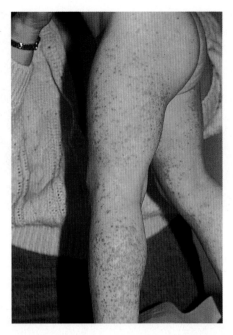

Fig. 20-8 Fixed drug eruption. Bullous reaction to tetracycline. The lesions have a necrotic, hyperpigmented epidermis with sharp demarcation of normal and involved skin.

Fig. 20-9 Vasculitis. Amoxicillin-induced lesions on legs.

Box 20-3	**Drugs Associated With Fixed Drug Eruptions***

Trimethoprim-sulfamethoxazole
Acetaminophen
Barbiturates
Sulfonamides
Carbamazepine
Phenolphthalein
Tetracycline
Trimethoprim
Ciprofloxacin
Oral contraceptives

*First four listed are most frequent

Box 20-4	**Drugs Associated With Vasculitis**

Allopurinol
Barbiturates and hydantoins
NSAIDs
Azithromycin
Gold
Penicillins, including ampicillin
Sulfonamides
Diuretics, including thiazides and furosemide
Cimetidine
Thioureas
Coumadin

Uncommon Drug Reaction Patterns
Vasculitis

Palpable purpuric lesions associated with cutaneous necrotizing vasculitis can be associated with drugs. The vasculitis is usually on the lower extremities in dependent areas but can occur anywhere on the body (Fig. 20-9). The lesions may begin as soft, small erythematous or urticarial papules that blanch when pressure is applied over the skin. Over several hours to days the lesions become firm and dark red-blue or purple. Box 20-4 lists drugs associated with vasculitis.

The exfoliative dermatitis/fever/hepatitis/lymphadenopathy syndrome

Progressively widespread erythema with scaling accompanied by fever, elevated liver enzymes, and finally generalized lymphadenopathy are seen in the

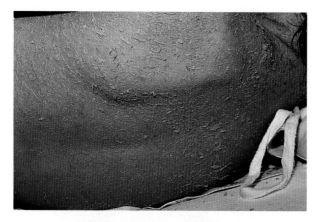

Fig. 20-10 The exfoliative dermatitis/fever/hepatitis/lymph-adenopathy syndrome. Diffuse erythema and marked desquamation in an adolescent on dilantin, misdiagnosed as lymphoma.

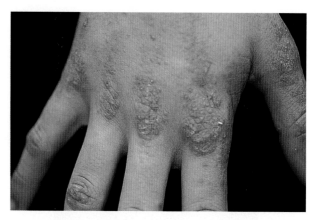

Fig. 20-11 Lichenoid eruption of the hand in a child treated with thiazide diuretics.

Box 20-5   Drugs Associated With Exfoliative Dermatitis/Fever/Hepatitis/Lymphadenopathy Syndrome

Hydantoins
Carbamazepine
Allopurinol
Barbiturates
Penicillins
Phenazone derivatives (phenylbutazone)
Sulfonamides
NSAIDs, including sulindac

Box 20-6   Drugs Associated With Acute Generalized Erythematous Pustulosis (AGEP)

Antibiotics, particularly amoxicillin, azithromycin, and erythromycin, and rarely, the cephalosporins
Anticonvulsants, such as carbamazepine
NSAIDs
Sulfonamides

Box 20-7   Drugs Associated With Lichenoid Eruptions

Diuretics, such as furosemide and thiazides
Beta-blockers
Antimalarials
Phenothiazine

---

exfoliative dermatitis/fever/hepatitis/lymphadenopathy syndrome (Fig. 20-10). This may mimic lymphoma or chronic infections. Often the drug is not suspected because the child has been receiving it for 1 or 2 months. Discontinuation of the drug slowly results in reversal of symptoms. The hydantoin anticonvulsants are the most frequently implicated (Box 20-5).

Acute generalized erythematous pustulosis

A rapid onset of widespread truncal redness with thousands of pinpoint (0.1 mm) pustules, followed by waves of desquamation, characterizes the distinct uncommon reaction pattern of acute generalized erythematous pustulosis (AGEP). It may begin within hours of starting the drug and certainly within a few days. The child appears toxic and may have fever.

Rapid reversal occurs with discontinuation of the drug. AGEP is particularly associated with amoxicillin, macrolide antibiotics, and anticonvulsants (Box 20-6).

Lichenoid drug eruptions

Slowly developing purple-red plaques characterize lichenoid eruptions (Fig 20-11). The onset is often 1 to

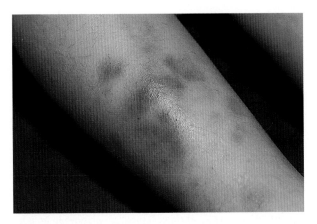

Fig. 20-12 Erythema nodosum on the leg of a child taking NSAIDs.

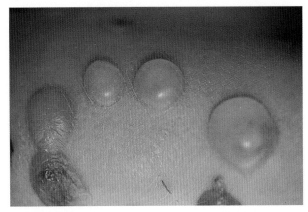

Fig. 20-13 Tense bullae in a child treated with vancomycin.

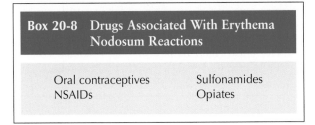

Box 20-8	**Drugs Associated With Erythema Nodosum Reactions**	
Oral contraceptives	Sulfonamides	
NSAIDs	Opiates	

Box 20-9	**Drugs Associated With Widespread Bullous Reactions**	
Vancomycin	NSAIDs	

3 months after starting the drug. The skin lesions may mimic lupus erythematosus or dermatomyositis. Diuretics and beta blockers are most responsible (Box 20-7).

Erythema nodosum reactions

Tender, ill-defined, red to dusky-red nodules are seen on the legs in erythema nodosum (Fig 20-12). The onset is abrupt and begins 2 to 5 weeks after starting the drug. Oral contraceptives are most frequently implicated, but infectious causes are far more likely than drug reactions (Box 20-8).

Bullous drug reactions

In bullous drug reactions, tense bullae develop, usually on the extremities but often widespread (Fig. 20-13). They often begin within 2 weeks of starting the drug. Vancomycin is the most common cause of there eruptions (Box 20-9).

Photosensitive drug eruptions

Drug photosensitivity reactions can be either phototoxic or photoallergic. In either situation a combination of topical or systemic medication and exposure to light is necessary.

Photoallergic reactions are less common than phototoxic reactions. The photoallergic reaction involves an immunologic response to a chemical (drug) that is altered by ultraviolet light. The body recognizes the altered form as a foreign antigen and develops an immunologic delayed hypersensitivity response. This process requires sufficient drug and light to produce adequate antigen for immunization.

Phototoxic reactions involve direct cutaneous injury by a drug after the drug is changed by light energy. Increased light energy or an increased amount of drug increases the risk of a phototoxic reaction.

Photosensitive eruptions are characterized by more intense dermatitis in the areas of greatest sun exposure. Often the face, upper trunk, and extensor surfaces of the arms are involved. The lesions are usually erythematous and edematous, with associated papules, vesicles, or oozing, weeping lesions. Increased skin fragility and scarring may be seen. Lesions may resolve with marked hyperpigmentation that may remain for months.

Phototoxic reactions are often painful, similar to a severe sunburn (Figs. 20-14 and 20-15). Drugs responsible for phototoxic reactions are listed in Box 20-10.

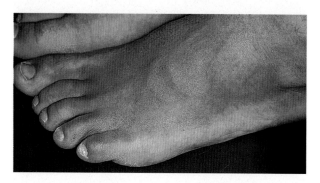

Fig. 20-14 Acute sunburn phototoxic reaction in an adolescent receiving tetracycline.

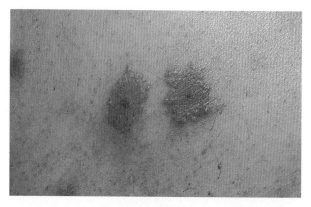

Fig. 20-16 Sweet's syndrome. Tender red plaques in an adolescent treated with Neupogen.

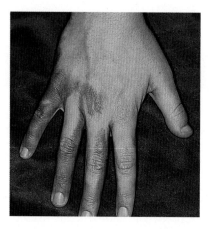

Fig. 20-15 Phototoxic reaction to psoralen-containing plant that caused marked hyperpigmentation of the hand.

Box 20-11 Drugs Associated With Photoallergic Reaction

Fragrances and perfumes   Phenothiazines
PABA esters   Sulfonamides

Box 20-12 Drugs Associated With Sweet's Syndrome

Granulocyte colony stimulating factor
Granulocyte-macrophage colony stimulating factor

Box 20-10 Drugs Associated With Phototoxic Reactions

Coal tar derivatives
Furocoumarins found in plants
Furosemide
Griseofulvin
Ibuprofen
Methotrexate
Naproxen
Nifedipine
Para-aminobenzoic (PABA) esters
Phenothiazines
Psoralen
Sulfonamides
Tetracycline
Thiazides
Tretinoin

Photoallergic reactions may be painful or have severe pruritus in the areas of the most intense sun exposure. Phototoxic reactions are dependent on both the amount of drug and the amount of light exposure. In addition to sunlight, fluorescent lamps or sunlight that comes through window glass may produce photosensitive drug reactions. Drugs responsible for photoallergic reactions are listed in Box 20-11.

Sweet's syndrome reactions

Acute febrile neutrophilic dermatosis (Sweet's syndrome) is characterized by the abrupt onset of tender red plaques on the skin (Fig. 20-16). It is rare, but with the increasing use of recombinant granulocyte stimulating factors the drug-induced eruption is far more frequent than the spontaneous disease (Box 20-12).

DIFFERENTIAL DIAGNOSIS
Commonly Seen Types of Drug Reactions
Morbilliform drug eruptions

The onset of the eruption may occur after the offending drug is stopped. Morbilliform eruptions may fade over time, even with continuation of the responsible medication. Morbilliform drug eruptions caused by antimicrobial agents are often a diagnostic dilemma because the eruption may be a viral illness misdiagnosed as bacterial infection and treated with antibiotics. The morbilliform rash may be a viral exanthem.

Urticarial drug eruptions

Urticarial lesions are usually pruritic, and at times it is difficult to separate an urticarial eruption from a morbilliform eruption early in the course of the condition (see Fig. 20-4). Urticarial lesions may occur immediately after exposure to the drug, or within several days. The individual urticarial lesions usually resolve over 24 hours, with new lesions arising. In the morbilliform drug eruption, individual lesions expand over several days, giving more of a confluent, macular-type eruption, whereas urticarial plaques are raised and indurated. Urticarial lesions commonly occur in children and are most often not associated with drugs (see Chapter 13). The serum-sickness–like reaction to drugs is not usually associated with circulating immune complexes, proteinuria, and lymphadenopathy, which are seen in a true serum-sickness reaction. The eruption usually begins 7 or more days after the drug is first given.

Fixed drug eruptions

Erythema multiforme, traumatic skin bruising, and pigmented lesions may be confused with fixed drug eruptions. Biopsy of the fixed drug lesion will often help to confirm the diagnosis.[13] A history of a previous episode with the drug should be sought. Rechallenge with the suspected medication may cause recurrences of similar lesions in the identical spot. The area of residual macular hyperpigmentation may take several months to resolve.

Uncommon Drug Reaction Patterns
Vasculitis

Drug-induced vasculitis can occur quickly after drug exposure or prolonged drug use. Because drugs are one of many causes of cutaneous vasculitis, other conditions inducing these lesions must be considered. Sepsis with bacterial emboli, and many viruses, can cause palpable purpura with very similar cutaneous appearances. Biopsy of an individual lesion can confirm the small-vessel vasculitis, and immunofluorescence examination of the biopsy should be negative in drug-related conditions; however, IgA or other immunoreactants may be found in infectious vasculitis.

The exfoliative dermatitis/fever/hepatitis/ lymphadenopathy syndrome

Atopic dermatitis, severe contact dermatitis, or psoriasis may mimic the initial lesions. As the disease progresses, lymphoma, Epstein Barr virus, human immunodeficiency virus (HIV) infections, or other chronic infections are often considered. A skin biopsy will sometimes differentiate.[13] Improvement after withdrawal of the suspected drug is definitive.

Acute generalized erythematous pustulosis

Pustular psoriasis may demonstrate the same gross morphology as AGEP, but the presence in skin biopsy samples of interstitial and angiocentric neutrophils in the drug reaction will distinguish.[13]

Lichenoid drug eruptions

The skin lesions may mimic lichen planus, lupus erythematosus, or dermatomyositis. The findings of skin biopsy will mimic other lichenoid eruptions, but immunofluorescent examinations are negative in drug reactions.[13]

Erythema nodosum reactions

Erythema nodosum reactions caused by infections are far more likely than those related to drug reactions. The histology is the same.

Bullous drug reactions

Immunobullous disorders or porphyrias may mimic drug-induced disease. Diuretics and nonsteroidal antiinflammatory drugs (NSAIDs) may produce a pseudoporphyria syndrome that mimics porphyria cutanea tarda. Examination of plasma or urinary porphyrins will distinguish the porphyrias.

Biopsy for immunofluorescent examination will be negative in most drug-induced reactions and positive in immunobullous disorders. The exception is vancomycin-induced bullae in which linear IgA deposits are found along the dermal-epidermal junction, as found in linear IgA dermatosis. Improvement after withdrawal of the drug is definitive.

Photosensitive drug eruptions

Childhood dermatomyositis, lupus erythematosus, idiopathic photodermatosis, and erythropoietic protoporphyria may mimic photosensitive drug reactions.

A skin biopsy for immunofluorescence is negative in drug reactions and often positive in collagen vascular diseases.

Sweet's syndrome reactions

Acute febrile neutrophilic dermatosis caused by acute myelogenous leukemias are rare and may be distinguished on skin biopsy by the presence of atypical myelogenous cells in the dermal infiltrate.

PATHOGENESIS

Drug reactions can occur secondary to immunologic or nonimmunologic reactions. Immunologic reactions require host immunologic pathways and are called *drug allergies*. The ability of a drug to elicit an immune reaction depends on many characteristics. Most drugs are small organic molecules with molecular weights less than 1000 daltons. Because of their size, they are unable to elicit immune responses unless they bind to a larger molecule, which is usually a protein macromolecule. In this situation the drug functions as a hapten. Most drugs have little ability to form covalent bonds with macromolecules and are unable to form this type of immunologic antigen.

The host reacts to drugs in different manners. The body may respond differently to a drug given intravenously than to one applied topically. Patients may have variation in their ability to absorb or metabolize a given drug. The patient with infectious mononucleosis may be more likely to develop a morbilliform eruption to ampicillin.

The body's immunologic response to drugs may be immunoglobulin E (IgE)–dependent, which can be associated with pruritus, urticaria, bronchial spasm, and laryngeal edema. Drug eruptions may be associated with serum sickness caused by circulating immune complexes. Cytotoxic drug reactions can occur where the drug combines with the tissue, and that combination then becomes the target for antibodies or cellular-mediated cytotoxicity.

Most morbilliform reactions are not reproducible and are believed to be nonimmunologic. Nonimmunologic drug reactions can result through various modalities. Aspirin, opiates, and radiocontrast medications may directly release mast cell mediators, resulting in urticaria. Overdosage of a medicine may cause adverse cutaneous side effects by direct injury to cutaneous cells. Genetic inability to detoxify certain chemical compounds results in toxic metabolites that can also damage cutaneous cells. Direct activation of granulocytic cells by colony stimulating factors is responsible for Sweet's syndrome.

Secondary side effects of chemotherapy can include alopecia or particular types of rashes secondary to thrombocytopenia, or it can target specific areas of skin, as in acral erythema seen with cytotoxic agents. Antibiotics can destroy the normal bacterial flora, allowing overgrowth of other organisms.

Drugs may interact to compete for binding sites or cause metabolic changes. In addition, certain drugs, such as lithium, can exacerbate acne and psoriasis by activating neutrophils. Treatment with NSAIDs of a child with urticaria can exacerbate the urticaria.

Drug-induced urticaria can also be caused by IgE mechanisms, anti-IgE receptor antibodies, or circulating immune complexes. The IgE-dependent urticaria reactions usually occur within 36 hours of drug exposure, but they can occur within minutes. The eruption associated with circulating immune complexes is a type of serum-sickness reaction. It usually begins 4 to 12 days after exposure to the drug, at which time an equilibrium has been achieved between antibody and drug antigen, allowing for the formation of immune complexes. The serum-sickness–type reaction is often accompanied by fever, hematuria, and arthralgia. Liver and neurologic injury may occur.

The pathophysiology of drug-associated cutaneous vasculitis is not clear, but immune complexes may be responsible. The lesions usually begin to resolve several days or weeks after the offending drug is removed.

The histologic picture for photoallergic contact dermatitis and phototoxic reaction is similar, with associated epidermal spongiosis, dermal edema, and inflammatory response. True phototoxicity is pathologically more like sunburn than a dermatitis.

The photosensitivity may be confirmed by a photopatch test in which the drug is readministered and multiple intensities of ultraviolet light exposure are given. Photosensitive reactions are usually in the ultraviolet A range. Photosensitive reactions often resolve with marked hyperpigmentation that may take several months to resolve.

TREATMENT

Removal of the offending drug is the usual first therapy. Drug eruption is easily diagnosed when one can identify a specific pattern of drug eruption with a known timely exposure to only a single medication, and that medication has been frequently associated with that specific type of eruption. The infant or child exposed to multiple medications over a short period offers a more difficult diagnostic and therapeutic dilemma. Depending on the severity of the drug reaction, none of the drugs, the most likely drug, or all of the drugs may need to be removed.

Morbilliform eruptions may fade with time, without drug removal, especially when associated with amoxicillin or ampicillin. Urticarial eruptions may respond to antihistamine therapy.

Anaphylaxis associated with urticarial eruptions and angioedema is a medical emergency. Immediate therapy should be started with 1:1000 aqueous epinephrine, 0.2 to 0.5 ml given subcutaneously, and intravenous fluids. Antihistamines and systemic steroids may also be required to maintain an adequate airway while the symptoms subside.

Early referral to the appropriate center may be lifesaving for children with Stevens-Johnson syndrome or toxic epidermal necrolysis (see Chapter 11).

PATIENT EDUCATION

The parents of the affected child should be informed of the possible association of the cutaneous eruption and the specific drugs involved. The risk for the child from subsequent exposure to the specific or similar medications needs to be explained. For a severe reaction, the child may be instructed to wear a bracelet or necklace to alert examining health care workers to the suspected allergy. The parents should be informed of alternative forms of therapy that would avoid the offending agent.

The cause of the photosensitivity should be fully described to the family and child. If the drug that caused a phototoxic reaction is required, it may be continued if the ultraviolet light intensity can be decreased to a level that is not adequate to cause significant dermatitis. Children who develop a phototoxic reaction to psoralen-containing plants, such as celery or limes, should avoid the combination of plant exposure and sun exposure. If possible, the photosensitizing drug should be totally withdrawn. If hyperpigmentation occurs, it may require months to resolve.

FOLLOW-UP VISITS

Follow-up visits are necessary to confirm the resolution of the eruption and recognize the response of the original illness that required drug therapy. The frequency and timing of the visits will depend on the severity of the original illness and the drug eruption.

The patient's medical records should document the possible drug-associated eruption to attempt avoidance of future exposures to the drug or related compounds. For penicillin-associated reactions, skin testing may be indicated to attempt to predict the future possibility of hypersensitivity reactions to the penicillins.

In children with photosensitive drug eruptions, additional follow-up visits for photopatch testing to confirm the diagnosis may be considered.

REFERENCES

1. Litt JS: *Drug eruption reference manual 2000,* New York, 2000, Parthenon.
2. Knowles S, Shapiro L, Shear NH: Drug eruptions in children, *Adv Dermatol* 14:399, 1999.
3. Wolkenstein P, Revuz J: Allergic emergencies encountered by the dermatologist: severe cutaneous adverse drug reactions, *Clin Rev Allergy Immunol* 17:497, 1999.
4. Ibia EO, Schwartz RH, Wiedermann RL: Antibiotic rashes in children, *Arch Dermatol* 136:849, 2000.
5. Romano A: Recognizing antibacterial hypersensitivity in children, *Paediatric Drugs* 2:101, 2000.
6. Park J, Matsui D, Rieder MJ: Multiple antibiotic sensitivity syndrome in children, *Can J Clin Pharmacol* 7:38, 2000.
7. Lazarou J, Pomeranz BH, Corey PN: Incidence of adverse drug reactions in hospitalized patients: a meta-analysis of prospective studies, *JAMA* 279:1200, 1998.
8. Morelli JG et al: Fixed drug eruptions in children, *J Pediatrics* 134:365, 1999.
9. Mahboob A, Haroon TS: Drugs causing fixed eruptions: a study of 450 cases, *Int J Dermatol* 37:833, 1998.
10. Diaz Jara M et al: Allergic reactions due to ibuprofen in children, *Pediatr Dermatol* 18:66, 2001.
11. Cribier B et al: Erythema nodosum and associated diseases: a study of 129 cases, *Int J Dermatol* 37:667, 1998.
12. Kakourou T et al: Erythema nodosum in children: a prospective study, *J Am Acad Dermatol* 44:17, 2001.
13. Crowson AN, Magro CM: Recent advances in the pathology of cutaneous drug eruptions, *Dermatol Clin* 17:37, 1999.
14. Pruszkowski A et al: Neonatal and infantile erythrodermas, *Arch Dermatol* 136:875, 2000.

CHAPTER TWENTY-ONE

Skin Diseases In Newborns

Skin lesions appearing in the first month of life usually prompt parents to seek medical advice. A thorough knowledge of fetal skin biology (see Chapter 1) and of cutaneous lesions of newborns is expected of those providing neonatal care.

This chapter is divided into five sections: neonatal skin care, transient skin disease in the newborn, birthmarks, common congenital malformations, and miscellaneous skin conditions in the newborn period. Many of the transient disorders of the newborn will be considered by their clinical features, differential diagnosis, and pathogenesis only because no treatment is required of these self-limited problems. Acne neonatorum is also discussed in Chapter 3, miliaria in Chapter 11, and pigmentary changes in Chapter 17.

NEONATAL SKIN CARE

The full-term newborn's skin feels very soft and smooth. The smooth texture and softness is related to the hydration of the epidermis and condition of the collagen and dermal matrix substances. At birth the full-term infant's skin is functionally mature. The barrier portion of the epidermis, the stratum corneum, is intact and effectively protects the infant.

Even though the infant's barrier function may be normal at birth, he or she is at increased risk for systemic toxicity of topically applied compounds (Box 21-1). The infant's surface area is great when compared to body mass. The infant's metabolism, excretion, distribution, and protein binding of chemical agents may be different from those of an adult. The premature infant is at much greater risk. The premature infant has markedly decreased epidermal barrier function and an even greater body surface area to body volume ratio. In addition, the immature organs of the premature infant may greatly change the metabolism, excretion, distribution, and protein binding of chemical agents. Local or systemic toxicity can occur in the premature infant from soaps, lotions, or other cleansing solutions that may not cause problems for the term infant.

The skin of the mature infant often appears dry and cracked soon after birth (Figs. 21-1 and 21-2).

The stratum corneum, which has been accumulated in utero, has not yet shed. Fissures and bleeding may occur on the ankles and wrist. During this time topical care should include moisturizing lotions or creams. The goal of therapy is to retain the soft flexible texture of the infant's skin by hydrating and lubricating the epidermis. For infants in a dry environment, the moisturizers may need to be used indefinitely. Infants from a more humid environment may need only intermittent use of moisturizers.

The skin care of the premature infant is much more difficult and complex (Box 21-2).[1-5] Not only is the barrier portion of the epidermis absent or defective, but the skin has markedly increased fragility. Because of epidermal and dermal injury, the infant may have significant cutaneous pain that is accentuated by routine handling. The infant is at risk for developing sepsis from skin-associated organisms.[6] Maintaining a humid environment will decrease the infant's transepidermal water loss and assist in skin hydration.[7] This can be done by using a humidity-controlled isolette or thin, plastic tents over infants under infrared warmers.

Dry, flaking, fissured skin of premature infants should be treated with moisturizing creams or ointments.[2,3] Petrolatum-based ointments with little or no preservatives appear to offer the greatest benefit and lowest risk. Ointments placed on an infant's skin under an infrared warmer will not cause cutaneous burns.

Box 21-1 Reasons for Increased Risk of Systemic Toxicity From Topically Applied Agents in Infants

Increased surface area to body weight ratio
Differences in drug excretion
Differences in drug metabolism
Differences in drug protein binding
Differences in drug distribution

Fig. 21-1 Dry, flaking skin on term infant 36 hours old.

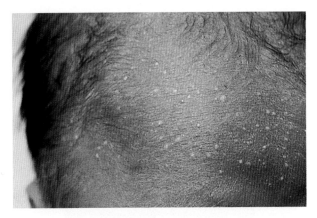

Fig. 21-3 Milia. Multiple white papules seen over the forehead of an infant.

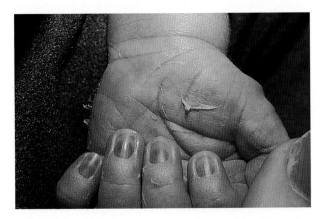

Fig. 21-2 Postmature infant. Long fingernails and peeling of the palms can be seen this 2-day-old infant.

Semipermeable wound dressings may offer additional cutaneous pain relief and protection, but additional studies must be done to analyze the potential for associated risk with bacterial growth under the dressings.[4]

TRANSIENT SKIN DISEASE
Milia
Clinical features

Milia are multiple, white, 1- to 2-mm papules seen over the forehead, cheeks, and nose of infants (Fig. 21-3). They may be present in the oral cavity as well, where they are called *Epstein's pearls*. Approximately 40% of newborns have milia on the skin, and 60% on the palate.[8] The cystic spheres rupture onto the skin surface and exfoliate their contents within a few weeks of birth.

Differential diagnosis

Molluscum contagiosum, an acquired viral infection, may mimic milia but does not usually appear in the

---

Box 21-2   Care of the Premature Infant's Skin

GENTLE HANDLING
Use adhesive tape sparingly, in the smallest possible area
Infrequent cardiac monitor changes
Sparing use of antibacterial cleansing solutions
Avoid frictional trauma to the skin

INTERVENTION
Humidify infant environment
Skin lubrication with awareness of possible absorption of preservatives and emulsifiers within the product used
Localized use of semipermeable wound dressings

---

immediate neonatal period. Sebaceous gland hyperplasia also occurs over the nose and cheeks of infants, but it is yellow rather than whitish.

Pathogenesis

On histologic examination, milia appear as superficial epithelial cysts in the upper dermis, just beneath the epidermis. The cyst cavity is filled with keratin.

Sebaceous Gland Hyperplasia
Clinical features

Tiny (1 mm) yellow macules or yellow papules are seen at the opening of each pilosebaceous follicle over the nose and cheeks of newborns (Fig. 21-4). These occur in about 50% of infants.[8] They recede completely by 4 to 6 months of age.

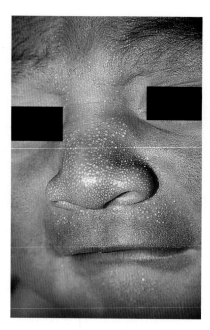

Fig. 21-4 Sebaceous gland hyperplasia on the nose and upper lip of a neonate.

Differential diagnosis

Milia may mimic sebaceous hyperplasia but are white and cystic in appearance.

Pathogenesis

Maternal androgenic stimulation is responsible for the increase in sebaceous gland volume, sebaceous cell size, and the total number of sebaceous cells.

Mottling
Clinical features

A lacelike pattern of dusky erythema appears over the extremities and trunk of neonates when exposed to a temperature decrease. This phenomenon may be sensitive to small increments of temperature change. The mottling disappears on rewarming. Mottling that persists beyond 6 months of age may be a sign of hypothyroidism or the vascular malformation *cutis marmorata telangiectatica congenita*, which can be associated with musculoskeletal or vascular abnormalities.[9,10]

Differential diagnosis

Certain birthmarks, such as cutis marmorata telangiectatica congenita, may mimic mottling, but the color change will not disappear with rewarming. Similarly, the livedo reticularis seen with collagen vascular diseases, such as neonatal lupus erythematosus, will persist when the skin is warmed.

Pathogenesis

Immaturity of the autonomic control of the skin vascular plexus is believed to be responsible for mottling, with constriction of the deeper plexus and opening of the superficial plexus.

Harlequin Color Change
Clinical features

When a low-birth-weight infant is placed on one side, an erythematous flush with a sharp demarcation at the midline develops on the dependent side. The upper half of the body becomes pale. The color change usually subsides within a few seconds of placing the baby in the supine position, but may persist for as long as 20 minutes.

Differential diagnosis

The color change is seldom confused with other vascular problems.

Pathogenesis

The exact mechanism of this unusual phenomenon is not known, but the immaturity of autonomic vasomotor control is believed to be responsible.

Subcutaneous Fat Necrosis
Clinical features

In subcutaneous fat necrosis of the newborn, firm, sharply circumscribed, reddish or purple nodules appear over the cheeks, buttocks, arms, and thighs (Fig. 21-5).[11] The lesions usually begin within the first 2 weeks of life and resolve spontaneously over several weeks to months. Occasionally the lesions can heal with atrophy, leaving a skin depression. Infrequently, hypercalcemia can occur with or without associated irritability, vomiting, weight loss, and failure to thrive.[11,12] Serum calcium evaluations should be repeated weekly until the lesions have totally resolved for a month or more in infants who have multiple large plaques of involved skin or have renal disease.

Differential diagnosis

Bacterial cellulitis or septicemic lesions may be confused with subcutaneous fat necrosis at the onset. The infant with fat necrosis appears healthy and nurses vigorously, in contrast to those with bacterial infections. Several separate lesion sites are often

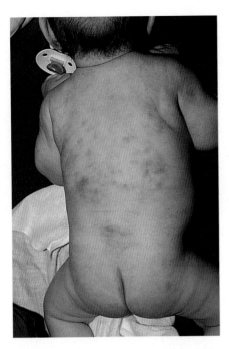

Fig. 21-5 Subcutaneous fat necrosis. Multiple firm indurated nodules on the back of an infant.

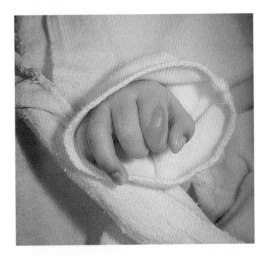

Fig. 21-6 Sucking blister. Oval noninflammatory blister on the finger of a newborn.

seen with subcutaneous fat necrosis and would be extremely unusual with cellulitis.

Pathogenesis

Cold injury is believed to be responsible for subcutaneous fat necrosis. The fat of the neonate contains more saturated fatty acids, which have a higher melting point.[13] Once the temperature of the skin drops below the melting point of the fat, crystallization occurs within the fat of the subcutaneous fat cells and is followed by a granulomatous reaction.

Sclerema
Clinical features

Premature newborns that suffer hypothermia are susceptible to the development of sclerema, a diffuse hardening of the skin. The skin becomes tight, immobile, yellow, and shiny. Sclerema appears in severely ill newborns that have suffered sepsis, hypoglycemia, metabolic acidosis, or other severe metabolic abnormalities.[13] Temperature control, nutritional replacement, correction of metabolic acidosis, and possibly repeated exchange transfusions will arrest the process. Infant mortality in sclerema is high.

Differential diagnosis

The thickening and hardening of the skin are so characteristic of sclerema that it is not confused with other disorders.

Pathogenesis

The susceptibility of the subcutaneous fat to cold injury is believed to be the cause of sclerema. Edema of fibrous septa surrounding fat lobules, without fat necrosis, is found.

Sucking Blisters
Clinical features

Sucking blisters are usually solitary intact oval blisters or erosions on noninflamed skin in the newborn.[14] They occur on the forearms, wrists, fingers (Fig. 21-6), or upper lip and resolve within a few days.

Differential diagnosis

Herpesvirus infection or bullous impetigo should be considered when sucking blisters are encountered, but these lesions appear on an erythematous base. In incontinentia pigmenti, multiple linear blisters are present, in contrast to the solitary sucking blister.

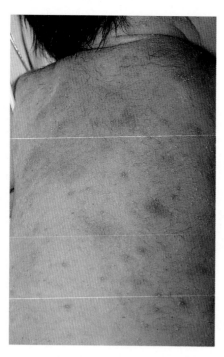

Fig. 21-8 Erythema toxicum. Closer view demonstrating the vesicles and pustules, which are with or without an erythematous base.

Fig. 21-7 Erythema toxicum. Blotchy erythematous macules and plaques with multiple papules and pustules.

Epidermolysis bullosa usually presents with multiple new blisters that develop after birth.

Pathogenesis

Vigorous sucking in utero has been postulated as the cause of these blisters.

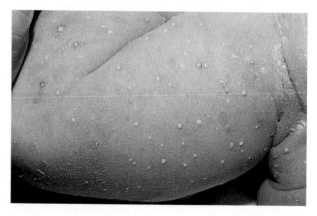

Fig. 21-9 Transient neonatal pustular melanosis. Multiple papules present at birth on the arm of an infant.

Erythema Toxicum
Clinical features

Blotchy, erythematous macules 2 to 3 cm in diameter, with a tiny 1- to 4-mm central vesicle or pustule, are seen in erythema toxicum (Figs. 21-7 and 21-8). They usually begin at 24 to 48 hours of age. They occur in about 50% of term infants and less commonly in premature infants.[15,16] Lesions are seen on the chest, back, face, and proximal extremities, sparing the palms and soles. The individual lesions clear in 4 to 5 days, and new lesions may occur from birth to the tenth day of life. Smear of the central vesicle or pustule contents will reveal numerous eosinophils on Wright-stained preparations. A peripheral blood eosinophilia up to 20% may accompany the tissue eosinophil accumulation, particularly in infants with numerous lesions.

Transient Neonatal Pustular Melanosis
Clinical features

The lesions of transient neonatal pustular melanosis present at birth as vesicles, pustules, or ruptured vesicles or pustules with a collarette of surrounding scale (Fig. 21-9).[17] Pigmented macules are also often present at birth, or they develop at the sites of resolving pustules or vesicles (Fig. 21-10).[18] The vesicles and pustules usually disappear by 5 days of age, whereas the pigmented macules resolve over 3 weeks to 3 months. These lesions are more common on black infants, and they can occur on the palms and soles. Smear of the vesicle or pustule contents will reveal numerous neutrophils and an occasional eosinophil on Wright-stained preparations.

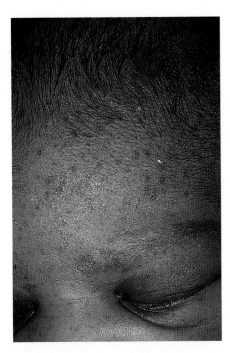

Fig. 21-10 Transient neonatal pustular melanosis. Multiple macules at sites of previous pustules on a 10-day-old infant.

Differential diagnosis

Miliaria rubra is frequently confused with erythema toxicum. The erythema around miliaria rubra is small in area (1 to 2 mm versus 20 to 30 mm in erythema toxicum). The central vesicle or pustule may mimic herpes simplex or bacterial folliculitis lesions. A Gram's stain of the pustules of erythema toxicum or transient neonatal pustular melanosis will be negative. The Wright-stained slide from a pustule of erythema toxicum will show a predominance of eosinophils, whereas the slide of a pustule of transient neonatal pustular melanosis will usually show a predominance of neutrophils.

Pathogenesis

Erythema toxicum is believed to be associated with obstruction of the pilosebaceous orifice. The cause of transient neonatal pustular melanosis is not known.

Pustules in the Newborn
Clinical features

Pustules are discrete, yellow, 1- to 9-mm raised lesions that frequently display a red base. The appearance of pustules in the newborn should immediately bring to mind the possibility of bacterial sepsis. Pustules on the newborn skin in association with other signs or symptoms of sepsis, or when prolonged rupture of maternal membranes has occurred, should make one suspect bacterial sepsis. Bacterial culture of pustules of other body fluids, such as blood, urine, and cerebrospinal fluid, should be performed. There is no rapid, completely reliable method of determining whether a baby has bacterial sepsis, and one should always maintain a high index of suspicion. The incidence of bacterial sepsis is higher in the preterm infant than in the full-term infant, and overall sepsis is an uncommon cause of pustules in the newborn. However, the high mortality rate of unrecognized bacterial sepsis makes it imperative for the clinician to consider this possibility.

Differential diagnosis

Other causes of pustules in the newborn may be considered after bacterial sepsis is eliminated as a possibility. Erythema toxicum may occasionally be pustular, particularly if skin involvement is extensive. Transient neonatal pustular melanosis mimics erythema toxicum and is characterized by pustules present at birth. Herpes simplex skin infections may be pustular but are usually vesicular. Acne neonatorum is usually not present in the first 14 days of life, and evolution to the pustular stage may require several more weeks. Candidiasis, particularly of the diaper area or of other intertriginous areas, may be pustular, and satellite pustules are characteristically found at a distance from the margins of confluent areas of candidiasis. Congenital candidiasis, acquired in utero, may also be pustular, with discrete pustules at birth and subsequent development of diffusely eczematous skin. Infantile acropustulosis may begin at birth or within the newborn period and present with discrete pustules limited to the distal extremities, with prominent involvement of the palms and soles. Nevus comedonicus is a birthmark consisting of patulous follicular openings in which pustule formation, or even deeper abscesses, may occur, but not usually in the newborn period. Psoriasis rarely occurs in the newborn period, but it also may be extensive and pustular.

Pathogenesis

In bacterial infections, pustules arise as the result of accumulation of neutrophils within the skin after dissemination of bacteria from the blood to the skin or direct bacterial invasion of the skin.

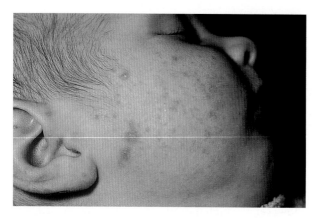

Fig. 21-11 Acne neonatorum. Multiple small inflammatory papules on the face of a 1-month-old infant.

Acne Neonatorum

Clinical features

Neonatal acne (see also Chapter 3) is rarely present at birth but may appear as multiple, discrete papules at 2 to 4 weeks of age. The face, chest, back, and groin are the usual areas for cutaneous lesions (Fig. 21-11). Papules evolve into pustules after a few weeks. Neonatal acne may persist up to 8 months of age. There is some suggestion that infants with extensive neonatal acne may experience severe acne as adolescents.

Differential diagnosis

The differential diagnosis of acne neonatorum is the same as for pustules in the newborn.

Pathogenesis

Neonatal acne may be a part of the so-called *miniature puberty of the newborn*. Neonatal sebaceous glands are hyperplastic, and hydroxysteroid dehydrogenase activity in these structures is high in the 2 months just before birth and at birth. There is evidence that newborns with acne experience transient increases in circulating androgens.

Treatment

Neonatal acne usually resolves spontaneously without treatment. If the involvement is severe, topical therapy with 2.5% benzoyl peroxide gel can be used.

Acropustulosis of Infancy

Clinical features

Acropustulosis of infancy presents as pustules or vesicles on the palms and soles (Fig. 21-12). The lesions may be present at birth or occur up to age 3.[19] The le-

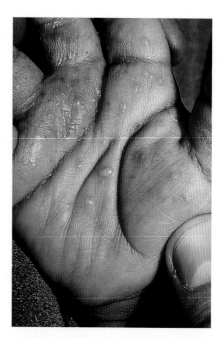

Fig. 21-12 Pustules, scaling, and lichenification on the hand of an infant with infantile acropustulosis.

sions occur in recurrent crops of erythematous papules that rapidly become pruritic pustules.[20] Pruritus in the neonate or infant may be expressed as an irritable, fretful child who does not demonstrate the coordination to scratch. The pustules resolve with scale, and eventually lichenification may develop in the affected area. The lesions may recur until 2 to 3 years of age.

Differential diagnosis

Lesions caused by scabies can be very similar to the lesions of acropustulosis of infancy.[21] All infants should be examined for scabies by scraping the involved area and looking for mites. A history of pruritus in family members is strongly suggestive for scabies, and if mites are not found on the infant, the family members should be examined and scraped. Dyshidrotic eczema usually occurs in older children and adults and presents with smaller vesicles.

Pathogenesis

Bacterial cultures of the lesions should be sterile. The histology will demonstrate edema between keratinocytes and an infiltrate of mononuclear cells, neutrophils, or possibly eosinophils. The cause of this condition is unknown, and once scabies is excluded, biopsy or culture is unnecessary because of the characteristic presentation of the lesions.

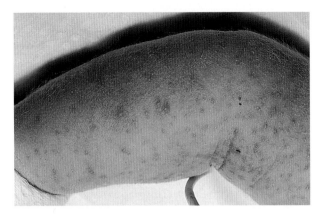

Fig. 21-13 Pustules and erythematous papules noted at birth in an infant with congenital cutaneous candidiasis.

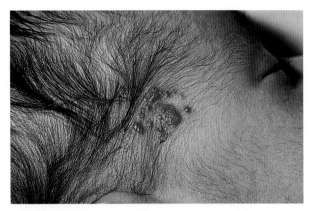

Fig. 21-14 Neonatal herpes simplex. Grouped vesicles on an erythematous base in this 9-day-old infant.

Treatment

Moderate potency topical steroids may be required to decrease the intensity of pruritus. Occasionally, oral antihistamines (hydroxyzine 2 mg/kg/day) may also be required. The lesions continue to recur until 2 to 3 years of age.

Patient education

Reassessment and continued suspicion of scabies is important because of the long-term nature of this condition. Long-term therapy for the pruritus should be monitored on a quarterly basis.

Congenital and Neonatal Candidiasis
Clinical features

Candida albicans can present in the neonate as a congenital infection acquired before birth or as a neonatal infection acquired during the birth process.[22,23] Infants with congenital cutaneous candidiasis present have scaling lesions, erythematous papules, and pustules at birth (Fig. 21-13). A skin scraping prepared with potassium hydroxide (KOH) should document the pseudohyphae and/or budding yeast, and a skin culture should document *C. albicans*. Infants with neonatal candidiasis will develop lesions several days or weeks after birth. The infants may have a diffuse scaling dermatitis or present with typical satellite pustules in the intertriginous areas. The KOH preparation and cutaneous culture should document the cause of the cutaneous eruption.

Differential diagnosis

Erythema toxicum, miliaria, transient neonatal pustular melanosis, and herpesvirus infections can cause blisters and pustules in the neonate. The KOH preparation will document a yeast infection, and a cutaneous culture will confirm *Candida albicans*. Low-birth-weight infants may develop systemic candidiasis.[23-25]

Pathogenesis

C. albicans can penetrate through the amnion and chorion to cause congenital infections. The neonatal infection appears to be acquired during the birth process through the vagina colonized with candida.

Treatment

Topical treatment with an antifungal such as nystatin, miconazole, or ketoconazole is effective for infants with only cutaneous lesions. Systemic infections in low-birth-weight infants require intensive antifungal intravenous therapy.

Herpes Simplex Infection
Clinical features

Grouped vesicles on an erythematous base should bring to mind neonatal herpes simplex virus infection (Fig. 21-14). Any area of skin may be involved, but vesicles on the scalp or buttock are particularly common. Monitoring electrodes may produce sufficient skin trauma on involved skin sites to allow invasion by the virus and to induce herpes simplex virus skin lesions.[26] Vesicles may be present immediately at birth, but the onset after birth is more likely, with 6 days as the mean age of onset. Some infants with neonatal herpes simplex virus will not have skin lesions, but about half of all infants infected with herpes simplex virus display lesions.[27]

Mucous membrane involvement is common. Sixty to eighty percent of neonatal herpes simplex infections are type 2.[27,28]

Differential diagnosis

Other blistering diseases of the newborn, such as congenital varicella, bullous impetigo, and incontinentia pigmenti, may be considered in a differential diagnosis. A Wright-stained smear of cells scraped from a vesicle base will demonstrate multinucleated giant cells and balloon cells in herpes simplex virus infection. Fluorescein-tagged anti-herpes simplex virus–specific antibody may be used to examine vesicle smears or snap-frozen biopsy sections of skin to make a rapid diagnosis. Viral culture of herpes simplex virus requires 12 to 120 hours to grow, and in all infected or suspected neonates, cultures of skin lesions, urine, nasopharynx, eyes, and cerebrospinal fluid are indicated. Serum antibodies for herpes simplex virus are of little assistance in making the diagnosis accurately. Rapid diagnosis of herpes simplex virus is essential, and a high index of suspicion should be maintained.

Pathogenesis

Herpes simplex virus is usually related to maternal infection in the birth canal.[29-31] Infected infants are likely to have had a premature birth, may have signs that mimic bacterial sepsis, and may develop psychomotor retardation even if obvious signs of dissemination of herpes simplex virus are not evident in the newborn period.[27] Infants born to mothers with a primary herpes genital infection at the time of delivery are more likely to develop neonatal herpes simplex than infants born to mothers with recurrent genital lesions.[32]

Treatment

Adenosine arabinoside, or acyclovir, administered intravenously, has been demonstrated to be efficacious.[27] Early recognition and early therapeutic intervention appear to lead to an improved outcome in the infected infant. Cesarean delivery may not be effective in prevention of neonatal herpes simplex infections.[33] Prevention of infection of pregnant women with an unsuspected risk of a primary infection during pregnancy will be the therapy of the future.[32,34]

Varicella
Clinical features

Congenital varicella is quite rare but may mimic herpes simplex virus in the newborn (see Chapter 8). This infection is associated with maternal chickenpox 2 to 3 weeks before delivery. Lesions appear as crops of macules and papules that evolve into vesicles and then crust. Age of onset is within the first 10 days after birth, and mortality has been reported in infants who develop skin lesions between 5 and 10 days of age. A Wright-stained smear of cells from a blister base or a skin biopsy demonstrates the same changes seen in herpes simplex virus. Maternal history of varicella and cutaneous lesions in the infant compatible with varicella are most useful in making the diagnosis. Varicella can also develop in neonates infected postnatally. This could result in a severe infection, especially in premature infants.[35]

Differential diagnosis

Herpes simplex virus infection and bullous impetigo are the two most important considerations in the differential diagnosis of congenital varicella. Fluorescein-tagged anti-herpes zoster virus-specific antibody may be used to examine vesicle smears or snap-frozen biopsy sections of skin to make a rapid diagnosis. Culture identification of the virus from the vesicles may require 7 to 14 days.

Pathogenesis

Maternal infection with varicella-zoster virus results in dissemination of the virus to the newborn. Maternal infection may be unrecognized.

Treatment

Immediate administration of zoster immune globulin to the infant is recommended if maternal infection is present from 5 days before to 2 days after delivery.[36] Infected infants require therapy with intravenous acyclovir. Passive immunization with varicella-zoster immunoglobulin should be considered for premature and term infants that have had postnatal exposure to varicella.

Impetigo
Clinical features

Bacterial impetigo may be observed in the newborn period (see Chapter 5). Flaccid, well-demarcated bullae may be seen that evolve into erosions. Any area of skin may be involved, but the scalp, face, and diaper areas are the most common sites of infection. A collarette of scale around the erosion is characteristic of *Staphylococcus aureus* (Fig. 21-15).[37]

Differential diagnosis

Bacterial culture of skin lesions and culture of the nasopharynx will yield the organism within 24 hours.

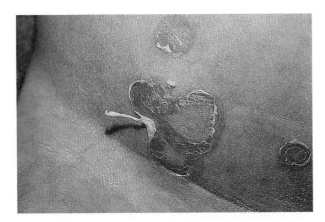

Fig. 21-15 Impetigo over the suprapubic area of a neonate. A collarette of scale around erythematous erosions is characteristic of *Staphylococcus aureus* impetigo.

Smear of vesicle contents and a Gram's stain will demonstrate the bacteria.

Pathogenesis

S. aureus is a predominant organism producing impetigo, including those strains capable of producing the staphylococcal scalded skin syndrome (SSSS); therefore prompt recognition and treatment are necessary. Occasionally group A streptococci or gram-negative bacteria can cause impetigo in the newborn period.

Treatment

The appropriate systemic antibiotic should be administered promptly to prevent sepsis and diminish spread of bacteria to other patients and hospital personnel.

Staphylococcal Scalded Skin Syndrome (Ritter's Disease)
Clinical features

Infants 2 to 30 days old may develop an abrupt onset of generalized erythema followed in 24 hours by bullae, with subsequent exfoliation of large sheets of skin within 48 hours. The lesions are commonly around the head, neck, buttocks, groin, axillae, and periumbilical area of the abdomen.[38]

Differential diagnosis

Toxic shock syndrome (TSS) and toxic epidermal necrolysis (TEN) should be considered in the differential diagnosis of SSSS. However, these conditions are rarely observed in the newborn period.

Pathogenesis

Skin injury in SSSS is the result of an intraepidermal cleavage through the granular layer of epidermis caused by circulating exotoxin produced by *S. aureus*. Small amounts of staphylococci, less than 10^8 organisms, may produce enough toxin to exfoliate a human. Culture of the nasopharynx, rectum, and blisters are likely to yield the organism.

Treatment

Isolation of the affected newborn to prevent nursery epidemics is essential. Antistaphylococcal antibiotics should be administered systemically, and fluid and electrolyte replacement provided, much like that provided for burn therapy. Topical lubrication will decrease the pain and associated discomfort.

Breast Abscess
Clinical features

Swelling, erythema, and fluctuance in one breast of a newborn infant may signify a breast abscess. Onset usually begins 5 to 20 days after birth. Fever may be present, but the infant is usually asymptomatic otherwise.

Differential diagnosis

Breast hyperplasia caused by miniature puberty of the newborn may produce asymmetric enlargement of one breast. The breast is not red or fluctuant to the feel in breast hyperplasia, in contrast to abscess.

Pathogenesis

S. aureus and gram-negative organisms are the most likely pathogens for breast abscess. A needle aspiration of the infection may be necessary to obtain a positive bacterial culture.

Treatment

Systemic antibiotic therapy with the appropriate antistaphylococcal agent is usually necessary.

Omphalitis
Clinical features

Redness and induration of the umbilical region is characteristic of omphalitis. Often, the redness is not well localized and diffusely spreads beyond the umbilicus.

Differential diagnosis

An irritant dermatitis produced by treatment of the umbilicus with various bacteriostatic agents may sometimes mimic omphalitis.

Pathogenesis

Bacterial infection through the cut surface of the umbilical cord is the usual cause of omphalitis. It is predominantly caused by *S. aureus* and, if untreated, may progress to bacterial sepsis.

Treatment

Prophylactic bacteriostatic agents applied to the cord in the newborn period have reduced the likelihood of this infection in many nurseries. Administration of systemic antistaphylococcal antibiotic is the treatment of choice.

Caput Succedaneum and Cephalohematoma
Clinical features

Caput succedaneum is subcutaneous edema over the presenting part of the head. Cephalohematoma is a subperiosteal collection of blood. Edema or hemorrhage of the scalp appears as deep swelling, with or without purpura. The swelling occurs primarily in vertex deliveries, particularly those with prolonged labor, and resolves spontaneously in 7 to 10 days. If the purpura is extensive, it can serve as a source of hyperbilirubinemia. Secondary bacterial infection of cephalohematoma may rarely occur, resulting in cellulitis.

Differential diagnosis

The caput succedaneum tends to feel soft and lacks a well-defined outline. The cephalohematoma is bounded by the suture lines of the skull and often feels fluctuant. Both lesions can mimic cellulitis or bacterial abscess. Appropriate cultures may assist in the differential diagnosis.

Pathogenesis

Both lesions are caused by shearing forces on the scalp skin and skull during labor.

Petechiae and Purpura
Clinical features

Petechiae and purpura may be presenting features of congenital infection, particularly when the newborn is small for gestational age and has hepatosplenomegaly. An acronym used for these infections is the *TORCH syndrome*. Petechiae and purpura are the most common cutaneous symptoms for this group of congenital infections and may be important clues to the diagnosis. Newborns with congenital infection may also demonstrate other features, such as microphthalmia, congenital heart defects, cataracts, and psychomotor retardation.

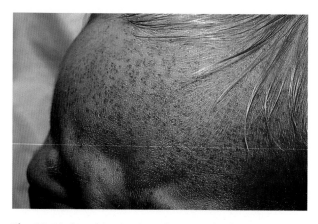

Fig. 21-16 Petechiae in a newborn. Multiple petechiae on the forehead of a neonate after a difficult vertex delivery.

Differential diagnosis

Toxoplasmosis, syphilis (see also Chapter 5), rubella, cytomegalovirus, and congenital herpes simplex virus infections are the usual congenital infections responsible for the production of petechiae and purpura. Serologic tests and viral cultures for these infections should be performed. Other causes of petechiae and purpura in the newborn include trauma, with face and scalp petechiae common in difficult vertex deliveries or in deliveries by cesarean section (Fig. 21-16). Neonatal thrombocytopenia caused by maternal autoantibodies, as in idiopathic thrombocytopenic purpura or systemic lupus erythematosus, may also produce neonatal petechiae a few hours after birth. Hypoprothrombinemia may result in purpura in the newborn older than 2 or 3 days because of vitamin K deficiency. Protein C deficiency can also cause severe purpura in the neonate. Neonatal petechiae and purpura are unusual in the hemophilias, but bleeding from circumcision sites may be the first manifestation of hemophilia in the newborn period. Neonatal purpura secondary to platelet dysfunction may be observed in von Willebrand's disease or Wiskott-Aldrich syndrome.

BIRTHMARKS

Birthmarks represent an excess of one or more of the normal components of skin per unit area: blood vessels, lymph vessels, pigment cells, hair follicles, sebaceous glands, epidermis, collagen, or elastin. Birthmarks are collections of highly differentiated cells in tissue. Vascular birthmarks are the most common.

Congenital malformations are most frequently observed in skin. The two most commonly seen are the

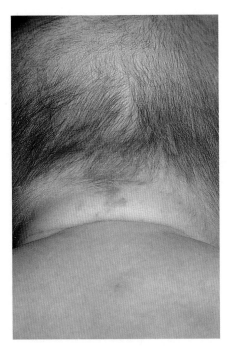

Fig. 21-17 Salmon-patch lesion on the nape of the neck. Also called a *stork bite* because in mythology this is where the stork carries the baby before it is delivered.

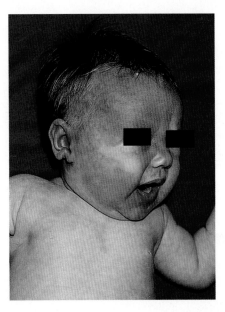

Fig. 21-19 Port-wine stain on infant who subsequently developed seizures associated with Sturge-Weber syndrome.

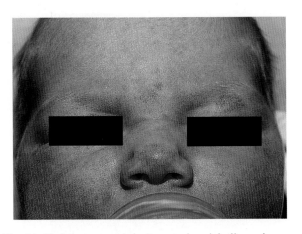

Fig. 21-18 Salmon-patch lesion on the glabella and upper eyelids.

so-called *salmon patch* and *Mongolian spots*. Salmon patches are observed in about 70% of white infants and 60% of black infants.[39] Mongolian spots are more frequently observed in Asian infants (80%) and black infants (95%) but are less common in white infants.[40] Mongolian spots and salmon patches are observed at least 100 times more frequently than any other skin birthmark.[39]

Vascular Birthmarks: Salmon Patches and Port Wine Stains

See Chapter 13 for detailed description of diagnosis and treatment of the individual conditions.

The salmon patch appears as a light-red macule over the nape of the neck, the upper eyelids, and the glabella (Figs. 21-17 and 21-18). A salmon patch is present over the back of the neck in over 40% of infants. Salmon patches fade with time, but remnants may persist well into adult life. Generally, the eyelid lesions fade by 6 to 12 months of age and the glabellar lesions by 5 or 6 years of age. Lesions on the nape of the neck are more likely to persist.

Port wine stains appear as deep-red or purple-red macules over the face or extremities (Fig. 21-19). They are usually unilateral (Fig. 21-20). Occasionally, they are extensive and cover large areas of skin. Port wine stains over the face or an extremity may be associated with soft tissue and bony hypertrophy. A port wine stain over the face may be a clue to Sturge-Weber syndrome.

Vascular Birthmarks: Hemangiomas

Hemangiomas may not be observed at birth (see Chapter 13), but a circumscribed area of blanched skin with a few fine telangiectases may be present,

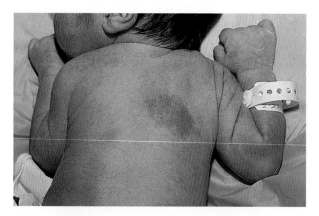

Fig. 21-20 Port-wine stain lesion on the back of a neonate.

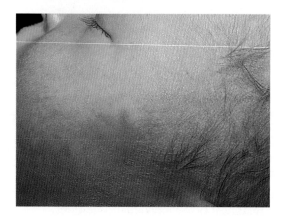

Fig. 21-21 Precursor to raised hemangioma. Blanched skin with fine telangiectasia is present at birth. Later the lesion will become raised.

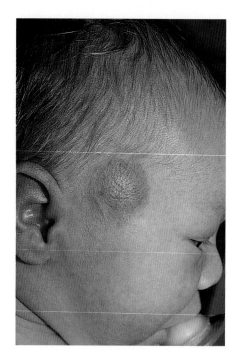

Fig. 21-22 Hemangioma on a 2-week-old. This lesion is raised with a blue-red color.

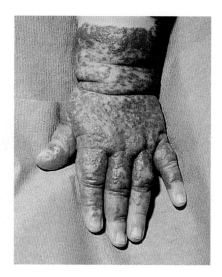

Fig. 21-23 Hemangioma developing on the hand, wrist, and fingers of an infant.

representing a developing hemangioma (Fig. 21-21). By 2 to 4 weeks of age, the skin becomes raised, with red nodules (Figs. 21-22 and 21-23). The lesions grow out of proportion to the baby for the first 8 to 12 months of life. Hemangiomas begin to show signs of involution around 15 months of age, when pale gray areas appear within the red nodule. Soon the first sign of flattening appears. In hemangiomas, ulceration of the epithelial surface may be associated with secondary S. aureus bacterial superinfection (Fig. 21-24).

Cutis Marmorata Telangiectatica Congenita

In cutis marmorata telangiectatica congenita, a mottled pattern of blue or dusky-red erythema is seen from birth (see Chapter 13). Often, a single extremity is involved, but the lesions may occur bilaterally on the extremities or on the trunk. The skin surface overlying such areas may be depressed. A gradual increase in the size of lesions is expected over the first few years of life, but most fade by adult life. Rigorous natural history studies of cutis marmorata telangiectatica congenita are not available. Associations with

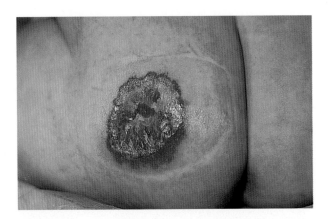

Fig. 21-24 Ulcerated hemangioma on the buttock of an infant.

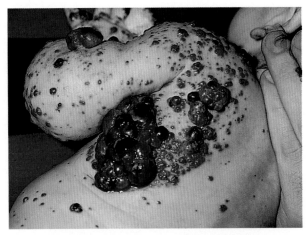

Fig. 21-26 Infant in Fig. 21-25 at 30 days of age. Note rapid enlargement of the size of the lesions and the multiple lesions on the back and arm.

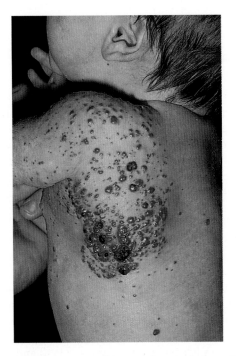

Fig. 21-25 Diffuse neonatal hemangiomatosis in an 18-day-old infant.

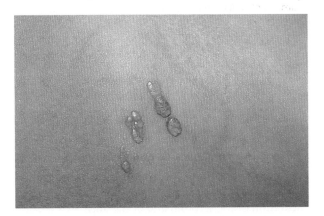

Fig. 21-27 Lymphangioma circumscriptum. Grouping of gelatinous skin-colored papules on the abdomen.

musculoskeletal or vascular abnormalities occur and are discussed in Chapter 13.

Diffuse Neonatal Hemangiomatosis

In the rare syndrome called *diffuse neonatal hemangiomatosis* (see Chapter 13), multiple, small, raised, cutaneous hemangiomas are noted that may be associated with hemangiomas in the liver, lungs, gastrointestinal tract, and central nervous system (Figs. 21-25 and 21-26). The raised hemangiomas may be present at birth and more develop with time. The hemangiomas vary from 2 to 15 mm in diameter. Spontaneous involution of the lesions has been reported. Bleeding may occur into the gastrointestinal tract.

Lymph Vessel Birthmarks: Lymphangiomas

Lymphangiomas may be circumscribed, superficial skin papules (Figs. 21-27 and 21-28) or deep, cavernous nodules (see Chapter 13). Circumscribed lymphangiomas appear as a solitary group of 2- to 4-mm, gelatinous, skin-colored papules limited to a skin area

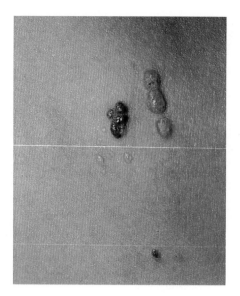

Fig. 21-28 Lymphangioma circumscriptum. After minor trauma the lesions may darken secondary to bleeding into the lesion.

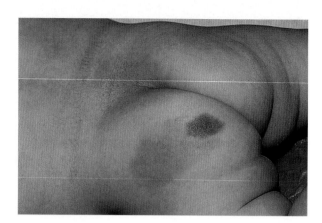

Fig. 21-29 Mongolian spot on the buttock of a neonate.

less than 10 cm. They are often connected to underlying venous channels, and hemorrhage into one or more papules may occur, producing sudden darkening. They may be present at birth, but are often not noticed until late infancy or childhood.

Pigment Cell Birthmarks: Mongolian Spots

An infant's skin is always light at birth and becomes progressively darker with increasing age. Hyperpigmentation of the scrotum and of the linea alba is common in dark-skinned infants at birth. The most commonly observed pigmentary abnormality of infants is the Mongolian spot (see Chapter 17).

Mongolian spots are blue-black macules commonly located over the lumbosacral area (Fig. 21-29). They are occasionally noted over the shoulders and back and may extend over the buttocks and extremities. Mongolian spots fade somewhat with time, and the difference in pigmentation from normal skin pigment becomes less obvious as the newborn's pigment darkens. Some traces of Mongolian spots may persist into adult life.

Pigment Cell Birthmarks: Cafe-au-lait Spots

Light-brown oval macules that may appear more dark brown on black skin are found anywhere on the body and are called *cafe-au-lait spots*. Black infants are far more likely (12%) than white infants (0.3%) to have a solitary cafe-au-lait spot.[41] Cafe-au-lait spots persist through childhood and may increase in number with age (see Chapter 17).

Pigment Cell Birthmarks: Junctional Nevocellular Nevi

Dark-brown or black macules with distinct borders represent clones of melanocytes found at the junction of the epidermis and dermis and are called *junctional nevocellular nevi*. As an infant ages, these nevi may become slightly raised and papular and develop intradermal melanocytes, creating a compound nevus. Often, the surface of the lesion at birth is slightly irregular.

Pigment Cell Birthmarks: Raised Nevocellular Nevi

Skin-colored to tan or brown solitary papules with smooth surfaces represent intradermal nevi (see Chapter 17). Most nevi are small, measuring less than 1.5 cm at their greatest diameter. When these localized, raised pigment cell lesions are greater than 10 or 20 cm at their greatest diameter, there is a concern about their cancer potential (Figs. 21-30 and 21-31).

Hypopigmentation: Phenylketonuria
Clinical features

Newborns with phenylketonuria have blond hair, blue eyes, and light-colored skin. Routine screening tests for the presence of excessive amounts of phenylalanine in the blood will help detect this syndrome.

Differential diagnosis

Phenylketonuria should be distinguished from albinism and Chediak-Higashi syndrome. Analysis of

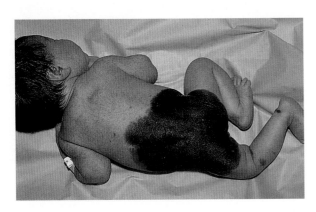

Fig. 21-30 Giant congenital nevus in a bathing-trunk distribution.

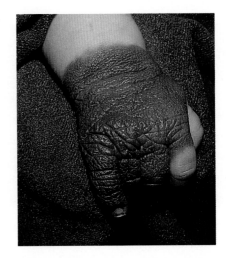

Fig. 21-31 Congenital nevus on the hand of an infant.

blood for phenylalanine is the most useful differentiating test.

Pathogenesis

Patients with phenylketonuria lack the enzymes needed to utilize phenylalanine. Their hypopigmentation is thought to be related to the tight binding of phenylalanine to the receptor sites of tyrosinase such that the enzyme cannot oxidize phenylalanine to melanin.

Epidermal Birthmarks: Epidermal Nevi

Increases in mature epidermal cells, hair follicles, or sebaceous glands may appear as birthmarks. The majority of lesions are present at birth but new lesions can develop into adolescence.

Clinical features

Epidermal nevi have a warty surface and appear anywhere on the body (Fig. 21-32). They are often linear or oval, with the long axis of the lesion parallel to the long axis of the dermatome (Fig. 21-33). The majority of lesions are present at birth and up to 95% of the lesions are present by 7 years of age.[42] Initially the lesion is barely palpable and may be a confluence of smooth-topped papules. In time the lesion becomes more wart-like and scaly (Fig. 21-34). Most are 2 to 5 cm in length, but occasionally they may appear as long, unilateral streaks involving an entire extremity or one side of the trunk (nevus unius lateris). The lesions may be so extensive as to involve most of the body. The terms *ichthyosis hystrix* or *benign congenital acanthosis nigricans* have been applied to such extensive epidermal

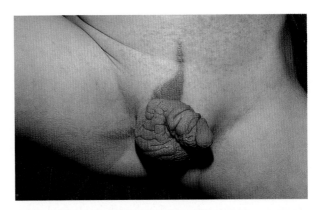

Fig. 21-32 Epidermal nevus. Unilateral lesion on the right side of the penis, scrotum, and pubic skin.

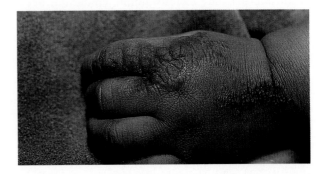

Fig. 21-33 Epidermal nevus. Linear hyperpigmented lesion on the dorsum of the hand. Some areas of lesion are smooth with a waxlike appearance.

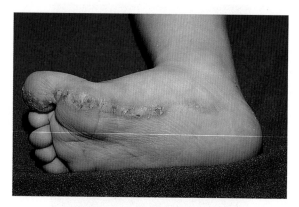

Fig. 21-34 Epidermal nevus on the plantar aspect of foot.

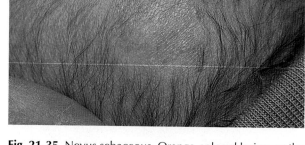

Fig. 21-35 Nevus sebaceous. Orange-colored lesion on the scalp of an infant.

nevi. Epidermal nevi may become erythematous and itchy, with episodes of redness and inflammation, and may be called *inflammatory linear verrucous epidermal nevi (ILVEN)*.

Patients with epidermal nevi may have associated abnormalities. They have an increased number of cutaneous lesions, including cafe-au-lait spots, congenital hypopigmented macules, and congenital nevocellular nevi. They may have associated skeletal defects, seizure disorders, mental retardation, and ocular abnormalities.[43] Patients with more extensive skin involvement have a higher association of other abnormalities than those with limited skin involvement.

Differential diagnosis

Warts are commonly confused with epidermal nevi. The presence from birth and the linear arrangement will help distinguish epidermal nevi from warts. Extensive lesions may be confused with ichthyosis, and certain features of congenital bullous ichthyosiform erythroderma may exactly mimic epidermal nevi. Some epidermal nevi may have keratin abnormalities as seen in epidermolytic hyperkeratosis.[44] Inflammatory linear epidermal nevi may be confused with the warty stage of incontinentia pigmenti, with lichen striatus, or with a dermatitis.

Pathogenesis

Epidermal nevi show thickening of the epidermis and hyperkeratosis. In some lesions, a peculiar vacuolization of the granular layer appears, with separation of the cells in that layer, resulting in a microscopic blister cavity. This process is called *epidermolytic hyperkeratosis* and it may be associated with genetic mo-saicism.[44] In inflammatory lesions, dermal accumulation of inflammatory cells and alternating bands of parakeratosis are described. Overgrowth of sebaceous glands and apocrine glands may be found underlying the epidermal proliferation.

Treatment

For small lesions, surgical excision is the best treatment. Extensive lesions may be improved with the use of mild keratolytics (see Chapter 22) or with bland lubricant therapy. The lesions revert to their hyperkeratotic state when treatments are discontinued.

Patient education

It should be emphasized to parents that this birthmark may be a clue to internal problems. Infants with extensive lesions should have careful neurologic examinations and bone radiographic studies to detect skeletal lesions. A birth defect clinic may be a good referral source for a multidisciplinary approach to such infants. Most infants have no other abnormalities.[42]

Follow-up visits

The frequency of follow-up visits is determined by the severity of the associated problems.

Epidermal Birthmarks: Sebaceous Nevi
Clinical features

Jadassohn's sebaceous nevus appears at birth as a slightly raised oval or linear area with a yellow or orange color (Figs. 21-35 to 21-37). These nevi are common on the scalp and are devoid of hair, producing a congenital circumscribed hair loss. They may be seen on the face as well. Sebaceous nevus

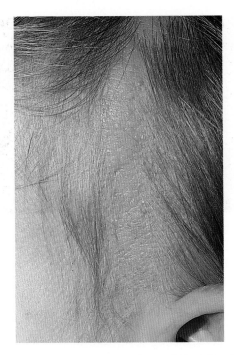

Fig. 21-36 Nevus sebaceous. Linear, yellow-colored lesion on the scalp of an infant.

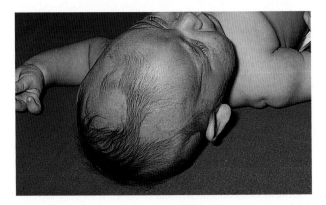

Fig. 21-37 Nevus sebaceous. Large orange lesions on the scalp of a newborn.

may be contiguous with an epidermal nevus and constitute part of the epidermal nevus syndrome. At puberty, or with androgenic stimulation, the nevi enlarge and become warty on the surface and raised (Fig. 21-38). Basal cell carcinomas arise in these tumors. Recent studies have suggested that trichoblastoma can be confused with basal cell carcinoma in a sebaceous nevi. Basal cell carcinomas and other types of benign tumors occur in about 15% of these lesions.[45,46]

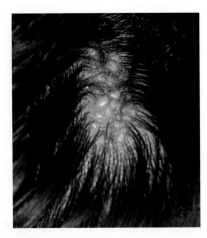

Fig. 21-38 Nevus sebaceous after puberty. Warty, raised growth in the scalp.

Differential diagnosis

Juvenile xanthogranulomas and xanthomas are yellow or orange lesions that may mimic sebaceous nevus. Skin biopsy will distinguish these lesions.

Pathogenesis

Sebaceous nevus is a birthmark with an increased number of sebaceous glands without hair follicles. Such lesions often have an increased number of apocrine glands as well.

Treatment

Surgical excision is often the treatment of choice for these lesions because of the potential for tumor growth. For lesions in the scalp, the excision can often be done after puberty with local anesthesia. Cosmetically less attractive lesions on the face may require earlier excision.

Patient education

The nature of this birthmark should be explained. The possibility of future benign or malignant skin growth should be explained.

Follow-up visits

Follow-up visits should be as usual for newborn care.

Epidermal Birthmarks: Nevus Comedonicus
Clinical features

In nevus comedonicus, linear or oval groups of widely dilated follicular openings plugged with keratin are present at birth on the face and scalp (Fig. 21-39).

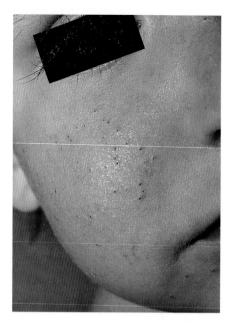

Fig. 21-39 Nevus comedonicus on the cheek of a child.

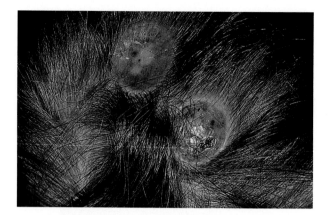

Fig. 21-40 Aplasia cutis congenita. Two oval lesions on the scalp of a child.

They may become inflamed and pustular as the child ages and mimic acne. Bilateral and widespread lesions occur rarely.

Differential diagnosis

In contrast to nevus comedonicus, neonatal acne begins at 1 month of age and involves discrete, single lesions rather than grouped arrangements of lesions.

Pathogenesis

Nevus comedonicus is a birthmark consisting of pilosebaceous follicles with patulous openings.

Treatment

In small lesions, simple surgical excision is the treatment of choice. Large or extensive lesions may be controlled with the application of topical retinoic acid cream once or twice daily.

Patient education

The clinician should explain to the family that this is a birthmark containing pilosebaceous follicles and it is not necessarily related to acne.

Follow-up visits

Follow-up can be made on routine neonatal care visits.

Aplasia Cutis Congenita
Clinical features

In aplasia cutis congenita, oval, sharply marginated, 1- to 2-cm depressed areas are seen primarily in the midline of the posterior scalp (Fig. 21-40). They are hairless, may appear as an ulcer, or are covered by a smooth, finely wrinkled epithelial membrane. Ulcerated defects heal with scar formation. Aplasia cutis congenita is a developmental defect rather than a true birthmark.[47] It occurs in about 1 per 5000 live births.[39] Aplasia cutis most commonly appears as an isolated lesion without associated defects. Other developmental defects, such as cleft palate or lip, syndactyly absence of digits, and congenital heart disease may be associated. It may be seen as an autosomal dominant trait in some families. Although the majority of lesions appear on the scalp, lesions may be found on the trunk, face, or proximal extremities. Medical evaluation should include imaging studies when suspicion exists of underlying bone or brain involvement.

Differential diagnosis

Scalp ulcers at birth may be mistaken for obstetric trauma, although a careful history will distinguish between the two. Other forms of congenital circumscribed hair loss should be considered.

Pathogenesis

Aplasia cutis congenita represents a developmental failure of skin fusion. Dermis, epidermis, and fat all may be missing, or single layers may be absent.

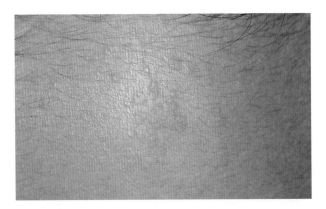

Fig. 21-41 Connective tissue nevus. Raised, skin-colored papules grouped over the sacrum.

Treatment

If the lesion is small, surgical excision, with mobilization of the scalp and simple closure, will correct the hairless defect. Hair transplantation has been successful into large defects.

Patient education

Explanation of the failure to form certain layers of skin will help parents understand that this lesion does not represent mishandling of the child during the birth process.

Follow-up visits

Follow-up visits as necessary for routine newborn care are advised.

Connective Tissue Birthmarks

Connective tissue nevi are skin lesions consisting predominantly of the elements of extracellular collagen tissue and products of fibroblasts, such as collagen, elastin, and proteoglycans.[48] All connective tissue nevi are quite rare, although the precise incidence is not known.

Clinical features

Connective tissue nevi are localized areas of thickened skin appearing as multiple skin-colored papules and plaques (Fig. 21-41). Stretching the overlying skin will give a yellowish discoloration to the areas. They may occasionally have increased vascularity and appear red. Collagenomas are localized areas of thickened skin with multiple skin-colored papules or plaques. They may be solitary or appear in a zosteri-

form segmental pattern. Elastomas are solitary plaques that are present at birth and contain increases in both elastic tissue and proteoglycans. Elastomas may be solitary or they may be multiple in the Buschke-Ollendorff syndrome. This autosomal dominant syndrome appears as symmetrically distributed skin-colored papules or nodules with a predilection for the lower trunk or for the extremities. Lesions may assume a thickened appearance of skin and develop a lacy pattern over the trunk. Radiographs may show sclerotic densities of the ends of long bones, pelvis, and hands, although such lesions are often asymptomatic. The shagreen patch of tuberous sclerosis is a connective tissue nevus. The nevi are subtle at birth and may go unnoticed. They tend to persist throughout life.

Differential diagnosis

The lesions of connective tissue birthmarks are so characteristic that they are seldom misdiagnosed. Examinations for possible associated systemic disease may be necessary.

Pathogenesis

Connective tissue nevi show thickened, abundant collagen bundles with or without associated increases in elastic tissue. Such histologic changes are difficult to appreciate unless the skin biopsy includes adjacent normal skin for comparison.

Treatment

Treatment is unnecessary.

Patient education

Connective tissue nevus is a birthmark consisting of collagen and/or elastin, and it should be emphasized that such lesions may be related to systemic or genetic disease. In the absence of associated disease the connective tissue nevus does not represent a serious problem.

Follow-up visits

Follow-up visits are unnecessary except for routine neonatal visits.

COMMON CONGENITAL MALFORMATIONS THAT INVOLVE SKIN

Congenital malformations involving the skin are frequently observed in newborns. They are observed in 7 per 100 live births.

Ear Anomalies

Minor abnormalities in the formation of the ear constitute the most common congenital malformations. Loss of the fold of the skin in the superior part of the helix is the most common abnormality. Low-set ears that angle away from the eye, periauricular skin tags (Fig. 21-42), accessory tragi, auricular or preauricular pits, or auricular sinuses and/or small ears are less common. Deafness may accompany congenital malformations of the external ear, or they may be associated with hemifacial microsomia (Goldenhar's syndrome).

Digital Abnormalities

A single crease on one or both upper palms, called a *simian crease*, occurs in 2 per 100 live births. It is one feature of Down syndrome, but it also may be observed in a variety of other syndromes, including trisomy 13, Cornelia de Lange syndrome, Seckel's syndrome, and cri du chat syndrome. Clinodactyly with inward curvature of a digit is often observed in the fifth finger, and overlapping of the second and third toes is also a frequently observed malformation. Partial or complete fusion (syndactyly) of the second or third toes and clubfoot also occur with relative frequency.

Genital Abnormalities

Hydrocele of one testis and hypospadias are the most common genital anomalies and malformations observed. Malformations of the external genitalia may be clues to urinary tract anomalies, and investigation of the urinary tract may be indicated. They may also be clues to chromosomal abnormalities and may be associated with undescended testes.

Epicanthal Folds

Epicanthal folds of skin on the inner aspect of each eye are frequently observed. They are present in chromosomal abnormalities such as Down, Turner's, and Klinefelter's syndromes.

Supernumerary Nipples

Supernumerary nipples occur in approximately 2.5% to 4% of newborns.[49,50] These lesions may enlarge during puberty. In the past an association with renal abnormalities has been suggested, but recent studies suggest that supernumerary nipples are not associated with renal abnormalities.[50]

Neural Tube Defects

Primary defects in neural tube closures, such as meningomyelocele, encephalocele, and anencephaly are fortunately rare congenital malformations. Occult spinal dysraphism can be missed if a cutaneous clue to an underlying neural tube defect is not noticed. The clue is a midline lipoma, dimple, hairy patch, or vascular abnormality.[51] Early diagnosis by ultrasound or magnetic resonance imaging (MRI) may identify a surgically correctable lesion before neurologic damage.

Abnormalities of the Lip and Mouth

Pits in the lips have been described in 2 per 100 live births. Cleft lip and palate, or cleft lip alone, are less common. The finding of lip pits or cleft lips and/or cleft palate may be a clue to the so-called *first arch syndrome*, which includes a small jaw and ocular hypertelorism. A number of syndromes are associated with first arch syndrome, including Pierre Robin syndrome, orodigitofacial syndromes, and Treacher Collins syndrome.

Skin Dimpling

Infants may develop small dimplelike depressed scars secondary to injury during amniocentesis procedures. The skin over the lesion appears to be pulled in by absent dermis. The lesion may not be noticed until the infant is several months old and has developed additional subcutaneous fat. Midline dimpling is of more serious concern, as mentioned above.

MAJOR CHROMOSOMAL ABNORMALITIES

Chromosomal abnormalities occur in 1 of 200 live births, in a higher percentage of births resulting in perinatal death, and in up to 50% of spontaneous abortions.

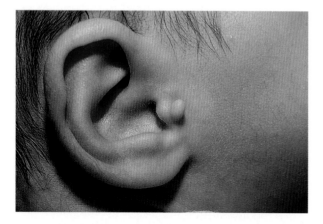

Fig. 21-42 Preauricular skin tag on an infant.

Trisomy 21 (Down Syndrome)

Trisomy 21 is seen in 1 per 800 live births. Mothers over 40 years of age have an increased chance of giving birth to a child with Down syndrome. Cutaneous features are most useful in the recognition of this syndrome. These include prominent epicanthal folds, eyes slanting upward, small ears, simian palmar crease, excessive skin over the back of the neck, and clinodactyly of the fifth fingers. The presence of these cutaneous features, plus muscular hypotonia and evidence of congenital heart disease, are the major clinical characteristics. Chromosomal analysis will confirm the diagnosis. Mental retardation may be severe, and growth failure associated with congenital heart disease makes the prognosis poor.

Trisomies 18 and 13-15

Trisomy 18 is observed in 1 per 3000 live births; trisomy 13-15 occurs in 1 per 5000 live births. In both of these chromosomal abnormalities, increased parental age has been an associated feature. Babies with trisomies 18 or 13-15 are small for gestational age, have low-set ears, simian creases, congenital heart disease, and severe mental retardation. The presence of a cleft lip and palate associated with these features makes trisomy 13-15 more likely, whereas rocker-bottom feet and flexion contractures of the fingers make trisomy 18 the more likely diagnosis. Chromosomal analysis is required for precise diagnosis.

Turner's Syndrome

The most common sex chromosome anomaly is Turner's syndrome, in which only one X chromosome is present (XO). Newborns with Turner's syndrome exhibit webbing of the neck and marked edema of the hands and feet. The neck is often quite short. Coarctation of the aorta may be associated. Chromosomal analysis is necessary to confirm the diagnosis.

Klinefelter's Syndrome

Extra sex chromosomes are characteristic of Klinefelter's syndrome (XXY, XXXY, XXXXY). A low birth weight, undescended testes, and a small penis lead to suspicion of this syndrome. Hypotonia and a variety of other anomalies may also be observed. Mental deficiency is usually severe in this syndrome, and chromosomal analysis is required to confirm the diagnosis.

MISCELLANEOUS SKIN CONDITIONS IN THE NEWBORN
The Red, Scaly Newborn
Physiologic scaling and redness

A scaling and often red newborn may be an enigma to the inexperienced observer.[52] A postmature baby may exhibit desquamation that is marked over the hands, feet, and lower trunk, and, if observed during the first day of life when the newborn skin is quite red, may result in an erroneous diagnosis of one of the ichthyoses. Similarly, preterm infants born at 32 weeks of gestational age or earlier will have red or glistening skin that similarly may be confused with ichthyosis. Such changes are transient and are often resolved within the newborn period.

Collodion baby

Newborns with an encasement of shiny, tight, inelastic scale are said to have a *collodion membrane* (Fig. 21-43). The membrane is composed of greatly thickened stratum corneum that has been saturated with water. As the water content evaporates in extrauterine life, large fissures appear in the membrane and the membrane is shed, revealing red skin underneath. The presence of a collodion membrane does not allow one to predict that the affected baby will necessarily develop ichthyosis, and spontaneous healing may occur.[53,54] Skin biopsy of the collodion membrane is usually not diagnostic. Most collodion babies do have a form of ichthyosis, and the majority of them develop features of lamellar ichthyosis. Infants with bullous ichthyosis, X-linked ichthyosis, Netherton's syndrome, or Gaucher's disease have also been reported to present as collodion babies. Collodion babies should be observed closely for dehydration associated with high transepidermal water loss.[55]

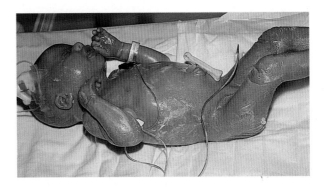

Fig. 21-43 Collodion baby. Erythematous, tight, shiny skin that has been treated with a thick covering of white petrolatum.

Harlequin fetus

Although harlequin fetus has been considered a more severe form of lamellar ichthyosis, most authorities now believe that it represents a distinct, rare autosomal-recessive disease.[56] Harlequin fetus is usually incompatible with extrauterine life; infants have massive, dense, platelike scales, which produce severe deformities of skeletal and soft tissues that restrict respiration. This has been associated with defects in both lipid and protein metabolism. Recently, infants treated with oral retinoids have survived, with residual severe ichthyosis.

Atopic Dermatitis and Seborrheic Dermatitis

Atopic dermatitis is said to have its onset after the newborn period, with the most frequently observed age of onset being 2 to 3 months. If a dermatitis begins within the newborn period, many authorities designate it *seborrheic dermatitis*. It has now become clear, however, that infants who later develop typical atopic dermatitis may have the onset of their skin eruption within the newborn period. There is significant overlap in infants who have seborrheic and atopic dermatitis, both in distributions of the lesions, which involve the scalp, diaper area, and extensor area, and in the history of pruritus, feeding patterns, food intolerance, and family members with atopic disease. Physiologic overproduction of sebum occurs in the newborn period, giving any dermatitis a greasy feel to the skin surface. It is advisable to designate dermatitis seen in newborns as simply *dermatitis* (see also Chapter 4).

Diaper Dermatitis

Diaper dermatitis occurring in the newborn period is primarily perianal in location and is related to the irritant substances found in stool.[57] Superinfection with *C. albicans* is frequent in any diaper dermatitis present for more than 72 hours.

Scabies

Infants with scabies may present with a generalized dermatitis. They may have only a few or as many as thousands of lesions. Infants usually have involvement of the head and neck. Individual burrows may be obscured and difficult to detect because of the confluence of dermatitis. The scabies mite can be recovered from papules or burrows, with the hands and feet the best sites of recovery.

Histiocytosis X

A generalized dermatitis, particularly that with purpuric papules or petechiae within the dermatitis and involvement of the head and neck, is characteristic of histiocytosis X. The skin eruption may be present at birth, and the presence of chronic draining ears and enlargement of the liver and spleen are useful additional clues in the diagnosis. Skin biopsy will demonstrate the characteristic infiltration with histiocytic cells containing Langerhans-like granules (see also Chapter 12).

REFERENCES

1. Lund C et al: Neonatal skin care: the scientific basis for practice, *JOGNN* 28:241, 1999.
2. Lane AT, Drost SS: Effects of repeated application of emollient cream to premature neonates' skin, *Pediatrics* 92:415, 1993.
3. Nopper AJ et al: Topical ointment therapy benefits premature infants, *J Pediatr* 125(5):660, 1996.
4. Mancini AJ et al: Semipermeable dressings improve epidermal barrier function in premature infants, *Pediatr Res* 36:306, 1994.
5. Darmstadt GL, Dinulos JG: Neonatal skin care, *Pediatr Clin North Am* 47(4):757, 2000.
6. Hall SL: Coagulase-negative staphylococcal infections in neonates, *Pediatr Infect Dis J* 10:57, 1991.
7. Hammarlund K et al: Transepidermal water loss in newborn infants, *Acta Pediatr Scand* 66:553, 1977.
8. Rivers JK, Frederiksen PC, Dibdin C: A prevalence survey of dermatoses in the Australian neonate, *J Am Acad Dermatol* 23:77, 1990.
9. Gerritsen MJ et al: Cutis marmorata telangiectatica congenita: report of 18 cases, *Br J Dermatol* 142(2):366, 2000.
10. Amitai DB et al: Cutis marmorata telangiectatica congenita: clinical findings in 85 patients, *Pediatr Dermatol* 17(2):100, 2000.
11. Cook JS, Stone MS, Hansen JR: Hypercalcemia in association with subcutaneous fat necrosis of the newborn: studies of calcium-regulating hormones, *Pediatrics* 90:93, 1992.
12. Burden AD, Krafchik BR: Subcutaneous fat necrosis of the newborn: a review of 11 cases, *Pediatr Dermatol* 16(5):384, 1999.
13. Fretzin DF, Arias AM: Sclerema neonatorum and subcutaneous fat necrosis of the newborn, *Pediatr Dermatol* 4:112, 1987.
14. Murphy WF, Langley AL: Common bullous lesions—presumably self-inflicted—occurring in utero in the newborn infant, *Pediatrics* 32:1099, 1963.
15. Carr JA et al: Relationship between toxic erythema and infant maturity, *Am J Dis Child* 112:129, 1966.
16. Marchini G et al: Erythema toxicum neonatorum: an immunohistochemical analysis, *Pediatr Dermatol* 18(3):177, 2001.
17. Ramamurthy RS et al: Transient neonatal pustular melanosis, *J Pediatr* 88:831, 1976.
18. Wyre CHW, Conder MO, Murphy MC: Transient neonatal pustular melanosis, *Arch Dermatol* 115:458, 1979.
19. Dromy R, Raz A, Metzker A: Infantile acropustulosis, *Pediatr Dermatol* 8:284, 1991.
20. Vignon-Pennamen MD, Wallach D: Infantile acropustulosis, *Arch Dermatol* 122:1155, 1986.

21. Mancini AJ, Frieden IJ, Paller AS: Infantile acropustulosis revisited: history of scabies and response to topical corticosteroids, *Pediatr Dermatol* 15(5):337, 1998.

22. Stuart SM, Lane AT: Candida and Malassezia as nursery pathogens, *Semin Dermatol* 11:19, 1992.

23. Darmstadt GL, Dinulos JG, Miller Z: Congenital cutaneous candidiasis: clinical presentation, pathogenesis, and management guidelines, *Pediatrics* 105(2):438, 2000.

24. Baley JE, Silverman RA: Systemic candidiasis: cutaneous manifestations in low birth weight infants, *Pediatrics* 82:211, 1988.

25. Faix RG et al: Mucocutaneous and invasive candidiasis among very low birth weight (<1500 grams) infants in intensive care nurseries: a prospective study, *Pediatrics* 83:101, 1989.

26. Parvey LS, Ch'ien LT: Neonatal herpes simplex virus infection introduced by fetal-monitor scalp electrodes, *Pediatrics* 65:1150, 1980.

27. Whitley R et al: A controlled trial comparing vidarabine with acyclovir in neonatal herpes simplex virus infection, *N Engl J Med* 324:444, 1991.

28. Sullivan-Bolyai J et al: Neonatal herpes simplex virus infection in King County, Washington, *JAMA* 250:3059, 1983.

29. Arvin AM et al: Failure of antepartum maternal cultures to predict the infant's risk of exposure to herpes simplex virus at delivery, *N Engl J Med* 315:796, 1986.

30. Prober CG et al: Low risk of herpes simplex virus infections in neonates exposed to the virus at the time of vaginal delivery to mothers with recurrent genital herpes simplex virus infections, *N Engl J Med* 316:240, 1987.

31. Prober CG et al: Use of routine viral cultures at delivery to identify neonates exposed to herpes simplex virus, *N Engl J Med* 318:887, 1988.

32. Kulhanjian JA et al: Identification of women at unsuspected risk of primary infection with herpes simplex virus type 2 during pregnancy, *N Engl J Med* 326:918, 1992.

33. Randolph AG, Washington AE, Prober CG: Cesarean delivery for women presenting with genital herpes lesions, *JAMA* 270:77, 1993.

34. Jacobs RF: Neonatal herpes simplex virus infections, *Semin Perinatol* 22(1):64, 1998.

35. Lipton SV, Brunell PA: Management of varicella exposure in a neonatal intensive care unit, *JAMA* 261:1782, 1989.

36. Committee on Infectious Diseases: Varicella-zoster infections. In Pickering L, editor: 2000 Red book: report of the Committee on Infectious Diseases, ed 23, Elk Grove Village, Ill, 2000, American Academy of Pediatrics.

37. Darmstadt GL, Lane AT: Impetigo: an overview, *Pediatr Dermatol* 11:293, 1994.

38. Ladhani S et al: Clinical, microbial, and biochemical aspects of the exfoliative toxins causing staphylococcal scalded-skin syndrome, *Clin Microbiol Rev* 12(2):224, 1999.

39. Alper JC, Holmes LB: The incidence and significance of birthmarks in a cohort of 4641 newborns, *Pediatr Dermatol* 1:58, 1983.

40. Jacobs AH, Walton RG: The incidence of birthmarks in the neonate, *Pediatrics* 58:218, 1976.

41. Alper J, Holmes LB, Mihm MC: Birthmarks with serious medical significance: nevocellular nevi, sebaceous nevi, and multiple café-au-lait spots, *J Pediatr* 94:696, 1979.

42. Rogers M, McCrossin I, Commens C: Epidermal nevi and the epidermal nevus syndrome, *J Am Acad Dermatol* 20:476, 1989.

43. Hodge JA, Ray MC, Flynn KJ: The epidermal nevus syndrome, *Int J Dermatol* 30:91, 1991.

44. Paller AS et al: Genetic and clinical mosaicism in a type of epidermal nevus, *N Engl J Med* 331:1408, 1994.

45. Cribier B, Scrivener Y, Grosshans E: Tumors arising in nevus sebaceus: a study of 596 cases, *J Am Acad Dermatol* 42(2 Pt 1):263, 2000.

46. Jaqueti G, Requena L, Sanchez Yus E: Trichoblastoma is the most common neoplasm developed in nevus sebaceus of Jadassohn: a clinicopathologic study of a series of 155 cases, *Am J Dermatopathol* 22(2):108, 2000.

47. Frieden IJ: Aplasia cutis congenita: a clinical review and proposal for classification, *J Am Acad Dermatol* 26:646, 1986.

48. Uitto J, Santa Cruz DJ, Eisen AZ: Connective tissue nevi of the skin, *J Am Acad Dermatol* 3:441, 1980.

49. Mimouni F, Merlob P, Reisner SH: Occurrence of supernumerary nipples in newborns, *Am J Dis Child* 137:952, 1983.

50. Jojart G, Seres E: Supernumerary nipples and renal anomalies, *Int Urol Nephrol* 26:141, 1994.

51. Enjolras O, Boukobza M, Jdid R: Cervical occult spinal dysraphism: MRI findings and the value of a vascular birthmark, *Pediatr Dermatol* Sep;12(3):256, 1995.

52. Glover MT, Atherton DJ, Levinsky RJ: Syndrome of erythroderma failure to thrive, and diarrhea in infancy: a manifestation of immunodeficiency, *Pediatrics* 81:66, 1988.

53. Frenk E, Techtermann F: Self-healing collodion baby: evidence for autosomal recessive inheritance, *Pediatr Dermatol* 9:95, 1992.

54. Pongprasit P: Collodion baby: the outcome of long-term follow-up, *J Med Assoc Thailand* 76:17, 1993.

55. Buyse L et al: Collodion baby dehydration: the danger of high transepidermal water loss, *Br J Dermatol* 129:86, 1993.

56. Hashimoto K, De Dobbeleer G, Kanzaki T: Electron microscopic studies of harlequin fetuses, *Pediatr Dermatol* 10:214, 1993.

57. Lane AT, Rehder PA, Helm K: Evaluations of diapers containing absorbent gelling material with conventional disposable diapers in newborn infants, *Am J Dis Child* 144:315, 1990.

| # Dermatopharmacology and Topical Formulary

A great variety of topical preparations are available to treat the skin of pediatric patients. However, the majority of these preparations have not been rigorously investigated as to their efficacy and risk-benefit ratio in infants and children. This chapter contains an abbreviated formulary of the most useful topical preparations and the principles of and rationale for their use. Specific treatment programs are discussed in the other chapters on each skin disease.

Treatment should be simple and aimed at preserving or restoring the normal physiologic state of the skin. Topical therapy is often preferred because topical medication can be delivered in optimal concentrations at the exact site where it is needed, and effects on internal organs can be minimized. Compounding of preparations or adding medications to commercially available topical preparations is not advised because the ingredients may lose their bioavailability.[1]

PERCUTANEOUS ABSORPTION

Absorption of topical medications through the epidermal barrier into the dermis is a complex process.[2] However, for clinical purposes, percutaneous absorption may be simplified and related to skin hydration. In the normal state of hydration of the stratum corneum, the epidermal barrier may be penetrated only by medications passing through a tight lipid barrier between cells.

Hydration of the skin allows binding of water molecules to hydrophilic lipids between stratum corneum cells, so that water-soluble medications may pass between cells. Thus any of the factors that enhance hydration of the skin increase percutaneous absorption (e.g., plastic wrap, airtight occlusion, the use of oils or ointments, urea compounds, propylene glycol). The mechanism of action of occlusive substances is prevention of evaporation of the 200 to 300 ml of body water that normally moves through the stratum corneum daily and would ordinarily evaporate had it not been for those occlusive coverings. Urea compounds and propylene glycol interact with the lipids

between stratum corneum cells. The factors that enhance percutaneous absorption are listed in Box 22-1.

When choosing a topical medication for a child, one selects a preparation that contains two major components, the active medication and the vehicle. Each is important in determining the success or failure of the therapeutic regimen. Selection of the correct active medication and incorrect vehicle may cause failure of the treatment program.

Water and the Skin

The outermost layer of the epidermis, the stratum corneum, forms a barrier (the epidermal barrier) (see Chapter 1) to the penetration of active medication into the skin. Both excessive environmental humidity and low environmental humidity result in loss of the integrity of the epidermal barrier.

Excessive environmental humidity

Immersing the skin in water results in uptake of water by the stratum corneum cells and saturation of its intercellular spaces. This water uptake is so great that the stratum corneum triples in thickness from 15 microns at 60% humidity to 48 microns at 90%. Further water exposure results in replacement of lipid covalent bonds between the stratum corneum cells by weak hydrogen (water) bonds, and the stratum corneum cells separate. We see this clinically as maceration. Maceration occurs in naturally occluded areas in which evaporation of water is usually retarded, such as in the axillae, under the breasts, and in the perineum, scalp, and interdigital webs. Preventing evaporation of water from the skin surface with plastic occlusive wraps, ointments, or oils will also result in maceration.

Deficient environmental humidity

At less than 10% environmental humidity, excessive shrinking of the stratum corneum occurs, resulting in microscopic and macroscopic cracks in the stratum corneum. This is manifested by a dry feel to the skin

---

Box 22-1   Factors Enhancing Percutaneous Absorption

Epidermal injury
Heat
Increased water content of stratum corneum
Inflammation

Box 22-2   Function of Moisturizers

Impede water loss
Retain heat
Increase percutaneous absorption
Reduce scaling
Promote epidermal repair

Box 22-3   Useful Moisturizing Lotions

PETROLATUM BASED
Dermasil
DML Lotion
Moisturel Lotion
Nutraderm Lotion
Replenaderm Lotion

MIXTURES OF LANOLIN AND PETROLATUM
Eucerin Lotion
Lubriderm Lotion
Keri Lotion
Nivea Moisturizing Lotion

WITHOUT LANOLIN OR PETROLATUM
Complex 15 Lotion
Corn Huskers Lotion
Cetaphil Lotion

Box 22-4   Useful Moisturizing Creams

PETROLATUM BASED
DML Forte
Purpose Dry Skin Cream
Replenaderm Cream
Cetaphil Cream
Dermasil Cream
Keri Creme

MIXTURES OF LANOLIN AND PETROLATUM
Eucerin Creme

WITHOUT LANOLIN OR PETROLATUM
Neutrogena Norwegian Formula Hand Cream

Box 22-5   Useful Moisturizing Ointments

PETROLATUM BASED
White petrolatum (Petrolatum White, Vaseline Pure Petroleum Jelly)

MIXTURES OF LANOLIN AND PETROLATUM
Aquaphor Natural Healing Ointment

---

surface, thin scales with erythema around the borders (eczema craquelé), and dry, inspissated plugs of scale in follicular openings (keratosis pilaris).

Substances Designed to Retain Water on the Skin Surface (Moisturizers)

On dry, exposed areas of skin, such as the dorsum of the hands and arms, it is desirable to retain water in the stratum corneum. Moisturization is often all that is necessary to treat chronic dryness and inflammation of the skin successfully (Box 22-2).[3]

Moisturizers are complex mixtures designed to moisturize the skin surface, and they may be called either *moisturizers* or *lubricants*.[4] These preparations are complex mixtures of either water-in-oil emulsions or oil-in-water emulsions.[5,6] The individual ingredients are combined to make them more efficient at hydrating the skin and enable them to give a more pleasing cosmetic appearance when applied.[7] Ninety percent of the moisturizers sold are oil-in-water emulsions.[4] The vehicles that are used to provide skin lubrication are usually petrolatum based or are mixtures of lanolin and petrolatum. The vehicles that contain solids and little or no water are called *ointments*; those with 20% to 50% water are called *creams*. Lists of useful moisturizers are found in Boxes 22-3, 22-4, and 22-5. All moisturizers are best applied to wet skin.

Components of moisturizers and vehicles and their function

Petrolatum, the base for most moisturizers, is prepared from the residue remaining in stills after the distillation of petroleum. It usually is a colored solid and must be decolorized to make white petrolatum (petroleum jelly, white soft paraffin). Petrolatum contains a mixture of hydrocarbons, including triglycerides, and is insoluble in water. It retains heat, impedes water loss from the skin surface, and increases percutaneous absorption. It has minor vasoconstrictive activity when applied to the skin and may enhance reepithelialization of wounds. Petrolatum alone is cosmetically disagreeable, leaving a greasy film on the skin surface that frequently results in overheating of the skin and sweat obstruction. The mixing of substances to allow the addition of water to petrolatum will result in a more efficient moisturizing capacity of the skin with a less greasy feel and more cosmetic acceptance. Substances added to moisturizers to increase water-binding capacity include cetyl alcohol, stearyl alcohol, and other stearates. Addition of cetyl alcohol to petrolatum will increase its water-binding capability from 10% to 50%. Other additives include polyethylene glycol (PEG) of low molecular weight (PEG 300-400) or of high molecular weight (PEG 1540, 4000) (Carbowax) as an agent to uniformly disperse the mixture or for its solvent properties. Addition of cholesterol or polysaccharide macromolecules such as polysorbate (Tween 20 or 80) as emulsifiers and the addition of yellow or white wax (beeswax) for stiffness of the product are common practices. Glycerin, a fatty alcohol derived from triglycerides as a byproduct of the manufacture of soap, is a clear, colorless, sticky liquid that takes up water from the skin surface. Its role as an additive to certain creams is unclear.

Bacteriostatic and fungistatic agents are added to preparations that contain water to prolong the life of the product. Popular preservatives include parabens, formaldehyde, or formaldehyde-releasing agents (imidazolinylureas); oxyquinoline sulfate; organic quaternary ammonium compounds; chlorobutanol; and hexachlorophene. Fragrances are added to cover any unpleasant smell from the basic product. The added preservatives and fragrances can be responsible for irritant or allergic reactions to these moisturizers in children. The functions of frequently used ingredients of moisturizers and of medicated creams and lotions are listed in Table 22-1. One should not recommend a skin preparation unless he or she is familiar with its ingredients and its therapeutic indications.

Table 22-1	Components of Lubricants and Vehicles and Their Function
Component	**Function**
Cetyl alcohol, stearates, cholesterol	Additional water binding
Polyethylene glycol (Carbowax)	Dispersants
Yellow wax, white wax	Stiffness
Parabens, formaldehyde releasers	Preservatives
Propylene glycol, alcohol	Solvent
Essential oils	Fragrance
Cholesterol, polysaccharide polymers (Tween, Span)	Emulsifiers

Liquid petrolatum (mineral oil, liquid paraffin) is a fluid phase of petrolatum obtained by distilling the residual petroleum liquid at 330° F and decolorizing it. It is composed of 15 to 20 carbon hydrocarbons and, because it is in a fluid form at room temperature, it is added to skin preparations in which easy spread on the skin surface is desirable.

Lanolin is a purified fatlike substance obtained from the wool of sheep. It consists of cholesterol esters and oxycholesterol esters called *wool fat* or *wool wax alcohol.* Ordinary lanolin contains 25% to 30% water and is a yellowish-white solid. It must be mixed with other agents such as mineral oil or cetyl alcohol so that it can be spread smoothly on the skin. Lanolin is found in a number of skin moisturizers. Fragrance-, lanolin-, and preservative-free preparations are listed in Box 22-6.

Ointments. Ointments spread easily on the skin and are more cosmetically pleasing if they contain some water. White petrolatum, mineral oil, and liquid paraffin are completely water insoluble and have maximal water-retaining (occlusive) properties. However, they often leave a greasy film on the skin and cause excessive heat retention, which make them unacceptable to many patients.

Mixing ointments or oils with water and an emulsifier makes them spread on the skin more easily and give less of a greasy feel. The bulk of the moisturizers in clinical use are emulsified with water and contain mostly ointment, with a small amount of water. The

Box 22-6	Skin Lubricants That Are Fragrance, Lanolin, and Preservative Free

FRAGRANCE FREE
DML Lotion
Eucerin Creme and Lotion

FRAGRANCE FREE, LANOLIN FREE
Moisturel Lotion
Replenaderm Cream and Lotion

FRAGRANCE FREE, PRESERVATIVE FREE
Aquaphor Natural Healing Ointment

FRAGRANCE FREE, PRESERVATIVE FREE, AND LANOLIN FREE
White petrolatum (Vaseline Pure Petroleum Jelly, Petrolatum White)

and make the skin more pliable. Commercially available urea and alpha-hydroxy acid moisturizers are listed in the formulary at the end of this chapter.

The urea creams dissolve hydrogen bonds and add water-binding sites. To make a cream, the urea must first be dissolved in water before mixing with oil. High concentrations of urea (20% or more) or improper mixing may result in urea crystals in the preparation, causing severe irritation when applied to the skin.

Lactic acid is one of the alpha-hydroxy acids and may act as a moisturizer by loosening the dry surface layer of dead cells. Lactic acid–containing preparations, especially Lac-Hydrin, may frequently burn or sting when applied to the skin, limiting their usefulness in children. Combinations of lower concentrations of lactic acid and urea may decrease the incidence of discomfort and increase effectiveness as a moisturizer.

Caution must be observed if using a urea or lactic acid–containing product when treating large surface areas in children. Both products can be absorbed and can be toxic.[8,9]

water stays in droplet form in the ointment phase, making such moisturizers water-in-oil emulsions.

These preparations should be applied to wet skin two or three times per day for maximal lubrication. Patients are instructed to wet the skin with a 5- or 10-minute bath, then apply the moisturizers to the wet skin before drying it. These preparations are used successfully on most regions of the skin except the scalp and axillae.

Creams and lotions (oil-in-water emulsions). When environmental humidity is high and in naturally occluded areas, the use of moisturizers that contain more water than oil is desirable. These are the lubricating creams and lotions, which contain oil in droplet form in water (oil-in-water emulsions). Creams are viscous and do not pour, whereas lotions are less viscous and pour slowly.[5] Such preparations are easily washed from skin surfaces and are cosmetically pleasing. Lubricant creams and lotions must be applied more frequently to achieve the same lubricant effect obtained with every 12-hour application of ointment.

Skin-hydrating agents. Certain chemicals act as skin-hydrating agents by adding extra water-binding sites to the skin rather than by simple occlusion. Alpha-hydroxy acids and urea remove excess adherent scales

Gels. Gels are colorless semicolloids that liquefy on contact with the skin. Because of their alcoholic base, they may burn and sting. They permit good penetration of steroids and other medications and are useful in medications applied to the scalp and in acne preparations. They are the most effective delivery system for benzoyl peroxides for use in acne (see Chapter 3) and the clear, colorless, odorless tar preparations used for psoriasis.

Amount to dispense and patient education

Therapy often fails because patients apply the topical medication incorrectly. In a comparison of medication application by trained technicians and by patients, it was found that trained technicians applied 1.8 g/m^2 of body surface, but the self-application group averaged 16.3 g/m^2, with a range of 0.4 to 44.3 g/m^2.[10] Over-medication is common and expensive for the patient.

Table 22-2 presents guidelines for the amount of topical therapy to dispense. Box 22-7 lists important rules for prescribing topical medication that will result in therapeutic success when followed by the patient. One way to estimate the amount of topical therapy to apply is to use the fingertip unit (FTU).[11] Most topical prescription preparations have a tube orifice of about 5 mm. One FTU is the amount of ointment that is expressed from a tube, which reaches from the distal tip

Table 22-2   Amount to Dispense in Grams

	One Application (g)	Approximate Twice-Daily Application for 2 Weeks (g)
3- TO 6-MONTH OLD		
Face and neck	½	15
Arm and hand	½	15
Leg and foot	¾	20
Chest and abdomen	½	15
Back and buttocks	¾	20
1- TO 2-YEAR-OLD		
Face and neck	¾	20
Arm and hand	¾	20
Leg and foot	1	30
Chest and abdomen	1	30
Back and buttocks	1½	45
3- TO 5-YEAR-OLD		
Face and neck	¾	20
Arm and hand	1	30
Leg and foot	1½	45
Chest and abdomen	1½	45
Back and buttocks	1¾	50
6- TO 10-YEAR-OLD		
Face and neck	1	30
Arm and hand	1¼	35
Leg and foot	2¼	65
Chest and abdomen	1¾	50
Back and buttocks	2½	70

Box 22-7   Rules for Prescribing Topical Medication

1. Prescribe enough medication
2. Demonstrate to the patient how to apply the medication
3. Apply lubricants liberally to wet skin
4. Substitute lubricant therapy for topical steroids whenever possible; do not allow the patient to use the steroid for the lubricant properties of the vehicle when the vehicle alone would suffice
5. Apply ointments to exposed dry areas, creams to naturally occluded moist areas
6. Use medications twice daily
7. Avoid superpotent steroids in prepubertal children
8. Use only hydrocortisone in diaper area
9. Monitor growth parameters in children who have used steroids for long periods

of an adult finger to the crease on the skin over the distal interphalangeal (DIP) joint. Two FTUs are equivalent to about 1 g of ointment. In addition, one FTU covers the approximate area of two times the surface area of one flat adult hand with the fingers held together.[11] As a result of these calculations, we have a relationship of four adult hands equal two FTUs, which equals 1 g of topical product. Table 22-2 is based on estimates of the amount of product to dispense for different ages of children using the FTU.[11]

ANTIINFLAMMATORY AGENTS
Wet Dressings

Water is an important therapeutic tool, but it is often forgotten that it is also an antiinflammatory agent. The evaporation of water from the skin surface results in vasoconstriction, relief of pruritus, and debridement of crusts from the skin surface. Water is also the active ingredient in the drying lotions; the antiinfective medications added to these preparations are of little benefit. Infected dermatitis should be treated with systemic antibiotics and dressings wet with tap water. Wet dressings can be used in acute dermatitis from any cause. Pruritus is relieved by placing the skin in an environment in which the humidity is 90% and allowing it to evaporate to 60%. This slow evaporation of water from the skin surface occurring over a 4- to 6-hour period is the basis of the wet-dressing technique. The methods for wet dressings are described in Box 4-6 (see Chapter 4) and in the patient education handouts.

Relief of pruritus is dramatic, as is reduction of erythema. After 24 hours the patient is greatly improved, with maximal benefit occurring at 48 to 72 hours. Treatment beyond this period is of little benefit. Topical steroid creams applied to the skin before the application of wet dressings enhances the wet-dressing technique considerably.

Topical Glucocorticosteroids

Topical glucocorticosteroids are the mainstay of therapy of many inflammatory and hyperproliferative skin diseases.[12,13] Glucocorticosteroids applied to the skin reduce inflammation by causing vasoconstriction and preventing the egress of inflammatory cells (neutrophils, lymphocytes, monocyte/macrophages, eosinophils) from the bloodstream to tissue sites. Maximal glucocorticosteroid penetration is achieved from ointment vehicles, followed by gels and creams. Penetration is poor with lotions or sprays. A cutaneous antiinflammatory effect can be achieved with topical glucocorticosteroids without

---

Box 22-8   Potency of Topical Glucocorticosteroids

LOW POTENCY

Hydrocortisone 1%, (Nutracort, Penecort, Hytone, OTC)
Desonide 0.05% (Desowen, Tridesilon)

MODERATE POTENCY

Aclometasone dipropionate 0.05% (Aclovate)
Betamethasone valerate 0.1% (Valisone)
Fluocinolone acetonide 0.01% (Synalar, Fluonid)
Hydrocortisone valerate 0.2% (Westcort)
Mometasone furoate 0.1%, (Elocon)
Triamcinolone acetonide 0.025% , 0.1% (Kenalog, Aristocort)

HIGH POTENCY

Amcinonide 0.1% cream (Cyclocort)
Betamethasone dipropionate 0.05% (Diprosone, Diprolene)
Desoximetasone 0.25% cream (Topicort)
Fluocinonide 0.05% cream, ointment (Lidex, Lidex-E)
Halcinonide 0.1% cream (Halog)

HIGHEST POTENCY

Betamethasone dipropionate (in optimized vehicle) (Diprolene)
Clobetasol propionate 0.05% (Temovate)
Diflorasone diacetate 0.05% (Psorcon)
Halobetasol propionate 0.05% (Ultravate)

---

adrenal suppression, which is not the case with systemic steroids. Many parents are fearful of topical steroid use.[14] Better information needs to be given regarding the safety, potency, and appropriate use of topical corticosteroids. Moderate-potency topical steroids used daily in infants and children for months to years are efficacious and safe.[15]

Potency of topical steroids

The potency of a topical steroid is evaluated by vasoconstriction (blanching) of the skin, which roughly correlates with its antiinflammatory effects. Although glucocorticosteroid potency can be subdivided further, it is convenient to divide it into four categories (Box 22-8). Numerous moderate-potency glucocorticosteroids are available, with little difference in their

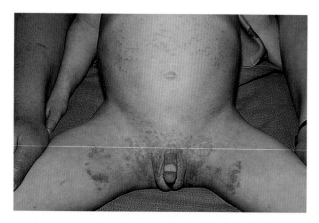

Fig. 22-1 Steroid atrophy secondary to long-term application of a moderate-potency steroid (triamcinolone) and mycostatin combination (Mycolog).

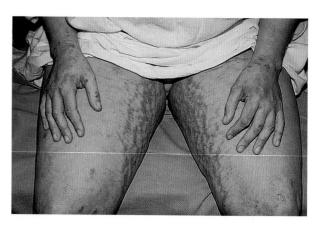

Fig. 22-2 Steroid atrophy secondary to long-term use of topical steroids for atopic dermatitis.

effectiveness. The different products are often available in creams, ointments, and possibly lotions and gels. Some vehicles may increase the potency of a cortico-steroid by increasing penetration through the epidermis. The clinician should select one low-potency and one moderate-potency preparation from the list in Box 22-8 to use for children with inflammatory skin diseases.

Guidelines for use of topical steroids

For most acute, subacute, and chronic dermatitides, the physician should select a preparation from the moderate-potency list and instruct the patient and family to apply twice daily for 3 to 10 days until symptoms have subsided. At that time, bland moisturizers should be applied twice daily, with topical glucocorticosteroids applied once daily. Topical glucocorticosteroid use should be eliminated as soon as possible. There are no indications for high-potency topical glucocorticosteroid use in children, except for pulse-dose therapy under the direction of an experienced dermatologist.

On the face and scrotum, only low-potency glucocorticosteroids (hydrocortisone 1%) should be used, because the epidermis is thin in these areas and the side effects may be severe (Figs. 22-1 and 22-2) (Box 22-9).

When applied to the skin, high-potency glucocorticosteroids and some moderate-potency glucocorticosteroids may cause tachyphylaxis. That is, after 1 to 3 days of application, maximal vasoconstriction has been achieved and further application results in a rebound vasodilation, manifested by diffuse erythema

Box 22-9 Side Effects of Topical Steroids

LOCAL
Striae (especially in genital area and axillae)
Persistent erythema and telangiectasia (face)
Pustular acneiform eruption (face) (steroid rosacea)
Atrophic, shiny, erythematous skin
Telangiectasia, purpura
Granuloma gluteal infantum
Folliculitis, miliaria
Hypertrichosis
Steroid addiction syndrome
Allergic contact dermatitis

SYSTEMIC
Suppression of hypothalamic-pituitary-adrenal axis
Stunted growth in children
Cataracts and glaucoma
Glycosuria
Cushing's syndrome

on the child's face. This is particularly true with the superpotent topical steroids. The clinician should simply substitute bland moisturizers for such patients, and their skin will return to normal in 1 to 2 weeks.

Systemic side effects have been noted with the short-term use of potent topical glucocorticosteroids and the long-term use of moderately potent glucocorticosteroids over 50% of body surface.

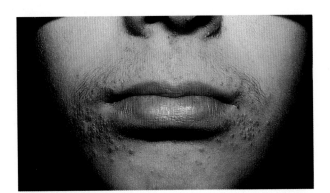

Fig. 22-3 Steroid addiction appearing to be acne. This condition was caused by long-term application of a moderate-potency steroid (triamcinolone) and mycostatin combination (Mycolog).

Topical steroid addiction

Because potent and superpotent topical glucocorticosteroids have become available, a syndrome of topical steroid addiction has been recognized (Fig. 22-3). The syndrome is the result of chronic daily application for greater than a 1-month period of a potent or moderately potent glucocorticosteroid preparation to the facial skin. As treatment continues the patient experiences a rebound vasodilation of the facial skin 2 to 6 hours after the application. The face becomes red, and the patient applies the steroid more frequently. Soon, burning of the skin is experienced and is only relieved by further steroid applications. Permanent redness of the facial skin eventuates, with thinning and fine wrinkling of the skin observed. It is difficult to withdraw the steroid because the patient cannot tolerate the burning sensation, which is relieved only by topical steroids. Substitution of a bland ointment for the topical steroid, plus administration of oral antihistamines, will result in progressive improvement over a 4-week period.

In susceptible infants and children, application of potent or moderately potent glucocorticosteroid preparations to the facial skin may also result in redness and acneiform papules and pustules located on the nose, chin, cheeks, and lower eyelids. This is known as acne rosacea. Abruptly stopping the topical steroid preparation will result in increased numbers of papules and pustules over the subsequent 7 days. Treatment is the same as that recommended for acne, with severe forms requiring systemic antibiotics.

Coal Tar Preparations

Coal tars are byproducts of the destructive distillation of coal. They contain 48% hydrocarbons and benzene, toluene, naphthalene, anthracene, xylene, phenol, cresols, pyridine ammonia, peroxides, and other aromatic compounds. They are black, stain the skin and clothing, and are malodorous. Their mechanism of action is unknown, but they restore normal keratinization in eczematous and hyperplastic epidermis.

Most tar compounds are derived from coal tars, but oil shale tars (ichthammol), juniper tars (cade oil), or pine tars are sometimes used.

Crude coal tar, 1% to 10% in petrolatum, was commonly used in the past for hospitalized patients or in outpatient psoriasis daycare centers. Because of the staining properties, usually commercial preparations listed in the formulary are used.

Tars are applied twice daily and always with a downward motion rather than a circular or up-and-down motion, to avoid tar folliculitis. The tar may concentrate in follicular openings, resulting in a superficial chemical folliculitis. Such chemical folliculitis is rapidly responsive to benzoyl peroxide gels applied twice daily. New colorless and relatively odorless tar preparations have increased the acceptability of tar therapy and made it a viable alternative to topical steroids. The tar gels are clear and colorless vehicles that allow penetration into the skin. They are applied twice daily and are immediately covered with a lubricant because gels are drying. Tar gels are equivalent to crude coal tar 5%. Coal-tar shampoos are useful on the scalp to treat scalp psoriasis. Coal-tar solution, liquor carbonis detergens (LCD), is an alcoholic extract of coal tar. LCD 5% equals crude coal tar 1% in potency. It is used as a shampoo in tincture of green soap or as a bath additive.

Calcipotriene

Calcipotriene is a synthetic analog of vitamin D_3, which is helpful in treatment of psoriasis. Applied twice a day, it improves the majority of patients who use it. The side effects include burning and itching, and its high cost is detrimental when used to treat large surface areas of involved skin. The safety of calcipotriene in children has not been documented.

Nonsteroidal Topical Immunomodulators

Many new pharmacologic agents are being developed to modulate the immune response in disease conditions.[16] Topical tacrolimus is currently available for use in children over 2 years of age with atopic dermatitis. Tacrolimus is a potent immunosuppressive agent that suppresses cytokine production. In some children, the topical preparation is irritating to the skin. Topical tacrolimus may be useful as a second-line or adjunctive therapy in pyoderma gangrenosum, immunobullous disorders of childhood, and resistant cases of atopic dermatitis. Many additional pharmacologic agents are currently under study.

FORMULARY FOR COMMON PEDIATRIC DERMATOLOGY CONDITIONS

This formulary is designed to provide information regarding a number of useful skin preparations, but it is not intended to be encyclopedic. Formulas for compounding skin mixtures are omitted because low-cost and high-quality preparations from pharmaceutical manufacturers are readily available and are often superior to compounded mixtures.[17,18]

I. Skin moisturizers and cleansers

Creams and lotions contain water, requiring the addition of preservatives, which are potential allergens. They must be applied more frequently than ointments but are aesthetically more pleasing to apply. Many different products are available and the ingredients of the brand-name products may change. Many brand-name manufactures market several products that may have properties that are fragrance free, preservative free, or lanolin free, whereas other products with a similar name will have different ingredients. Boxes 22-3, 22-4, 22-5, and 22-6 list commonly used products.

A. Urea creams and lotions
1. Cream 10% (Aquacare, Nutraplus)
2. Cream 20% (Carmol 20)
3. Lotion 10% (Aquacare, Nutraplus, Carmol 10)
B. Lactic acid–containing lotions
1. 5% (LactiCare)
2. 12% (Lac-Hydrin) (prescription product)
Lac-Hydrin is a prescription moisturizer that contains 12% lactic acid. Lactic acid–containing preparations, especially Lac-Hydrin, may frequently burn or sting when applied to the skin, limiting usefulness in children. By combining lower concentrations of lactic acid and urea, moisturizers may reduce the incidence of discomfort and increased effectiveness.
C. Lactic acid and urea
1. Eucerin Plus Cream and Lotion
2. Ureacin-20 Cream and Ureacin-10 Lotion

D. Soaps and soap substitutes[19]
NOTE: For children with sensitive skin, soap substitutes are preferred. If soap is to be used, it should be neutral pH.
1. Cetyl alcohol cleanser (Cetaphil lotion, Aquanil lotion)
2. Moisturel Sensitive Skin Cleanser
3. Purpose Gentle Cleansing Wash
4. Dove 4.75 oz. bar
II. Hair and scalp preparations
The therapeutic shampoos are generally massaged for several minutes into a wet scalp. The shampoo should remain in contact with the scalp for several minutes before it is rinsed out with water.
A. Antimicrobial shampoos
1. Selenium sulfide suspension 1% (Selsun Blue), 2.5% (Exsel, Selsun)
2. Zinc pyrithione (Denorex, Head & Shoulders, Sebulon)
B. Tar shampoos 0.5% to 2% (Sebutone, T-Gel, DHS-T, Zetar)
C. Keratolytic shampoos (salicylic acid-sulfur) (Sebulex, Ionil, Vanseb) (salicylic acid 2%, sulfur 2% in detergent shampoo)
D. Keratolytic scalp preparation
P & S (phenol and saline solution) is valuable in the management of severe scaling of the scalp, which commonly occurs in psoriasis. The P & S solution can be massaged into the scalp and allowed to remain in place for several hours. Often, a thick application can be placed into the scalp at bedtime and a shower cap can occlude the treated area overnight. Shampooing of the hair containing the P & S solution will remove large quantities of scale from the scalp.
NOTE: All keratolytic agents are irritating to the skin and mucous membranes, and contact with eyes, nose, and mouth should be avoided. Sunburn may occur more readily after use of the agents, and areas greater than 10% of the skin surface should not be treated because of possible percutaneous absorption. Skin lubricants are useful adjuncts when keratolytics are used.
E. Detergent shampoos
A large variety of commercial over-the-counter shampoos are available. Their main ingredients are water, sodium lauryl sulfate as an emulsifier and dispersing agent, and fragrance. The sodium lauryl sulfate may act as

an irritant. For dry scalp or cradle cap, such preparations may be used daily. Massage the shampoo in for 20 minutes, then rinse out.

III. Keratolytic agents

These preparations are used for excessive thickening of the palms and soles, the ichthyoses, and follicular plugging states. The mechanism of action is unknown, but faulty cell-to-cell adherence is the major effect.

A. Retinoic acid, tretinoin (Retin-A)

Available in:

0.01%, 0.025% gel; 15-g, 45-g tubes

0.025%, 0.05%, 0.1% cream; 20-, 45-g tubes

B. Lactic acid (see I. B and 1.C above)

C. Salicylic acid: 3%-6% ointment

1. Whitfield's Ointment USP (salicylic acid 3%, benzoic acid 6% in polyethylene glycol ointment)

2. Keralyt Gel (salicylic acid 6%, propylene glycol 60% in alcohol)

IV. Agents that reduce sweating

A. Aluminum chloride solutions

1. Aluminum chloride hexahydratein alcohol (20%, Drysol or 6.25%, Xerac AC)

2. Aluminum chlorohydrate spray (Arrid Extra Dry, Unscented)

B. Glutaraldehyde 10% solution (must be compounded)

Note: Restricted for use on feet only. Stains skin brown. Allergic contact dermatitis may occasionally result.

V. Sunscreens

The potency of sunscreens is determined by a sun protection factor (SPF), which represents the multiples of time to sunburn. At least SPF 15 or higher should be recommended. A large number of sunscreens are available. Sunscreens that are fragrance free and nonstinging to children's skin are preferred. As with moisturizers, the manufacture may change ingredients of a given sunscreen brand, or a given brand name may have variations of ingredients with different SPF factors.

VI. Coal tars

A. Coal tar 1% ointment USP and 5% lotion

B. Tar gels (Estar [5%], PsoriGel [17.5%])

REFERENCES

1. Metry DW, Hebert AA: Topical therapies and medications in the pediatric patient, *Pediatr Clin North Am* 47(4):867, 2000.
2. Rawlings AV et al: Stratum corneum moisturization at the molecular level, *J Invest Dermatol* 103:731, 1994.
3. Hannuksela A, Kinnunen T: Moisturizers prevent irritant dermatitis, *Acta Derm Venereol* 72:42, 1992.
4. Jackson EM: Moisturizers of today, *J Toxicol Cut Ocular Toxicol* 11:173, 1992.
5. Jackson EM: Latest information on how moisturizers work, *Cosmetic Dermatol* 5:35, 1992
6. Orchard D, Weston WL: The importance of vehicle in pediatric topical therapy, *Pediatr Ann* 30(4):208, 2001.
7. Draelos ZD: Therapeutic moisturizers, *Dermatol Clin* 18(4):597, 2000.
8. Goldsmith LA: Salicylic acid, *Dermatology* 18:32, 1979.
9. Abdel-Magid EHM, Ahmed FEA: Salicylate intoxication in an infant with ichthyosis transmitted through skin ointment: a case report, *Pediatrics* 94:939, 1994.
10. Schlagel CA, Sanborn EC: The weights of topical preparations required for total and partial body inunction, *J Invest Dermatol* 42:253, 1964.
11. Long CC, Mills CM, Finlay AY: A practical guide to topical therapy in children, *Br J Dermatol* 138(2):293, 1998.
12. Yohn JJ, Weston WL: Topical glucocorticosteroids, *Curr Probl Dermatol* 11:31, 1990.
13. Hepburn D, Yohn JJ, Weston WL: Topical steroid treatment in infants, children, and adolescents, *Adv Dermatol* 9:225, 1994.
14. Charman CR, Morris AD, Williams HC: Topical corticosteroid phobia in patients with atopic eczema, *Br J Dermatol* 142(5):931, 2000.
15. Ellison JA et al: Hypothalamic-pituitary-adrenal function and glucocorticoid sensitivity in atopic dermatitis, *Pediatrics* 105(4:Pt 1):794, 2000.
16. Paller AS: Use of nonsteroidal topical immunomodulators for the treatment of atopic dermatitis in the pediatric population, *J Pediatr* 138(2):163, 2001.
17. Drugs Facts and Comparisons, St. Louis, 1995, Facts and Comparisons Inc.
18. Arndt KA: Manual of dermatologic therapeutics, ed 6, New York, 2001, Lippincott Williams & Wilkins.
19. Morelli JG, Weston WL: Soaps and shampoos in pediatric practice, *Pediatrics* 80:634, 1987.

Patient Instructions

Acne

Every teenager has some acne. One of three will require medication. Acne occurs in skin with abundant oil glands, such as the face, chest, and back. Cells made to proliferate by androgen hormones block off the oil glands. The blockage occurs within the middle layer of skin, and scrubbing your face will not get deep enough to remove the blockage. When oil glands are first blocked, they produce tiny white bumps called *whiteheads* or *closed comedones*. Bacteria may then grow in the blocked oil gland and produce red bumps or even pus bumps.

Your doctor will try to treat your acne from both the inside and the outside. To open up the blocked oil glands, your doctor will prescribe tretinoin (Retin-A) cream or gel, Differin cream or gel, or benzoyl peroxide gels. In the beginning, these treatments may be applied every third or fourth night, with the frequency gradually increased so they are eventually used nightly. They may dry the skin and make it red during the first 10 to 14 days of use, but then they are tolerated better.

If you have many red bumps and pus bumps, an oral antibiotic will be used. Tetracycline, erythromycin, doxycycline, and minocycline are the drugs most often used. They should be taken by mouth twice a day. To improve acne significantly, 6 to 8 weeks of treatment are required. You should not take tetracycline with food because it binds to calcium in dairy products. Stomachache, exaggerated sunburn, and vaginal yeast infections can occur with the use of tetracycline. Erythromycin may also cause stomach upset. Minocycline can cause dizziness and headaches or blue-gray spots on your skin and mucous membranes. You should discontinue the antibiotic and notify your doctor if side effects occur.

Oil glands respond very slowly, and nothing will speed the response. Try not to get too frustrated with your slow response. Remember no one has a medicine that will prevent you from ever having another pimple. After a good response, your doctor may wish to stop the oral antibiotics and substitute antibiotics in a solution or cream. If you do not respond to this treatment after 6 to 12 weeks, your doctor may wish to try another strategy. Many over-the-counter preparations are advertised to treat acne but are unproven therapies, and some may make the acne worse.

One in 20 boys and 1 in 200 girls will develop painful deep acne or cystic acne. Deep acne often responds to oral antibiotics and topical retinoids, but a few individuals will require Accutane pills. This is a strong medication that requires careful monthly monitoring by your doctor.

May be duplicated for use in clinical practice. From Weston WL, Lane AT, Morelli JG: *Color textbook of pediatric dermatology,* ed 3, St Louis, 2002, Mosby.

Atopic Dermatitis (Eczema)

Eczema, *atopic dermatitis*, and *atopic eczema* are terms that describe a genetic disorder resulting in "sensitive skin." All children with eczema have slightly immature, dry skin with an inability to retain water on the skin surface. In a child with sensitive skin there are many external factors that may influence eczema on a day-to-day basis because the skin barrier to irritation is inadequate. There may be someone else in the family with eczema, asthma, or hay fever, but this is not always the case.

INITIAL TREATMENT FOR ATOPIC DERMATITIS

The first steps in the treatment of atopic dermatitis should be to make your child better as safely and quickly as possible. The mainstay of treatment will be a medium-strength steroid ointment. Although many parents are concerned about steroid ointments, your doctors will prescribe ones that have been used daily for 2 or 3 years on children's skin without ill effects. Steroid ointment is the best method of relieving itching and restoring the skin to normal. You should apply the ointment twice daily. If your child's skin is particularly bad, your doctor may instruct you to use "wet dressings" at bedtime (see instructions on "how to do wet dressings"). Steroid ointment treatment will be for at least 2 weeks and if your child's skin is thickened, for 4 weeks. If your child is not sleeping well because of itching, an antihistamine such as hydroxyzine may be given 1 hour before bedtime. Excessive scratching of the skin may lead to skin infection with staphylococcal bacteria. Open sores on your child's skin, pus, or enlarged lymph nodes may be clues to infection. If skin is infected, the eczema will not respond well to treatment unless antibiotics are used. An antistaphylococcal antibiotic such as cephalexin may be prescribed for the infection. Treatment may be for 10 to 14 days with the antibiotic.

KEEPING YOUR CHILD'S SKIN HEALTHY

After your child's skin is healed, it is essential to moisturize the skin daily or twice daily. Use of Vaseline, Eucerin, Aquaphor, or similar lubricants should become part of the routine care. Sensitive skin is easily chapped. Excessive bathing and soaping of the skin may make the skin red and itchy. There are two ways to avoid this. In one method, bathing should be reduced to a 5-minute bath every third or fourth day. A soap substitute or liquid synthetic soap such as Dove should be used instead of soap. These are massaged into skin, then patted dry. Do not rinse off with water. The second method, a 5-minute bath twice a day with water only is used. After the bath, towel off the beads of water quickly and apply the topical prescription ointments to the areas that are red and irritated. Quickly apply the lubricant to the entire skin surface and over the topical medication.

If your baby drools while teething, don't wash the face, but pat dry and apply ointment. There is no "cure" for eczema, and an occasional flareup may occur. Simply re-treat with the steroid ointment again for 1 to 2 days until the skin clears. Allergy tests, restriction diets, and environmental hypoallergenic changes will not cure your child's eczema. All attention should be devoted to treating the skin. Soft, loose-fitting, mostly cotton clothing to avoid overheating of skin and keeping the child's nails trimmed short are recommended.

The tendency for sensitive skin will remain with your child even into teenage years. However, your child's skin will usually mature and the eczema will gradually improve as the child gets older. The age at which eczema ceases to be a problem varies, but many children show a significant improvement by the age of 5 years, and most will have only occasional trouble by the time they are teenagers. Only a few continue to have troublesome eczema in adult life, especially those children that suffer from hay fever and eczema.

Creams and Ointments

HOW TO APPLY

Creams and ointments are best applied to wet skin for optimal absorption. They are active when simply placed on the skin surface and do not have to be massaged into the skin. To avoid clogging hair follicles, ointments should always be applied to the skin in a downward direction and should never be applied in a circular motion.

Most people apply far too much cream or ointment to a child's skin. Only a thin layer is required to achieve good results. The amount of cream or ointment that covers one adult fingertip is considered a Finger Tip Unit (FTU). One FTU provides a thin film for a surprisingly large area of skin and is a good guideline for how much to use. Two FTUs equals 1 g of cream or ointment.

HOW MUCH CREAM OR OINTMENT PER APPLICATION

Number of Finger Tip Units Per Age and Skin Area to be Treated

Skin Area to be Treated	AGE OF CHILD			
	0-6 Months	6 Months- 2 Years	2-5 Years	5-10 Years
One arm, face, or chest	1	1.5	2	2.5
One leg or entire back	1.5	2	3	5

If the cream or ointment used is potentially irritating, especially to the skin near the eyes or lips, apply the FTU elsewhere first, then apply the thin amount remaining on your finger to the skin around the eyes or lips.

May be duplicated for use in clinical practice. From Weston WL, Lane AT, Morelli JG: *Color textbook of pediatric dermatology*, ed 3, St Louis, 2002, Mosby.

Dry Skin

Dry skin is a common problem secondary to low environmental humidity or removal of water-binding ceramides from the skin surface. Excess water loss causes red, dry, cracked skin. Soaps aggravate dry skin by removing the natural water-binding substances from your skin surface, and a soap substitute, such as Cetaphil or Moisturel cleanser, should be used. It is important to massage these into skin and then pat dry with a soft cloth. Do not rinse off.

Moisturizing creams or ointments need to be used daily. They should be applied to wet skin after every shower or bath and as many other times during the day as possible. Ointments are greasier but are better moisturizers and need to be applied less often. A room humidifier is also helpful. Sometimes dry skin is so severe that dermatitis develops, and treatment for 1 week with a topical steroid ointment may be necessary.

May be duplicated for use in clinical practice. From Weston WL, Lane AT, Morelli JG: *Color textbook of pediatric dermatology,* ed 3, St Louis, 2002, Mosby.

Head Lice

Lice are blood-sucking insects and about ⅛ inch in length. They may be seen crawling on the child's scalp or as white spots tightly attached to the child's hair. Many things can mimic lice on the scalp, including clothing fibers, airborne particulates that land on the scalp, or hair casts. Hair casts are small white material that surrounds the hair and can be moved down the hair, whereas nits cannot. Sharing clothing, including scarves, caps, hats, and other headgear, may help spread lice. Crowded living conditions also help spread lice.

There are very effective lice shampoos available for the cure of head lice. For head lice infestations, 1% permethrin shampoo (Elimite) or 0.3% pyrethrin shampoo (Rid or Nix) applied for 10 minutes and then rinsed out results in an 80% cure rate. Malathion 0.5% lotion, left on for 8 to 12 hours, is also effective. Resistance of head lice to permethrins, pyrethrins, and malathion has been reported but is rare. You should ask your doctor if it is a problem in your area. Using greasy ointments on the scalp is thought by some to smother the lice.

Shampoo treatments other than malathion lotion will not, however, remove the gelatinous nits. The use of a warm damp towel for 30 minutes on the scalp will loosen the nits and allow their mechanical removal with a fine-toothed comb (nit comb). Most pediculocide shampoos are supplied with a nit comb. Retreatment in 7 days is recommended. Boiling of clothing, bedding, and other possible fomites is ovicidal, lousicidal, and necessary because nits may be attached to clothing.

It is tempting for some persons to use pediculicides repeatedly in children with lice infestations. We do not recommend this because of the hazards of central nervous system and other toxicity posed by such usage. All contacts should be identified and treated simultaneously. Students should be readmitted to school the morning after the first treatment. "No-nit" policies for return to school cannot be justified. Cutting the child's hair short should be discouraged because it does not eradicate the head lice. Schoolmates should be examined by the school nurse or other health care provider to determine if other children are infested.

May be duplicated for use in clinical practice. From Weston WL, Lane AT, Morelli JG: *Color textbook of pediatric dermatology*, ed 3, St Louis, 2002, Mosby.

Insect Repellents for Children

Insect repellents should be accompanied by the use of protective clothing. Repellents that have a high concentration (more than 15%) of DEET should not be used on an infant's skin because of toxicity. Spray repellents that are designed to be used on clothing only should not be used on your child's skin. The table below lists some insect repellents and their ingredients that are available in the United States.

Insect Repellents and Their Ingredients

Brand	Manufacturer	% DEET
PLANT-BASED REPELLANTS		
Bite Blocker (geranium oil)	Consep, Inc	
Avon Skin-So-Soft Bug Guard spray (citronella 0.10 %)	Avon	
DEET-CONTAINING REPELLENTS		
Skedaddle for children	Minnetonka	6.5
Skeddadle for children with sunscreen SPF 15	Minnetonka	6.5
Off! Skintastic for Kids spray	Johnson Wax	5.0
Cutter Just for Kids	United Industries	5.0
Cutter Pleasant Protection with sunscreen SPF 15	United Industries	7.0
Repel Camp Lotion for Kids	Wisconsin Pharmacal	10.0
Repel Soft Unscented gel	Wisconsin Pharmacal	7.0
PERMETHRIN INSECTICIDE SPRAYS (For clothing only! Not to be applied on skin.)		
Cutter Outdoorsman Gear Guard spray (Permethrin 0.5%)	Cutter	
Repel Permanone	Wisconsin Pharmacal	

Keratosis Pilaris

Keratosis pilaris is a very common skin disorder that presents as small, scaly, white or red, pinpoint bumps on the arms, legs, buttocks, and cheeks. It is caused by plugging of the hair follicles with dry scale. It is a very difficult problem to cure, but treatment will help control the condition. Dry skin makes this condition much worse, and the instructions on the "Dry Skin" handout should be followed. Also, the application of an alpha-hydroxy acid–containing lotion will be useful. The alpha-hydroxy acids are lactic, glycolic, and citric. Many companies make alpha-hydroxy acid–containing lotions, and there is no evidence that one is superior to another for treating keratosis pilaris. Moisturizing creams that contain 10% urea will also be helpful if applied at a different time of day than the alpha-hydroxy acid moisturizers.

Molluscum Contagiosum

Molluscum contagiosum is a virus that infects the outer layer of skin, causing tiny white bumps. The center of the bump has an opening filled with rough material that makes the bumps look like tiny volcanoes. Molluscum is contagious, but most older children and adults are immune. Infants and toddlers are most susceptible to catching molluscum. Dozens or hundreds of bumps may be seen. Involvement of the groin, thighs, and armpits is common, but bumps can appear anywhere, including the face and eyelids.

Molluscum may be difficult to treat. The molluscum contagiosum virus effectively hides from the child's immune system. If untreated, molluscum may last 2 or 3 years. Usually it causes no harm, but your child can scratch or pick at the bumps and infect them with bacteria. Your doctor may try to destroy the molluscum by freezing, scraping, or applying a chemical to the surface. The new interferon-inducing cream imiquimod may be applied daily to help the child develop immunity. Imiquimod cream should be applied with a toothpick or cotton-tip applicator (Q-tip) to each molluscum. Once the molluscum bump turns red, stop treating that molluscum. Overtreating results in a tender, scabbed spot. It usually takes several visits to the doctor to eliminate molluscum, and if you decide to begin treatments, you must be compliant or the treatments are unlikely to work.

Around each molluscum bump the skin may get red. This is a sign that immunity to molluscum is starting and is called *molluscum dermatitis*. Your doctor may recommend treating the redness with a cortisone ointment. Some large molluscum spots may get scabbed and heal with a scar.

Papular Urticaria

Each itchy bump your child develops represents a site of an insect bite. The condition is called *papular urticaria* and is quite common, especially in toddlers. It is frustrating to most families because usually the toddler is the only family member affected. The reason your child reacts when others in the household do not is because the child is allergic to the insect. Fortunately, this allergy is temporary and will clear in 6 months, even if not treated.

Each itchy skin bump represents delayed hypersensitivity reactions to a variety of biting or stinging arthropods. Dog and cat fleas are the usual offenders. Less commonly, mosquitoes, lice, scabies, fowl mites, and grain or grass mites are responsible.

The logical therapy is to remove the offending insect. Often an obvious source initially is not evident and a thorough search should be made for the source, including inquiries into daycare, preschool, and visits to neighbors, friends, and relatives. If a pet is suspected, dogs or cats should be treated for fleas or mites by a veterinarian. The child should be kept away from the pet. Protective clothing, such as long sleeves, may be useful. The prophylactic use of an oral antihistamine, such as cetirizine (Zyrtec), may reduce the reactions. Use of insect repellents (see "Insect Repellents for Children" handout) may make the child less attractive to the insect. The most successful repellent is Bite Blocker, with DEET-containing insect repellents almost as efficacious. Fleas or mites living in carpets or furniture may be eliminated by treatment with a commercial insecticide. Window casings should be treated in the case of bird mites. Symptomatic relief may sometimes be obtained with topical mid-potency cortisone creams or ointments applied three times daily.

Perioral Dermatitis

Perioral dermatitis is a scaly, bumpy rash that occurs around the mouth, around the nose, and sometimes on the eyelids. In some families it is related to acne rosacea. Cortisone creams and ointments make the condition worse while seeming to initially make it less red. Use of these creams and ointments must be stopped for the skin to clear. Comedogenic moisturizers or makeup also make this type of dermatitis worse, and their use should also be stopped.

Your doctor will recommend an oral or topical antibiotic to be used daily for 4 to 6 weeks. If you have been applying a cortisone previously, stopping the cortisone will make the rash worse for 7 to 10 days before it gets better.

Psoriasis

Your child's psoriasis is not contagious but it is believed to be hereditary. It is a very common disease, with 4 to 6 million people in the United States affected. Most people with psoriasis have a very mild skin condition, often with a few scaly skin spots in the scalp or on the elbows and knees. Some affected family members do not realize they have psoriasis.

SITUATIONS THAT MAKE PSORIASIS WORSE

1. Sore throats caused by streptococcal infections may result in dozens of small skin spots of psoriasis. A throat culture, and prompt antibiotic treatment if the culture is positive for streptococcus, is recommended for every sore throat or exposure to streptococcal bacteria.
2. Injury to the skin from abrasions, scratches, or picking off the scale will bring out more psoriasis. This is called the *Koebner phenomenon.* Have your child put extra moisturizer on the skin. This will help your child avoid picking the skin.
3. Certain prescription medications may make psoriasis worse, such as cortisone shots or pills, beta-blockers, or lithium. Try to avoid having your child take these.

TREATMENTS FOR PSORIASIS

There is no cure for psoriasis, but there are many very effective treatments that control the problem. The treatments often require 4 to 6 weeks to show improvement or clearing of the psoriasis, and the best success requires paying careful attention to the details of the treatment program.

Steroid Creams and Ointments

For limited areas of psoriasis, steroid creams or ointments are the most common treatment. Over-the-counter (OTC) cortisones are ineffective, and your doctor may prescribe a medium- or high-strength steroid.

Vitamin D3 Cream and Ointment

For many psoriasis patients, twice-daily application of a vitamin D3 cream or ointment (Dovonex) helps clear psoriasis. It can be irritating to the skin in some children, and a few complain of stinging on application. The cost is expensive.

Anthralin

Antralin is an old but good treatment for stubborn patches of psoriasis. The cream is left on for 5 to 10 minutes, then washed off with Dove soap (pH 7.0). This is called *"short-contact anthralin therapy"* or *SCAT.* The soap neutralizes changes in the medicine after exposure to air. Leaving anthralin on too long will result in red and sometimes tender skin.

Coal Tars

Coal-tar ointments have been used to treat psoriasis for 150 years. They are effective but smelly and stain the skin, clothing, and bathtub. Your doctor can recommend a product and a treatment routine. They are usually used at bedtime and washed off in the morning. Using the same pair of sleep wear is recommended.

Retinoid Creams and Ointments

Tazorac ointment may be applied to the skin once daily for the treatment of psoriasis. It is effective when a few thick areas of psoriasis are present. It can be quite irritating, and use of daily lubrication is helpful to counteract the drying and irritating action of the drug.

Sunlight and Ultraviolet Light Treatments

Sunlight has been known to improve psoriasis since the ancient Greek civilization. Using mineral oil on the skin just before light exposure allows the light to uniformly penetrate the skin. The scale of psoriasis normally reflects light rather than absorbing it. Light treatments work slowly. Usually, sunbathing three times a week or using artificial UVB sunlamps three times a week requires 25 to 30 treatments for clearing the skin. Newer narrow-band UVB lights are not widely available but will clear the skin in a shorter period of time. Too much sunlight can cause sunburn, premature aging of skin, eye damage, and, later in life, skin cancers. For safety, ultraviolet light must be used in a medically supervised situation.

Photochemotherapy

Long-wave ultraviolet light (UVA) can be used when the person is given a pill (psoralen) that makes him or her very sensitive to long-wave ultraviolet light (PUVA). The pill often makes children nauseated, and the child must avoid sunlight for 24 hours after taking the pill. Twice weekly treatments are recommended. This therapy has a risk of promoting skin cancer and should rarely be used in children.

Methotrexate

Methotrexate is a strong anticancer drug that is used for children with the most severe forms of psoriasis. It requires periodic blood tests and is taken once weekly.

Psoriasis Scalp Care

Thick, adherent scales may pile up on your child's scalp. This makes it difficult for topical medications to reach the scalp skin. The thick scales are difficult to remove, and scalp psoriasis may respond much more slowly than psoriasis in other areas, requiring special treatment. A useful three-step strategy for daily scalp treatment in psoriasis is as follows:

1. At bedtime, massage in a scale-softening and removing solution (this can be Baker's Phenol and Saline, or T-sal, or the pharmacist can mix 3% salicylic acid in mineral oil). Your doctor may recommend a preparation that is also antiinflammatory, such as Derma-Smoothe-FS.

2. In the morning, shampoo with a commercial shampoo or Baker's P & S shampoo, followed by a conditioner. (Your doctor may recommend a medicated shampoo instead.)

3. While the hair is still wet, massage the prescription solution (fluocinolone 0.01% solution, fluocinonide 0.05% solution, or calcipotriene 0.005% solution) thoroughly into the scalp skin.

After all of the scale is gone, this strategy can be done three times a week. If washing the hair in between treatment days is desired, the use of a commercial shampoo followed by conditioner is recommended. Do not attempt to remove scales by excessive brushing, scrubbing, or combing. This may result in sufficient skin injury to bring out more psoriasis.

May be duplicated for use in clinical practice. From Weston WL, Lane AT, Morelli JG: *Color textbook of pediatric dermatology,* ed 3, St Louis, 2002, Mosby.

Scabies

Scabies is caused by a microscopic human mite, not visible to the naked eye, but only seen with magnification. It is transmitted only from humans, not from animals. It is easily transmitted because during the first 3 weeks that people have scabies they do not itch or have itchy bumps. You should ask if any household members or persons in contact with your child have itchy bumps.

Application of a scabicide, such as 5% permethrin creme, is curative. In children and adolescents, application of 5% permethrin creme for 8 to 14 hours produces a 98% cure rate. Ivermectin in a pill form in a single oral dose has also been demonstrated to be curative. However, permethrin cream or lotion may be superior to single-dose ivermectin. In children under 5 years of age, or in pregnant or lactating women, ivermectin is not recommended. Permethrin creme is approved for use for those 2 months of age or older. In any infant or toddler, covering the hands with clothing to prevent licking the scabicide from the skin is recommended. For children with only a few lesions, routine retreatment is not necessary. Babies have dozens or hundreds of itchy bumps, and several retreatments 7 or 8 days apart may occasionally be required. Boiling of clothing and bedding is not helpful because scabies mites are not heat sensitive.

May be duplicated for use in clinical practice. From Weston WL, Lane AT, Morelli JG: *Color textbook of pediatric dermatology,* ed 3, St Louis, 2002, Mosby.

Scalp Ringworm (Tinea Capitis)

Scalp ringworm is largely caused by infections with either *Trichophyton tonsurans* or *Microsporum canis*. *T. tonsurans* is transmitted from human to human, is currently epidemic in North America, and accounts for more than 95% of scalp ringworm. It is most prevalent in areas of crowding and accounts for virtually all tinea capitis in inner-city children in North America. Transmission is predominantly from sharing hats, caps, scarves, combs, or brushes with infected individuals.

A bald patch in the scalp is a regular feature of tinea capitis. Some infections are quite mild, with only scales in the scalp or a few pus bumps. The presence of enlarged lymph nodes on the back of the head or the back of the neck in association with hair loss should make one consider first the diagnosis of tinea capitis. When there is hypersensitivity to the infection a red, tender scalp lump called a *kerion* may appear.

Scalp ringworm infections caused by *M. canis* are seen as one or several patches of broken-off hairs that appear thickened and white. Cats, dogs, and certain rodents harbor *M. canis*, and children handling such animals are susceptible to infection. Humans appear to be a terminal host for *M. canis*, and human-to-human transmission does not occur.

To treat scalp ringworm, your doctor will select an oral medicine that is taken for 1 to 3 months. Griseofulvin used for a minimum of 2 months, or terbinafine for 1 month is the best treatment. Topical antifungal creams and lotions cannot reach the hyphae within the hair shaft and are ineffective. Griseofulvin is a safe drug in children. Absorption of griseofulvin is enhanced by a fatty meal and your doctor may suggest taking griseofulvin once or twice a day with ice cream or whole milk. In addition to oral griseofulvin, many doctors suggest an antifungal shampoo such as selenium sulfide 2.5% shampoo or ketoconazole 2% shampoo to be applied twice weekly to the scalp to reduce infectivity and to hasten your child's return to school or child-care setting. The child may return to school once treatment is started.

Children should not share combs, brushes, or head wear. School and daycare contacts should be referred for evaluation if they have scaling hair loss. Screening of contacts with a Wood's lamp is of no value because the epidemic strains in North America are not fluorescent. Hair regrowth even with treatment is slow, often taking 3 to 6 months. If a hypersensitivity kerion is present, some scarring and permanent hair loss might result.

May be duplicated for use in clinical practice. From Weston WL, Lane AT, Morelli JG: *Color textbook of pediatric dermatology*, ed 3, St Louis, 2002, Mosby.

Sun Protection

All children should practice good sun protection. Babies under 6 months of age should be kept out of the sun. Babies' sweat glands easily get blocked with sun exposure, resulting in a reduced sweating rate and fever. For your baby, you should practice sun avoidance (see below).

There are three main strategies of sun protection. The best is sun avoidance, the next best is protective clothing, and the weakest strategy is the use of sunscreens. If your child has sun sensitivity, sun avoidance should be practiced.

SUN AVOIDANCE

Keep your child out of the sun between the hours of 10 AM and 4 PM. These hours are when the damaging sun rays reaching the Earth's surface are the strongest. Your doctor may have to write an excuse for school recess or other outdoor activities that occur during those hours. Keep your child in the shade of an umbrella or tree if possible.

PROTECTIVE CLOTHING

Clothing is better at sun protection than sunscreens. Wearing protective swim wear, a shirt, and a wide-brimmed hat are recommended.

SUNBLOCKS AND SUNSCREENS

A sun protection factor (SPF) of 30 is recommended when using sunblocks and sunscreens. Remember that all sunscreens and sunblocks wash off with sweating or swimming. Reapplication every hour while exposed may be necessary. The amount of sunlight may be underestimated on the first sunny days of Spring. Reflection of sun off of snow (160% of sunlight), water (130%), and sand (120%) may provide extra sunlight. Do NOT use sunscreens to increase the time spent in the sun.

Warts

Warts are caused by a virus that infects the outer layer of skin. Warts can occur anywhere on the skin. The most common type is a raised, rough bump on the hands. Some children will get only a few warts, whereas others will get dozens. In most children, the wart virus evades the child's immune system and it may take 1 to 2 years to get immune.

The more warts a child has, and the larger the wart, the harder they are to treat. Warts on the bottom of the foot are called *plantar warts*. Sometimes warts are not as raised and rough; these are called *flat warts* and are often seen on the face. Warts last 1 to 2 years if untreated. Although they may spread and be unsightly, they are harmless.

There is no treatment that specifically kills the wart virus. There are many treatments for warts because no single treatment is very effective. Common treatments include freezing the wart, burning it with a laser, or applying chemicals. The goal of treatment is to kill the skin that contains the wart virus. It may take many treatments to eliminate warts and you must be very compliant or the treatments are unlikely to work. Warts that are frozen will often develop a blister or blood blister within 1 or 2 days. If a blister develops, soak the skin in warm soapy water, then gently open the blister. Sometimes a ring of warts will grow around a wart that is treated. Wart liquids and plasters frequently turn the skin white. Every 2 or 3 days, soak the wart in warm water for 30 to 60 minutes, then rub off the dead white skin with a washcloth. Cutting the wart is likely to spread the wart. If a vascular laser is available, it is less painful for the child than freezing and equally as effective.

Imiquimod (Aldara) cream will cause the skin cells to make interferon, the body's natural wart virus–fighting chemical. Daily application to each wart is required, often for 4 to 8 weeks. When the wart gets red, stop treating that wart with the cream.

Wet Dressings

Your health care provider wishes to use wet dressings to treat your child's itchy skin condition. Wet dressings are safe, and their effect is in the relief of itching and healing of the skin. Three major benefits result from the use of wet dressings:

1. Constant evaporation from the skin surface stimulates a cooling sensation and interferes with any itchy sensation.
2. The water restores the optimum moisture to the skin surface.
3. The child has restricted access to the skin and finds it difficult to scratch.

HOW TO APPLY WET DRESSINGS

Wet dressings can be used with or without steroid ointments or creams. Following the seven steps listed below will ensure the wet dressings are properly applied.

STEP ONE: If your child is prescribed a steroid ointment or cream, apply it to the itchy skin.

STEP TWO: Use two pair of pajamas, sleepers, or long underwear. It is preferable if they are at least 40% cotton. The more cotton, the better. If you are treating arms or legs, you may use long stockings.

STEP THREE: Soak one pair of pajamas or other clothing in warm water.

STEP FOUR: Wring out the wet clothing until it is damp.

STEP FIVE: Put the damp clothing on the child.

STEP SIX: Put dry clothing over the wet.

STEP SEVEN: Make certain the room is warm, but not hot. Make certain that the damp dressing remains damp. Do not let it dry out.

Wet dressings can be used overnight for 7 nights or may be changed every 8 hours around the clock for 72 hours. When doing continuous wet dressings, take off the clothing every 8 hours, then reapply the ointment or cream, redampen the damp clothing, and place the dry clothing over it. When using wet dressings overnight, apply the topical steroid preparation in the morning after removing the wet dressings.

For a severe flare-up of the rash, wet dressings can again be used overnight for one or two nights.

Index

Page numbers followed by b indicate boxes; f, figures; t, tables.

Continued from inside front cover.

Vascular Lesions

Newborns

A. *Blanching*
1. Mottling, 300, 310-311
2. Flat hemangioma, 187-193
3. Urticaria, 202-210
4. Erythema toxicum, 302-303
5. Harlequin color change, 300
6. Port-wine stain, 194-195, 196-198, 309-310
7. Other vascular birthmarks, 309-311
8. Neonatal lupus, 134

B. *Nonblanching (purpuric)*
1. Congenital infection, 334-338
   a. Toxoplasmosis, 308
   b. Enterovirus, 71, 109
   c. Rubella, 92-93, 308
   d. Cytomegalovirus, 308
   e. Herpes simplex, 305-306
   f. Syphilis, 57-59
2. Coagulation defects, 217-218
3. Autoimmune disorders
   a. Idiopathic thrombocytopenic purpura, 308
   b. Systemic lupus erythematosus (SLE), 308
4. Hemangioma with platelet trapping syndrome, 190, 191
5. Epidermolysis bullosa, 274-280

Infants and Children

A. *Blanching*
1. Hemangioma, 187-193
2. Urticaria, 202-210
3. Livedo reticularis, 132, 135, 136, 137
4. Angiofibroma, 243
5. Pyogenic granuloma, 178-179
6. Spider telangiectasia, 199-200
7. Telangiectasis of connective tissue disease
8. Erythema multiforme, 155-157
9. Erythema infectiosum, 94-96
10. Kawasaki disease, 160-161
11. Morbilliform viral exanthems, 89-101
12. Scarlet fever, 49-50
13. Toxic shock syndrome, 54-55
14. Drug eruptions, 287-297
15. Urticarial lesions of juvenile rheumatoid arthritis, SLE, periarteritis nodosa, dermatomyositis, rheumatic fever, Crohn's disease, ulcerative colitis, aphthous stomatitis, Behçet's disease, thyroiditis
16. Erythema chronicum migrans (Lyme disease), 56-57, 81-82
17. Early lesions of pityriasis rosea, 125-127
18. Early lesions of guttate psoriasis, 119, 123, 124, 125
19. Syphilis, 57-59

B. *Nonblanching (purpuric)*
1. Coagulation disorders
   a. Idiopathic thrombocytopenic purpura, 308
   b. Leukemia, 184
   c. Hemophilia, 308
2. Trauma, 219
3. Progressive pigmentary purpura, 218-219
4. Erythema nodosum, 212-213
5. Meningococcemia, 54
6. Rocky Mountain spotted fever, 218
7. Atypical measles, 90-91
8. Herpes simplex purpura, 101-106
9. Gonococcemia, 215
10. Staphylococcal sepsis, 215
11. Subacute bacterial endocarditis, 215
12. Pseudomonas sepsis, 52, 215
13. Infectious mononucleosis, 97-98
14. Echovirus, 96-97

Papulosquamous Disorders

Newborns

1. Candidiasis, 73-75, 305
2. Epidermal nevus, 313-314
3. Tinea corporis, 67-68
4. Ichthyosis, 270-274
5. Psoriasis, 119-125, 304
6. Congenital rubella, 92-93, 308
7. Pityriasis rubra pilaris, 140-142
8. Dermatitis, 26-42

Infants and Children

1. Pityriasis rosea, 125-127
2. Psoriasis, 119-125
3. Tinea corporis or tinea faciei, 67-68, 69
4. Lupus erythematosus, 132-136
5. Parapsoriasis, 128-130
6. Keratosis pilaris, 41-42
7. Secondary syphilis, 57-59, 128-129
8. Darier's disease, 178, 209, 284
9. Scabies, 77-80
10. Lichen planus, 130-132
11. Dermatitis, 26-42
12. Ichthyosis, 270-274
13. Pityriasis rubra pilaris, 140-142
14. Porokeratosis of Mibelli, 139-140
15. Dermatomyositis, 136-138

Eczematous Disorders

Newborns

1. Diaper dermatitis, 34-35, 320
2. Atopic dermatitis, 26-33, 320
3. Seborrheic dermatitis, 39-40, 320
4. Contact dermatitis, 33-39
5. Acrodermatitis enteropathica, 284-285
6. Leiner's disease, 39
7. Multiple carboxylase deficiency, 39
8. Severe combined immunodeficiency, 39
9. Histiocytosis X, 183, 320
10. Scabies, 77-80, 320
11. Candidiasis, 73-75, 305
12. HIV, 110-111

Infants and Children

1. Atopic dermatitis, 26-33
2. Contact dermatitis, 33-39
3. Nummular eczematous dermatitis, 40-41
4. Polymorphous light eruption, 147-149
5. Drug eruption, 287-297
6. Tinea corporis, 68-69
7. Scabies, 77-80
8. Sunburn, 144-147
9. Juvenile plantar dermatosis, 35-36
10. Candidiasis, 73-75
11. HIV, 110-111
12. Seborrheic dermatitis, 39-40
13. Histiocytosis X, 183
14. Lichen planus, 130-132
15. Dermatitis herpetiformis, 165